Pediatric Critical Care

The Essentials

Edited by

Joseph D. Tobias, MD

Director, Pediatric Critical Care/Pediatric Anesthesiology
Professor of Pediatrics and Anesthesiology
The University of Missouri School of Medicine
Columbia, Missouri

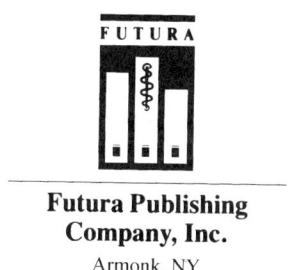

Futura Publishing Company, Inc.
Armonk, NY

Library of Congress Cataloging-in-Publication Data

Pediatric critical care : the essentials / edited by Joseph D. Tobias.
    p.   cm.
  Includes bibliographical references and index.
  ISBN 0–87993–428–X (alk. paper)
  1. Pediatric intensive care—Handbooks, manuals, etc.
2. Pediatric emergencies—Handbooks, manuals, etc. I. Tobias, Joseph D.
    [DNLM: 1. Critical Care—in infancy & childhood handbooks.
2. Intensive Care Units, Pediatric handbooks. WS 39 H2353 1999]
RJ370.H354 1999
618.92′0028—DC21
DNLM/DLC
for Library of Congress   98–54112
                                                      CIP

Copyright © 1999
Futura Publishing Company, Inc.

Published by
Futura Publishing Company
135 Bedford Road
Armonk, New York 10504

LC#: 98–54112
ISBN#: 0-87993-428-x

Every effort has been made to ensure that the information in this book is as up to date and accurate as possible at the time of publication. However, due to the constant developments in medicine neither the author, nor the editors, nor the publisher can accept any legal or any other responsibility for any errors or omissions that may occur.

All rights reserved.

No part of this book may be translated or reproduced in any form without written permission from the publisher.

Printed in the United States on acid-free paper.

Dedication

This book is dedicated to those who have taken the time and made the extra effort to teach me so much about not only the science but also the art of medicine. I will always be grateful to those who made the extra effort to teach and to nurture:

Dr. Charles Wurrey
Dr. Charles Pratt
Dr. Joseph Garcia-Prats
Dr. Alan Percy
Dr. David Nichols

Contributors

Rosaleah V. Bernardo MD Section of Pediatric Critical Care Medicine, Department of Pediatrics and Adolescent Medicine, University of South Dakota School of Medicine, Sioux Falls, SD

Thomas V. Brogan, MD Assistant Professor, Departments of Anesthesiology and Pediatrics, Children's Hospital and Regional Medical Center, University of Washington School of Medicine, Seattle, Washington

Kevin B. Churchwell MD Division of Pediatric Critical Care and Anesthesia, Departments of Pediatrics and Anesthesiology, Vanderbilt Children's Hospital, Vanderbilt University Medical Center, Nashville, TN

R. Blaine Easley, MD Chief Resident/Clinical Instructor, Department of Child Health, University of Missouri Hospitals and Clinics, Columbia, MO

Ted Groshong, MD Interim Chairman, Department of Child Health, Associate Professor of Child Health, Director of Pediatric Nephrology, University of Missouri, Columbia, MO

J. Steven Hata, MD Director of Surgical Intensive Care, Assistant Professor, Department of Anesthesiology, University of Iowa Hospitals and Clinics, Iowa City, IA

Steven E. Haun, MD Section of Critical Care Medicine, Department of Pediatrics and Adolescent Medicine, University of South Dakota School of Medicine, Sioux Falls, SD

Jessica Klekamp MD Division of Pediatric Critical Care, Department of Pediatrics, University of Iowa Hospitals and Clinics, Iowa City, IA

Lynn D. Martin, MD Assistant Professor of Anesthesiology and Pediatrics, Departments of Anesthesiology and Pediatrics, Children's Hospital and Regional Medical Center, University of Washington, Seattle, Washington

David G. Nichols, MD Director, Division of Pediatric Critical Care and Anesthesiology, Professor, Departments of Anesthesiology/Critical Care Medicine and Pediatrics, The Johns Hopkins Hospital, Baltimore, MD

Sayonara Pérez Mato, MD Fellow, Section of Pediatric Infectious Diseases, Department of Pediatrics, Tulane University School of Medicine, Louisiana State University School of Medicine, New Orleans, LA

Marcus S. Schamberger, MD Department of Pediatrics, Division of Pediatric Cardiology, Riley Children's Hospital, Indianapolis, IN

Joseph E. Segeleon, MD Section of Critical Care Medicine, Department of Pediatrics and Adolescent Medicine, University of South Dakota School of Medicine, Sioux Falls, SD

Joseph D. Tobias, MD Director, Pediatric Critical Care/Pediatric Anesthesiology, Professor of Pediatrics and Anesthesiology, University of Missouri School of Medicine, Columbia, MO

Adalberto Torres Jr., MD   Assistant Professor of Pediatrics, Division of Pediatric Critical Care, University of Illinois College of Medicine at Peoria, Peoria, IL

Sara S. Viessman, MD   Assistant Professor, Residency Program Director, Department of Child Health, University of Missouri School of Medicine, Columbia, MO

Pat Wiggins MS, RD, CS   Clinical Coordinator, Arkansas Children's Hospital Nutrition Center, Little Rock, AR

William R. Wilson, Jr., MD   Director, Pediatric Cardiothoracic Surgery, Associate Professor of Surgery and Pediatrics, University of Missouri, Columbia, MO

Contents

Contributors v

Foreword ix
William A. Altemeier, MD

Preface xi

Chapter 1. **Airway Management** 1
Joseph D. Tobias, MD

Chapter 2. **Cardiovascular Physiology, Shock, Inotropic Agents,
and Invasive Hemodynamic Monitoring** 17
Joseph D. Tobias, MD

Chapter 3. **Croup, Upper Airway Obstruction, and Status Asthmaticus** 37
Joseph D. Tobias, MD and David G. Nichols, MD

Chapter 4. **Mechanical Ventilation, Respiratory Monitoring,
and the Basics of Pulmonary Physiology** 57
Lynn Martin, MD

Chapter 5. **Alternative Modes of Respiratory Support** 107
Thomas V. Brogan, MD and Lynn D. Martin, MD

Chapter 6. **Acute Respiratory Distress Syndrome in Children** 137
J. Steven Hata, MD

Chapter 7. **Congenital Heart Diseases/Arrhythmias** 155
Marcus S. Schamberger, MD

Chapter 8. **Postoperative Cardiac Care** 181
Joseph D. Tobias, MD and William R. Wilson Jr., MD

Chapter 9. **Status Epilepticus** 207
Joseph E. Segeleon, MD and Steven E. Haun, MD

Chapter 10. **Increased Intracranial Pressure/Intracranial Pressure Monitoring** 223
Steven E. Haun, MD and Joseph E. Segeleon, MD

Chapter 11. **The Use of Sedative/Analgesic and Neuromuscular Blocking
Agents in Children in the Pediatric Intensive Care Unit** 241
Joseph D. Tobias, MD

Chapter 12. **Traumatic Injury and Burns** 273
Joseph D. Tobias, MD

Chapter 13. **Fluid and Electrolyte Issues, Metabolic Disorders, Tumor Lysis Syndrome** 287
Rosaleah V. Bernardo MD, Joseph E. Segeleon MD, and Steven E. Haun, MD

Chapter 14. **Nutrition in the Pediatric Intensive Care Unit Patient** 311
Adalberto Torres Jr, MD and Pat Wiggins, MS, RD, CS

Chapter 15. **Blood Product Administration and Coagulation Function** 333
Joseph D. Tobias, MD

Chapter 16. **Acute Renal Failure and Renal Replacement Therapy** 349
R. Blaine Easley, MD and Ted Groshong, MD

Chapter 17. **Diabetic Ketoacidosis** 367
Jessica Klekamp MD and Kevin B. Churchwell, MD

Chapter 18. **Hypertensive Emergencies in the Pediatric Intensive Care Unit Patient** 377
Ted D. Groshong, MD

Chapter 19. **Infectious Disease Issues in the Pediatric Intensive Care Unit Patient** 389
Sayonara Pérez Mato, MD and Sara S. Viessman, MD

Chapter 20. **Poisonings and Toxic Ingestions** 413
R. Blaine Easley, MD and Joseph D. Tobias, MD

Chapter 21. **Gastrointestinal Tract Disorders in the Pediatric Intensive Care Unit Patient** 439
Joseph D. Tobias, MD

Index 455

Foreword

This is my kind of book. I have always enjoyed mixing critical care, in controlled doses (maybe 10% but no more than 20% time), with general pediatrics. Critical care on inpatient units or in the emergency center gives meaning to general pediatrics, and vice versa. The variety is stimulating and it sets you apart from those who cannot care for seriously ill patients. But doing critical care as a generalist is not easy and requires some adjustments and commitment. The following is a description of some ways I have used to handle this, the tricks to keep you going. They may or may not apply to you.

First, you have to confront your own doubts. Being on the spot as the physician responsible for a seriously ill child is usually frightening for a general pediatrician. There is so much at stake—for the child, the family, and you. It helps for me to admit that this fear is normal, and to confront rather than deny it. This way you can resist the possibility of being paralyzed by it and can fight the impulse to dump the responsibility on someone less trained or too far away; or to say, "I can't . . . " or, "I won't take care of this child." Of course, being overconfident or unrealistically optimistic is also a problem. Besides, there are not that many jobs where you can completely avoid being on the spot for critical care. You may think you have one, but be sure this is rationalization—that you are counting on good luck to keep the disasters away when you are on call. The question is more "how soon and how often?" rather than "will it happen?" The key, then, is to change the anxiety from a negative to a positive, by using it to motivate readiness for critical care.

The single most important step is to get and keep (by recertifying every 2 years) certification in Pediatric Advanced Life Support (PALS). This is a 1-day course that totally immerses you into the basics of recognizing and managing respiratory distress and failure, shock from septic, cardiogenic, or hypovolemic origins, acid-base imbalances, electrolyte and fluid disturbances, arrhythmias, newborn resuscitation, and trauma. Although designed primarily for emergencies, much of PALS also applies to the ongoing in-patient management of the critically ill child. PALS emphasizes the ABCs (airway, breathing, and circulation) method for prioritizing critical care.

Second, have an emergency minilibrary at hand for quick reference, close to where your critical care experience is likely to occur. This book, *Pediatric Critical Care: The Essentials,* should be there, as should the PALS guidebook, produced by the American Heart Association and the American Academy of Pediatrics. Some basic pediatric texts and the poison control phone number may also be included.

Third, check your emergency equipment. Make sure you have a crash cart and know where it is and what it contains. Break the seal (with permission) and become familiar with the drugs, the equipment, and how it works. Adult crash carts do not automatically have all the right pediatric equipment. Is there a system to make sure the cart is routinely checked for completeness? Is everything there that you will need? If not, recommend adding pediatric sizes and drugs.

The pediatric emergency or critical care physician can generally relax and take the emergencies as they come. The generalist must do more to achieve the best outcomes in these situations. Here are some suggestions for ways to do this. When a sick patient is on the way, you often have 5 to 30 minutes to get ready. The warning may come from another physician, by communication with the ambulance en route, or from the family. Make the best of this. Get to the emergency center in plenty of time. If possible, there should be several minutes before the patient arrives. Why would you not get there immediately? Because sometimes the subconscious wish that you were "anywhere else" slows you down. If you have time, check and set up the crash cart, oxygen, and suction equipment. Next, think about who you should call on for help. One way the generalist compensates for a lack of everyday experience is by drawing heavily on consultations. Call them in when you know you will or probably will need them. Put them on alert when you think you might need help. Respiratory therapy and the best pediatric nurse available should always be there. A surgeon or anesthesiologist may help with arterial or venous access. Having anesthesiology there is usually the best help if the patient needs intubation. Often the anesthesiologist will stand by to guide and advise while you intubate, but will take over if you don't get it right away. Think about letting the critical care unit where you refer these patients know that you are expecting an emergency. You can use the excuse of alerting them about a possible transfer to present what you know about the child and to get some last minute tips.

Decide who will be in charge. One person, the most experienced in critical care or the one with the broadest pediatric training, must be "called" or identified to take charge in an emergency. Fight the tendency to turn this over to someone with less training or less pediatric experience, just because that individual is more aggressive. If you are in charge, you can still assign duties to any and all of those present. Delegate freely. A nurse should be designated to record, by the clock, everything that happens: who did what, what drugs were given, what doses were given, and when. Another nurse (or whomever is available) should also be asked to bring back a history from the family or ambulance personnel when you do not have one.

When the patient is stabilized, the next question will be whether to keep the child under your care, or to refer. This has been one of the most difficult critical care decisions, at least for me. Objectivity is the challenge, and besides medical knowledge, ego may inappropriately push you to keep a child, or fear may inappropriately push you to refer. Conferring with an objective individual that you trust, perhaps at your referral PICU, can clear the air for you to make the right choice for the child. Nursing care and equipment are also part of this equation. If you keep the patient, use diligence, attention to detail, reading, the free use of consults, and anticipation of problems to compensate for a lack of everyday experience.

Do the best you can. Remember that things may go bad even in the best of circumstances. These episodes are a time when you have to draw on everything you learned in medical school and since. You have to rely on your wits, but these events and their anticipation define a real and affirming part of pediatrics, at least for me. The pediatrician who never has to care for sick patients or be prepared for emergencies is not living up to his or her training. In the day and age of managed care, the pediatrician needs to be a specialist in the care of children.

William A. Altemeier, MD
Associate Dean for Medical Education
Professor, Department of Child Health
The University of Missouri
Columbia, MO

Preface

The practice of critical care medicine has seen a dramatic increase in the technology and pharmacology available for the care of the critically ill patient. While much of the care provided to critically ill patients is directed by physicians formally trained in pediatric ICU medicine, pediatricians and primary care physicians are frequently faced with caring for the critically ill during the initial diagnosis and stabilization of the patient, either in the office setting or in the emergency room. Additionally, due to manpower issues and hiring constraints, some pediatric ICUs are not staffed 24 hours a day with physicians formally trained in pediatric critical care medicine. This may be particularly true in nonurban settings.

Even when transport to another facility is contemplated, stabilization must occur prior to transport to a tertiary care facility. As such, these physicians represent the first line of care for these critically ill children. Numerous studies have demonstrated that effective treatment in the first few hours of a critical illness can have significant impact on the patient's eventual outcome.

Although there are several outstanding pediatric critical care texts, these are primarily directed at those of us who practice pediatric critical care medicine on a daily basis. The purpose of the current book, *Pediatric Critical Care: The Essentials,* is to provide a preliminary overview or introduction to critical care medicine. It is not meant as an exhaustive text dealing with all of the intricacies and controversies of pediatric critical care medicine. Rather it is provided as an introductory overview for those who may be periodically faced with caring for critically ill children. Its primary objective is to provide useful and practical information that can be used during the initial stabilization and management of the critically ill child, and to provide an overview of the day-to-day management of such patients during their PICU course.

Additionally, I would hope that this text would serve as an introduction to the pediatric ICU for house staff of various disciplines, for medical students, and for nursing staff. I have frequently been asked by people during their rotations in the pediatric ICU, for a text that outlines some of the basic concepts of pediatric ICU medicine and is presented in a format that can be easily read during a night on call or during rotations in the pediatric ICU. I would hope that this text would accomplish this purpose. It is of a length that should permit it to be read in its entirety during a resident's 2- to 3-month tour in the pediatric ICU.

Joseph D. Tobias, MD

Chapter 1

Airway Management

Joseph D. Tobias, MD

Introduction

The most immediate concern in the management of pediatric resuscitation and medical emergencies is an assessment of the airway and respiratory function. Regardless of the etiology of respiratory failure, further attempts at resuscitation or treatment of the underlying condition will fail if airway control with restoration of ventilation/oxygenation is delayed or ineffective. Emergency airway management may be fraught with difficulties, as there may be limited time to prepare for the problem; thus there is an emphasis on the need for prior preparation and appropriate training of all essential personnel.[1]

An added concern with airway management in the trauma setting is the protection of the cervical spine. Until proven otherwise, it is assumed that all pediatric trauma patients have a cervical spine injury. Although a thorough physical examination and a radiologic investigation can be used to exclude an injury, in the emergent setting there is frequently inadequate time to embark on such investigations. Therefore, the airway is managed with the assumption that there is an injury, and techniques are used to control the airway and to intubate the trachea (see below) that will not be harmful if an injury is found during the subsequent evaluation. The issues of airway management in the trauma setting, the radiologic evaluation of the cervical spine, and the techniques used to prevent cervical spine injury during airway management are reviewed in greater depth elsewhere in this volume.[2]

Airway Management

The goals of airway management are: 1) to relieve anatomic obstruction; 2) to prevent the aspiration of gastric contents; and 3) to promote adequate gas exchange. All patients should receive 100% oxygen (delivered by a nonrebreathing system) until the initial assessment of respiratory function is made, even if the oxygen saturation is adequate. The administration of 100% oxygen provides an alveolar oxygen tension of 600 to 700 mm Hg so that there is a significant reservoir of oxygen in the lungs to provide an adequate supply of oxygen during periods of respiratory compromise. With an alveolar oxygen tension of 600 to 700 mm Hg, a patient with a normal, functional residual capacity can tolerate periods of apnea of 5 to 10 minutes without a significant drop in the hemoglobin oxygen saturation.

Airway management may be as simple as relieving soft tissue obstruction of the airway by proper positioning of the head. Several factors predispose the pediatric patient to airway obstruction. Airway obstruction most commonly occurs because the tongue and/or pharyngeal soft tissues collapse into

---

From: Tobias JD (ed): *Pediatric Critical Care: The Essentials.* ©Futura Publishing Co., Inc., Armonk, NY, 1999.

the airway. Alterations in the level of consciousness that are related to closed-head injury or cardiovascular compromise with inadequate cerebral perfusion can lead to relaxation of pharyngeal musculature with soft tissue obstruction of the airway. The proportionately larger head of the child, when compared to the rest of the body, promotes neck flexion. The oral cavity is relatively small and the tongue is relatively large. All of these factors make upper airway obstruction a likely occurrence in children.

Simple measures to relieve airway obstruction include proper positioning of the head with avoidance of neck flexion (head tilt), anterior displacement of the mandible (jaw thrust), lifting the anterior portion of the mandible (chin lift), and placement of an oral airway. These three maneuvers are collectively referred to as the triple airway maneuver. An additional option is placement of an oral airway (Fig. 1) to provide anterior movement of the tongue. This maneuver should be avoided in combative or semiconscious patients, as it may be poorly tolerated and may lead to vomiting. The head tilt is avoided in the trauma setting because of the possibility of aggravating a cervical spine injury.

Decisions that must be made regarding endotracheal intubation include the route (oral versus nasal) and whether the patient should be awake or anesthetized. These decisions are based on the assessment of the normalcy of the airway and the ability to successfully perform endotracheal intubation (see below for management of the abnormal airway). In most cases, the preferred route for endotracheal intubation is oral. Attempts at nasal intubation can result in bleeding, which can obstruct visualization and make further attempts at endotracheal intubation impossible. Awake nasal intubation can lead to significant increases in intracranial pressure (ICP) and is absolutely contraindicated in patients with closed-head injuries. Nasal intubation is also contraindicated in patients who have evidence of facial trauma, cerebrospinal fluid leaks, or physical findings suggestive of basilar skull fracture (ie, Battle's sign, raccoon eyes, hemotympanum). Any of the above are suggestive of disruption of the cribriform plate and the usual barrier between the nasopharynx and the intracranial vault.

Prior preparation is an absolute requirement to ensure that endotracheal intubation is accomplished in an expedient manner. The available equipment should include a resuscitation bag and oxygen source (it is important to double check that the oxygen flow is turned on), appropriately sized masks, laryngoscopes, endotracheal tubes (ETTs), stylets, suction, and drugs. Various sizes and shapes of laryngoscopes are available, but they can most simply be classified are either straight (Miller) or curved blades (Macintosh) (Fig. 2). During laryngoscopy, the straight blade is placed on the laryngeal side of the epiglottis while the curved blade is placed on the pharyngeal side of the epiglottis in the vallecula. This author's preference is to use straight blades for children who weigh 10 kg or less, and curved blades for older patients. Suggested sizes and types of laryngoscopes are listed in Table 1.

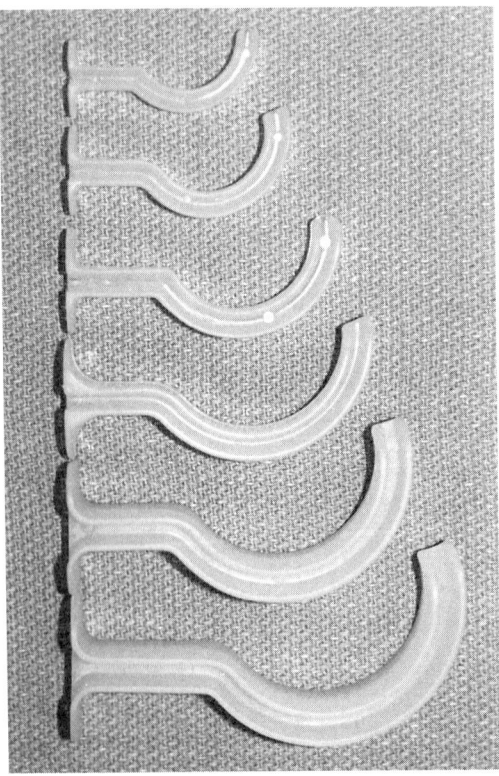

Figure 1. Photograph of various sizes of oral airways for the pediatric patient.

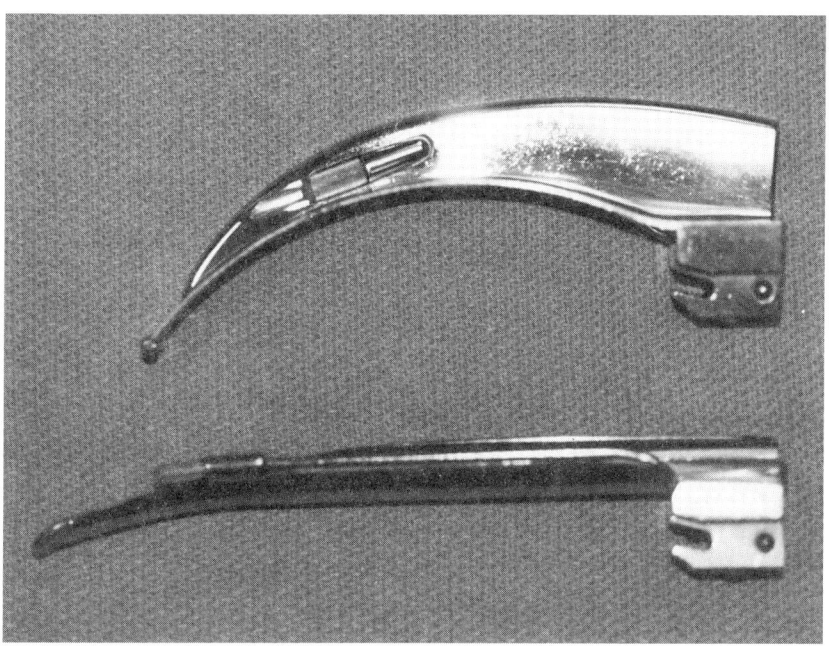

Figure 2. Photograph of the two basic types of laryngoscopes. The curved or Macintosh blade (above) and the straight or Miller blade (below) come in various lengths to accommodate patients of all sizes and weights.

The appropriate size for the ETT is based on the patient's age. A 3.0- or 3.5-mm ETT should be used in a term neonate, while a 4.0-mm ETT is appropriate for an infant who is 2 to 6 months of age. Beyond 6 months of age, the appropriately sized tube (mm) can be estimated using the rule:

$$\frac{AGE + 16}{4}$$

Maximum 7–7.5 mm ETT in patients greater that 14 years of age.

Table 1

Suggested Laryngoscope Sizes Based on Patient Weight

Patient weight	Laryngoscope
0–3 kg	Miller 0
3–5 kg	Miller 0,1
5–12	Miller 1, Wis-Hipple 1.5
12–20 kg	Wis-Hipple 1.5, Macintosh 2
20–30 kg	Macintosh 2, Miller 2
>30 kg	Macintosh 3, Miller 2

Another method of estimating ETT size is to use an ETT whose outside diameter approximates that of the patient's little finger. The formulas used to estimate ETT size are only starting guidelines; the real test is during laryngoscopy and passage of the ETT through the glottis. Excessive force must be avoided. The ETT should pass through the cords easily without undue force. Following placement, there should be a minimal airleak heard around the ETT with inflating pressures of 20 to 30 cm H_2O. The latter number was chosen because pressures above this exceed the perfusion pressure of the tracheal mucosa and may result in tissue necrosis, edema, scarring, and postextubation problems.

While cuffed ETTs are not routinely recommended for patients younger than 6 to 8 years of age, it is important to note that it is the pressure from cuff inflation and not the cuff itself that causes the damage. In specific circumstances it may be appropriate to use a cuffed ETT in younger patients. With severe pulmonary parenchymal disease, high peak inflating pressures may be needed to provide adequate oxygenation and ventilation. Without a sealed airway with a cuffed ETT, it may not be feasible to deliver these high pressures.

As the formulas are only starting guidelines, it is possible that the chosen uncuffed ETT will be too small, causing a need to change the ETT because of the excessive airleak. In the trauma setting, repeated laryngoscopies and changes of the ETT are not desirable and it may be appropriate to use a cuffed ETT the first time and inflate the cuff if necessary. If a cuffed ETT is used, a tube that is a half size smaller should be chosen, and the cuff should be inflated with the least amount of air necessary to prevent an excessive airleak.

The appropriate equipment and drugs should be prepared prior to the patient's arrival. It is frequently best to have a specific dedicated area or room in which all emergencies are handled, or a cart in which the equipment is kept. This allows for the collection of all of the appropriate equipment in one area.

An additional issue with emergency patients is the risk of aspiration during intubation. Unlike endotracheal intubation performed for elective surgical cases in the operating room, patients who present with acute medical emergencies are frequently not "nothing by mouth" (NPO). During sedation and paralysis for endotracheal intubation, passive or active regurgitation of stomach contents may occur. Trauma, pain, and anxiety all delay gastric emptying; therefore, regardless of when the patient last ate, he or she is still considered to have a "full stomach." Hence, techniques to minimize the risks of regurgitation of stomach contents are necessary.[3,4]

The risks of pulmonary damage following acid aspiration are related to both the volume and pH of the fluid. The risks are greatest with volumes in excess of 0.4 mL/kg and with a pH less than 2.5. In emergency airway management, there is not adequate time for pharmacologic management of either the volume or the pH of the fluid. The techniques used to prevent acid aspiration include cricoid pressure and rapid neuromuscular blockade/anesthesia (rapid-sequence induction and intubation).

Attempts at emptying the stomach with an orogastric tube are not recommended, as this does not effectively empty the stomach and it may also induce vomiting.

The goals of a rapid-sequence intubation are to secure the airway and to protect the lungs from acid aspiration. Cricoid pressure (Sellick's maneuver) is a technique that prevents the passive regurgitation of stomach acid. The upper esophagus is compressed against the cervical vertebral column by the application of anteroposterior pressure on the cricoid cartilage. The cricoid cartilage is the only complete ring of the trachea, and it can be used to compress the esophagus without interfering with the ability to pass an ETT. Cricoid pressure should be maintained from the time consciousness is lost until proper placement of the ETT is confirmed or, if intubation is unsuccessful, until the patient reawakens.

The second key to a successful endotracheal intubation is the appropriate use of rapidly acting neuromuscular blocking agents (see also chapter 11) and anesthetic agents. With rapid neuromuscular blockade and anesthesia, the possibility of vomiting at the time of intubation is reduced. Rapid-sequence intubation should always be preceded by the administration of 100% oxygen via a tight-fitting face mask. With full denitrogenation, the typical adult, without pulmonary parenchymal disease and/or abnormalities of functional residual capacity, can sustain approximately 5 to 10 minutes of apnea without developing hypoxemia. The period of apnea to the development of hypoxemia may be significantly less in infants and children, due to their increased metabolic rate for oxygen and decreased functional residual capacity. The use of a pulse oximeter during endotracheal intubation provides an added margin of safety and alerts the physician performing the intubation when the attempt should be aborted and bag/mask ventilation started. Gentle assisted ventilation with cricoid pressure can be applied following the administration of anesthetic agents and neuromuscular blocking agents to maintain oxygenation and ventilation until the onset of full neuromuscular blockade that is adequate for endotracheal intubation. The latter technique may also be used to provide hyperventilation prior to intubation in patients with altered intracranial compliance who are at risk for increases in ICP.

The Normal Airway

Sedative and neuromuscular blocking agents are contraindicated if the airway is judged to be abnormal and there is a question of the ability to successfully complete endotracheal intubation. In this situation, other techniques to secure the airway are needed (see below). If the airway is assessed as normal, one can proceed with neuromuscular blocking agents and sedative/analgesic agents for endotracheal intubation (Table 2).

The neuromuscular blocking agent used may be either a depolarizing agent such as succinylcholine or a nondepolarizing agent (pancuronium, vecuronium, rocuronium). The advantages of succinylcholine include a rapid onset of action (30 to 45 seconds) as well as a short duration of action (4 to 5 minutes). The latter may be particularly important in patients with head trauma or suspected cervical spine injury, so that immediate reassessment of their clinical status is possible. The short duration also provides a margin of safety should the clinician be faced with the "cannot intubate" scenario. If successful bag/mask ventilation can be provided, it may be most appropriate to allow the effects of the succinylcholine and the sedative agent to dissipate and then attempt endotracheal intubation using another approach (see below).

Extensive burns, crush injuries, and various neurologic and neuromuscular diseases remain contraindications to succinylcholine, as an exaggerated hyperkalemic response may be seen (Table 3). Succinylcholine is also contraindicated in patients with open-globe injuries, since the contraction of the extraocular muscles may lead to expulsion of the intraocular contents and permanent loss of vision.

Succinylcholine has been demonstrated to cause a modest increase (5 to 10 mm Hg) in ICP.[5] However, with its rapid onset of neuromuscular blockade, endotracheal intubation can be accomplished sooner with the restoration of adequate oxygenation and ventilation. The latter are the primary determinants of cerebral blood flow and ICP. Because of the effect of succinylcholine on ICP, its use in patients with altered intracranial compliance remains controversial. In the emergency setting, regardless of the age of the patient, a small dose of an anticholinergic agent such as atropine (5 to 10 µg/kg; up to 0.4 mg) is suggested prior to the administration of succinylcholine to prevent bradycardia.

Nondepolarizing muscle relaxants should be used in situations or with underlying conditions that contraindicate suc-

Table 2

Intubating Drugs and Doses

Neuromuscular blocking agents	
succinylcholine	2 mg/kg
pancuronium	0.15 mg/kg
vecuronium	0.1–0.3 mg/kg
rocuronium	1.0 mg/kg
Amnestic/analgesic agents	
ketamine	0.5–2 mg/kg
pentothal	2–6 mg/kg
propofol	2–3 mg/kg
etomidate	0.2–0.3 mg/kg
midazolam	0.2 mg/kg
Miscellaneous medications	
lidocaine	1–1.5 mg/kg
atropine	0.01 mg/kg
glycopyrrolate	0.005–0.01 mg/kg

Table 3

Contraindications to Succinylcholine

1. Hyperkalemia
2. Muscular dystrophies
3. Burns
4. Metabolic acidosis
5. Paraplegia/quadriplegia
6. Denervation injury
7. Metastatic rhabdomyosarcoma
8. Parkinson's disease
9. Disuse atrophy
10. Polyneuropathy
11. Degenerative central nervous system diseases
12. Purpura fulminans

cinylcholine. Several different nondepolarizing agents are available (Table 4). Their primary differences include onset and duration of action, metabolic rate, and cardiovascular effects. Significant histamine release can occur with several of the agents, including curare, atracurium, and mivacurium, thereby limiting their use in the emergency setting. Pancuronium (0.15 mg/kg) will provide acceptable conditions for intubation in 90 to 120 seconds, with paralysis lasting from 45 to 90 minutes. Mild histamine release and an increase in heart rate related to its vagolytic effects may be seen. Pancuronium is primarily (70% to 80%) dependent on renal excretion, with a significantly prolonged effect in patients with renal insufficiency/failure. A more rapid onset of paralysis can be achieved with either vecuronium or rocuronium. As vecuronium is devoid of cardiovascular effects, increased doses can be used to speed the onset of neuromuscular blockade. Doses of 0.3 mg/kg will provide acceptable conditions for endotracheal intubation in 60 to 90 seconds with a duration of blockade of 60 to 90 minutes. Priming may also be used to speed the onset of vecuronium. For this, 0.01 mg/kg is administered, followed in 2 to 3 minutes by the remainder of the intubating dose of 0.15 mg/kg. In the emergency setting, a priming dose is generally not recommended because it may induce significant amounts of neuromuscular blockade. It is also generally recommended that the intubating dose be given 2 to 3 minutes after the priming dose. This delay may not be practical during emergency airway management. Because of these problems, this practice is not recommended for emergent airway management.

The problem of the delayed onset with nondepolarizing muscle relaxants has been somewhat alleviated with the introduction of rocuronium.[6] Acceptable intubating conditions are achieved within 60 seconds in the majority of patients treated with rocuronium, making it the most rapidly acting of the nondepolarizing neuromuscular blocking agents. Like vecuronium, it is relatively devoid of cardiovascular effects. The duration of action following an intubating dose of 0.6 to 1.2 mg/kg is 30 to 60 minutes.

One must also select the drugs used to provide amnesia/analgesia during rapid-sequence induction (Table 2). The drugs chosen are based on two factors: the patient's hemodynamic status and the presence/absence of increased ICP (Table 5). In the hemodynamically stable patient (with or without a closed-head injury), standard induction doses of thiopental (4 to 6 mg/kg) or propofol (2 to 3 mg/kg) can be used. In addition to providing anesthesia for the procedure of endotracheal intubation, both agents also provide central nervous system protection. Both propofol and thiopental decrease the cerebral metabolic rate for oxygen, leading to reflex cerebral vasoconstriction and a lowering of ICP.[7,8] Lidocaine (1.5 mg/kg), 1 to 2 minutes prior to endotracheal intubation, can also be used to blunt the increase in ICP that can occur during laryngoscopy.

In the hemodynamically unstable patient without closed-head injury, etomidate (0.2 to 0.3 mg/kg) or ketamine (0.5 to 1 mg/kg) may be used to provide amnesia/analgesia.[9,10] Neither agent will significantly affect cardiovascular function. Although ketamine has direct negative inotropic properties, it causes a release of endogenous catecholamines, which generally overshadows its direct negative inotropic effects on myocardial contractility. The end result is generally an increase in heart rate and mean arterial pressure. Ketamine increases ICP and is contraindicated in patients with altered intracranial compliance. Ketamine is also the drug of choice

Table 4

Nondepolarizing Muscle Relaxants

Aminosteroid compounds:
　pancuronium
　vecuronium
　rocuronium
　pipecuronium

Benzylisoquinolinium compounds:
　tubocurarine
　metocurine
　atracurium
　mivacurium
　doxacurium

Table 5
Suggested Anesthetic Agents for Airway Management

Normal ICP/normal CV:	Normal ICP/abnormal CV:
pentothal/propofol	ketamine
Increased ICP/normal CV:	**Increased ICP/abnormal CV:**
pentothal/propofol	etomidate

ICP = intracranial pressure; CV = cardiovascular function.

during the endotracheal intubation of patients with increased airway reactivity. The release of endogenous catecholamines may be beneficial in patients with bronchospastic disorders.

In the hemodynamically unstable patient with a closed-head injury, etomidate can be used to provide amnesia and to lower ICP without deleterious effects on cardiac output and systemic vascular resistance. Etomidate, like propofol and thiopental, decreases ICP by decreasing the cerebral metabolic rate for oxygen and cerebral blood flow.

Once endotracheal intubation is accomplished, correct tube placement can be confirmed by one of several means, including direct visualization of the tube passing through the vocal cords, auscultation of breath sounds, mist in the ETT, carbon dioxide in the exhaled gases, fiber optic documentation of tracheal rings, or subsequent chest x-ray. Capnography or documentation of end-tidal carbon dioxide ($ETCO_2$) serves as a useful adjunct to ETT placement and should be considered routine in any setting in which endotracheal intubation occurs. Many of the newer $ETCO_2$ devices are compact and portable, allowing for their easy transport to any locale in which endotracheal intubation is necessary (Fig. 3). Alternatively, disposable, one-time use devices are available to document the presence of carbon dioxide in exhaled gases (Fig. 4). These devices rely on a chemical reaction

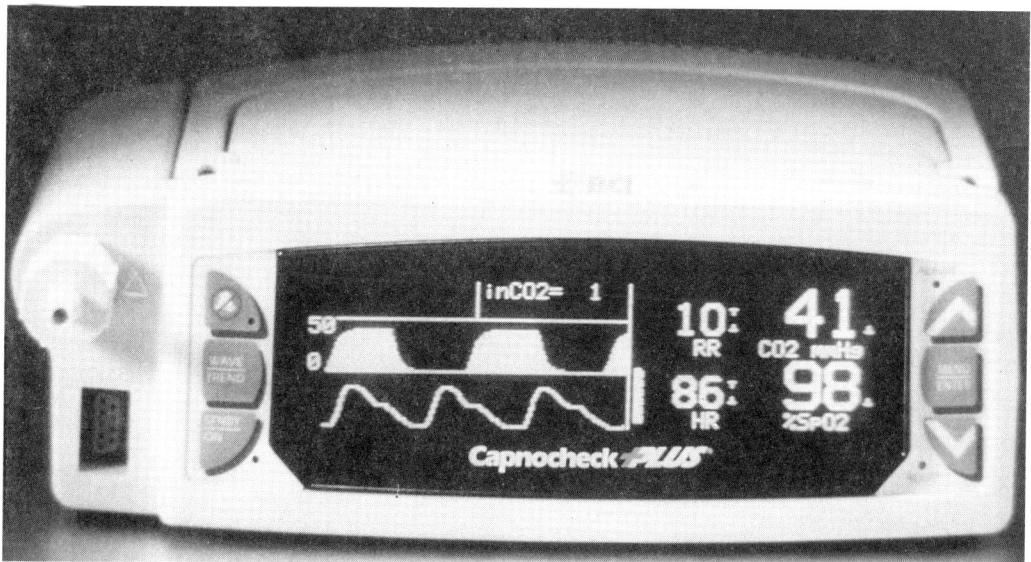

Figure 3. Photograph of the Capnocheck Plus Monitor (BCI International, Waukesha, WI). The monitor allows for sidestream sampling of end-tidal carbon dioxide from either an endotracheal tube or a nasal cannula, as well as continuous pulse oximetry.

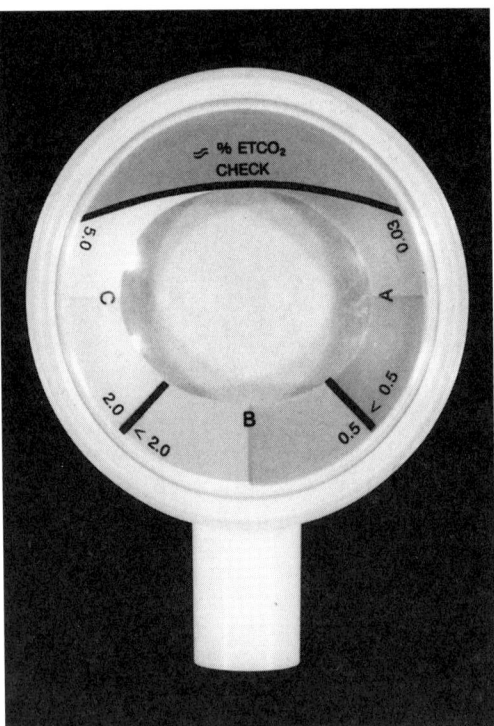

Figure 4. Disposable end-tidal carbon dioxide monitor. The device can be attached to an endotracheal tube to document the presence of exhaled CO_2 following successful endotracheal intubation. The presence of CO_2 in expired gases results in a color change of the device.

between the substrate in the paper and the carbon dioxide, resulting in a color change that demonstrates the presence of carbon dioxide.

Once correct ETT placement is identified, the tube is taped securely in position, bilateral breath sounds are auscultated again (after taping the ETT), and a chest x-ray is obtained. When the ETT is secured, the stomach is decompressed with an orogastric or nasogastric tube.

Failed Endotracheal Intubation

If the trachea cannot be intubated after paralysis and sedative agents have been given, an immediate decision must be made as to how to handle the failed intubation. A second attempt at intubation may be made after changing the patient's head position and the laryngoscope blade or after adding pressure on the larynx to help visualize the glottis. If these maneuvers fail, 100% oxygen should be administered through a tight-fitting face mask and assisted ventilation should be initiated. Cricoid pressure should be maintained until the patient awakens. At this point, the alternatives to be considered should follow the algorithm for failed intubation provided by American Society of Anesthesiologists (ASA) (Fig. 5). If bag/mask ventilation is successful, there is time to consider alternative routes of securing the airway, such as fiber optic intubation, performance of a tracheostomy using local anesthesia, or retrograde intubation techniques. Such techniques should only be performed by physicians skilled in pediatric airway management. If the trachea cannot be intubated but bag/mask ventilation is adequate, the most prudent maneuver is to allow the effects of the neuromuscular blocking/sedative agents to dissipate and for the patient to resume spontaneous ventilation.

If bag/mask ventilation cannot be accomplished, it is necessary to move quickly along the ASA algorithm to prevent hypoxemia, hypoxia, and central nervous system sequelae. The options at this point include placement of a laryngeal mask airway (LMA), use of the Combitube (Kendall-Sheridan, Argyle, NY), or needle cricothyrotomy. The use of any of these devices without proper training is not recommended. Of the three, the LMA is the easiest to become facile with and has the highest incidence of success and the lowest incidence of adverse sequelae. Placement and use of the LMA is a skill that anyone who may be involved in airway management may want to take the time to learn.[11] Training with the LMA has recently been incorporated in some advanced pediatric life support courses. Reference 12 provides a more in-depth review of the use of the LMA in the emergency setting.

The LMA is available in seven sizes to accommodate all sizes of patients from infancy through large adults (Table 6). It con-

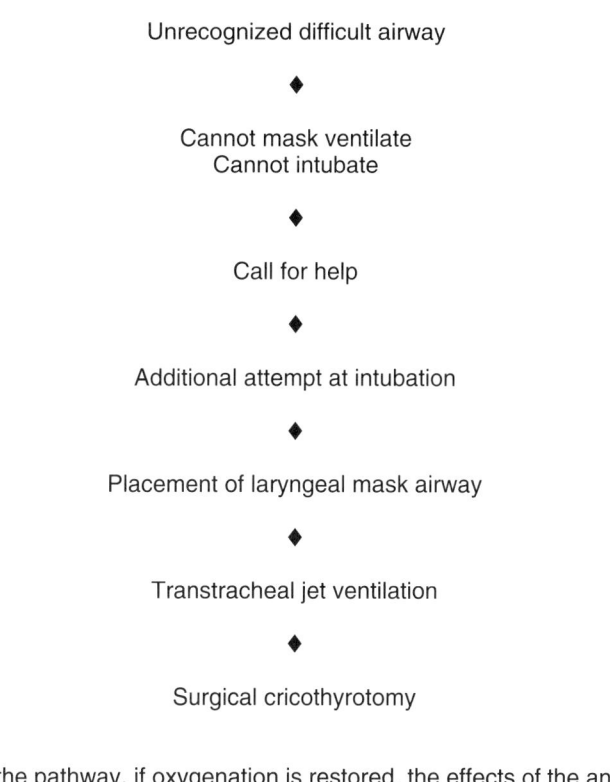

Figure 5. Modification of the American Society of Anesthesiologists algorithm for management of the "cannot intubate/cannot ventilate" scenario. LMA = laryngeal mask airway.

sists of a silicone rubber tube connected to a bowl-shaped mask with an inflatable rubber cuff (Fig. 6). The LMA is designed to sit in the hypopharynx directly over the glottis. It is passed without direct visualization into the oropharynx until resistance is felt. Placement can be accomplished with the neck in a neutral position, making it is suitable for use in the trauma patient. Following placement, the cuff is inflated and the 15-mm adapter is connected to an Ambu bag or to the anesthesia circuit, allowing for either spontaneous or positive pressure ventilation. In the "cannot intubate/cannot ventilate" algorithm (Fig. 5), placement of the LMA is the initial maneuver recommended following failed intubation.

Using one of several techniques,[13–15] the LMA can also be used as a guide for endotracheal intubation. As the distal opening of the correctly positioned LMA sits superior to the glottic opening, blind passage of an ETT through the LMA and into the trachea is possible. During insertion and passage through the LMA, the ETT is rotated 90° so that the tip of the ETT passes through the bars at the distal opening of the LMA. Due to the similar lengths of the LMA and the ETT, a limited amount of the ETT protrudes beyond the end of the LMA

Table 6

Description of the Different Sizes of Laryngeal Mask Airways

Mask Size	Pt Weight (kg)	Internal Diameter (mm)	Cuff Vol (mL)
1	<6.5	5.25	2–5
1.5	6.5–10	6.0	5–7
2	10–20	7.0	7–10
2.5	20–30	8.4	10–15
3	30–70	10	15–20
4	70–90	10	25–30
5	>90	11.5	30–40

Pt = patient.

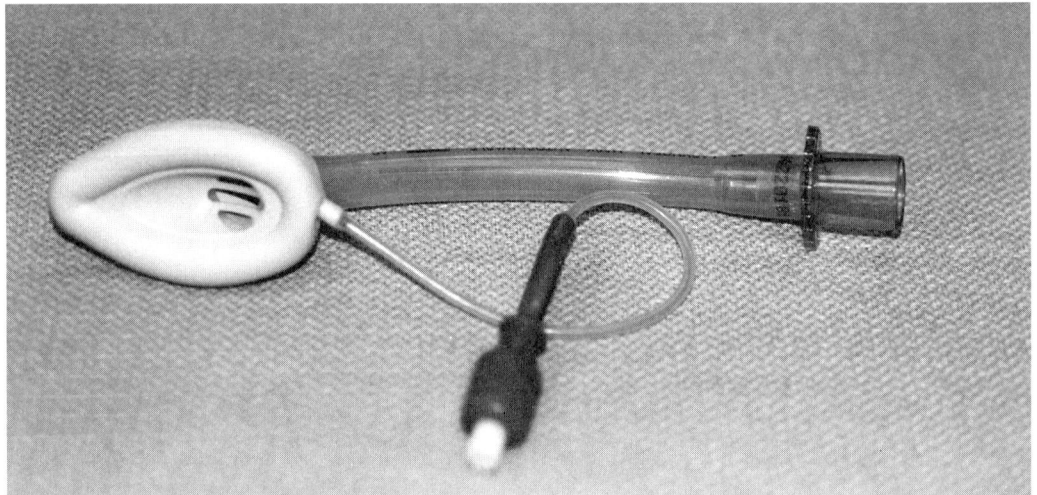

Figure 6. Photograph of a laryngeal mask airway (LMA).

following correct positioning in the trachea (Fig. 7). It is therefore recommended that the LMA and ETT be left in place, since removal of the LMA may dislodge the ETT. Success rates of up to 90% have been reported with blind passage of an ETT through the LMA.

Although use of cricoid pressure is recommended to prevent aspiration during airway management in the pediatric trauma patient, it has been demonstrated that the application of cricoid pressure may interfere with successful LMA placement and/or blind intubation through the LMA. Cricoid pressure increases the angle between the shaft of the LMA and the trachea. Therefore, cricoid pressure should be temporarily released during LMA placement or blind intubation through the LMA.

Alternatively, a gum elastic bougie (GEB), or intubating stylet, can be passed through the LMA and into the trachea.[16] This is a narrow cylindrical device, 3 to 4 mm in diameter and 50 to 70 cm in length (Fig. 8). As the GEB is passed into the trachea, a characteristic click is felt as the tracheal rings are engaged. After the GEB is passed into the trachea, the LMA is removed, and an ETT is passed over the GEB into the trachea. Rotation of the ETT 90° in either direction may facilitate passage of the ETT into the trachea. Success rates of up to 80% have been reported with this technique.

The LMA can also be used as a guide

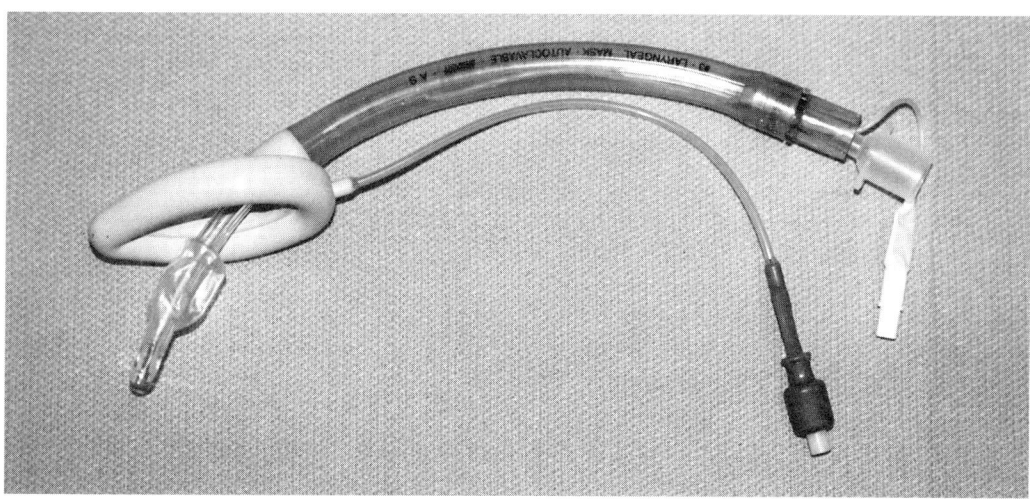

Figure 7. Photograph of an endotracheal tube that has been passed through a laryngeal mask airway (LMA). This technique can be used to provide endotracheal intubation if conventional techniques using direct laryngoscopy fail. Since the distal end of the endotracheal tube does not extend much past the end of the LMA, it is generally recommended that the LMA be left in place, as its removal may result in inadvertent removal of the endotracheal tube.

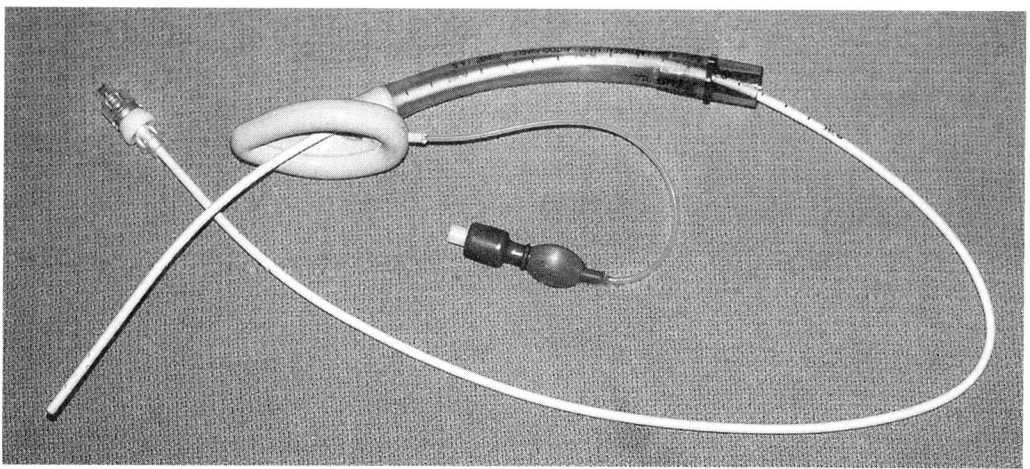

Figure 8. Following placement of the laryngeal mask airway (LMA), it may be possible to pass an intubating stylet through the LMA and into the trachea. The LMA is then removed and the endotracheal tube (ETT) is passed over the stylet and into the trachea. Placement of the ETT can be facilitated by performing direct laryngoscopy in the usual manner as the ETT is passed over the stylet and into the trachea.

during oral fiber optic bronchoscopic guided endotracheal intubation. Following LMA placement, the fiber optic bronchoscope (FOB) can be passed through the LMA past its distal opening and directly into the trachea. An ETT that has been previously placed over the FOB can then be guided into the trachea.

The LMA does not seal the airway; therefore the patient is still at risk for aspiration. It is used as a temporizing measure to reestablish ventilation and oxygenation or as an adjunct to guide endotracheal intubation. Despite these limitations, it may be life-saving in the "cannot intubate/cannot ventilate" scenario.

Needle cricothyrotomy is accomplished by inserting a 14- or 16-gauge intravenous catheter through the cricothyroid membrane into the trachea. The catheter is advanced through the skin into the trachea with a syringe that is filled with air or air/saline. Constant pressure is maintained on the plunger as the syringe is advanced, and air bubbles can be seen in the saline when the trachea is entered. The plastic catheter is then advanced over the needle into the trachea. The plastic catheter should advance without resistance off the needle and into the trachea. Once the catheter is positioned in the trachea, the syringe is attached again and the aspiration is repeated to ensure the correct placement of the catheter. An alternative means includes the use of a syringe and needle as previously described, but with the passage of a guidewire into the trachea followed by a dilator and a catheter. The latter may ensure that the catheter is not advanced off the needle into a false tract. A more recently described technique for ensuring the intratracheal location of the catheter includes the attachment of an $ETCO_2$ detector to the syringe or needle.[17] As the trachea is entered, carbon dioxide will be detected.

Identification of the trachea and correct catheter placement may be quite difficult in younger patients or in patients with distorted anatomy. The importance of ensuring that the catheter is in the trachea prior to instituting jet ventilation cannot be overemphasized. Jet ventilation through a catheter that is not in the trachea is disastrous, as subcutaneous emphysema and distortion of the anatomy may preclude further airway maneuvers, resulting in significant morbidity and mortality.

Once the catheter is placed in the tra-

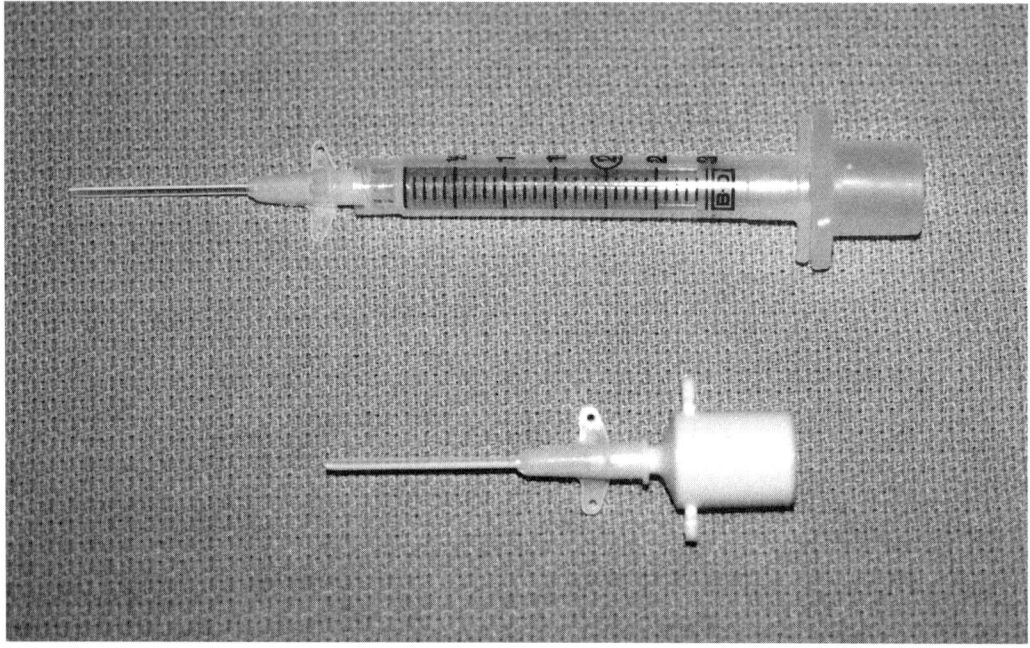

Figure 9. Techniques of jet ventilation. The small end of the 15-mm adapter from a 3.0-mm endotracheal tube fits directly into the intravenous catheter. Alternatively, the small end of the 15-mm adapter from a 7.0-mm endotracheal tube can be inserted into the barrel of a 3-mL syringe and the luer lock end attached to the catheter. The 15-mm adapter allows connection to an oxygen supply such as a standard resuscitation bag.

chea, oxygenation is maintained by intermittent jets from a high-pressure system. An oxygen line and toggle valve originating at a 50-psi oxygen source can be attached directly to the intravenous catheter. If this is not readily available, the small end of the 15-mm adapter from a 3.0-mm ETT will fit into the intravenous catheter (Fig. 9). Alternatively, the small end of the 15-mm adapter from a 7.0-mm ETT can be inserted into the barrel of a 3-mL syringe, and the luer lock end attached to the catheter (Fig. 9). The 15-mm adapter allows connection to the oxygen supply, such as a standard resuscitation bag. Any of the above mentioned techniques can be used to provide oxygenation, although their efficacy in providing ventilation and carbon dioxide removal is somewhat limited. The latter is not a problem, as most patients tolerate hypercarbia without significant adverse physiologic effects.

The Abnormal Airway

Occasionally, a patient's airway is abnormal due to an underlying condition (ie, Pierre-Robin sequence) to suggest that endotracheal intubation may be difficult. Table 7 lists other clues noted on physical examination that suggest that direct laryngoscopy and endotracheal intubation may be difficult. In these situations, alternatives to standard rapid-sequence intubation with muscle paralysis/anesthesia are required to ensure patient safety. An attempt at blind nasal intubation may be indicated in patients without facial trauma, signs of basilar skull fracture, and normal ICP.

Awake intubations are generally difficult in younger patients due to their age, level of understanding, and inability to cooperative. Awake intubation (of any route) is contraindicated in patients with increased ICP, penetrating neck wounds, and open-globe injuries. However, in the cooperative patient with a suspected difficult airway, there is generally nothing to lose by attempting a careful awake intubation. Awake intubation may be made easier by the combination of small doses of intravenous sedation (midazolam 0.03 to 0.5 mg/kg) and topical anesthesia of the airway with a local anesthetic solution. This may be accomplished by aerosolization of a local anesthetic, topical application of local anesthetic to the mucosa of the oropharynx, or by the direct blockade of the innervation of the airway. The latter method should be attempted only by those trained in this technique. A review of these techniques is provided in References 2 and 18. Consultation with a pediatric anesthesiology specialist or with other subspecialists trained in difficult airway management is suggested when one is confronted with such patients.

The structures of the oropharynx can be quickly anesthetized by topical spray (4% lidocaine or benzocaine). A second option is the use of a nebulizer (the same as that used for nebulizing β-adrenergic agonists) for the administration of 3 to 5 mL of 2% or 4% lidocaine, depending on the size of the patient. The total dose of lidocaine should not exceed 5 to 7 mg/kg (0.25 to 0.35 mL/kg of a 2% solution). Either of the above mentioned choices will provide adequate anesthesia of the airway above the level of the vocal cords. More distal anesthesia may be obtained with the aerosolized administration of lidocaine.

After the airway is topically anesthetized, several options exist for its management. The first is direct laryngoscopy with oral endotracheal intubation. Despite the anticipation of difficult oral endotracheal intubation, this technique is frequently successful. The technique can be safely performed in patients with documented or suspected cervical spine injuries. Meschino et al[19] noted no exacerbation of neurologic injury in their series of 165 trauma patients who underwent awake, oral endotracheal intubation.

Table 7

Physical Features Suggestive of Difficult Intubation

1. Short neck
2. Limited neck mobility
3. Limited mouth opening
4. Micrognathia
5. Large tongue
6. Small mouth

In addition to direct laryngoscopy with oral endotracheal, the options for oral endotracheal intubation in the awake patient include the Bullard laryngoscope, the light wand, fiber optic guided endotracheal intubation, and wire-guided retrograde intubation.[20] The majority of experience with any of these techniques has been in the adult population, and their use in the awake state, as with awake oral endotracheal intubation, requires an alert, cooperative patient.

The Bullard laryngoscope (Circon ACMI, Stamford, CT) is an anatomically shaped laryngoscope that uses fiber optic technology to view the larynx.[21,22] As such, direct visualization is not required and the need for lining up the oropharynx and larynx is eliminated. The blade is in the shape of a curved L. Once the blade has been rotated around the base of the tongue, force is applied superiorly (in a plane perpendicular to the axis of the patient) to visualize the larynx. While visualization of the larynx is usually excellent, passage of the ETT into the glottis may be difficult. The current design has an intubating style that is incorporated into the laryngoscope and lies along the right, posterolateral aspect of the blade in an attempt to correctly align the ETT and the airway. The Bullard laryngoscope can be used in the awake patient or following the induction of general anesthesia with spontaneous ventilation or following the provision of neuromuscular blockade. As there is limited movement of the cervical spine with both placement and subsequent use, it has been recommended as a useful tool for managing the airway in patients with suspected or confirmed cervical spine injury.

The light wand is a malleable illuminating stylet that can be used for blind oral intubation. The illuminating stylets can be inserted into an ETT of 5.0 mm or greater. As such, the technique can be used in patients as young as 5 to 6 years of age. The distal end of the stylet and ETT are bent 90° to facilitate entry into the trachea. The preparation of the patient for awake oral intubation using the light wand is the same as for other awake techniques and can include topical anesthesia or direct nerve blockade. Alternatively, the device can be used after the induction of general anesthesia with either spontaneous or controlled ventilation. If awake, the patient is instructed to protrude the tongue, and the stylet with ETT are inserted blindly into the oropharynx. As the device passes around the posterior aspect of the tongue and into the larynx, the light can be visualized in the anterior aspect of the neck at the level of the thyroid cartilage. Observation of the light may be facilitated by turning down the room lights. The light can be followed into the suprasternal notch if entry into the trachea occurs while the light disappears as a result of the tube passing into the esophagus. Once the ETT enters the trachea, the usual procedure is followed to confirm correct positioning. Successful use of the technique has been described in patients with normal and abnormal airways, in children, and in the trauma setting.[22,23] Since neck movement is not required for successful placement, it can be used in patients with cervical spine injuries, and it has also been suggested as a back-up or alternative means of intubating the trachea when direct laryngoscopy fails.

Recent advances in technology have significantly improved the quality of fiber optic devices as well as decreasing their size, thus making them suitable adjuncts to airway management in children. Fiber optic guided endotracheal intubation may be used via the oral or nasal route to aid in endotracheal intubation of the difficult airway. However, certain problems exist surrounding their use in the emergency setting. Most importantly, significant practice and experience may be required to become facile with these techniques, especially in smaller children. Once they are learned, ongoing practice is required to maintain the skills. Blood or secretions in the airway can significantly interfere with airway visualization. Important as they are, fiber optic techniques can be time consuming or impossible in the uncooperative patient.

Respiratory Function Following Endotracheal Intubation

Following successful endotracheal intubation, confirmation of correct ETT placement is mandatory and should begin with the auscultation of bilateral breath sounds. No method of confirming the intratracheal location of an ETT is 100% sensitive except for the direct observation of tracheal rings when a bronchoscope is passed through the ETT. $ETCO_2$ monitoring is suggested whenever airway management is performed as an additional means of confirming correct ETT placement. The $ETCO_2$ monitor may also be useful during transport, to identify inadvertent endotracheal extubation, should it occur, and to ensure that the desired arterial carbon dioxide range is maintained.[24] The latter may be particularly important if hyperventilation is instituted as a means of controlling ICP.

Once endotracheal intubation is performed and confirmed, the attention should focus on providing oxygenation and ventilation. Initial tidal volumes of 8 to 12 mL/kg are suggested, with respiratory rates adjusted according to the patient's age and the desired arterial carbon dioxide. Once the initial tidal volume is set, the peak inflating pressure (PIP) should be noted. PIPs greater than 35 to 40 cm H_2O suggest altered compliance with the need for appropriate investigation (see below). The initial FiO_2 should be 1.0. Moderate periods of time, even up to 10 to 12 hours of the high FiO_2, are not detrimental to pulmonary function. An FiO_2 of 1.0 is generally continued during the initial stabilization and transport of the patient. An adequate oxygen supply must be ensured prior to starting transport. An extra tank should be brought along if there is any question that the transport time will be prolonged.

If poor ventilation or abnormal pulmonary compliance is noted, an immediate evaluation is necessary. The first step should be auscultation of breath sounds to rule out mainstem intubation. This is more likely to be a problem in younger patients. A suction catheter should be passed through the ETT to ensure that the ETT is not kinked or that secretions/blood have not blocked the tube. A chest x-ray is indicated to rule out a pneumo/hemothorax. If a pneumothorax is suspected, either because of lack of movement of the chest wall or absence of breath sounds, needle aspiration should be carried out followed by thoracostomy tube placement. There may not be time to obtain a chest film if the child's ventilatory or cardiovascular function is deteriorating. Even with adequate airway management and effective ventilation, there may still be hypoxia and arterial desaturation due to pathologic right-to-left shunting through damaged pulmonary tissue, or due to acid aspiration, pneumonia, or lung contusion. Although these latter problems will require subsequent evaluation and treatment, the initial approach is the same: secure the airway and maintain adequate ventilation with 100% oxygen.

Summary

Several factors increase the difficulty and urgency of airway management in children in the emergency setting. Early and appropriate airway management are of prime importance in improving the eventual outcome of such patients. The major decision points of airway management include the assessment of the airway and the ability to successfully perform endotracheal intubation. If the airway is judged to be normal, oral endotracheal intubation following sedation and neuromuscular blockade is suggested. Rapid-sequence intubation to prevent acid aspiration should be employed. While the medications for airway management are generally administered intravenously, it should be kept in mind that the intraosseous route is an acceptable alternative for the administration of several different agents, including those used for endotracheal intubation.[25]

If the airway cannot be secured following the administration of anesthetic and neuromuscular blocking agents, the ASA algorithm for the "cannot intubate/cannot ventilate" scenario should be followed (Fig. 5). When the airway is judged to be abnormal, one of the above described awake techniques may be employed. While there is ample literature concerning these techniques in adults, their use in children has been limited. Most importantly, considerable practice may be required to become and stay facile with these "alternative techniques" of airway management. In certain circumstances, surgical cricothyrotomy should be considered as an alternative to airway management. Regardless of the technique chosen, appropriate personnel and preparation are mandatory to ensure the safe and effective management of the airway in the pediatric emergency patient. Due to the various skills and expertise of different subspecialists, a multidisciplinary approach to such patients is recommended. Such an approach may involve pediatricians, emergency room physicians, surgical subspecialists, anesthesiologists, and critical care physicians.

References

1. Nakayama DK, Gardner MJ, Rowe MI. Emergency endotracheal intubation in pediatric trauma. *Ann Surg* 1990;211:218–223.
2. Tobias JD. Airway management in the pediatric trauma patient. *J Intensive Care Med* 1998;13:1–14.
3. Davies JAH, Howell TH. The management of anaesthesia for the full stomach case in the casualty department. *Postgrad Med J* 1973;49:58–62.
4. Hastings RH, Marks JD. Airway management for trauma patients with potential cervical spine injuries. *Anesth Analg* 1991;73:471–482.
5. Minton MD, Grosslight K, Stirt JA, Bedford RF. Increases in intracranial pressure from succinylcholine: Prevention by prior nondepolarizing blockade. *Anesthesiology* 1986;65:165–169.
6. Magorian T, Flannery KB, Miller RD. Comparison of rocuronium, succinylcholine, and vecuronium for rapid sequence induction of anesthesia in adult patients. *Anesthesiology* 1993;79:913–918.
7. Wechsler RL, Dripps RD, Kety SS. Blood flow and oxygen consumption of the human brain during anesthesia produced by thiopental. *Anesthesiology* 1951;12:308–314.
8. Sebel PS, Lowdon JD. Propofol: A new intravenous anesthetic agent. *Anesthesiology* 1989;71:260–277.
9. Brussel T, Theissen JL, Vigfusson G, et al. Hemodynamic and cardiodynamic effects of propofol and etomidate: Negative inotropic properties of propofol. *Anesth Analg* 1989;69:35–40.
10. Bergen JM, Smith DC. A review of etomidate for rapid sequence intubation in the emergency department. *J Emerg Med* 1997;15:221–230.
11. Pennant JH, White PF. The laryngeal mask: Its uses in anesthesiology. *Anesthesiology* 1993;79:144.
12. Tobias JD. The laryngeal mask airway: A review for the emergency room physician. *Pediatr Emerg Care* 1996;12:370–373.
13. Inada T, Fujise K, Tachibana K, Shingu K. Orotracheal intubation through the laryngeal mask airway in paediatric patients with Treacher-Collins syndrome. *Paediatric Anaesthesia* 1995;5:129–132.
14. Heath ML, Allagain J. Intubation through the laryngeal mask: A technique for unexpected difficult intubations. *Anaesthesia* 1991;46:545–548.
15. Brimacombe J. Cricoid pressure and the laryngeal mask airway (letter). *Anaesthesia* 1991;46:986–987.
16. Allison A, McCrory J. Tracheal placement of a gum elastic bougie using the laryngeal mask airway (letter). *Anaesthesia* 1990;45:419–420.
17. Tobias JD, Higgins M. Capnography during transtracheal needle cricothyrotomy. *Anesth Analg* 1995;81:1077–1078.
18. Benumof JL. Management of the difficult adult airway with special emphasis on awake tracheal intubation. *Anesthesiology* 1991;75:1087–1110.
19. Meschino A, Devitt JH, Koch JP, et al. The safety of awake tracheal intubation in cervical spine injury. *Can J Anaesth* 1992;39:114–117.
20. Saunders PR, Giesecke AH. Clinical assessment of the adult Bullard laryngoscope. *Can J Anaesth* 1989;36:S118–S119.
21. Borland LM, Casselbrandt M. The Bullard laryngoscope: A new indirect oral laryngoscope (pediatric version). *Anesth Analg* 1990;70:105–108.
22. Ellis DG, Jakymec A, Kaplan RM, et al. Guided orotracheal intubation in the operating room using a lighted styles: A comparison with direct laryngoscopic technique. *Anesthesiology* 1986;64:823–826.
23. Holzman RS, Nargozian CD, Florence FB. Lightwand intubation in children with abnormal upper airways. *Anesthesiology* 1988;69:784–787.
24. Tobias JD, Garrett J, McDuffee A, Lynch A. End-tidal carbon dioxide monitoring during intra-hospital transport of children. *Pediatr Emerg Care* 1996;12:249–251.
25. Tobias JD, Nichols DG. Intraosseous succinylcholine for orotracheal intubation. *Pediatr Emerg Care* 1990;6:108–110.

Chapter 2

Cardiovascular Physiology, Shock, Inotropic Agents, and Invasive Hemodynamic Monitoring

Joseph D. Tobias, MD

Introduction

The cardiovascular system is responsible for the delivery of oxygen and nutrients to the tissues and for the removal of the end products of catabolism. Disturbances in cardiovascular function can result from several different factors that derange the controllers of cardiovascular function including the filling volume of the heart (left ventricular end-diastolic volume [LVEDV] or preload), myocardial contractility, or vascular tone. Alterations of these parameters can significantly impair tissue perfusion, oxygen delivery, and the removal of catabolic products. Early and aggressive intervention with correction of these problems is required to restore perfusion before there is irreparable damage to end organs. This chapter reviews basic cardiovascular physiology, the hemodynamic derangements of the various types of shock, the treatment of shock states including fluid resuscitation, the use of inotropic agents, and invasive hemodynamic monitoring.

Cardiovascular Physiology: The Basics

One problem in treating abnormalities of cardiovascular function is the lack of a simple and quick clinical tool to measure cardiac output. Even in the intensive care unit (ICU), such measurements require placement of invasive vascular monitors and the use of sophisticated equipment (see below). The regulation of cardiovascular function and blood pressure is dependent on the interactions of cardiac output and vascular tone. This relationship implies that blood pressure is a poor indicator of cardiac output. This is especially true in the pediatric population, since children are capable of maximizing their systemic vascular resistance (SVR) to maintain blood pressure even with significant decreases in intravascular volume and cardiac output. Cardiac output can be four to five times that of normal and yet the patient can be hypotensive, or the cardiac output can be one fourth to one fifth of normal while the blood pressure remains normal. The regulation of vascular tone, either endogenously by the renin-angiotensin system or exogenously by vasoactive medications, controls blood pressure relatively independent of cardiac output.[1] Therefore, the clinician must use other signs to assess cardiac output. These may include peripheral perfusion and temperature, capillary refill, urine output, mentation, and acid-base status. The latter may be a particularly valuable way of assessing the ade-

From: Tobias JD (ed): *Pediatric Critical Care: The Essentials.* ©Futura Publishing Co., Inc., Armonk, NY, 1999.

quacy of resuscitation and the ongoing treatment of shock. With inadequate tissue perfusion, anaerobic metabolism occurs with the accumulation of lactic acid leading to a base deficit. While many laboratories cannot quickly perform lactate assays, the base deficit on a routine arterial or venous blood gas analysis can be used to assess the adequacy of the ongoing resuscitation and the need for further base administration or volume resuscitation.

There are two additional relationships that are crucial for an understanding of the physiologic control of the cardiovascular system and its subsequent pharmacologic manipulation. The first is:

$$\text{cardiac output} = \text{heart rate} \times \text{stroke volume}$$

The volume of blood leaving the heart every minute (cardiac output) is equal to the heart rate times the amount ejected with each beat (stroke volume). In the majority of patients, the primary mechanism for controlling cardiac output is stroke volume. If the heart rate drops, the stroke volume increases to maintain cardiac output. However, specific patient populations may be unable to alter stroke volume. In this setting cardiac output is dependent on heart rate. If the ventricular muscle is noncompliant, the stroke volume cannot change and cardiac output falls when heart rate falls. Various disorders of the myocardium may lead to a noncompliant state. Examples can be seen in patients who have had multiple myocardial infarctions, patients with chronic cardiomyopathies, immediately following cardiopulmonary bypass for the correction of congenital cardiac lesions, and the neonatal population. The latter group is especially important to consider, as neonates do not tolerate bradycardia well because the drop in heart rate results in a precipitous fall in cardiac output.

The second basic relationship of cardiovascular physiology is that there are three variables that control stroke volume:

1. preload
2. afterload
3. myocardial contractility

Preload is determined by the volume of blood in the left ventricle at the end of diastole (prior to contraction) or LVEDV. Preload generally reflects the volume status of the patient. In the clinical arena, LVEDV is not measured, but rather inferred from measurements of filling pressures such as central venous pressure (CVP) or pulmonary capillary wedge pressure (PCWP).[2]

The LVEDV determines cardiac output according to the relationship originally described by Starling. Starling demonstrated that increasing the resting muscle strip length prior to excitation increases the tension and subsequently the force of contraction. This relationship holds true until the muscle fiber is overstretched, at which point the tension or force of contraction decreases. In the clinical arena, increasing the precontraction muscle fiber length by increasing LVEDV through volume administration results in an increase in the force of contraction and, therefore, the cardiac output.

The second variable that regulates cardiac output is afterload. Afterload is the impedance or resistance to ventricular ejection. It is primarily determined by two variables: vascular tone and changes in intrathoracic pressure. When contractility and preload are kept constant, cardiac output decreases as the afterload increases. Increasing afterload can be thought of as an increased resistance or force inhibiting flow of blood out of the heart. In the normal state, the vascular resistance is the primary determinant of afterload; however, with patients in acute respiratory distress, large increases in the negative interpleural pressure occur. The marked increase in interpleural pressure increases afterload and can adversely affect cardiac output, especially in patients with decreased preload or compromised myocardial contractility. This relationship is one of the reasons for the early institution of airway control and mechanical ventilation in patients with shock (see below).

Cardiac output is determined by heart rate and stroke volume. Stroke volume, in turn, is controlled by preload, afterload, and myocardial contractility. These relationships are particularly important to keep in mind when treating shock states and when considering the use of fluid versus inotropic agents. Identification of the cause of shock and the physiologic alterations related to it will help guide subsequent therapy and hopefully improve the eventual outcome.

Classification of Shock States

Shock is an acute disruption of circulatory function leading to the inadequate delivery of nutrients to the tissue. Shock cannot be diagnosed based on blood pressure. As stated previously, the body's response to a drop in cardiac output is to activate the renin-angiotensin and sympathetic nervous systems to increase vascular tone (systemic vascular resistance [SVR]) and to maintain blood pressure even as the cardiac output falls. Therefore, a patient in shock can have low, normal, or even high blood pressure.

Shock is the end result of several different physiologic disturbances. The various etiologic factors responsible for the disruption of circulatory function leading to shock can have markedly different effects on the three determinants of cardiac output: preload, afterload, and myocardial contractility. Shock can be further classified, according to its cardiovascular features, as cardiogenic, septic, hypovolemic, and distributive. The classification is useful in that it may give some information about the physiologic alterations involved, including the changes in preload, afterload, and contractility (Table 1). These cardiovascular changes should be kept in mind as therapy is instituted. The underlying etiology, when known, can be used to guide the appropriate therapy (fluid versus inotrope as well as which inotropic agent). While the fist four types of shock require varying degrees of fluid administration and inotropic agent titration, obstructive shock is a different story. The possibility of obstructive shock must be kept in mind whenever dealing with the patient with cardiovascular compromise. Obstructive shock includes anatomic factors which impede left ventricular filling and emptying (Table 2). The most important type of obstructive shock in the neonate and infant remains obstructive left-sided cardiac lesions including critical aortic stenosis, interrupted aortic arch, and hypoplastic left heart syndrome. Although the treatment of such problems includes the basic ABCs (airway, breathing, and circulatory support) along with correction of metabolic abnormalities (see below), paramount in the successful resuscitation of patients with these problems is the prompt administration of prostaglandin E in an attempt to reestablish patency of the ductus arteriosus, and provision of systemic blood flow from the pulmonary artery (PA) across the duct to the aorta. Although this is deoxygenated blood, the flow of deoxygenated blood is superior to the no-flow state that exists with the duct closed.

The remaining four types of shock require fluid and inotrope administration based on the etiology of the cardiovascular disturbance. Distributive shock describes a constellation of physiologic findings that occur with a long list of disorders (Table 3). The underlying cardiovascular alteration is a marked decrease in SVR resulting in hypotension and inadequate perfusion pressure. The drop in vascular tone can also affect the venous side, leading to a decrease in venous return/preload. From Table 1, it is

Table 1

Cardiovascular Changes in Shock			
Type of Shock	Preload	Afterload	Contractility
Cardiogenic	increased	increased	decreased
Hypovolemic	decreased	increased	normal
Septic:			
early	decreased	decreased	increased
late	increased	increased	decreased
Distributive	decreased	decreased	increased

Table 2
Etiology of Obstructive Shock
Left-sided obstructive cardiac lesions:
critical aortic stenosis
interrupted aortic arch
aortic coarctation
hypoplastic left heart syndrome
Cardiac tamponade
Pneumothorax
Hemothorax
Chylothorax

Table 3
Etiology of Distributive Shock
Anaphylaxis
Anaphylactoid reactions
Spinal cord injury/spinal shock
Head injury
Sepsis: early stage
Drug intoxication:
barbiturates
phenothiazines
antihypertensive agents

apparent that the cardiovascular changes seen with early septic shock are the same as those of distributive shock and, in fact, early septic shock is the most common cause of distributive shock in children.

The physiologic changes caused by septic shock are dependent on the stage of the disease. Early in the process, there is a marked vasodilatation with a drop in SVR and a decrease in venous tone and preload. These changes result in hypotension with tachycardia, increased cardiac contractility, and increased cardiac output. Clinically, the patient is frequently febrile with a bounding, rapid pulse with warm and vasodilated extremities. This can rapidly progress to late septic shock with myocardial failure. The hemodynamic changes of late septic shock are the same as those of cardiogenic shock with decreased myocardial contractility and increased SVR as the body attempts to maintain mean arterial pressure (MAP) in the setting of decreased cardiac output.

Cardiogenic shock is broadly defined as acute circulatory failure caused by inadequate myocardial function. In the pediatric age range, this occurs most commonly following cardiopulmonary bypass and surgery for congenital heart lesions or in the late stages of septic shock. In the child who presents to the emergency department with cardiogenic shock, the differential diagnosis is more extensive (Table 4). The most likely diagnoses include congestive heart failure from a congenital cardiac lesion, idiopathic myocarditis, or late septic shock.

Aside from the previously mentioned classification of shock, three additional etiologic possibilities must be kept in mind when facing the neonate or young infant with shock. These include congenital adrenal hyperplasia (CAH), inherited metabolic disorders with hyperammonemia, and obstructive left-sided cardiac lesions. Infants with CAH may present in the neonatal period with profound alterations of cardiovascular function, shock, metabolic acidosis, and hyperkalemia. While some children in shock will have hyperkalemia related to ongoing acidosis and alterations in renal blood flow, the diagnosis of CAH should be considered in the seriously ill child with metabolic acidosis and hyperkalemia. If the appropriate assay to diagnosis CAH is not readily available, blood can be stored for later investigations and a corticosteroid (methylpred-

Table 4
Etiology of Cardiogenic Shock
Congenital heart disease
Arrhythmias
Ischemic heart disease
anomalous origin of the left coronary artery
Kawasaki's disease
anoxic injury
Myocarditis
Myocardial contusion/traumatic injury
Acute drug toxicities
Chronic drug toxicities:
chemotherapeutic agents
radiation
Late septic shock
Infiltrative diseases:
mucopolysaccharidoses
glycogen storage diseases
Thyrotoxicosis
Pheochromocytoma

nisolone: 2 mg/kg, or hydrocortisone: 10 mg/kg) can be administered. While mild elevations of serum ammonia are sometimes seen with shock and acidosis, patients with inborn errors of protein metabolism (ie, urea cycle defects, organic acidemias) will generally have elevations of serum ammonia levels in excess of 1000 mg/dL.

The last of the triad of diseases that must be ruled out when faced with the neonate in shock is an obstructive left-sided cardiac lesion (see above). A group of acquired and congenital cardiac lesions including aortic stenosis, hypoplastic left heart syndrome, coarctation of the aorta, and interrupted aortic arch can present as shock in the neonatal period. Infants with these lesions are dependent on the ductus arteriosus for perfusion of all or part of the systemic circulation. Since blood cannot be ejected from the left side of the heart (aortic stenosis, hypoplastic left heart syndrome) or cannot reach the lower half of the body (coarctation of the aorta, interrupted aortic arch), blood flows from the PA across the duct into the systemic circulation. Although this is deoxygenated blood, the oxygen content is sufficient to meet the metabolic needs of the tissues. As the duct closes, the flow ceases and circulatory failure and tissue hypoxia occur.

Treatment of Shock States

Initial Management: Airway and Breathing

The approach to and treatment of shock in infants and children will vary somewhat based on the etiologic classification. However, regardless of the cause, the primary resuscitative efforts must include the basic ABCs. During the initial assessment, supplemental oxygen should be administered via a high-flow, nonrebreathing system. Even if the patient is well saturated, supplemental oxygen should be administered until the initial assessment is completed. There are few, if any, deleterious effects of administering 100% oxygen for brief periods.

If there is certainty of a diagnosis of a "ductal-dependent" lesion such as aortic stenosis or hypoplastic left heart syndrome, the administration of a high FiO_2 may have deleterious physiologic effects. The high alveolar oxygen may lead to excessive pulmonary vasodilation. In patients with obstructive left-sided lesions who are receiving prostaglandin E, as the blood leaves the ventricle, it may travel out the PA to the lungs or across the ductus arteriosus to the aorta to provide systemic circulation. The ideal situation is a 1:1 ratio of blood traveling to the pulmonary circulation to blood traveling to the systemic circulation. The ratio of the flow is controlled by the differential resistance of the two vascular beds (pulmonary versus SVR). The administration of high doses of oxygen by increasing the alveolar oxygen tension will dilate the pulmonary vascular bed, leading to more pulmonary blood flow and less systemic flow. Although the infant looks pink and the oxygen saturation is 85% to 95%, the systemic circulation is decreased and tissue hypoxia may develop. In these patients, the administration of oxygen should be titrated to maintain a systemic saturation of 75% to 80% to ensure a relatively constant 1:1 ratio of pulmonary to systemic blood flow. Control of $PaCO_2$ is equally important, as excessive minute ventilation can lead to pulmonary vasodilation and excessive pulmonary blood flow.

The initial physical examination should focus on the pertinent findings that can be used to assess cardiovascular function and attempt to determine the etiology of the cardiovascular disturbance. These should include an initial set of vital signs, auscultation of the cardiorespiratory system, examination of peripheral perfusion/pulses/capillary refill, and an assessment of liver size. The physical examination combined with the history may give clues as to the underlying etiology that can be used to direct further therapy.

The importance of early airway management cannot be overemphasized (see chapter 1). Early endotracheal intubation and control of ventilation may be indicated even in patients with a normal $PaCO_2$ and acceptable oxygen saturations. If there is any indication of impending respiratory failure or airway compromise, endotracheal intubation and controlled ventilation are suggested. Airway control should be based on the clinical state of the patient and not the numbers on the arterial blood gas (ABG). Early endotracheal intubation allows for control of ventilation with mild hyperventilation to partially compensate for metabolic acidosis. A decrease of $PaCO_2$ of 10 mm Hg results in an increase in the pH of 0.08 units. The administration of 100% oxygen improves oxygenation and maximizes the oxygen content of blood and oxygen delivery (see below). In patients with severe respiratory distress, the increases in negative intrathoracic pressure that occur with breathing may significantly increase afterload and may further compromise cardiovascular function. This effect is eliminated with controlled ventilation. Most importantly, although the patient may look stable, patients with shock have decreased oxygen delivery to all muscles, including the diaphragm, which can result in progressive respiratory fatigue and failure.[3] An additional indication for airway control is the apnea that can be caused by the administration of prostaglandin E.

Cardiovascular Resuscitation and Fluid Management

After the assessment and management of "airway and breathing," one's attention should next be focused on "circulation." The resuscitation of the cardiovascular system is dependent on the underlying etiology of shock. Treatment is based on the presumed alterations of preload, afterload, and myocardial contractility. These factors can be used to guide initial fluid and inotrope administration prior to the placement of invasive hemodynamic monitoring (see below).

Before appropriate fluid resuscitation can be accomplished, vascular access must be established. The simplest, safest, and often the most rapid means of obtaining venous access is by percutaneous peripheral vein cannulation. Because of the smaller size of veins in children and the fact that veins usually collapse during shock, percutaneous peripheral cannulation may be difficult and time-consuming. If peripheral venous cannulation cannot be accomplished within 60 to 90 seconds, initial access to the circulation can be rapidly obtained by placement of an intraosseous cannula. The preferred site for placement of an intraosseous needle is the medial aspect of the tibia, 2 to 4 cm below the anterior tibial tuberosity. While there are several commercially available intraosseous needles, a 16- or 18-gauge spinal needle can also be used. Fluid and medications can be administered through the intraosseous needle. The intraosseous route provides rapid and direct access to the central circulation. Once appropriate fluid resuscitation has been carried out, cannulation of a peripheral vein is often possible.

One area of active debate in shock resuscitation is the type of fluid that should be used: crystalloid or colloid.[4,5] Only 25% of the volume of crystalloid that is administered remains in the intravascular compartment while the remainder fills the interstitial and extracellular fluid compartments. The tendency for crystalloids to leave the vascular compartment along with the dilution of plasma proteins may theoretically predispose patients to the development of pathologic extravascular fluid such as pulmonary edema. While this theoretically makes sense based on the Starling forces that control fluid movements across the vascular compartment, clinical studies do not provide any evidence for the superiority of colloid over crystalloid for volume expansion in shock resuscitation. Additionally, there is a marked cost reduction when using crystalloids compared to colloids. The cost of 1 L of 5% albumin is as much as 50 times that of a vasoactively equivalent amount (4 L) of normal saline.

The commercially available colloid solutions include 5% albumin, 6% hydroxyethyl starch, and low molecular weight dextran (dextran 40 and 70). Adverse effects including platelet dysfunction, interference with crossmatching of blood, anaphylactoid reactions, and renal failure limit the use of dextran 40 and 70. Albumin is a naturally occurring plasma protein that provides approximately 80% of the intravascular colloid oncotic pressure in normal subjects.[6] The albumin molecule has a molecular weight of 69,000 and, under normal conditions, is relatively impermeable to the vascular membrane. The vascular membrane may be disrupted following sepsis and shock, thereby allowing albumin to pass into the interstitial spaces. The intravascular half-life of albumin is 24 hours with hemodynamic improvement persisting for up to 36 hours after administration.[7] As albumin is heat-treated, there are no infectious disease risks with its use. Another protein product derived from blood (plasma protein fraction or Plasminate) is not recommended for resuscitation in shock, as it can occasionally cause hypotension due to the presence of activated mediators of the kininogen pathway that are present in the solution.

Hydroxyethyl starch is a synthetic colloid that consists of a hydroxyethyl-substituted, branched-chain amylopectin with a molecular weight similar to that of albumin. Although its elimination half-time is 17 days, its clinical effects generally persist for only 24 to 36 hours.[8] Adverse effects include inhibition of platelet aggregation following the administration of more than 15 to 20 mL/kg.

Controversy also remains as to which particular crystalloid is most appropriate for volume expansion (Table 5). For volume expansion, in all cases, an isotonic fluid should be used. This includes normal saline, Ringer's lactate, or Plasmalyte. Ringer's lactate has a chloride concentration (109 mEq/L) that is roughly equivalent to the plasma chloride, while the lactate provides a source of buffer. The lactate of Ringer's lactate is converted into bicarbonate. One problem with Ringer's lactate is that the sodium concentration of 130 mEq/L is somewhat hypotonic compared to normal plasma, perhaps making it inappropriate for patients who are at risk for increased intracranial pressure.

While the sodium concentration of normal saline (154 mEq/L) is isotonic with normal serum, the high chloride concentration of 154 mEq/L can lead to the development of hyperchloremia acidosis. A third alternative is Plasmalyte, which has a more physiologic concentration of sodium and chloride (Table 5). Its buffers include both gluconate and acetate.

Aside from the isotonic crystalloids, recent attention has shifted to the possible beneficial effects of hypertonic crystalloids with or without the addition of colloid. These agents were initially used in clinical practice as early as World War I. The principle behind their use is to restore effective circulating blood volume with a lower volume of fluid (4 to 5 mL/kg). This can be accomplished, since the hypertonic saline increases serum osmolarity and promotes the movement of endogenous fluid from the extravascular space into the intravascular space. Additional effects demonstrated in laboratory animals include an increase in inotropic function of the heart, constriction of capacitance vessels, decrease in resistance vessels, and dilatation of precapillary sphincters.[9-11] The initial clinical studies in humans have shown similar beneficial effects. Holcroft et al[12] and Vassar et al[13] have demonstrated successful resuscitation of trauma patients with hypertonic saline (250 mL of 7.5% sodium chloride) without adverse effects except for transient hypokalemia. The initial clinical studies in adult trauma victims have demonstrated improved survival following resuscitation with hypertonic saline as compared with Ringer's lactate.[14,15] These agents may be particularly

Table 5

Composition of Crystalloid Solutions*						
Solution	Na+	Cl−	K+	Ca++	Mg++	Buffer
Normal saline	154	154	0	0	0	none
LR**	130	109	4	3	0	lactate 28 mEq/L
Plasmalyte	140	98	5	0	3	acetate 27 mEq/L gluconate 23 mEq/L

*concentrations are all expressed in mEq/L; **LR = lactated Ringer's.

beneficial for patients with associated closed-head injuries and those at risk for cerebral edema. As with other crystalloid solutions, the hypertonic solutions are inexpensive and have a long shelf life. Studies are needed in the pediatric population to determine whether similar beneficial effects will be seen in pediatric resuscitation.

At present, clinical studies do not support any advantage of colloids over crystalloids. Blood and blood products are administered only when replacement of hemoglobin or coagulation products is necessary. Appropriate fluids for intravascular resuscitation include normal saline, Ringer's lactate, and Plasmalyte. Dextrose-containing fluids should not be used for volume expansion.

The second question concerning the fluid resuscitation of shock is, how much fluid should be administered? This will depend on the type of shock. For cardiogenic shock, fluids may initially improve cardiac output and peripheral perfusion; however, the delayed effects may be deleterious, with the accumulation of extravascular fluid and pulmonary edema. In the setting of cardiogenic shock, inotropic agents are generally required to improve the underlying problem: defective myocardial contractility and increased SVR (see below).

For hypovolemic shock, the treatment is singular and straightforward: fluid. In this setting, fluid should be administered to restore cardiovascular function, peripheral perfusion, and urine output, and to correct metabolic abnormalities including lactic acidosis. Inotropic agents and vasoactive drugs should not be used in lieu of appropriate fluid administration to maintain blood pressure. In septic shock and distributive shock, the decrease in intravascular volume (preload) may be a direct problem related to fluid loss, but may also be an indirect effect due to venodilatation. Correcting these problems may require not only fluid, but also the use of an inotropic agent with vasoconstricting properties to increase the vascular tone.

In sepsis, decreased intravascular volume may result from increased insensible losses (fever, tachypnea), decreased intake, and increased losses (vomiting, gastrointestinal losses). The increased loss may be further compounded by a breakdown in the normal integrity of the vascular wall, with the transudation of fluid from the intravascular to extravascular spaces further decreasing the functional intravascular volume. The initial fluid requirements in these patients may be quite large, including up to 80 to 120 mL/kg during the initial resuscitative phase. Carcillo et al[16] examined the fluid requirements and eventual outcome, including the subsequent development of adult respiratory distress syndrome (ARDS), in children. The patients were divided into three groups based on the amount of fluid administered during the initial 60 minutes of therapy: group 1 received 20 mL/kg, group 2 received 20 to 40 mL/kg, and group 3 received more than 40 mL/kg of fluid. Patients in group 3 received 69±19 mL/kg of fluid at 1 hour and 117±29 mL/kg of fluid at 6 hours. The authors noted improved survival, decreased occurrence of persistent hypovolemia, and no increased incidence of cardiogenic or noncardiogenic pulmonary edema in group 3. The study demonstrates the large fluid requirements that may be present in patients with septic shock and the need to aggressively replete the intravascular volume to improve eventual outcome. The rapid repletion of the intravascular space does not increase the incidence of ARDS while the delayed or slow administration of fluid increases eventual mortality. While the use of inotropic agents is not suggested as a replacement for fluid therapy, agents that increase vascular tone are sometimes needed while restoration of the intravascular volume is provided (see below).

Fluids and inotropic agents are generally used in the treatment of distributive shock. While the primary problem is a decrease in SVR, alterations in the integrity of the vascular endothelium can lead to a transudation of fluid from the intravascular to the extravascular space with a decrease in the effective intravascular volume. The decrease in intravascular volume is further compounded by the increase in the vascular space due to vasodilatation. The combination of these problems generally requires fluid plus an adrenergic agent with vasoconstrictor properties.

In addition to fluid therapy, correction

of the metabolic abnormalities may improve cardiac output and may correct shock. With tissue hypoperfusion, metabolic acidosis frequently develops. This can be partially compensated for by endotracheal intubation and controlled ventilation. While fluid administration and cardiovascular resuscitation is mandatory to eliminate the ongoing anaerobic processes that lead to lactate production, buffer administration is frequently required to rapidly correct the problem. Persistent acidosis (pH <7.20) not only profoundly depresses myocardial contractility, but also impairs the effectiveness of exogenous catecholamines. The adverse effects of sodium bicarbonate must be weighed against the beneficial effects of restoring pH (Table 6). Sodium bicarbonate should be administered slowly, in doses calculated to correct the base deficit. One method of estimating the amount of sodium bicarbonate that should be administered for a half correction of pH is:

$$\text{mEq sodium bicarbonate} = 0.3 \times \text{weight (kg)} \times \text{base deficit}$$

A less cumbersome method may be to administer 1 mEq/kg for a base deficit of −1 to −5, 2 mEq/kg for a base deficit of −5 to −10, and 3 mEq/kg for a base deficit of greater than −10. In neonates and infants, half-strength sodium bicarbonate (0.5 mEq/mL) is recommended in order to avoid the deleterious effects of the administration of a hyperosmolar solution. If half-strength is not readily available, the standard concentration (1 mEq/kg) can be diluted 1:1 with sterile water. Note that this must be sterile water and not normal saline as is commonly used for i.v. flushes; the use of normal saline will not decrease the osmolarity of the solution. Sodium bicarbonate should not be given until effective ventilation is ensured. As the bicarbonate buffers the hydrogen ion, CO_2 is produced. An inability to remove the CO_2 load can result in hypercarbia or a paradoxical decrease in intracellular pH following the administration of sodium bicarbonate.

The rapid administration of sodium bicarbonate may abruptly increase pH and lower ionized calcium levels due to alterations in protein binding. Since many patients in shock may have low ionized calcium levels, measurement and correction of this cation may be indicated.[17] Hypocalcemia impairs cardiac contractility and limits the pressor effect of catecholamines. Since the free or ionized fraction is the physiologic active moiety, measurement of ionized calcium is suggested. Hypocalcemia is treated by the administration of either calcium chloride or calcium gluconate. Calcium chloride is administered in a dose of 0.1 to 0.2 mL/kg of a 10% solution, and spontaneously dissociates in the serum to release the free calcium ion. Calcium gluconate is administered in a dose of 0.2 to 0.4 mL/kg of a 10% solution. The larger dose is required, because on a milliliter-per-milliliter basis, the gluconate solution contains less calcium since the gluconate molecule has a greater molecular weight. Calcium gluconate is degraded in the liver to release the calcium ion. When given in equivalent amounts based on the calcium ion, both agents result in an equivalent rise in the serum ionized calcium level. If these agents are administered via a peripheral infusion, the calcium gluconate solution is suggested, since it may cause less tissue irritation should extravascular extravasation occur. Calcium solutions should be administered over 10 to 15 minutes in order to prevent bradycardia. In addition to repeated bolus administration, either calcium chloride or calcium gluconate can be added to maintenance i.v. fluids in concentrations of 10 to 20 mEq/L. Magnesium levels should be checked in patients with significant or persistent hypocalcemia. Magnesium is required for the release of parathormone in response to low serum calcium levels and is also required for the end-organ effects of parathormone. Hypomagnesemia can be corrected by the administration of a magnesium sulfate in a dose of 50 mg/kg

Table 6

Adverse Effects of Sodium Bicarbonate

Hyperosmolarity
Acute decrease in intracellular pH
Hypernatremia
Decreased ionized calcium concentration
Leftward shift of oxyhemoglobin dissociation curve

(maximum 2 grams) over 30 minutes. Magnesium should be administered over 20 to 30 minutes in order to avoid the effects of hypermagnesemia, including peripheral vasodilation and skeletal muscle weakness.

During the initial evaluation, a quick check of serum glucose is suggested with a rapid, bedside analyzer. The value can be confirmed by formal laboratory evaluation of serum glucose. Children, especially toddlers and infants, have limited glycogen stores and rapidly develop hypoglycemia during periods of stress. Severe hypoglycemia with subsequent central nervous system damage may occur if hypoglycemia is not identified and treated promptly. There is also some evidence to suggest that severe hypoglycemia may impair cardiovascular function. Serum glucose levels less than 60 mg% should be promptly treated with the administration of 1 mL/kg of 25% glucose or 2 mL/kg of 10% glucose. The latter agent is preferred in neonates and infants due to the concerns of hyperosmolarity with the rapid administration of concentrations of glucose greater than 10%. If 10% glucose is not readily available, 50% glucose can be diluted with sterile water to a 10% concentration.

Additional laboratory evaluation should include serum electrolytes, especially looking for hyperkalemia, blood urea nitrogen, and creatinine to evaluate renal function. While blood urea nitrogen generally rises out of proportion to creatinine with hypovolemia, significant elevations in creatinine may occur with isolated hypovolemia without underlying renal disease. Hemoglobin, hematocrit, and platelet count should also be checked. Shock, regardless of the etiology, can lead to disseminated intravascular coagulation and thrombocytopenia. Repeat determinations of hemoglobin and hematocrit may be indicated, as significant drops may occur after volume resuscitation.

Inotropic Agents

Endogenous and exogenous adrenergic agents exert their effects by binding to specific cell membrane-bound receptors. Several subclasses of adrenergic receptors exist including α_1, α_2, β_1, and β_2. Binding of the catecholamine to the beta receptor activates a stimulatory G protein which subsequently activates the enzyme, adenylate cyclase. This leads to the conversion of adenosine triphosphate to cyclic adenosine monophosphate (cAMP). cAMP is degraded by the enzyme phosphodiesterase (PDE). The increase of intracellular cAMP leads to the phosphorylation of intracellular enzymes that govern excitation-contraction coupling and intracellular calcium levels.

Activation of the α_1-adrenergic receptor and its associated G protein activates the enzyme phospholipase C with the hydrolysis of membrane-bound phospholipids with the release of inositol triphosphate (IP_3) and diacylglycerol. IP_3 stimulates the release of calcium from the sarcoplasmic reticulum. The increase in intracellular calcium increases excitation-contraction coupling with an increase in tone of the vascular smooth muscle (vasoconstriction) or an increase in contractility of myocardial cells (inotropy). The actual cardiovascular effects vary from inotrope to inotrope based on the dose used and their interaction with the various adrenergic receptors.

Dopamine is an intermediate product in the catecholamine pathway that ends in the production of epinephrine and norepinephrine. With exogenous administration, its cardiovascular effects are dose-dependent. In doses of 1 to 4 µg/kg/min, renal dopaminergic receptors are activated with an increase in glomerular filtration rate, renal vasodilatation, and increased sodium excretion by the renal tubules. These effects lead to an increase in urine output. Doses ranging from 4 to 8 µg/kg/min lead to predominantly β_1 activation with increased inotropic function of the myocardium. Doses in excess of 8 to 10 µg/kg/min activate α_1 receptors with vasoconstriction.

As it increases both inotropy and vascular tone, dopamine may be indicated in shock states with depressed inotropic function associated with decreased vascular tone such as early septic shock or distributive shock (see below). The β_1 effects, including increased chronotropic function with tachycardia and increased arrhythmogenicity, may limit its use in older patients. These latter effects are dose-dependent and more common with doses greater than 8 to 10 µg/kg/min.

Dobutamine is a synthetic catecholamine that exists as a mixture of the two optically active isomers. The (−) isomer is an α-agonist that results in vasoconstriction while the (+) isomer is a β-agonist that results in increased inotropic effects as well as peripheral β-agonism with vasodilatation that antagonizes the alpha effects of the (−) isomer. As a result, dobutamine causes an increase in inotropic function with a decrease in SVR, making it an appropriate agent for shock states that result in decreased inotropy and increased SVR (cardiogenic shock, late septic shock). Moderate tachycardia may also be seen with dobutamine, although the increase in heart rate and the arrhythmogenic potential are less than with dopamine. Doses range from 5 to 20 µg/kg/min.

Like dobutamine, the PDE inhibitors (amrinone, milrinone) lead to increased inotropic function with peripheral vasodilation. The PDE inhibitors are nonadrenergic agents that do not act via cell surface receptors, but rather inhibit PDE III, the enzyme responsible for the degradation of cAMP. The resultant increase in intracellular cAMP leads to an increase in the intracellular calcium concentration and an increased force of contraction. As the PDE inhibitors have a significantly longer half-life than the adrenergic agents such as dopamine, a loading dose is recommended prior to starting a continuous infusion. The recommended loading dose for amrinone in adults is 0.75 mg/kg over a period of 5 to 15 minutes; however, the limited studies in pediatric patients have suggested that higher loading doses (2 to 4 mg/kg) are needed.[18] The loading dose is followed by a continuous infusion of 5 to 10 µg/kg/min. Dosing regimens for milrinone include 50 µg/kg as a loading dose followed by 0.5 to 1 µg/kg/min. The loading dose of either amrinone or milrinone can cause significant vasodilation and a decrease in MAP. These effects can be minimized by increasing the duration of time over which the loading dose is administered.

While the cardiovascular actions are similar to those of dobutamine, the PDE inhibitors have a greater effect on the pulmonary vasculature and may be particularly beneficial in patients with increased pulmonary vascular resistance (PVR). These agents also are less arrhythmogenic than dobutamine and may be beneficial in patients that experience dysrhythmias with dobutamine administration. An additional benefit of the PDE inhibitors over conventional adrenergic agonists is their effect on the diastolic function of the heart. Diastole is an active, energy-dependent process during which calcium is taken up into the sarcoplasmic reticulum to allow the myocardium to relax. During this relaxation, ventricular filling occurs. This is known as the lusitropic function of the heart. With many pathologic states, diastolic function is impaired and ventricle relaxation is not effective. Diastolic dysfunction may occur in patients with chronic cardiomyopathies, congestive heart failure, and following cardiopulmonary bypass. In these states, the compliance of the ventricle is abnormal, thus requiring a higher than normal filling pressure to allow for adequate ventricular filling. While dopamine and dobutamine may make the diastolic dysfunction worse, the PDE inhibitors allow for improved ventricular relaxation and improve the lusitropic function of the heart.

Although the cardiovascular effects of amrinone and milrinone are similar, thrombocytopenia may occur following amrinone administration resulting from the production of an active metabolite. The thrombocytopenia may be particularly pronounced following cardiopulmonary bypass. This effect is not seen with milrinone.

Other adrenergic agents used for the treatment of shock states include epinephrine, phenylephrine, and norepinephrine. Epinephrine's cardiovascular effects are dependent on the dose used. Lower infusion rates of 0.05 to 0.2 µg/kg/min result primarily in stimulation of β_1 and β_2 receptors with increased inotropy, chronotropy, and peripheral vasodilatation. Infusion rates greater than 0.2 µg/kg/min lead to increased peripheral resistance through α-adrenergic stimulation. The effects of epinephrine are also age-dependent, so that tachycardia is more common and may limit the doses used in older patients. Infusion rates of 0.01 to 0.05 µg/kg/min may be effective in older patients.

Norepinephrine stimulates only α and β_1 receptors, leading to increased contractility and increased SVR. The increase in SVR limits the tachycardia that occurs via β_1 stimulation. Infusion rates vary from 0.05 to 0.2 µg/kg/min. Phenylephrine is a pure α-agonist that causes vasoconstriction. A significant problem with any agent that primarily causes increased SVR is that perfusion can be sacrificed at the expense of maintaining blood pressure. As mentioned previously, an adequate blood pressure does not ensure an adequate cardiac output. Monitoring of peripheral perfusion is mandatory when these agents are used. They should not be used at doses that result in peripheral vasoconstriction that leads to cold extremities and decreased urine output. Invasive hemodynamic monitoring should be considered when these agents are used (see below). Dopamine, in doses of 2 to 3 µg/kg/min, may be added to offset their detrimental effects on renal blood flow.

Isoproterenol has limited utility in the treatment of shock states. It is a pure β-agonist with effects at both the β_1 and β_2 receptors leading to increased heart rate, increased contractility, and peripheral vasodilatation. Its major role is in the treatment of refractory bradycardia that is unresponsive to anticholinergic agents such as atropine. Due to its β_2 effects with resultant bronchodilatation, it is also used for refractory status asthmaticus.

When selecting an inotropic agent for the treatment of shock, two important concepts should be kept in mind:

1. Inotropic agents should be not used instead of appropriate fluid resuscitation.
2. There is not a natural progression of one inotrope to another (ie, dopamine, dobutamine, epinephrine) based on how sick the patient is.

The inotropic agents have different cardiovascular actions, and different inotropic agents are used based on the type of shock and the underlying cardiovascular parameters (contractile state, SVR).

The primary problems associated with early septic shock include decreased preload and decreased SVR. Initial therapy includes aggressive fluid management; however an inotropic agent with vasoconstrictor properties may also be needed. These may include dopamine (doses of 8 to 20 µg/kg/min), norepinephrine, or phenylephrine. The latter agents are not used in place of fluid, but to increase the pathologically low SVR to normal levels. The same pathologic process occurs in distributive shock with an abnormally low SVR. In that setting, vasoconstrictor agents are also indicated.

In patients with late septic shock or cardiogenic shock, there is decreased cardiac contractility with an increase in SVR. Inotropic agents to treat these problems must produce increased inotropy with vasodilatation. This may include dobutamine, amrinone/milrinone, or epinephrine for refractory cases. The latter agent is used in doses of 0.05 to 0.2 µg/kg/min to provide pure beta receptor stimulation.

Mixing the Infusions

Various formulas have been suggested for the mixing of inotropic infusions. Fixed concentrations of drugs premixed in bags or vials in a set concentration (mg/mL) may be provided by the pharmacy. In this case, the infusion rate is adjusted according to the patient's weight, the concentration of the solution, and the desired infusion rate. Alternatively, the final concentration of the drug in solution can be calculated using the rule of 6's:

The final concentration of drug in solution (mg/100 mL) =

$6 \times$ patient's weight $\times$ y
y = the dose (µg/kg/min) delivered when the infusion is set at 1 mL/h

If one wants a dopamine infusion mixed so that 1 mL/h delivers 5 µg/kg/min for a 15-kg patient:

$6 \times 15 \times 5 = 450$
450 mg of dopamine are placed in 100 mL.
1 mL/h will deliver dopamine at 5 µg/kg/min.

Alternatively, in an emergency situation, fixed concentrations of inotropic agents can be added to solution. For this purpose it may be useful to keep the following dilutions in mind:

600 mg of dopamine or dobutamine can be mixed in 100 mL.

0.1 mL/kg/h delivers 10 µg/kg/min for either drug.

6 mg of epinephrine, norepinephrine, prostaglandin E, or isoproterenol are added to 100 mL.

0.1 mL/kg/h delivers 0.1 µg/kg/min of drug

Invasive Hemodynamic Monitoring

As mentioned previously, there is a poor correlation between mean arterial blood pressure and cardiac output. Although physical assessment and evaluation of factors such as capillary refill, skin temperature, and urine output can be used to gauge cardiac output, in specific circumstances a more accurate determination of the data may be required. Invasive hemodynamic monitoring may start with placement of a central venous line and CVP monitoring. The CVP can be measured from one of many sites including the subclavian, internal/external jugular, or the femoral vein. When placed via the femoral route, a frequently chosen site due to simplicity of placement and lack of significant adverse effects, the catheter can be used to accurately estimate CVP even when the tip is not in close proximity to the right atrium. In the absence of intra-abdominal processes increasing intra-abdominal pressure, there tends to be a close correlation along the entire lower venous system so that a catheter low in the inferior vena cava or femoral vein can provide an accurate reflection of CVP.

The CVP line can be used for venous access, and also for hemodynamic monitoring. CVP is measured from the distal port at the end of the catheter, while the proximal port or ports are used for drug and fluid administration. The CVP reflects right ventricular preload or right ventricular end-diastolic volume (RVEDV). The latter is a very rough estimate of LVEDV or left ventricular preload. However, significant problems exist with the use of the CVP for the estimation of the LVEDV. While a low CVP generally reflects low left-sided filling pressures, with a high CVP, the LVEDV can be low, normal, or high. In the patient with poor cardiac output, low urine output, and a high CVP, the most accurate means of obtaining further information to guide subsequent therapy is placement of a flow-directed PA or Swan-Ganz catheter. The PA catheter provides information concerning left heart function, right heart function, and pulmonary function including the shunt fraction (see below).

PA catheters come in several lengths and sizes (Fig. 1). Most pediatric intensive care units (PICUs) use two general sizes: a 5.0F or 5.5F catheter for patients 10 to 25 kg and a 7.0F or 7.5 F catheter for patients greater than 25 kg. The extra 0.5F in size includes the addition of the fifth lumen—the mixed venous oxygen sensor. The PA catheter has four or five ports. Port 1 is the proximal port or CVP port. Once the catheter is properly placed, the CVP or proximal port should sit in the right atrium and provide a CVP measurement. It is also through this port that saline is injected for determination of cardiac output. The CVP port is 30 cm from the end in the standard 7.0F or 7.5F PA catheter. In patients who weigh 25 to 45 kilograms, the proximal port may sit high in the vena cava and thereby not provide an accurate route for the administration of saline for cardiac output determination. Many of the adult-sized PA catheters (7.0F or 7.5F) provide an additional "right ventricular" access port for transvenous pacing or for the administration of vasoactive substances. If this additional port is present, this port and the standard CVP port can be connected to a transducer. If a CVP waveform is obtained from the "right ventricular" port, this port may be preferable for the injection of saline for cardiac output determination.

Port 2 is the distal port. This port provides an estimate of PA pressure and PCWP when the balloon is inflated. During placement ("floating") of the PA catheter, the distal port is monitored and the waveform is noted as the catheter is advanced from the right atrium to the right ventricle to the PA

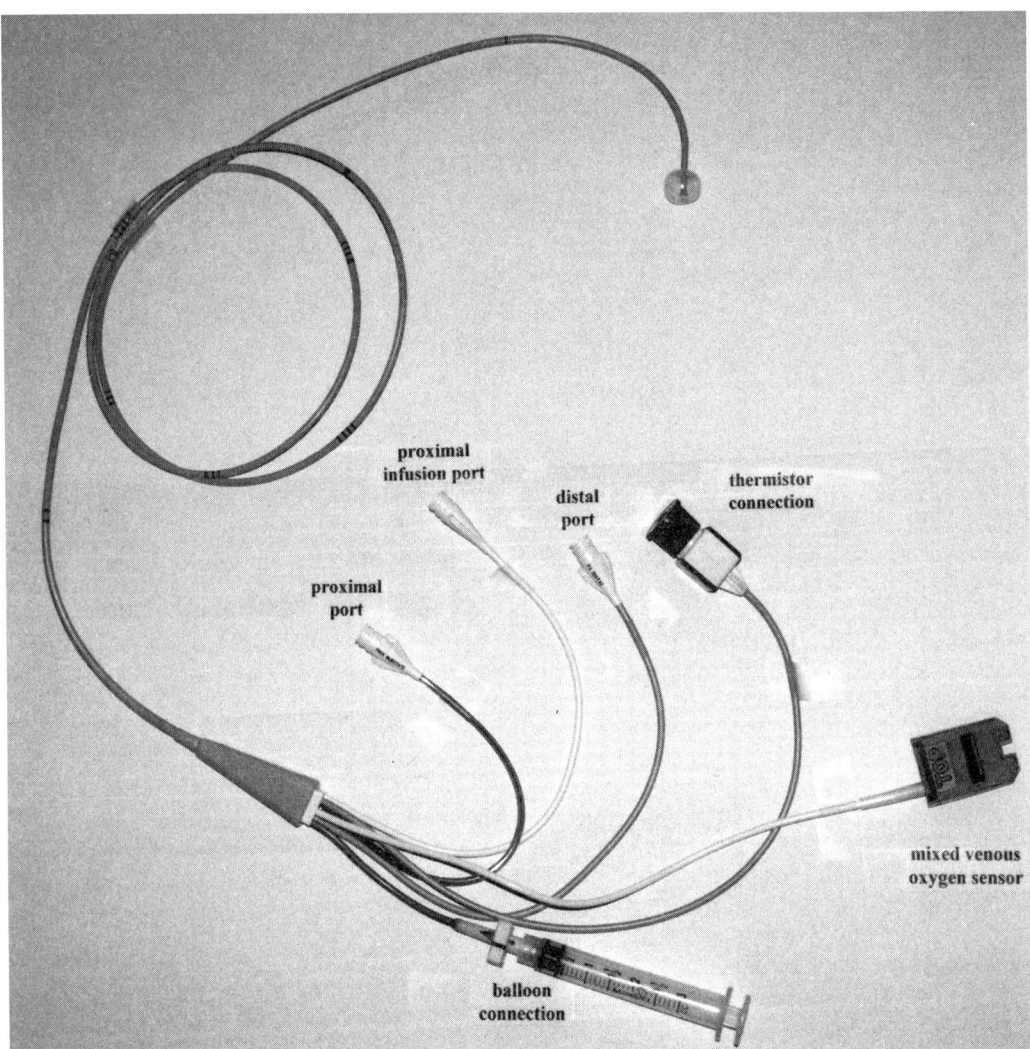

Figure 1. Photograph of a standard 7.5F thermodilution catheter with mixed venous oxygen sensor. The five lumens are identified and include the following: 1) the proximal port for central venous pressure (CVP) measurement and injection of saline for cardiac output determination; 2) the distal port for pulmonary artery pressure measurement—this is the port that is transduced to determine the pressures and observe the waveform during catheter placement; 3) the balloon port; 4) the thermistor that is connected to the computer to measure the blood temperature and determine the cardiac output; 5) the mixed venous oxygen sensor. The catheter also has a sixth port (the proximal infusion port) with an exit point 25 cm from the tip of the catheter. This port can be used for the administration of vasoactive substances. Additionally, in patients who weigh less than 45 kilograms, the proximal infusion port may sit in the right atrium while the proximal or standard CVP port, whose exit point is 30 cm from the tip of the catheter, is in the vena cava. In this setting, a more accurate cardiac output may be obtained by using the proximal infusion port for the room temperature saline injection.

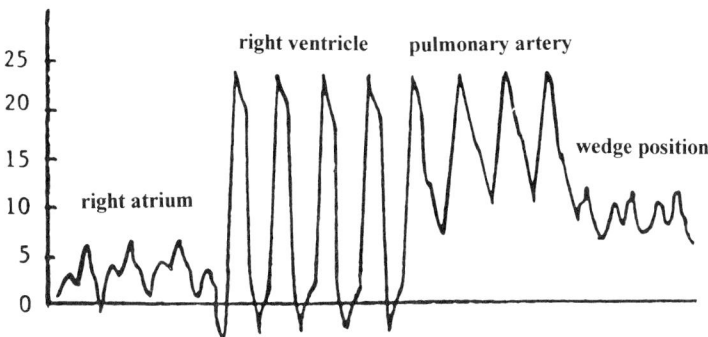

Figure 2. Drawing of the characteristic waveforms that are seen as the pulmonary artery catheter is advanced from the central circulation to the right atrium to the right ventricle to the pulmonary artery and then into the wedge position. The pulmonary artery waveform should reappear when the balloon is deflated.

and then to the wedge position (Fig. 2). Port 3 is for balloon inflation, and port 4 connects to the thermistor, which measures blood temperature used for the calculation of cardiac output. The optional fifth port available on both the 5F and 7F catheters provides a continuous estimation of mixed venous oxygen saturation measured from the PA at the tip of the PA catheter.

Mixed venous oxygen saturation provides an ongoing assessment of cardiac output. Mixed venous oxygen is the oxygen that the body does not need that is returned to the right atrium. It is determined by the difference between oxygen delivery and oxygen consumption. Normally the body uses only 25% of the delivered oxygen, resulting in a mixed venous oxygen saturation of 75%. Oxygen delivery to the tissues is determined by the oxygen content of the blood multiplied by the cardiac output. The oxygen content of the blood equals the amount of oxygen bound to hemoglobin plus that dissolved in the blood:

$$\text{arterial } O_2 \text{ content (vol \%)} = (1.39 \times \text{grams hgb} \times O_2 \text{ saturation}) + (0.003 \times PaO_2)$$

During the baseline state, O_2 consumption does not usually change abruptly unless the patient increases baseline activity by shivering, agitation, or fever. Likewise, hemoglobin concentration does not usually abruptly change, while changes in oxygen saturation are readily apparent when monitoring the oxygen saturation by pulse oximetry. Therefore, alterations in the mixed venous oxygen saturation without changes in oxygen consumption, hemoglobin concentration, or arterial oxygen saturation reflect a change in cardiac output and signal the need to check cardiac output and other cardiovascular parameters (see below). As the cardiac output drops, the mixed venous oxygen saturation also falls. Although mixed venous oxygen saturation is generally measured from the PA, in the absence of a PA catheter, a sample of blood can be obtained from a CVP catheter as a rough measure of mixed venous oxygen saturation and the adequacy of cardiac output.

After successful placement of a PA catheter, data can be obtained concerning right/left heart function, oxygen delivery/consumption, and pulmonary function including shunt fraction. The PA catheter provides important data concerning left heart function, including a means of measuring or calculating the three factors that control cardiac output: LVEDV, myocardial contractility, and afterload (SVR). When the balloon on the distal end of the PA catheter is inflated, the catheter is drawn into the "wedge" position. At this point, the waveform of the PA disappears. The PCWP is used to estimate left ventricular preload or LVEDV. Inherent in this measurement are specific problems which may preclude an accurate assessment. The PCWP is measured in mm Hg or pressure, and is used to estimate a volume. Conditions that affect the compliance of the left ventricle can disturb the normal relationship of volume and pressure so that a slight increase in volume causes a significant increase in pressure.

The second problem with PCWP monitoring is that the catheter is placed in the distal branch of the PA and is used to measure pressures beyond the lung in the left atrium. For accurate measurements, one assumes a normal flow of blood from the PA to the alveolar capillaries to the pulmonary veins to the left atrium and to the left ventricle. In the normal state (West zone 3), the PA pressure is greater than the pulmonary venous pressure, which is greater than the alveolar pressure—and the PCWP reflects left ventricular end-diastolic pressure (LVEDP) and LVEDV. With excessive increases in positive end-expiratory pressure (PEEP) and mean airway pressure, the alveolar pressure may rise and affect the accuracy of the PCWP. Various methods have been suggested to overcome this problem, including taking measurements while the patient is disconnected from the ventilator (not a good idea!), using an esophageal balloon to measure the transpulmonary pressure, or subtracting one half of the level of PEEP above 10 from the PCWP. An additional method is to obtain a lateral x-ray. If the tip of the catheter is below the level of the left atrium, the correlation of PCWP with left atrial pressure is generally acceptable, but if the tip is above the left atrium, the catheter should be repositioned. Other factors that influence the accuracy of PCWP measurements include pulmonary vascular disease, obstruction to pulmonary venous drainage, and mitral valve disease. Despite such problems, with the current available technology, the use of PCWP is the most accurate, readily available means of estimating LVEDV.

The PA catheter can also be used to directly measure cardiac output, by use of a thermodilution technique. For this purpose, a fixed volume of saline at room tempurature is injected into the right atrium via the proximal port of the PA catheter. As the fluid enters the right atrium, the temperature change that occurs as the blood passes the distal end of the PA catheter is noted. The magnitude of the temperature change and the rapidity with which it occurs is used by the sensor and computer to determine the cardiac output. In the pediatric patient, the cardiac output is divided by the surface area to the given cardiac index, which is measured in liters/minute/square meters. Other values can also be indexed, meaning that the value is divided by the body surface area. The normal values for measured and derived PA catheter data are listed in Table 7.

When cardiac output is known, SVR can be calculated. Resistance equals the difference in pressures across a system, divided by the flow. To calculate SVR, the difference in pressure across the systemic bed is the MAP minus the right atrial pressure or the CVP. The pressure is divided by the flow or cardiac output (CO).

$$SVR = \frac{80(MAP-CVP)}{CO}$$

By measuring the PCWP and the cardiac index, and calculating the SVR, the appropriate management can be determined for patients in various types of shock. This treatment can include fluids, vasodilators, or agents with direct positive inotropic effects.

The PA catheter can also be used to garner useful information concerning the pulmonary vascular bed. In addition to measuring the PA pressure from the distal port of the catheter, PVR can be calculated. The latter information can be important for patients with primary pulmonary hypertension or for those with associated congenital heart defects that predispose to pulmonary hypertension. Direct measurements of the PA pressure may be indicated with treatments aimed at reducing PVR. These treatments may include newer agents such as nitric oxide (see also chapter 8). PVR is calculated as the driving pressure across the pulmonary vascular bed (mean PA pressure [MPAP] minus left atrial pressure or PCWP) divided by the flow or cardiac output.

$$PVR = \frac{80(MPAP-PCWP)}{CO}$$

With measurement of either SVR or PVR, the value is multiplied by 80 to convert to the commonly used units of dyne-seconds/

Table 7

Value	Calculation	Normal Range
Cardiac index	Cardiac output/BSA	3.0–5.5 L/min/m²
PCWP	—	4–8 mm Hg
CVP	—	0–5 mm Hg
Stroke volume	CO/HR	50–80 mL
Stroke index	CI/HR	30–60 mL/m²
SVR	80(MAP-CVP)/CO	800–1200 dyne-sec/cm⁵
SVRI	80(MAP-CVP)CI	800–1600 dyne-sec/cm⁵/m²
PVR	80(MPAP-PCWP)/CO	120–240 dyne-sec/cm⁵
PVRI	80(MPAP-PCWP)/CI	80–240 dyne-sec/cm⁵/m²
Arterial oxygen content	$1.39(SaO_2)(hgb) + 0.003\ PaO_2$	20 mL O_2/100 mL
Oxygen delivery	$(CI)(CaO_2)$	600–1100 mL O_2/min/m²
Oxygen consumption	$(CI)(avDO_2)$	120–200 mL O_2/min/m²
$avDO_2$	$CaO_2 - CvO_2$	5 mL O_2/100 mL
Mixed venous oxygen saturation	—	60%–75%

CI = cardiac index; CO = cardiac output; HR = heart rate; SV = stroke volume; SI = stroke index; SVR = systemic vascular resistance; SVRI = systemic vascular resistance index; MAP = mean arterial pressure; CVP = central venous pressure; PVR = pulmonary vascular resistance; PVRI = pulmonary vascular resistance index; MPAP = mean pulmonary artery pressure; PCWP = pulmonary capillary wedge pressure; SaO_2 = oxygen saturation; hgb = hemoglobin; PaO_2 = arterial partial pressure of oxygen; CaO_2 = arterial oxygen content; C_vO_2 = mixed venous oxygen content; $avDO_2$ = arterio-venous oxygen content difference.

The calculation of oxygen delivery and consumption must take into account the fact that oxygen content is measured in mL O_2/100 mL and CI is measured in liters/min/M². The oxygen content should be converted to mL/L by multiplying by 10.

cm⁵. When PVR is measured in the cardiac catheterization laboratory, conversion by multiplying by 80 may not be used. In this case, the PVR is given as "Woods' units." The normal PVR is 180 to 240 dyne-seconds/cm⁵ or 2.2 to 3.0 Woods' units.

In patients with severe pulmonary parenchymal disease, the PA catheter can also be used to measure the intrapulmonary shunt fraction (Qs/Qt). This value may be used to determine the optimal level of PEEP in patients with severe pulmonary parenchymal disease or ARDS. As the level of PEEP is slowly increased, cardiac output determinations are made to determine the effects of PEEP on cardiovascular function. High levels of PEEP may affect cardiac output by decreasing venous return (preload or RVEDV) as well as increasing PVR. The increase in PVR may lead to increases in right ventricular end-diastolic pressure (RVEDP) and a shift of the ventricular septum so that it bows into the left ventricular and compromises left ventricular filling due to ventricular interdependence. As the PEEP is increased, the shunt fraction is measured. Shunt fraction (that percentage of the cardiac output that is passing through unventilated areas of the lung) is calculated as:

$$\frac{(C_{pv}O_2 - C_aO_2)}{(C_{pv}O_2 - C_vO_2)}$$

where $C_{pv}O_2$ = the oxygen content of pulmonary venous blood; C_aO_2 = the oxygen content of arterial blood; and C_vO_2 = the oxygen content of venous blood. These oxygen content values are determined from the formula:

$$\text{oxygen content} = (1.39 \times \text{grams Hgb} \times O_2 \text{ saturation}) + (0.003 \times PO_2)$$

The oxygen content of arterial blood is determined by measuring an ABG. The saturation must be determined by co-oximetry. Many of the standard blood gas analyses do not actually measure oxygen saturation, but calculate it from a nomogram that assumes a normal pH, body temperature, and 2,3-DPG levels. Since critical illness affects many of these values, it is necessary to actually measure the saturation.

Mixed venous blood is obtained from the distal or PA port of the PA catheter. The values for the oxygen content of pulmonary venous (pv) blood are determined using the alveolar air equation. It assumes an equilibration between alveolar O_2 and pulmonary venous O_2.

$$\text{Alveolar } O_2 = (Pb-47)FiO_2 - PaCO_2/R$$

where Pb = barometric pressure (usually 760 mm Hg); 47 is the partial pressure of water at 37°C; and R is the respiratory quotient; usually 0.8.

The alveolar air equation is based on the physical law that states that gases in a closed space equal the barometric pressure. In the alveolus the gases include air (oxygen and nitrogen), water vapor, and carbon dioxide. When measuring the shunt fraction, some authorities recommend administration of an FiO_2 of 1.0 to increase the accuracy of the measurement. The shunt fraction can exceed 50% to 60% in patients with severe ARDS. The optimal PEEP may be that level which decreases the shunt fraction to 15% to 20% without significantly impairing cardiac output.

The final data that can be obtained from the PA catheter comprise information concerning oxygen delivery, consumption, and extraction. Oxygen delivery is the product of cardiac output and arterial oxygen content (see above). Oxygen consumption is the difference between oxygen delivery to the tissues and that returning to the heart. This can been determined by multiplying the cardiac output by the difference between the contents of arterial and mixed venous blood. This value is then divided by the body surface area to give oxygen consumption in $mL/min/m^2$. The latter value may be important in the assessment of resuscitation in patients with septic shock and systemic inflammatory response syndromes. In the normal state, oxygen consumption does not increase as the cardiac output is increased. In the basal state, there is an excess of oxygen delivery to the tissues; hence, as the oxygen delivery increases, the tissues do not require more oxygen, and therefore oxygen consumption does not increase. In the septic state, there may be a pathologic condition known as a flow-dependent oxygen consumption, so that despite apparently adequate oxygen delivery, if the oxygen delivery increases, the oxygen consumption also increases. In this setting, it has been suggested that maximizing oxygen delivery until there is no longer an increase in oxygen consumption may improve survival.

Despite the apparent benefits of the PA catheter, significant complications may arise with its use (Table 8). Initial problems include difficulties or adverse effects associated with the placement of any invasive line including infection, vascular damage, bleeding, and pneumothorax. During passage of the catheter through the heart, arrhythmias or heart block may occur. The latter may be problematic in patients with preexisting left bundle branch block. Since a right bundle branch block may develop during catheter placement, patients with preexisting left bundle branch block may develop complete heart block. Access to transcutaneous pacing or transvenous pacing is suggested in such patients. In older patients, the use of specialized PA catheters that have an additional right ventricular port to allow transvenous pacing is an addi-

Table 8

Complications Related to Pulmonary Artery Catheter Placement and Use

Vascular access:
  vascular damage
  thromboembolic phenomena
  infection
  bleeding
  pneumothorax
Pulmonary artery catheter placement:
  arrhythmias
  complete heart block (especially with pre-existing left bundle branch block)
  right bundle branch block
  catheter knotting or kinking
  valvular damage
  perforation of cardiac chamber
Prolonged use:
  thromboembolic phenomena
  infection
  pulmonary infarction
  pulmonary artery rupture
  air embolism (with balloon rupture)

tional possibility. Arrhythmias may be treated by withdrawing the catheter and administering lidocaine (1 to 1.5 mg/kg). Knotting or kinking of the catheter can occur if an excessive length is inserted. The catheter should always be inserted with the balloon up, and removed slowly with the balloon down. Damage to the right-sided valves may occur if the catheter is withdrawn while the balloon is inflated. With ongoing use, complications may occur including thrombus formation, infection, and PA rupture or infarction. The latter may occur if the catheter is left in the wedge position for a prolonged period. As the catheter is in place for hours, it will gradually become more flexible, and it may travel further out into the PA and wedge itself without balloon inflation. Ongoing monitoring of the tracing from the distal port is mandatory so that the catheter can be withdrawn to a position where a normal PA trace is obtained.

Summary

Significant morbidity and even mortality can result if early and aggressive resuscitation is not provide for children in shock. The initial therapy for such patients must include the basics of resuscitation, including airway management and assisted ventilation when indicated. Correction of metabolic abnormalities such as hypoglycemia, hypocalcemia, and acidosis may partially correct the cardiovascular dysfunction. Fluids and inotropic agents are chosen based on the underlying pathology and the associated cardiovascular parameters. When ongoing resuscitation is required and there is a question as to the patient's hemodynamic parameters, invasive hemodynamic monitoring may be indicated.

References

1. Burnstock G. Integration of factors controlling vascular tone: Overview. *Anesthesiology* 1993;79:1363–1380.
2. Rahko PS. Comparative efficacy of three indexes of left ventricular performance derived from pressure-volume loops in heart failure induced by tachypacing. *J Am Coll Cardiol* 1994;23:209–218.
3. Aubier M, Trippenback T, Roussos C. Respiratory muscle fatigue during cardiogenic shock. *J Appl Physiol* 1981;51:499–508.
4. Shoemaker WC, Hauser CJ. Critique of crystalloid versus colloid therapy in shock and shock lung. *Crit Care Med* 1979;7:117–121.
5. Skillman JJ. The role of albumin and oncotically active fluids in shock. *Crit Care Med* 1976;4:55–58.
6. Tullis JL. Albumen. *JAMA* 1977;237:355–362.
7. Rothschild MA, Bauman A, Yalow RS, Berson SA. Tissue distribution of I-131 labeled human serum albumin following intravenous administration. *J Clin Invest* 1955;34:1354–1358.
8. Metcalf W, Papadopoulos A, Tufaro R, Barth A. A clinical physiologic study of hydroxyethyl starch. *Surg Gynecol Obstet* 1970;131:255–259.
9. Wildenthal K, Mierzqiak DS, Mitchell JH. Acute effects of increased serum osmolarity on left ventricular performance. *Am J Physiol* 1969;216:898–904.
10. Rowe GG, Mckenna DH, Corliss RJ, et al. Hemodynamic effects of hypertonic sodium chloride. *J Appl Physiol* 1972;32:182–184.
11. Lundvall J, Mellander S, White T. Hyperosmolarity and vasodilation in human skeletal muscle. *Acta Physiol Scand* 1969;77:224–233.
12. Holcroft J, Vassar M, Perry C, et al. Use of a 7.5% NaCl/6% dextran 70 solution in the resuscitation of injured patients in the emergency room. *Prog Clin Biol Res* 1989;299:331–338.
13. Vassar M, Perry C, Holcroft J. Analysis of potential risks associated with 7.5% sodium chloride resuscitation of traumatic shock. *Arch Surg* 1990;125:1309–1315.
14. Holcroft J, Vassar M, Perry C, et al. 3% NaCl and 7.5% NaCl/dextran-70 in the resuscitation of severely injured patients. *Ann Surg* 1987;206:279–288.
15. Holcroft J, Vassar M, Perry C, et al. Perspectives on clinical trials for hypertonic saline/dextran solutions for the treatment of traumatic shock. *Braz J Med Biol Res* 1989;22:291–293.
16. Carcillo JA, Davis AL, Zaritsky A. Role of early fluid resuscitation in pediatric septic shock. *JAMA* 1991;9:1242–1245.
17. Cardenas-Rivero N, Chernow B, Stoiko MA, et al. Hypocalcemia in critically ill children. *J Pediatr* 1989;114:946–951.
18. Lawless S, Burckart G, Diven W, et al. Amrinone in neonates and infants after cardiac surgery. *Crit Care Med* 1989;17:751–754.

Chapter 3

Croup, Upper Airway Obstruction, and Status Asthmaticus

Joseph D. Tobias, MD and David G. Nichols, MD

Introduction

Normal respiratory function requires the presence of an intact upper and lower respiratory tract to allow for the unimpeded passage of gas during inspiration and expiration. Various disease processes of either the upper or lower conducting pathways of the respiratory system can interfere with gas movement thereby resulting in respiratory failure. The patient's symptomatology will vary depending on the rapidity with which the process develops, the site of involvement, and the degree of narrowing of the airway. Regardless of the area of narrowing, many of these disease processes can result in fatal asphyxia if not appropriately identified and treated. This chapter discusses the etiology and management of patients with upper airway obstruction related to various disease processes including epiglottitis, croup, foreign body aspiration, and lower airway obstruction related to status asthmaticus.

Upper Airway Obstruction

Acute upper airway obstruction is a life-threatening emergency. Rapid and effective therapy is required in such patients, to prevent hypoxia, hypercarbia, and their sequelae. The urgency of treatment will depend on the initial assessment of the patient's respiratory function. Patients with impeding respiratory failure require rapid transportation to the operating room, where the personnel and facilities are available to deal with upper airway emergencies such as foreign body aspiration or epiglottitis. Table 1 lists the differential diagnosis of upper airway obstruction in children. Any of the conditions listed can present with severe upper airway obstruction and impending respiratory failure. Clinical signs and symptoms that are helpful in the differentiation of croup from epiglottitis, two of the more common causes of stridor in toddlers and children, are listed in Table 2.

Upon arrival at the emergency department, a rapid evaluation is made of the child's respiratory effort and the suspected site of obstruction (see below for treatment of status asthmaticus). One-hundred percent oxygen is administered via a high-flow system or nonbreather device. Patients with impeding respiratory failure, suspected foreign body, epiglottitis, or other surgical conditions listed in Table 1 are transported to the operating room. The appropriate personnel, including otolaryngologists, anesthesiologists, and intensive care physicians, should be assembled. It is imperative that,

From: Tobias JD (ed): *Pediatric Critical Care: The Essentials.* ©Futura Publishing Co., Inc., Armonk, NY, 1999.

Table 1

Etiologies of Upper Airway Obstruction in Children

Epiglottitis
Laryngotracheobronchitis or croup
Bacterial tracheitis
Peritonsillar abscess
Tonsillar hypertrophy
Severe tonsillitis
Retropharyngeal abscess
Foreign body aspiration
Subglottic stenosis
Mass effect from:
   tumor
   hematoma
   hemangioma
   papilloma
   cyst
Vocal cord paralysis
Poor control of pharyngeal musculature (altered CNS function)
Macroglossia
Trauma
Postoperative
Anaphylactoid reactions/anaphylaxis

CNS = central nervous system.

Table 2

Differentiating Features of Epiglottitis and Croup

	Epiglottitis	Croup
Etiology	bacterial	viral
Age	1 year to adult	1 to 5 years
Obstruction	supraglottic	subglottic
Onset	hours	days
Fever	high	low grade
Drooling	yes	no
Posture	sitting	recumbent
Toxic appearance	yes	no
Phonation	muffled	hoarse
Cough, URI	no	yes

URI = upper respiratory infection.

as long as there is some air exchange and the child is not dangerously hypoxemic, manipulation of the airway not be performed except by experienced personnel. Minor manipulation of the airway can result in complete airway obstruction, the inability to bag/mask ventilate or perform endotracheal intubation, and death. Once in the operating room, the inhalational induction of anesthesia is performed with increasing concentrations of sevoflurane or halothane in oxygen. This allows for the induction and maintenance of anesthesia while maintaining spontaneous respiration. During spontaneous respiration, the airway structures are kept open thereby improving gas exchange. If there is a foreign body or other mass effect including epiglottitis, the loss of spontaneous ventilation with the use of neuromuscular blocking agents can result in total airway obstruction. Once a sufficiently deep level of anesthesia is obtained, direct laryngoscopy is performed while the patient is still breathing spontaneously. At this time, examination of the oropharynx, peritonsillar and retropharyngeal areas, as well as the supraglottic and subglottic structures frequently provides an answer as to the etiology of the airway obstruction, and guides further therapy (see below). If the glottic structures can be identified, an endotracheal tube (ETT) is placed and a thorough examination of the airway and surrounding structures performed by the otolaryngologist. If a foreign body is present, it can be removed using a rigid bronchoscope. If the glottic structures cannot be identified, the otolaryngologist can place a ventilating bronchoscope and attempt to identify the glottic structures. If this is impossible, or if at any time complete airway obstruction occurs with progressive hypoxemia, tracheostomy or cricothyrotomy is performed.

If the diagnosis is epiglottitis, bacterial tracheitis, or some other process that is impinging on the airway, endotracheal intubation is continued postoperatively for a variable period until the process has resolved (see below for further discussion concerning the treatment of the conditions listed in Table 1). In patients with severe upper airway obstruction, the ETT is left in place and mechanical ventilation is continued for a variable period. There remains controversy as to the best course of action to ensure that the ETT remains in place. Although sometimes necessary, the routine use of neuromuscular blocking agents is discouraged due to their adverse effect profile (see chapter 11 for a full discussion of neuromuscular blocking agents). Additionally, the results are obviously disastrous if inadvertent extubation occurs in a patient who has upper airway pathology and is also receiving a neuromuscular blocking agent. Because of this, the maintenance of spontaneous ventilation is desirable; however, it may be difficult to walk the fine line between an appropriate level of sedation to prevent inadvertent extubation and yet allow for spontaneous ventilation. Our current practice, as is with most patients requiring mechanical ventilation, is to allow spontaneous ventilation by the judicious use of a continuous infusion with as-needed boluses of a benzodiazepine with or without an opioid. Other clinicians have suggested allowing the patient to provide his or her own entire minute ventilation by placing the patient with the ETT in place in a croup tent and not connected to the ventilator or ventilator tubing.

Endotracheal intubation is continued for a variable period depending on the diagnosis. Most importantly, resolution of supraglottic edema and swelling should be demonstrated prior to removal of the ETT. This can be evaluated by a return trip to the operating room or by direct laryngoscopy in the pediatric intensive care unit (PICU) after the administration of a sedative and short-acting neuromuscular blocking agent. Our current practice is to administer a single dose of propofol (2 to 3 mg/kg) with mivacurium (0.2 mg/kg) and perform direct laryngoscopy. If the upper airway pathology has resolved, the patient's trachea is extubated once he or she has met extubation criteria. Determination of the appropriate time for direct laryngoscopy to evaluate the upper airway may be based on the appearance of an airleak around the ETT. With airway pathology such as subglottic edema, croup, or epiglottitis, an ETT that is smaller than normal for the patient's age may be placed. With appropriate sizing of an uncuffed ETT in a child, a small airleak around the ETT is generally noted at a sustained inflation pressure of 18 to 20 cm H_2O. In patients with upper airway pathology, the presence of an airleak should be documented. A self-inflating resuscitation bag with a pressure manometer is attached to the ETT. The pressure is allowed to slowly increase and a stethoscope is placed over the neck. When there is audible air escaping around the ETT, an airleak is said to be present and the pressure is checked. In patients with cuffed ETTs in place, the cuff should be deflated to check for the presence of an airleak. If there is an airleak at a pressure of less than or equal to 25 cm H_2O, it is likely that the upper airway pathology has resolved and it may be appropriate to perform a direct laryngoscopy to evaluate the resolution of supraglottic pathology.

Additional therapy following placement of the ETT may include antibiotics based on the presumed etiology and the usual pathogens involved. The incidence of epiglottitis has decreased dramatically with the advent of an effective vaccine against *Haemophilus influenza B*. However, cases still occur in unvaccinated patients including older children, adolescents, and adults,[1] with failures of the vaccine and with infections due to other bacterial (*Staphylococcus aureus, Streptococcus pneumoniae*, group A *streptococcus*), viral, and fungal agents. Once appropriate airway management has occurred, the patient's trachea should remain intubated for 24 to 48 hours until the supraglottic edema and swelling resolve. Appropriate broad-spectrum antibiotic coverage such as a third-generation cephalosporin is indicated until the results of cultures (blood and direct swabs from the epiglottis) are available. Vancomycin may be indicated if disease due to resistant *Streptococcus pneumoniae* is suspected. In the era of epiglottis due to *Haemophilus influenza*, 50% to 70% of patients had positive blood cultures.

Another possible infectious etiology of upper airway obstruction is membranous laryngotracheobronchitis, otherwise known as bacterial tracheitis.[2] Patients with bacterial tracheitis present with a clinical picture that resembles both croup and epiglottitis. Like epiglottitis, bacterial tracheitis represents a medical emergency because the disease process can progress rapidly, with the development of total airway obstruction, asphyxia, and death. Unlike epiglottitis, bacterial tracheitis can have a relatively slow initial onset, and the supraglottic structures are normal thereby allowing for a relatively normal approach to endotracheal intubation. However, since the presentation can resemble any of the causes of airway obstruction listed in Table 1, these patients are generally best managed in the operating room (see above). Bacterial tracheitis is a bacterial infection of the subglottic area with the development of an adherent subglottic membrane. The diagnosis can be made by the presence of a large purulent mass that is suctioned from the ETT following endotracheal intubation. Cultures may reveal *S. aureus, K. pneumoniae, H. influenzae,* or other gram-negative organisms. Initial antibiotic therapy should be directed toward these organisms.

Other bacterial infectious processes that involve the oropharynx include retropharyngeal and peritonsillar abscesses as well as tonsillitis. Retropharyngeal abscesses occur in the potential space between the posterior pharyngeal wall and the prevertebral fascia that contains several lymph nodes. The lymph nodes and the potential for infection in this space generally disappear by the fourth year of life. As with peritonsillar abscesses and tonsillitis, likely infectious agents include *S. aureus, group A streptococcus,* and occasionally primary or secondary infections with anaerobic organisms. Following identification of the process and drainage in the operating room, broad-spectrum antibiotic coverage for all of these suspected organisms may be indicated. Single drug therapy may include clindamycin or the newer combination of ampicillin or ticarcillin and a β-lactamase inhibitor. Antibiotic therapy is altered based on culture results.

Many times, a patient presents with upper airway obstruction of mild to moderate severity, thereby allowing sufficient time for a more thorough investigation before proceeding to the operating room. Following the initial history and physical examination, based on the presumed etiology of the problem, it may be most appropriate to obtain a lateral and anteroposterior film of the neck and a chest x-ray. These films should identify radio-opaque foreign bodies, subglottic narrowing suggestive of laryngotracheobronchitis, or retropharyngeal and prevertebral swelling suggestive of a peritonsillar or retropharyngeal abscess. Subsequent therapy for these patients will depend on the suspected etiology. Therapy may include operative drainage of an abscess, antibiotics, corticosteroids, inhalation therapy with racemic epinephrine, and/or heliox to decrease the work of breathing (see below). In addition to these therapeutic endeavors, ongoing monitoring of such patients is suggested because rapid progression of the disease process may occur, thereby necessitating endotracheal intubation. Depending on the underlying pathology, endotracheal intubation may be performed in the PICU or in the operating room as outlined above. Ongoing monitoring should include continuous electrocardiography and pulse oximetry in addition to some monitoring of ventilation. Our preference for the latter is transcutaneous CO_2 monitoring.[3] While the correlation with $PaCO_2$ is not always exact, the trend of the CO_2 is often a helpful indicator of the patient's status. Correlation with an arterial value is not always necessary or suggested.

An additional infectious etiology to be considered in patients with upper airway compromise is croup or laryngotracheobronchitis. The latter is generally of viral etiology with the majority of cases due to parainfluenza viruses. Patients with laryngotracheobronchitis generally present with a gradual onset of increasing respiratory compromise following 1 to 2 days of upper respiratory infection symptoms. As the upper airway obstruction increases, the stridor becomes continuous with a preference for the expiratory component. The diagnosis is based on the history and physical examination. Anteroposterior x-ray examination of the airway may reveal the classic radiographic finding of a "steeple" sign which is due to the subglottic inflammatory process. If there is a question concerning the etiology, direct laryngoscopy in the operating room, as for suspected epiglottitis, is indicated. Patients with progressive respiratory failure may require endotracheal intubation. As the process affects the lower airway, direct laryngoscopy will reveal a normal upper airway and placement of an ETT is not generally problematic. An ETT that is smaller than normal for the patient's age may be needed and should be readily available. In mild to moderate cases, the time-honored therapy includes cool mist (ie, a croup tent). Adjunctive therapy includes corticosteroids and, as needed, racemic epinephrine. Corticosteroid therapy may be indicated for several of the conditions listed in Table 1. One of the problems with the use of corticosteroids in patients with upper airway diseases is that, as with many other disease processes, their efficacy has not been demonstrated by prospective, randomized trials. For infectious croup and other causes of upper airway obstruction,[4] dexamethasone in doses ranging from 0.5 mg/kg to 1 mg/kg may be beneficial and, with short-term use, has a limited adverse effect profile. All patients receiving corticosteroids should be monitored for gastrointestinal bleeding; our current practice is to use H_2 antagonists or other forms of gastrointestinal prophylaxis.

The other pharmacologic agent frequently used in patients with laryngotracheobronchitis is racemic epinephrine. Racemic epinephrine is available as a 2.25% solution containing both forms of optical isomers of epinephrine. The active cardiac form of epinephrine is l-epinephrine. Racemic epinephrine was originally produced with the thought that it would have the same effects on airway edema through its vasoconstricting properties and yet have limited effects on cardiovascular function if absorbed systemically. This has not been shown to be true in randomized studies comparing racemic epinephrine to l-epinephrine. Racemic epinephrine is administered in aerosolized form in doses of 0.3 to 0.5 mL mixed in 3 mL of normal saline. Alternatively, l-epinephrine (5 mL of the 0.1% solution) can be used if racemic epinephrine is unavailable.[5] Although it is indicated for patients with infectious croup and postintubation subglottic edema, other forms of upper airway pathology including epiglottitis may temporarily respond to aerosolized epinephrine, thereby giving a false impression of the etiology of the airway obstruction.

The final therapy that should be considered in patients with upper airway obstruction is the use of a helium/oxygen mixture.[6] This is used only as a temporizing measure, as it has no intrinsic therapeutic effects but can decrease the work of breathing and delay respiratory failure while allowing therapeutic agents or time to reverse the pathologic processes. Helium can be used to prevent the need for initial endotracheal intubation or immediately following extubation in patients with upper airway obstruction. Alternatively, it can also be used to "buy time" while the appropriate personnel are gathered to treat the patient who needs direct laryngoscopy in the operating room. When used in the operating room during inhalational induction with sevoflurane, the increased air exchange and minute ventilation achieved with helium/oxygen mixtures may allow for an increased minute ventilation and may improve the delivery of sevoflurane, thereby speeding the rate of anesthetic induction.

Helium was first isolated from atmospheric air in 1895 by Ramsay. It is an inert, nonflammable gas that possesses the lowest density of any gas other than hydrogen. Hydrogen is flammable and therefore cannot be used in clinical practice. Helium may be of benefit in various disease processes associated with obstruction to gas flow involving the upper airway (croup) or the lower airway (asthma). The basic premise for the use of helium is that during turbulent flow, the movement of gas through a tube is inversely proportional to its density. Resistance to gas flow through an orifice is directly related to the density of the gas as described by the relationship (resistance = $8\eta l/\pi r^4$) where l is the length of the connecting tube, η is the density of the gas, and r is the radius of the tube. As the density of the inhaled gas decreases, flow increases for a given pressure gradient.

The possible therapeutic uses of helium were first recognized and investigated in 1935 by Barach, who suggested its use in the treatment of various disorders, including obstructive conditions of the trachea, larynx, and bronchi as well as asthma, emphysema, bronchiectasis, and pulmonary fibrosis. While the initial results were favorable, helium's popularity as a therapeutic agent diminished after the introduction of other therapies for bronchospasm, such as the β-adrenergic agonists, as well as the decreased availability of helium during World

War II. Recently there has been a renewed interest in the application of helium for various disorders of the upper and lower respiratory systems.[6]

Duncan[7] evaluated the efficacy of helium as a temporizing measure in seven children with viral and postintubation subglottic edema. A scoring system based on breath sounds, degree of stridor, cough, retractions, and cyanosis was used as an objective measure of the patients' response. Only patients whose conditions were deteriorating despite maximal medical therapy were included. When switched from air to 80% helium/20% oxygen, there was a decrease in the patient's respiratory distress as judged by the croup score (7.9±0.4 to 3.9±0.3; $P<0.001$), $PaCO_2$ (46.0±3.9 to 40.4±2.9 mm Hg), and respiratory rate (51.7±7.0 to 44.7±6.7 breaths/min). None of the patients required endotracheal intubation. The helium/oxygen mixture was continued for 12 to 96 hours in the seven patients. After discontinuation of helium administration, all patients continued to show gradual improvement in their respiratory status. Although the majority of cases reported in the literature concerning the efficacy of helium in both children and adults with upper airway obstruction are relatively anecdotal with limited numbers of patients, the author's clinical experience with this therapeutic maneuver supports its efficacy.[8]

To achieve its beneficial effects, helium must be administered in concentrations of 60% to 80%. Administration of helium is suggested even in patients initially requiring a high FiO_2 since the decreased work of breathing and improved air exchange with helium may allow for a much lower oxygen concentration than without its use. Even if the patient requires 70% to 100% oxygen, the helium can be administered and its concentration slowly increased while monitoring the patient's oxygen saturation.

Helium is available in both E and H cylinders at a cost three to four times that of oxygen. The larger H tank will last 12 to 18 hours depending on the flow rate (5 to 10 L/min). Helium is also available in tanks as a 100% concentration at a lower price than the tanks that contain mixtures of helium and oxygen. These tanks must be mixed with oxygen prior to administration. When this is done, there must be a mechanism to ensure that a hypoxic mixture is not delivered if the oxygen supply is cut off or runs out. Anesthesia machines are equipped with a "fail-safe" mechanism which shuts off other gases if the oxygen pressure falls below a specific level. However, when helium is administered outside of the operating room, care must be taken to ensure that hypoxic mixtures are not administered and that the oxygen tank does not run out. Due to these issues, our practice includes the use of tanks that contain helium/oxygen in an 80%/20% mixture. These are blended with 100% oxygen to achieve the final desired concentration. The blending may use a standard oxygen blender that normally blends oxygen and air to achieve the final concentration. In such a case, the air hose is modified to fit to the heliox tank. Although the tank normally blends air that is 21% oxygen with oxygen, even when the 80/20 heliox tank is connected, the oxygen dial will not accurately reflect the oxygen concentration, because the dial works by opening orifices of various sizes to allow the flow of oxygen and the second gas. As heliox is less dense than air, a greater amount of it will flow through the orifice and, therefore, the delivered oxygen concentration will be less than that indicated on the dial. Therefore, the inspired concentration of oxygen should be monitored in line as it is delivered to the patient. Alternatively, the oxygen and heliox can be mixed by connecting the tubing from the two tanks using a "Y" or "T" connector. The single tubing from the connector then flows to the patient.

Helium/oxygen mixtures are administered by using a tight fitting continuous positive airway pressure mask or a high-flow/nonbreathing system to limit the entrainment of room air. A tent or a hood cannot be used because the helium, which is lighter than oxygen, will preferentially fill the top of the tent/hood. As the thermal conductivity of helium is 4 to 6 times that of nitrogen, the inhaled gas mixture must be humidified and warmed to body temperature to prevent excessive heat loss from the patient. Weaning the patient from heliox therapy can be accomplished by either decreasing the concentration incrementally down to 40% to 50% or by just removing the face mask and observing the patient. If symptoms recur, the mask can easily be reapplied and the helium administration restarted. The effect of helium is almost instantaneous.

Respiratory monitoring during helium administration poses no significant difficulties provided some principles are kept in mind. Pulse oximetry and transcutaneous monitoring can be used effectively. Monitors of the inspired oxygen concentration function normally in the presence of helium. Although infrared monitors do not measure the helium concentration, they can still be used to accurately monitor end-tidal CO_2. Helium can be measured by mass spectroscopy, but only if the machines are calibrated and set up to measure helium. Most machines used in the operating room are set up to measure oxygen, nitrogen, carbon dioxide, and inhalational anesthetic agents including nitrous oxide. If helium is used by such machines, it will not be measured. Therefore, if 70% helium and 30% oxygen are administered, the mass spectroscopy will only measure oxygen and will report a concentration of 100%.

Lower Airway Obstruction: Status Asthmaticus

Introduction

Asthma is an obstructive pulmonary disease characterized by reversible and recurrent constriction of the airways. The airways narrow because of bronchial wall inflammation, smooth muscle hyperreactivity (bronchospasm), and excessive intraluminal mucus. Status asthmaticus is defined as acute bronchospasm that is resistant to bronchodilator therapy. Most children with status asthmaticus present with a history of gradual deterioration over days, but a small number of patients can suffer a very rapid decompensation over hours. An increasing incidence of fatal asthma attacks over the past 15 years highlights the importance of prompt recognition and treatment of status asthmaticus.[9,10] From 1978 through 1989, asthma mortality rates nearly doubled.

The circumstances surrounding a life-threatening asthma attack have certain common features. Most patients with fatal asthma are teenagers or young adults.[11] Among children younger than 14 years of age, fatal asthma is more likely to occur in boys. There is a circadian rhythm in the presentation such that these children usually come to medical attention at night. Their medical history is often remarkable for past episodes of respiratory failure, a significant reduction in corticosteroid use, and psychosocial problems. The reduction in inhaled corticosteroid use suggests the importance of airway inflammation in the pathophysiology of severe asthma. These patients may represent a distinct pathophysiologic subpopulation with abnormalities in the control of airway smooth muscle caliber and reactivity. Bronchial smooth muscle from these patients exhibits a greater maximal response to contractile agonists and impaired relaxation to β-agonists and theophylline.[12] Postmortem examination of the airways in sudden asphyxic asthma patients has demonstrated decreased numbers of eosinophils and increased neutrophils.

Initial Evaluation and Therapy

Initial therapy depends on the severity of airway obstruction and the rapidity of decompensation. The majority of patients with severe status asthmaticus deteriorate slowly, allowing ample time for evaluation by physical exam and a few simple tests. Useful physical findings include chest wall retractions, a decreased level of consciousness, and the presence of pulsus paradoxus (over 10 mm Hg change in systolic blood pressure between inspiration and expiration).[13] Wheezing does not correlate well with the severity of airway obstruction. A silent chest is an ominous finding since wheezing does not occur if there is little or no air exchange. If time permits, two noninvasive assessment devices should be applied to the symptomatic patient: pulse oximetry and peak expiratory flow rates. Pulse oximetry and oxygen saturation (SaO_2) quantify the degree of hypoxemia and predict patients who are likely to improve with therapy or progress to respiratory failure. Cook and Stone[14] found that clinical improvement is predicted if albuterol nebulization produces an increase in the oxygen saturation. In the adult population, respiratory failure (defined as a $PaCO_2$ >42 mm Hg) is rare (4.2%) if the SaO_2 is greater than 92% on presentation.[15] Given the common occurrence of hypoxemia, all children in status asthmaticus should receive supplemental oxygen and, therefore, it may not be possible or reasonable to measure room air oxygen saturations.

Simple, hand-held flow meters provide a useful assessment of the degree of initial airway obstruction as well as allowing an ongoing assessment of the response to therapy. If the peak expiratory flow rate is less than 40% of the expected mean for age, a severe attack is present and the likelihood of the need for hospitalization is high.[16] Extremely dyspneic patients should not be forced to carry out the peak flow maneuver because it may exacerbate bronchospasm.[17]

Controversy surrounds the need for and efficacy of obtaining chest x-rays in all patients who present with status asthmaticus. However, routine chest x-rays should be obtained in most patients who require hospital admission. While most asthma exacerbations are of viral etiology, community-acquired and atypical bacterial etiologies may be responsible for pulmonary deterioration. There are no clear criteria on which to base the decision of whether to initiate antibiotic therapy. Many patients with status asthmaticus will have opacifications on the initial chest x-ray that may be the result of atelectasis or viral processes that do not require antibiotic therapy. The initial white blood cell count is frequently inaccurate due to the use of β-adrenergic agonists and corticosteroids. In the nonintubated patient, induced sputum samples are frequently difficult to obtain and, when obtained, may be contaminated with oral secretions that negate their predictive value. Blood cultures are frequently negative even in patients with bacterial pneumonia. When empiric antibiotic therapy is started, appropriate coverage should be provided for community-acquired pneumonia including *Mycoplasma pneumoniae*. When antibiotic therapy is started, our preference is to start therapy with intravenous azithromycin and switch to oral therapy once the patient's condition has stabilized.

When a child requires assisted ventilation within the first 1 to 3 hours of presentation to the emergency department, "sudden asphyxic asthma" or "hyperacute asthma attack" is present by definition.[18] Children with sudden asphyxic asthma, even if they have not suffered a respiratory arrest, have a virtually silent chest on auscultation. Arterial blood gas analysis reveals a mixed respiratory and metabolic acidosis with extreme hypercapnia often greater than 100 mm Hg. The mechanism of the metabolic acidosis has not been clarified but may involve lactic acidosis from hypoxia or the increased work of breathing. Males suffer sudden asphyxic asthma attacks more frequently than females. Respiratory arrest and hypoxic central nervous system damage may occur if medical attention is not immediately available. For those patients who reach medical attention in time to receive assisted ventilation, recovery is generally rapid with mechanical ventilation required for only 24 to 48 hours. Conversely, the majority of asthmatic patients with respiratory failure, who have experienced a gradual deterioration, require mechanical ventilation for approximately 90 hours.

Prehospital Care

Prehospital care for the patient with status asthmaticus may significantly decrease the morbidity and mortality of the disease. The Emergency Medical Services (EMS) system must be prepared to evaluate and care for children with life-threatening asthma. Fisher and Vinci[19] reported that 63% of children requiring EMS transport did not have a physical examination documented. Other common deficiencies in care included failure to administer supplemental oxygen to hypoxemic asthmatic patients and inability or failure to administer β-adrenergic agonists. The management by the ambulance team should emphasize the following:

1. immediate and ongoing assessment of air exchange and vital signs;
2. supplemental oxygen administration to all patients;
3. assisted ventilation if breath sounds are absent;
4. subcutaneous terbutaline or epinephrine for patients who are unable to tolerate inhaled β-adrenergic agonists or for patients with severe symptoms and minimal air exchange;
5. inhaled albuterol therapy if the equipment and training of the ambulance team are appropriate.[20]

In-Hospital Therapy

The pharmacologic options for treatment of patients with status asthmaticus are outlined in Table 3. β-Adrenergic receptor stimulation results in the rapid onset of bronchial smooth muscle relaxation. Consequently, this class of drug forms the mainstay of rescue therapy during acute bronchospasm. There are several options regarding the specific agent, route of delivery, and frequency of administration. Although there are many inhaled β-agonist preparations, albuterol, terbutaline, and metaproterenol are the most commonly used agents. Each of these drugs is considered relatively selective in activity for the β_2-adrenergic receptor such that the bronchodilatory effect is more pronounced than myocardial stimulation (β_1 effect). Long-acting β-agonists such as salmeterol are not indicated during status asthmaticus.

Albuterol inhalation remains the first choice for bronchodilator therapy in most pediatric emergency departments. Standard therapy consists of albuterol 0.15 mg/kg to a maximum 5 mg or 0.03 mL/kg of the 0.5% solution diluted in 2.5 to 3 mL of normal saline and nebulized every 10 to 20 minutes. There is no advantage to using lower doses (0.05 mg/kg) because therapeutic efficacy is reduced while the incidence of side effects is not.[21] If the child has not improved after three nebulization treatments, intravenous corticosteroid (methylprednisolone 2 mg/kg/dose every 6 hours) is added to the therapeutic regimen. If there is no improvement after an additional three nebulization treatments, hospital admission is indicated. The child with obvious severe airflow obstruction and impending respiratory failure may receive continuous albuterol nebulization (0.6 to 1.0 mg/kg/h), which is continued until there is clear-cut improvement or until undesirable side effects, such as tachycardia or vomiting, develop. In the latter case, methylprednisolone is also administered immediately.

The effectiveness of aerosol treatment depends on the nebulization technique, since only approximately 10% of the drug actually reaches the distal tracheobronchial tree.[22] In order to maximize drug delivery, the albuterol solution should be diluted in saline (2.5 to 3 mL) to achieve a final total volume of approximately 4 mL. This final solution is then nebulized with an oxygen flow rate of 6 to 10 L/min, which results in a maximal aerosol output of small particle size.[23]

Subcutaneous administration of β-agonists has been used for many decades and is the therapy that was initially recommended, prior to the increased use of aerosol treatment and the availability of the selective β_2-adrenergic agonists. There are fewer indications for subcutaneous therapy since the advent of effective and painless inhaled therapy. Current indications for subcutaneous epinephrine or terbutaline include the following:

1. a very rapidly decompensating patient;
2. failure to respond to inhaled β-adrenergic agonists;
3. inability to cooperate with inhalational therapy.

The doses for epinephrine (1:1000 concentration or 1 mg/mL) and terbutaline (1:1000) are identical at 0.01 mL/kg (maximum dose 0.3 to 0.5 mL) subcutaneously. Although terbutaline is considered a more specific β_2 drug and has been suggested to be associated with fewer systemic adverse effects, in practice epinephrine and terbutaline are equivalent in efficacy and side effect profile.

Anticholinergic Agents

Several studies suggest that the combination of a nebulized anticholinergic agent

Table 3

Therapeutic Maneuvers for Status Asthmaticus

Inhalation therapy:
  albuterol—0.03 mL/kg (maximum 1 mL) of a 0.5% solution every 10 to 20 minutes
  ipratropium—250 μg in infants; 500 μg in older children, adolescents

Corticosteroids:
  prednisone—0.5 mg/kg by mouth
  methylpredisolone—2 mg/kg/dose i.v. every 6 hours
  hydrocortisone—8 mg/kg/dose i.v. every 6 hours

Subcutaneous therapy:
  terbutaline or epinephrine—0.01 mL/kg (maximum 0.3 to 0.5 mL) of a 1:1000 solution (1 mg/mL)

Aminophylline:
  no previous therapy—loading dose of 6 to 8 mg/kg followed by a continuous infusion of 0.6 to 1.0 mg/kg/h adjusted to maintain serum concentration of 10 to 20 μg/mL
  previous therapy—check level; bolus of 1 mg/kg will increase level by 2 μg/kg followed by a continuous infusion as outlined above

Magnesium:
  75 mg/kg (maximum 2 grams) i.v. over 20 minutes; repeat dose in 4 hours as needed after checking serum magnesium level (should be less than 3 mEq/L)

Intravenous β-adrenergic agonist therapy:
  isoproterenol—0.05 to 0.3 μg/kg/min: start at 0.05 μg/kg/min and increase in increments of 0.05 μg/kg/min every 10 minutes as needed; monitor heart rate
  terbutaline—loading dose of 2.5 to 10 μg/kg followed by a continuous infusion of 0.1 μg/kg/min; repeat bolus and increase infusion by 0.1 μg/kg/min every 15 to 20 minutes as needed

Helium:
  no therapeutic effect, decreased density of gas decreases work of breathing; can be used in spontaneously breathing and mechanically ventilated patients

Inhalational anesthetic agents:
  direct effect on airway smooth muscle; consider use in refractory cases with endotracheal intubation mechanical ventilation; logistic problems with delivery

Extracorporeal techniques:
  ECMO (extracorporeal membrane oxygenation) has been used in refractory cases in patients with impending mortality; can use either venoarterial or venovenous support

with a β-adrenergic agent produces more effective bronchodilation than either drug alone. Cholinergic blockade results in bronchodilation, although anticholinergic drugs alone are not as effective as β-adrenergic agonists. The rationale for the use of anticholinergic agents comes from the observation that viral respiratory infections may trigger life-threatening asthma attacks that result from reflex vagal stimulation.[24] The mechanism involves the interaction of muscarinic receptor subtypes. Stimulation of muscarinic receptors of the M_3 subtype located on bronchial smooth muscle produces smooth muscle contraction (bronchoconstriction). Muscarinic blockade prevents or reverses such bronchoconstriction. Conversely, the inhibitory muscarinic (M_2) receptors on the vagal nerve endings inhibit the release of acetylcholine thus preventing further smooth muscle contraction.[25] These M_2 receptors act as a negative feedback loop and prevent further acetylcholine release from the nerve ending. During a viral infection of the respiratory tract, M_2 receptors are defective and no longer inhibit the release of acetylcholine, leaving M_3 receptor activity (bronchoconstriction) relatively unopposed.[26] The commercially available anticholinergic agents (atropine, glycopyrrolate, and ipratropium) are nonselective, but in patients with acute bronchospasm and M_2 receptor dysfunction, the effect is predominately on M_3 receptors leading to bronchodilation.

Atropine was the first anticholinergic agent to be used as an inhaled bronchodilator. Although it is clearly effective as a bronchodilator, since atropine crosses the blood-brain barrier, systemic absorption can lead to anticholinergic side effects including central nervous system effects of dysphoria and confusion. Glycopyrrolate is an effective anticholinergic bronchodilator that has the chemical structure of a quaternary amine and, thus, has limited penetration of the blood-brain barrier. Ipratropium bromide represents the most effective anticholinergic bronchodilator with the fewest systemic side effects. Its bronchodilatory effect is primarily local and site-specific. When administered through the inhalational route, its peak effect appears in 30 minutes, with a duration of approximately 4 hours. The combination of ipratropium with a β-adrenergic drug is significantly more effective than either drug taken alone. The physiologic benefits of the addition of ipratropium as the second drug include reduction of hyperinflation (measured by decrease in functional residual capacity) and further improvement in forced expiratory volume in 1 second (FEV_1).[27,28]

The dose-response relationship for ipratropium is unknown in children. The drug is supplied as a premixed unit dose inhalational solution (0.5 mg in 2.5 mL normal saline). Dosing may include 0.25 mg in infants and 0.5 mg in children and adolescents. Although the effects of ipratropium last 4 hours, Schuh et al[28] reported a beneficial effect on respiratory therapy with the administration of ipratropium every 20 minutes. Albuterol and ipratropium can be mixed together in the nebulization chamber.

Corticosteroids

Airway inflammation plays a prominent role in severe status asthmaticus. Therefore, anti-inflammatory therapy with corticosteroids is essential in the emergency management of the refractory asthmatic child. Depending on the severity of the attack, corticosteroids may be administered either orally or intravenously. Oral prednisone is appropriate for the child with a moderately severe asthma attack who is fully conscious and unlikely to require endotracheal intubation. Singh and Kumar[29] showed that nebulized salbutamol (albuterol) combined with oral prednisolone resulted in greater improvement in clinical score, oxygen saturation, peak expiratory flow rate, as well as earlier discharge from the hospital than a similar group of asthmatics treated with intravenous hydrocortisone and aminophylline. In our practice, either prednisolone or prednisone 0.5 mg/kg by mouth every 6 hours (maximum dose 100 mg/24 hours for 3 to 5 days) is used in this setting.

The patient with life-threatening status asthmaticus should receive intravenous corticosteroids as outlined above. The use of corticosteroids has been shown to potentiate the effect of β-adrenergic agonists. Severely asthmatic patients who received a single dose of intramuscular methylprednisolone (4 mg/kg) in addition to inhaled albuterol showed dramatic improvement compared to a group that received only inhaled albuterol.[30] The beneficial effects of the addition of parenteral corticosteroid were evident as early as 3 hours after the dose. Additionally, the corticosteroid-treated group had a significantly lower hospital admission rate. These benefits are most pronounced in children younger than 24 months old.

There are three options for the patient with status asthmaticus: 1) oral corticosteroid therapy (0.5 mg/kg prednisone); 2) intramuscular methylprednisolone at the same time albuterol nebulization is begun; or 3) intravenous methylprednisolone (2 mg/kg) for the critically ill patient or if the patient has not improved after the first hour of albuterol nebulization. The first two approaches start corticosteroid therapy immediately. Oral therapy is not recommended in patients with severe status asthmaticus and impending respiratory failure. The disadvantage of the second technique is that the injection is painful. Option three, later intravenous corticosteroid administration, avoids the needle stick in some children, but delays the benefits of corticosteroids for those patients who are resistant to albuterol nebulization alone. On balance, we favor intravenous steroids after the first hour of albuterol nebulization, unless the child is deteriorating rapidly, in which case intravenous corticosteroids are given immediately upon arrival in the emergency department.

Theophylline

Theophylline is a xanthine derivative with a structure similar to caffeine, that has been used for more than 50 years in the treatment of acute exacerbations of asthma. Despite decades of research, the bronchodilator mechanism of theophylline remains unclear. Postulated mechanisms include phosphodiesterase inhibition, interaction with G proteins (guanine nucleotide regulatory proteins), adenosine antagonism, indirect catecholamine release, effects on phospholipid metabolism, and effects on calcium uptake and utilization. More recent data suggest that phosphodiesterase inhibitors in general, and theophylline in particular, have anti-inflammatory properties and reduce eosinophil infiltration into the airway.[31]

The aggressive use of inhaled β-adrenergic agents and intravenous corticosteroids has largely displaced theophylline from the therapeutic armamentarium for patients with status asthmaticus. Several controlled studies have demonstrated that the addition of theophylline does not provide any benefit over inhaled albuterol and intravenous methylprednisolone.[32,33] These studies have not addressed the role of theophylline in the asthmatic patient suffering respiratory failure, who requires endotracheal intubation and mechanical ventilation. There may be a continued role for an aminophylline infusion for patients who have been resistant to inhaled bronchodilators and corticosteroids or who have had difficulty weaning from mechanical ventilation.

Table 4

Interactions with Aminophylline/Theophylline Metabolism

Increased metabolism/decreased level
　barbiturates
　phenytoin
　isoproterenol

Decreased metabolism/increased level
　allopurinol
　carbamazepine
　erythromycin
　cimetidine
　propranolol
　ketoconazole
　oral contraceptive agents

If the patient has not taken theophylline previously, a loading dose of 6 to 8 mg/kg of aminophylline is administered intravenously followed by an infusion of 0.6 to 1 mg/kg/h. Theophylline levels should be checked after the loading dose, again 6 hours after the infusion is started, and then daily while the infusion continues. If an aminophylline infusion is planned for a patient receiving long-term theophylline preparations, the patient's theophylline level should be measured and a loading dose administered as needed. If the serum concentration is therapeutic, a maintenance infusion is started. In either case, the aminophylline infusion is adjusted to maintain serum concentrations of 10 to 20 μg/mL. A bolus dose of 1 mg/kg will raise the serum concentration by approximately 2 μg/mL. Although 10 to 20 μg/mL is the recommended therapeutic level, some patients will develop adverse effects with levels in the high therapeutic range and the infusion may need to be decreased. As theophylline is metabolized by the hepatic P450 system, several drug interactions can occur (Table 4).

Magnesium Sulfate

The role of magnesium sulfate is uncertain in pediatric status asthmaticus, the data on its effectiveness being based mostly on series in adult patients. Its mechanism of action is thought to be through the inhibition of acetylcholine release at the neuromuscular junction that prevents the release of acetylcholine, leading to smooth (bronchial) muscle relaxation. With the depolarization of the neuronal end plate, there is an inward movement of calcium that is necessary for the release of the neurotransmitter acetylcholine. The inward movement of calcium is antagonized by magnesium. The bronchodilator effects of magnesium occur approximately 20 minutes after intravenous administration.

Magnesium sulfate (2 grams intravenously) taken alone is less effective than inhaled albuterol alone.[34] In unselected patients with status asthmaticus, the addition of magnesium sulfate after prior receipt of nebulized albuterol and intravenous methylprednisolone has not resulted in further improvement in pulmonary function.[35] However, in patients with severe status asthmaticus, defined as an FEV_1 less than 25% of predicted, there was a significant improvement in FEV_1 120 minutes after receipt of intravenous magnesium sulfate in a dose of 2 grams.[35] Although magnesium does not offer a significant benefit to the majority of patients with status asthmaticus, it may be of value in patients with severe status asthmaticus and impending respiratory failure. As it can be administered intravenously, it offers the advantage of allowing parenteral therapy in patients with limited air exchange in whom inhalational therapy may be less effective.

If magnesium is chosen, an initial dose of 75 mg/kg (maximum 2 grams) of magnesium sulfate is infused over 20 minutes. The dose can be repeated in 3 to 4 hours if needed. More rapid administration may result in cardiovascular effects including hypotension from peripheral vasodilatation. Adverse effects related to magnesium administration include the inhibition of acetylcholine release at other neuromuscular junctions including the vasculature leading to hypotension, and the skeletal muscle leading to weakness and respiratory failure. If repeated dosing is contemplated, serum magnesium levels should be monitored. Levels greater than 5 to 6 mg/dL may result in toxicity. Magnesium toxicity is manifested by weakness, areflexia, respiratory depression, and cardiac conduction abnormalities. Magnesium therapy is contraindicated in renal failure, disturbances of cardiac conduction, and myasthenia gravis or other disorders or neuromuscular transmission.

Intravenous β-Adrenergic Agonist Therapy

Intravenous β-adrenergic therapy is indicated in patients with status asthmaticus who have received aggressive therapy with inhaled β-adrenergic agonists/anticholinergic agents and intravenous corticosteroids and have developed impending respiratory failure manifested by an increasing $PaCO_2$. When β-adrenergic therapy is administered intravenously, bronchodilatory effects are seen within 5 minutes, with reversal of respiratory failure and prevention of the need for mechanical ventilation in up to 80% to 90% of patients.[36,37] Dosing regimens include a starting infusion rate of 0.05 μg/kg/min with an increase of 0.05 μg/kg/min every 10 minutes. The dose limiting factor is usually the increase in heart rate. With the start of the infusion, an initial decrease in oxygenation may be noted, as isoproterenol also induces vasodilation and may inhibit hypoxic pulmonary vasoconstriction thereby increasing shunt fraction. Adverse effects of isoproterenol are related to its β-adrenergic effects elsewhere and include hypokalemia, tachycardia, arrhythmias, and most importantly alterations of the myocardial oxygen delivery-demand ratio, with the possibility of inducing myocardial ischemia even in children. The cardiovascular effects of β-adrenergic agonists such as isoproterenol lead to an increase in heart rate which increases myocardial oxygen consumption, as well as a shortening of diastole during which coronary blood flow occurs. Through its vasodilatory properties, there is a decline in diastolic blood pressure with a decrease in coronary perfusion pressure (coronary perfusion pressure = diastolic blood pressure minus left ventricular end-diastolic pressure). Recommendations for monitoring during isoproterenol therapy include daily creatine phosphokinase of muscle band (CPK-MB) levels or other cardiac enzymes and electrocardiograms.

Due to the concerns about the use of the nonspecific β-adrenergic agonist, isoproterenol, recent interest has focused on the use of intravenous terbutaline as a means of achieving the β-bronchodilator effects while limiting the $β_1$ cardiac effects. Dosing regimens for terbutaline include intravenous bolus dosing of 2.5 to 10 μg/kg followed by infusions of 0.1 to 0.5 μg/kg/min. To date, there are no prospective studies that directly compare the cardiac and respiratory effects of isoproterenol and terbutaline.

Endotracheal Intubation and Mechanical Ventilatory Support

The reader is referred to chapter 1 for a full discussion of airway management, and to chapters 4 and 5 for a full discussion of ventilatory support. Emergency endotracheal intubation of the patient with acute asphyxic asthma is one of the greatest challenges of the emergency medical system. The patient should receive bag/mask ventilation with 100% oxygen during preparation for endotracheal intubation. If the patient is unresponsive and in respiratory arrest, endotracheal intubation should be performed immediately without further drug administration, with the possible exception of 0.01 mg/kg of atropine, which can be administered intravenously, intramuscularly, or intraosseously.

If the patient is still conscious, some form of sedation and neuromuscular blockade will be necessary in order to prevent coughing, gagging, regurgitation, and worsening bronchospasm. While bag/mask ventilation continues, intravenous access should be established quickly. Ketamine (2 mg/kg i.v.) is the preferred sedative because of its bronchodilator properties. It must be combined with an anticholinergic drug (atropine, 0.01 mg/kg i.v. or glycopyrrolate, 0.005 mg/kg i.v.) to counteract the increase in oropharyngeal secretions caused by ketamine. Most practitioners also add a benzodiazepine such as midazolam, 0.1 mg/kg, to prevent the emergence phenomena such as hallucinations, which may occur with ketamine.

The choice of a neuromuscular blocking agent depends on several factors including the speed of onset, need for prolonged paralysis, and effect on airway resistance. In order to achieve a rapid onset (within 30 to 60 seconds) and a short duration of paralysis, succinylcholine 2 mg/kg i.v. remains the drug of choice provided there are no contraindications to its use (see chapter 11). Airway resistance does not increase after succinylcholine as long as an anticholinergic drug such as atropine or glycopyrrolate has been administered first. The "rapid sequence" technique is used with application of cricoid pressure to prevent regurgitation after ketamine and succinylcholine have been administered.

Worsening bronchospasm and hypotension constitute the major potential complications at the time of endotracheal intubation. Worsening bronchospasm is rarely encountered because these patients already have life-threatening bronchospasm despite aggressive medical therapy. Furthermore, they have had general anesthesia induced (ketamine) before intubation. Nevertheless, alveolar ventilation may deteriorate if the lungs become more hyperinflated after intubation. The risk of further hyperinflation depends on the level of sedation, paralysis, and the ventilatory pattern employed (see below).

Systemic hypotension is a more common problem resulting from preexisting hypovolemia and the combined effects of hyperinflation, increased intrathoracic pressure, systemic vasodilation from β-adrenergic agonists, and myocardial depression from sedative drugs. Extreme hyperinflation leads to alveolar overdistension and pulmonary capillary compression. The resultant increase in right ventricular afterload and pressure may shift the position of the interventricular septum leftward such that left ventricular cavitary volume and, hence, stroke volume are reduced. Positive pressure ventilation further aggravates the risk of decreased stroke volume by decreasing venous return. These effects are manifested clinically as pulsus paradoxus. Hemodynamic complications are best treated by a combination of isotonic fluid volume administration and a ventilatory technique designed to limit increases in intrathoracic pressure and hyperinflation.

Tension pneumothorax should be considered in the differential diagnosis of hypotension. The diagnosis of pneumothorax becomes more likely if the breaths are asymmetric, if deliberate hypoventilation (with permissive hypercapnia) and intravascular volume expansion fail to improve the hemodynamics, and if hypoxemia develops despite ventilation with 100% oxygen. Definitive diagnosis is made by chest radiograph.

Many patients in the emergency department or during transport will be ventilated manually. The objective of manual ventilation is to prevent hypoxemia, barotrauma, and hypotension rather than to achieve a rapid reduction in $PaCO_2$. Therefore, the patient is ventilated with 100% inspired oxygen concentration, low tidal volumes or pressure-limited ventilation designed to maintain peak inflating pressure less than 35 to 40 cm H_2O, and slow respiratory rates (8 to 12 breaths/min) with prolonged exhalation times (3 to 5 seconds) to allow for complete exhalation. Ideally, the peak inflating pressure should be monitored with a manometer. The proper respiratory rate and exhalation time will depend on how long it takes for the patient's lungs to empty, which, in turn, depends on the degree of hyperinflation, elastic recoil of the chest wall, and airway obstruction. Auscultation is the simplest way to assess whether exhalation is complete before initiating the next manual breath. If wheezing persists until the next breath is initiated, it is likely that exhalation is incomplete. In severe cases thoracic compression may be required to augment elastic recoil and exhalation. The reader is referred to chapter 4 for a full discussion of ventilatory strategies for use in patients with status asthmaticus.

Helium Administration

As outlined above, helium is used most commonly for patients with upper airway obstructive processes; however, it may also be beneficial in patients with more distal airway diseases such as status asthmaticus in both spontaneously breathing and mechanically ventilated patients.[6] Because helium is less dense than nitrogen, it improves gas movement during turbulent flow. In addition, helium may increase gas movement by converting turbulent flow to laminar flow. The Reynolds' number is the ratio of kinetic and viscous forces. It predicts whether flow will be laminar or turbulent (turbulent flow occurs with a Reynolds' number >2000). The Reynolds' number is calculated as 2 times the product of the radius, the average velocity, and the density, divided by the viscosity. When substituted for nitrogen, helium lowers the Reynolds' number and may convert turbulent flow to laminar flow. An additional effect of helium is an increase in the elimination of carbon dioxide, since carbon dioxide diffuses 4 to 5 times faster through a mixture of helium/oxygen than through nitrogen/oxygen. Therefore, for the same partial pressure of carbon dioxide, a greater amount of the gas is eliminated per unit of time. In spontaneously breathing patients, the decreased density of helium may decrease the work of breathing as well as improve air exchange. In mechanically ventilated patients, the decreased density may result in a decreased peak inflating as well as increased expiratory flow rates thereby limiting air trapping, both of which may limit the incidence of barotrauma.

In certain clinical situations, helium has also been shown to improve ventilation-perfusion matching. Since bronchoconstriction leads to areas of low ventilation-perfusion matching, an increased distribution of ventilation to areas of previously low ventilation may result in improved gas exchange. While flow is generally laminar in the more distal parts of the airway, certain pathologic conditions may occur that decrease the compliance and increase the resistance of these terminal airways and thereby lead to turbulent flow. In this situation, in areas of long time constants (low compliance and high resistance), helium may lead to decreased resistance to gas movement and better matching of ventilation and perfusion.

Clinical studies have demonstrated the beneficial effects of helium in patients with status asthmaticus during both spontaneous and controlled ventilation.[38–40] Kass and Castriotta[38] evaluated the therapeutic impact of helium/oxygen in 12 patients with status asthmaticus and respiratory acidosis (pH <7.35 and $PaCO_2$ >45 mm Hg). Five patients received helium/oxygen through the ventilator while the seven whose tracheas were not intubated received helium/oxygen via a nonrebreathing mask. When these 12 patients are considered together, helium administration resulted in a decrease in $PaCO_2$ from 57.9±8.3 to 47.5±4.3 mm Hg and an increase in pH from 7.23±0.07 to 7.32±0.04. The authors noted a significantly shorter duration of symptoms (17.8±8.9 versus 78±36 hours) in the responders (8 patients) versus the nonresponders (4 patients). Based on their findings, the authors recommended the use of helium as a temporizing measure in status asthmaticus until a therapeutic effect can be obtained from other agents such as β-adrenergic agonists and corticosteroids. Similar findings were reported by Shiue and Gluck.[39]

Manthous et al[40] noted improved peak expiratory flow rates and decreased pulsus paradoxus in 27 spontaneously breathing adult patients with status asthmaticus. Although they noted a decrease in pulsus paradoxus and an increase in peak expiratory flow rate over time in the control group, related to β-adrenergic agonist/corticosteroid therapy, the changes were significantly greater in patients who were breathing helium/oxygen when compared to the control group (room air).

Gluck et al[41] evaluated the effects of helium/oxygen during mechanical ventilation in patients with status asthmaticus and respiratory acidosis. They noted a decrease in peak inflating pressure for a given tidal volume from a mean of 86 cm H_2O to 53 cm H_2O, and a decrease in the $PaCO_2$ from a mean of 87 to 51 mm Hg. The change in peak inflating pressure was noted early (2.5 minutes) while the maximal decrease in $PaCO_2$ was noted in 22.2 minutes.

While there are limited outcome data, these studies demonstrate that helium/oxygen may have temporizing effects on status asthmaticus. While helium has no direct therapeutic effects, its low density facilitates improved gas movement with decreased work of breathing, which may limit or delay respiratory muscle fatigue and allow time for therapeutic agents such as corticosteroids or β-adrenergic agonists to take effect. The decreased density may also allow for gas flow to alveoli with long time constants with a better matching of ventilation and perfusion.

Anderson et al[42] have demonstrated an additional effect of breathing helium/oxygen mixtures for patients with status asthmaticus: the improved delivery of aerosolized medications. Ten subjects with asthma inhaled 3.6 μmol/L particles labeled with ^{111}In in air or in a helium/oxygen mixture. The lung retention of the ^{111}In was measured at baseline and after 24 hours. The percentage retained at 24 hours was taken to represent the fraction deposited in the alveoli. The retention was significantly greater at 24 hours with the helium/oxygen mixture compared with air at flow rates of either 0.5 or 1.2 L/s. The authors concluded that the more distal delivery achieved with helium/oxygen may improve the delivery and thereby the therapeutic effect of inhaled β-adrenergic agonists. With minor modifications of the equipment, helium/oxygen mixtures can be used during continuous albuterol nebulization.[43]

The techniques used for the delivery of helium to spontaneously breathing patients are outlined above in the section concerning upper airway obstruction. When helium is administered through the ventilator, the helium tank(s) can be connected to the air inlet by adapting the hose that normally connects to the high-pressure air inlet to connect to the helium tank. The dial that controls the FiO_2 will not be accurate since it is calibrated for air and oxygen. Therefore, the oxygen concentration must be measured from the breathing circuit. Another option is to blend the oxygen and helium to the desired concentration and administer the gas mixture via the auxiliary gas port of the ventilator. To do this, both the oxygen and air connections should be removed from the wall outlets. When this is done, the ventilator will be dependent on the pressure in the helium tanks to provide pressure for ventilation. If the tanks run out, the ventilator will not work.

During mechanical ventilation (volume-limited), the tidal volumes delivered and recorded by the ventilator are not accurate because the flow meter has been calibrated for oxygen and nitrogen instead of helium and oxygen. Therefore, our practice[6] is to use helium/oxygen through a Servo 900C ventilator (Siemens Inc., Stockholm, Sweden) in the pressure-limited mode. The exhaled tidal volumes recorded by the ventilator will not be accurate, so we would suggest following arterial blood gases or noninvasive monitors (pulse oximetry, transcutaneous CO_2, or end-tidal CO_2) to judge the therapeutic efficacy of the switch to helium/oxygen ventilation.

Inhalational Anesthetic Agents

The bronchodilatory effects of general anesthetic agents had been noted as early as the 1930s. Since then, numerous reports have appeared concerning the use of inhalational anesthetic agents to treat refractory status asthmaticus.[44-47] Despite the success of these agents, their mechanisms of action on airway reactivity remain controversial. Postulated mechanisms of action have included direct effects on airway musculature, interactions with β-adrenergic receptors, and endogenous catecholamine release. While ether and cyclopropane increase endogenous catecholamine levels, which may account for part of their bronchodilatory effects, catecholamine levels do not change with halothane. In all likelihood, their effects result from a direct effect on bronchial smooth muscle tone.

Despite their beneficial effects on airway reactivity, significant problems and adverse effects may be seen with the inhalational anesthetic agents (Table 5). Although the majority of experience to date is with halothane, concerns with its use include its depressant effects on myocardial contractility and the potential for arrhythmias. Halothane's negative inotropic properties, which may be further magnified in the setting of acidosis, hypercapnia, and hypoxemia, may limit the concentrations that can be used. Saulnier et al[48] evaluated the hemodynamic effects of 1% halothane in 12 patients with status asthmaticus. Contrary to concerns that had been previously expressed in the literature,[44-47] no deleterious hemodynamic effects were noted. Although mean arterial pressure and heart rate decreased, no episodes of hypotension were noted. Cardiac index, systolic stroke volume, and left ventricular stroke work index were unchanged. They postulated that the improvement in respiratory function with correction of acidosis, hypoxemia, and hypercapnia would have a beneficial effect on hemodynamic function. However, they did caution that all of their patients had normal baseline cardiovascular function.

Perhaps more important is the arrhythmogenic potential of halothane especially in the asthmatic patient who is receiving β-adrenergic agonists and/or aminophylline. These factors with associated electrolyte derangements, hypoxemia, and hypercarbia may predispose these patients to ventricular ectopy. Given these problems, the other inhalational anesthetic agents (enflurane or isoflurane) may be better choices. Animal research and clinical experience suggest no real advantage in regard to bronchodilatory effects when comparing halothane with the other inhalational anesthetic agents.[49,50]

Table 5

Advantages/Disadvantages of Inhalation Anesthetic Agents

Advantages:
  therapeutic agent in refractory cases
  convenient route of administration
  abundant clinical experience
  provides sedation/analgesia in addition to therapeutic effect

Disadvantages:
  adverse cardiovascular effects
  cerebral vasodilatation
  triggering agent for malignant hyperthermia
  fluoride release with metabolism
  agent and equipment are expensive
  additional equipment needed to deliver agent and monitor its inspired/expired concentration
  arrhythmias and hepatitis (Halothane)
  agents alter metabolism of other drugs
  prolonged use leads to tolerance with abstinence syndrome if the agent is abruptly discontinued

Metabolism of the anesthetic agent can also lead to problems, especially with prolonged use. Enflurane undergoes considerable metabolism with the release of fluoride. High fluoride levels (>50 μm/L) can result in nephrotoxicity and a nephrogenic diabetes insipidus. Levels are dependent on the concentration of agent administered and the length of administration. Isoflurane is the least metabolized (0.2%) of the inhalational anesthetic agents.

Based on the available data, we currently favor isoflurane over the other inhalational agents for treatment of status asthmaticus. Isoflurane has limited negative inotropic effects and is not arrhythmogenic. Although it may decrease blood pressure, its primary hemodynamic effect is peripheral vasodilatation with an increase in cardiac output. In equipotent concentrations, its bronchodilatory properties are similar to those of halothane. Despite such beneficial effects, significant logistical problems can be encountered with the administration of inhalational anesthetic agents outside of the operating room. It has been suggested that patients receiving such agents are best cared for in the operating room or recovery room. If the patient remains in the intensive care unit (ICU), arrangements must be made for the use of specialized equipment including monitoring of inspired and expired concentration of the agent. It is necessary also to decide whether to use an anesthesia machine to deliver the agent or a standard ICU ventilator. While the anesthesia machine is logistically easier to use, the ventilators on most anesthesia machines have limited options for manipulation of ventilatory parameters of positive end-expiratory pressure, mode of ventilation, inspiratory flow patterns, and inspiratory-to-expiratory ratios, as well as having a maximum working pressure of 60 to 70 cm H_2O. The inhalational anesthetic agents can also be administered through a commercially available ventilator (Servo 900D; Siemens, Inc.). However, unlike the other Servo ventilators, the 900D model only functions in the volume mode. The final option is to custom fit a vaporizer onto a standard Servo 900C ventilator. Once the problems concerning delivery of the anesthetic agent have been solved, monitoring of the patient and the anesthetic agent is still necessary. In addition to routine ICU monitoring, some method of monitoring the inspired and expired concentration of the anesthetic agent is needed. This can easily be accomplished with infrared spectroscopy, which is the method routinely use in most operating rooms. Some method to scavenge the exhaled agent must also be instituted. This is usually accomplished by attaching the exhaust of the ventilator to the standard wall suction.

Summary

Normal respiratory function requires the presence of a patent upper and lower airway to provide a path for the easy and nonimpeded movement of gas. Pathologic conditions that result in alterations of the normal flow of gas from the environment to the alveoli can result in life-threatening emergencies. An immediate assessment of the severity of the limitation of airflow and investigations into its etiology are necessary to allow for prompt and effective therapy. Therapeutic interventions will depend on the underlying etiology of the obstructive process and the level of the airway that is involved. With upper airway obstruction, immediate transportation to the operating room may be indicated in severe cases. In the operating room, once general anesthesia has been induced, direct laryngoscopy not only provides information into the etiology of the problem, but allows for placement of an ETT. In patients with status asthmaticus and lower airway obstruction, therapeutic maneuvers include the administration β-adrenergic agonists via the aerosol or subcutaneous route, inhaled anticholinergic agents, and parenteral corticosteroids. Severe cases may require more aggressive therapy with intravenous β-adrenergic agonists, mechanical ventilation, and, in refractory cases, inhalational anesthetic agents. Life-threatening, refractory cases may require extracorporeal support.[51,52]

References

1. Crosby E, Reid D. Acute epiglottitis in the adult: Is intubation mandatory? *Can J Anaesth* 1991;38:914–918.

2. Gallagher PG, Myer CM III. An approach to the diagnosis and treatment of membranous laryngotracheobronchitis in infants and children. *Pediatr Emerg Care* 1991;7:337–342.
3. Tobias JD, Meyer DJ. Noninvasive monitoring of carbon dioxide during respiratory failure in toddlers and infants: End-tidal versus transcutaneous CO_2 carbon dioxide. *Anesth Analg* 1997;85:55–58.
4. Anene O, Meert KL, Uy H, et al. Dexamethasone for the prevention of post-extubation airway obstruction: A prospective randomized, double-blind placebo-controlled trial. *Crit Care Med* 1996;24:1666–1669.
5. Waisman Y, Klein BL, Boenning DA, et al. Prospective randomized double-blind study comparing l-epinephrine and racemic epinephrine aerosols in the treatment of laryngotracheitis (croup). *Pediatrics* 1992;89:302–306.
6. Tobias JD. Helium: Applications in the practice of anesthesia and critical care. *Am J Anesth* 1997;24:194–200.
7. Duncan PG. Efficacy of helium-oxygen mixtures in the management of severe viral and post-intubation croup. *Can Anesth Soc J* 1979;26:206–212.
8. Tobias JD. Heliox in children with airway obstruction. *Pediatr Emerg Care* 1997;13:29–32.
9. Mao Y, Semenciw R, Morrison H, et al. Increased rates of illness and death from asthma in Canada. *Can Med Assoc J* 1987;137:620–624.
10. Evans R, Mullaby DI, Wilson RW, et al. National trends in the morbidity and mortality of asthma in the US. *Chest* 1987;91(suppl):65S–74S.
11. Arrighi HM. US asthma mortality: 1941 to 1989. *Ann Allergy Asthma Immunol* 1995;74:321–326.
12. Bai TR. Abnormalities in airway smooth muscle in fatal asthma. *Am Rev Respir Dis* 1990;141:552–557.
13. McFadden ER Jr, Kiser R, DeGroot W. Acute bronchial asthma: Relations between clinical and physiologic manifestations. *N Engl J Med* 1973;288:221.
14. Cook T, Stone G. Pediatric asthma: A correlation of clinical treatment and oxygen saturation. *Hawaii Med J* 1995;54:665–668.
15. Carruthers DM, Harrison BD. Arterial blood gas analysis or oxygen saturation in the assessment of acute asthma? *Thorax* 1995;50:186–188.
16. Taylor MR. Asthma: Audit of peak flow rate guidelines for admission and discharge. *Arch Dis Child* 1994;70:432–434.
17. Lim TK, Ang SM, Rossing TH, et al. The effects of deep inhalation of maximal expiratory flow during intensive treatment of spontaneous asthmatic episodes. *Am Rev Respir Dis* 1989;140:340–343.
18. Wasserfallen JB, Schaller MD, Feihl F, Perret CH. Sudden asphyxic asthma: A distinct entity? *Am Rev Respir Dis* 1990;142:108–111.
19. Fisher JD, Vinci RJ. Prehospital management of pediatric asthma requiring hospitalization. *Pediatr Emerg Care* 1995;11:217–219.
20. Fergusson RJ, Stewart CM, Wathen CG, et al. Effectiveness of nebulised salbutamol administered in ambulances to patients with severe acute asthma. *Thorax* 1995;50:81–82.
21. Schuh S, Parkin P, Rajan A, et al. High-versus low-dose, frequently administered, nebulized albuterol in children with severe, acute asthma. *Pediatrics* 1989;83:513–518.
22. Newhouse MT, Dolovich MB. Control of asthma by aerosols. *N Engl J Med* 1986;315:870–874.
23. Newman SP, Clarke SW. Therapeutic aerosols 1: Physical and practical considerations. *Thorax* 1983;38:881–886.
24. Aquilina AT, Hall WJ, Douglas RG Jr, Utell MJ. Airway reactivity in subjects with viral upper respiratory tract infections: The effects of exercise and cold air. *Am Rev Respir Dis* 1980;122:3–10.
25. Fryer AD, Maclagan J. Muscarinic inhibitory receptors in parasympathetic nerves in the guinea pig. *Br J Pharmacol* 1984;83:973–978.
26. Fryer AD, Jacoby DB. Parainfluenza virus infection damages inhibitory M2 muscarinic receptors on pulmonary parasympathetic nerves in the guinea pig. *Br J Pharmacol* 1991;102:267–271.
27. Greenough A, Yuksel B, Everett L, Price JF. Inhaled ipratropium bromide and terbutaline in asthmatic children. *Respir Med* 1993;87:111–114.
28. Schuh S, Johnson DW, Callahan S, et al. Efficacy of frequent nebulized ipratropium bromide added to frequent high-dose albuterol therapy in severe childhood asthma. *J Pediatr* 1995;126:639–645.
29. Singh M, Kumar L. Continuous nebulised salbutamol and oral once a day prednisolone in status asthmaticus. *Arch Dis Child* 1993;69:416–419.
30. Tal A, Levy N, Bearman JE. Methylprednisolone therapy for acute asthma in infants and toddlers: A controlled clinical trial. *Pediatrics* 1990;86:350–356.
31. Banner KH, Page CP. Acute versus chronic

administration of phosphodiesterase inhibitors on allergen-induced pulmonary cell influx in sensitized guinea-pigs. *Br J Pharmacol* 1995;114:93–98.
32. Needleman JP, Kaifer MC, Nold JT, et al. Theophylline does not shorten hospital stay for children admitted for asthma. *Arch Pediatr Adolesc Med* 1995;149:206–209.
33. DiGiulio GA, Kercsmar CM, Krug SE, et al. Hospital treatment of asthma: Lack of benefit from theophylline given in addition to nebulized albuterol and intravenously administered corticosteroid. *J Pediatr* 1993;122:464–469.
34. Noppen M, Vanmaele L, Impens N, Schandevyl W. Bronchodilating effect of intravenous magnesium sulfate in acute severe bronchial asthma. *Chest* 1990;97:373–376.
35. Bloch H, Silverman R, Mancherje N, et al. Intravenous magnesium sulfate as an adjunct in the treatment of acute asthma. *Chest* 1995;107:1576–1581.
36. Downes JJ, Wood DW, Harwood I, et al. Intravenous isoproterenol infusion in children with severe hypercapnia due to status asthmaticus. *Crit Care Med* 1973;1:63–67.
37. O'Connell MB, Iber C. Continuous intravenous terbutaline infusions for adult patients with status asthmaticus. *Ann Allergy* 1990;64:213–218.
38. Kass JE, Castriotta RJ. Heliox therapy in acute severe asthma. *Chest* 1995;107:757–760.
39. Shiue ST, Gluck EH. The use of helium-oxygen mixtures in the support of patients with status asthmaticus and respiratory acidosis. *J Asthma* 1989;26:177–180.
40. Manthous CA, Hall JB, Melmed A, et al. Heliox improves pulsus paradoxus and peak expiratory flow in nonintubated patients with severe asthma. *Am J Respir Crit Care Med* 1995;151:310–314.
41. Gluck EH, Onorato DJ, Castriotta R. Helium-oxygen mixtures in intubated patients with status asthmaticus and respiratory acidosis. *Chest* 1990;98:693–698.
42. Anderson M, Svartengren M, Bylin G, et al. Deposition in asthmatics of particles inhaled in air or in helium-oxygen. *Am Rev Resp Dis* 1993;147:524–528.
43. Kudukis TM, Manthous CA, Schmidt GA, et al. Inhaled helium-oxygen revisited: Effect of inhaled helium-oxygen during the treatment of status asthmaticus in children. *J Pediatr* 1997;130:217–224.
44. Schwartz SH. Treatment of status asthmaticus with halothane. *JAMA* 1984;251:2688–2689.
45. Bierman MI, Brown M, Muren O, et al. Prolonged isoflurane anesthesia in status asthmaticus. *Crit Care Med* 1986;14:832–833.
46. O'Rourke P, Crone R. Halothane in status asthmaticus. *Crit Care Med* 1982;10:341–345.
47. Raine J, Palazzo M, Kerr JL, et al. Near fatal bronchospasm after oral nadolol in a young asthmatic and response to ventilation with halothane. *Br Med J* 1981;282:548–550.
48. Saulnier FF, Durocher AV, Deturck RA, et al. Respiratory and hemodynamic effects of halothane in status asthmaticus. *Intensive Care Med* 1990;16:104–107.
49. Hirshman CA, Bergman NA. Halothane and enflurane protect against bronchospasm in asthma dog model. *Anesth Analg* 1978;57:629–633.
50. Katoh T, Kazuyuki I. A comparison of sevoflurane with halothane, enflurane, and isoflurane on bronchoconstriction caused by histamine. *Can J Anaesth* 1994;41:1214–1219.
51. Kirkpatrick BV, Krummel TM, Mueller DG, et al. Use of extracorporeal membrane oxygenation for respiratory failure in preterm infants. *Pediatrics* 1983;72:872–876.
52. Tobias JD, Garrett JS. Therapeutic options for severe, refractory status asthmaticus: Inhalational anaesthetic agents, extracorporeal membrane oxygenation and helium/oxygen ventilation. *Paediatr Anaesth* 1997;7:47–57.

Chapter 4

Mechanical Ventilation, Respiratory Monitoring, and the Basics of Pulmonary Physiology

Lynn D. Martin, MD

Introduction

The goals of mechanical ventilation in the pediatric intensive care unit (PICU) are directly related to the common ventilatory needs of the critically ill as well as the specific requirements of the growing and developing child. The maintenance of a patent airway is a prerequisite for the provision of mechanical ventilation, and the measures to achieve this objective are of primary importance (see also chapter 1 for a full discussion of the techniques of endotracheal intubation and airway management). The principal purpose of mechanical ventilation is the maintenance of sufficient gas exchange (ie, delivery of oxygen to and clearance of carbon dioxide from the body) to maintain cellular homeostasis. Alterations in mechanical ventilation designed to improve oxygenation may impact on carbon dioxide clearance or vice versa. Thus, the maintenance of oxygenation and the provision of adequate alveolar ventilation for carbon dioxide clearance are best considered as two separate goals. The third goal of mechanical ventilation is to preserve or return respiratory mechanics to their normal function. The final goal is to minimize the metabolic expenditures of the respiratory system (ie, work of breathing). This last goal is particularly important in critically ill children, so that the caloric needs of the muscles of respiration with chronic respiratory failure (ie, bronchopulmonary dysplasia) can be redirected for growth and development.[1,2]

Respiratory Physiology

Since their introduction into the modern ICU, there has been an explosion of new ventilatory techniques that present a complex array of alternatives for treatment of patients with respiratory failure (see chapter 5 for a discussion of alternative means of respiratory support). Physicians contemplating the use of mechanical ventilation must be familiar with these therapeutic options and their potential benefits and associated risks. Only by weighing the therapeutic benefits and the detrimental physiologic consequences will the clinician be able to establish a set of attainable goals for mechanical ventilation (Table 1).

Maintenance of Oxygenation

The partial pressure of oxygen in the alveolus (PAO_2) is one of the primary deter-

Table 1

Goals of Mechanical Ventilation

- Maintenance of systemic oxygen delivery
- Provision of adequate alveolar ventilation
- Preserve or return respiratory mechanics to their normal state
- Minimize metabolic expenditures of the respiratory system

minants of arterial oxygen tension and is the chief target of alterations in mechanical ventilation. The PAO_2 is determined by the alveolar gas equation: $PAO_2 = PiO_2 - PACO_2$, where PiO_2 is the partial pressure of inspired oxygen and $PACO_2$ is the partial pressure of alveolar carbon dioxide. The PiO_2 is determined by the fraction of inspired oxygen ($FiO_2 = 0.21$ when the patient is breathing room air), the barometric pressure ($P_b = 760$ mm Hg at sea level), and the partial pressure of water vapor ($P_{H2O} = 47$ mm Hg). Thus the $PiO_2 = FiO_2 (P_b - P_{H2O}) = 150$ mm Hg in room air at sea level. For clinical purposes, $PACO_2$ is assumed to equal the partial pressure of arterial carbon dioxide ($PaCO_2 = 40$ mm Hg) divided by the respiratory quotient (RQ; determined by the mix of metabolic substrates and usually estimated to be approximately 0.8) resulting in 50 mm Hg. Substituting these values for PiO_2 and $PACO_2$, respectively, into the previous equation yields the classic alveolar gas equation: $PAO_2 = FiO_2 (P_b - P_{H2O}) - PaCO_2/RQ$. The latter equation yields a PAO_2 of 100 to 120 mm Hg at room air and sea level. The alveolar gas equation reveals three etiologies for hypoxemia (Table 2): 1) low FiO_2 (ie, hypoxic gas mixture); 2) low barometric pressure (ie, high altitude); and 3) hypoventilation. Although the first two are rarely clinical causes of hypoxemia, an important principle of the alveolar gas equation can be revealed by closer inspection of the last cause of hypoxemia. A decrease in alveolar ventilation by 50% in room air at sea level will yield a PAO_2 of 50 mm Hg, a clinically significant level of hypoxemia. However, with the administration of 25% inspired oxygen, the PAO_2 increases to 78 mm Hg, a nonhypoxemic concentration. Thus, a very small increase in inspired oxygen tension will easily overcome hypoxemia due solely to hypoventilation.

The difference between the partial pressure of oxygen in the alveolus (PAO_2) and that in the pulmonary capillary (PaO_2), approximately 10 mm Hg under normal conditions, is caused by the diffusion barrier of the alveolar-capillary membrane and the overall ventilation-perfusion (V/Q) ratio of the lung. While the former is easily overcome by increasing inspired oxygen concentration and rarely is a cause for clinically significant hypoxemia, the same cannot be said for the latter. The principal etiology for clinically significant hypoxemia is pulmonary pathology associated with decreased lung volumes, reduced lung compliance, and an increased proportion of low V/Q compartments of the lung.[3] Under severe conditions, areas of the lung may become completely atelectatic and lead to right-to-left intrapulmonary shunting. One of the primary objectives of mechanical ventilation is to restore normal lung volumes and mechanics through the application of

Table 2

Alveolar Partial Pressure of Oxygen Under Various Conditions

Condition	$PAO_2 = FiO_2 (P_B - P_{H2O}) - PACO_2/RQ$	PAO_2 (mm Hg)
Normal	$PAO_2 = 0.21 (760 - 47) - 40/0.8$	$PAO_2 = 100$ (mm Hg)
Hypoxic gas mixture at sea level	$PAO_2 = 0.15 (760 - 47) - 40/0.8$	$PAO_2 = 57$ (mm Hg)
Normoxic, hypobaric pressure	$PAO_2 = 0.21 (560 - 47) - 40/0.8$	$PAO_2 = 58$ (mm Hg)
Normoxic, hypoventilation at sea level	$PAO_2 = 0.21 (760 - 47) - 80/0.8$	$PAO_2 = 50$ (mm Hg)
Hypoventilation with supplemental O_2	$PAO_2 = 0.25 (760 - 47) - 80/0.8$	$PAO_2 = 78$ (mm Hg)

continuous positive airway pressure (CPAP). A useful clinical index of the effect of changes of ventilation variables is mean airway pressure (P_{aw}).[4] Alterations in peak and end-expiratory pressure, ventilator rate, and inspiratory-to-expiratory (I:E) ratio are used to increase P_{aw}, which recruits atelectatic or poorly ventilated alveolar units thereby restoring normal V/Q matching and decreasing intrapulmonary shunting.[5] The restoration of lung volumes frequently allows a dramatic reduction in the inspired oxygen concentration as well as improving respiratory mechanics and decreasing the work of breathing. These improvements may allow for the partial or compete restoration of spontaneous ventilation, which is associated with several possible advantages (improved V/Q matching, decreased risk of barotrauma, diminished adverse effects of continuous positive pressure ventilation).[6]

From the previous discussion, the major etiologic factors producing hypoxemia can be listed as: 1) hypoxic gas mixture; 2) hypoventilation; 3) ventilation-perfusion mismatch; 4) diffusion abnormalities of the alveolar-capillary membrane; and 5) true shunt related to cyanotic, congenital heart diseases.

Maintenance of Alveolar Ventilation

A second goal of mechanical ventilation is to augment or control alveolar ventilation. Respiratory failure is frequently defined in terms of $PaCO_2$, which is inversely related to alveolar ventilation (V_A): $PaCO_2 \propto V_{CO_2} / V_A$, where V_{CO_2} is carbon dioxide production. Alveolar ventilation is also defined (at normal ventilatory frequencies) as: $V_A = f(V_T - V_D)$, where V_T is tidal volume, V_D is dead space volume, and f is the respiratory frequency. Alterations in V_T and/or f, which are the components of minute ventilation (V_E), will result in changes in $PaCO_2$. Clinicians may fail to account for the third component in these equations, namely V_D. The relationship between V_E and $PaCO_2$ can be described by the following: $PaCO_2 = 0.863\ V_{CO_2} / [V_E (1 - V_D/V_T)]$, where V_{CO_2} is the metabolically produced carbon dioxide at standard temperature and pressure.

Most of V_D in normal individuals is the result of the volume of the conducting airways (anatomic V_D). Since the anatomic dead space is relatively constant, with an increasing V_T, V_D/V_T tends to decrease and rarely exceeds 0.3. In patients with intrinsic lung disease undergoing mechanical ventilation, V_D/V_T has been found to exceed 0.6 and is primarily due to continued ventilation of poorly perfused regions of the lungs (alveolar V_D). In this setting, increases in V_T may not decrease V_D/V_T since higher alveolar pressures as a result of larger V_T may result in a further decrease in pulmonary perfusion and increase in alveolar V_D. The effect of increases in V_T on V_D/V_T can be facilitated by measurement of V_D/V_T using capnography: $V_D/V_T = (PaCO_2 - P_{et}CO_2) / PaCO_2$, where $P_{et}CO_2$ is the partial pressure of carbon dioxide in exhaled gas, commonly referred to as end-tidal carbon dioxide. In summary, three factors must be considered when changes in $PaCO_2$ occur: 1) changes in metabolic $\dot{V}_{CO_2}$; 2) alterations in V_E as a result of increases or decreases in V_T and f; and 3) modifications of V_D.

Mechanics of Ventilation

A simplified single-compartment model of the lungs composed of a single, cylindrical flow-conducting tube (ie, conducting airways) connected to a single, spherical elastic compartment (ie, alveoli) is frequently used to describe pulmonary mechanics (Fig. 1). In this model, the lungs are considered as a homogeneous assembly of units with uniform pressure-volume (compliance) and pressure-flow (resistance) characteristics derived from this single representative unit. To achieve inflation, a transrespiratory pressure (P_{tr}) composed of two components is required. The first component, the transthoracic pressure (P_{tt}), is defined as the pressure required to deliver the tidal volume against the elastic recoil of the lungs and chest wall, while the second component, the transairway pressure (P_{ta}), is the pressure necessary to overcome airflow resistance. This is described mathematically by the equation $P_{tr} = P_{tt} + P_{ta}$, where P_{tr} = airway minus body surface pressure, P_{tt} = alveolar minus body surface pressure, and

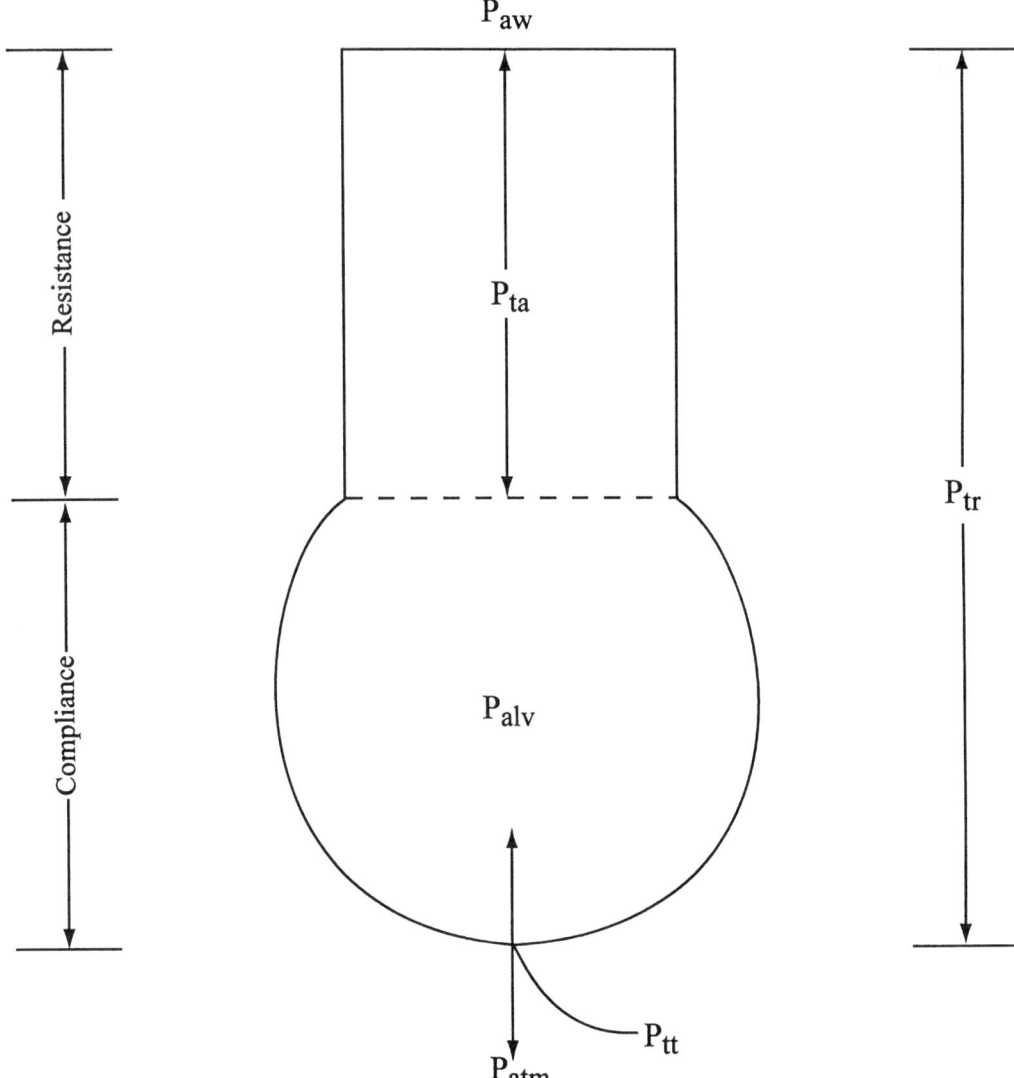

Figure 1. The simplified single compartment model of the lungs composed of a flow-resistive element adjoined in series with a compliance element. P_{aw} = airway pressure; P_{alv} = alveolar pressure; P_{atm} = atmospheric pressure; P_{ta} = transairway ($P_{aw} - P_{alv}$) pressure; P_{tt} = transthoracic ($P_{alv} - P_{atm}$) pressure; P_{tr} = transrespiratory ($P_{aw} - P_{atm}$) pressure. Ventilator manometers are equivalent to P_{tr}.

P_{ta} = airway minus alveolar pressure. The pressure required for inspiration may come from the respiratory muscles (P_{rm}) and/or the ventilator (P_{tr}): $P_{rm} + P_{tr} = P_{tt} + P_{ta}$. Since the ventilator measures pressure relative to atmosphere, P_{tr} is equal to P_{aw} displayed by the ventilator, allowing the substitution: $P_{rm} + P_{aw} = P_{tt} + P_{ta}$.

The single-compartment model assumes a linear relationship between pressure and volume and between pressure and flow. The change in P_{tr} is directly proportional to the corresponding change in lung volume and the constant of proportionality is the slope ($\Delta P/\Delta V$) of the pressure-volume curve (ie, reciprocal of compliance [C]). Similarly, the change in P_{ta} is proportional to the change in flow rate (F) and the constant of proportionality ($\Delta P/\Delta F$) is resistance (R). Substituting $\Delta P/\Delta V$ for P_{tr} and $\Delta P/\Delta F$ for P_{ta} yields the equation of motion of the respiratory system for inspiration: $P_{rm} + P_{aw} = V/C + (F)(R)$, where V is the volume inspired or expired, C is the compliance of the respiratory system, F is the inspiratory or expiratory flow rate, and R is the resistance of the respiratory system. For passive expiration, the equation of motion of the respiratory system is defined as: $V/C = -(F)(R)$, where the elastic components of the lungs ($P_A = V/C$) provides the pressure to drive expiratory flow rate. In situations where respiratory muscles are relaxed, measurement of pressure, volume, and flow allow calculation of total respiratory system compliance and resistance.

The relationships represented in the equation of motion can be graphically represented for both constant inspiratory flow (ie, volume-limited ventilation) and constant inspiratory pressure (ie, pressure-limited ventilation) as seen in Figure 2. During constant inspiratory flow ventilation (Fig. 2, left), the initial rise in pressure is related to the resistance and flow rate while the slope of the pressure rise is inversely proportional to compliance, tidal volume, resistance, and inspiratory flow rate. Lung pressure (P_L) is expressed as $P_L = (F)(t)/C$, where F is inspiratory flow rate, t is the inspiratory time, and C is the compliance of the respiratory system. Lung volume (V_L) can be represented as $V_L = (F)(t)$. During constant inspiratory pressure ventilation (Fig. 2, right), the P_L, V_L, and F during inspiration are exponential functions of time derived from the equation of motion as $P_L = \Delta P(1-e^{-t/\tau})$, $V_L = C(\Delta P)(1-e^{-t/\tau})$, and $F = \Delta P/R \times (e^{-t/\tau})$, where ΔP is equal to peak inspiratory pressure minus end-expiratory pressure, t is the inspiratory time, e is the natural logarithm (≈ 2.72), and τ is the time constant of the respiratory system. The time constant (τ) is the product of compliance (volume/pressure) and resistance (pressure x time/volume) and is measured in seconds. Exhalation during any form of mechanical ventilation is passive. Therefore, the P, V, and F can also be derived from the equation of motion as: $P_L = \Delta P (e^{-t/\tau})$, $V_L = C (\Delta P)(e^{-t/\tau})$, and $F = -\Delta P/R (e^{-t/\tau})$, where t is the expiratory time and τ is the expiratory time constant. Note that all variables are measured relative to their value at end-expiration, thus P_L is pressure above positive end-expiratory pressure (PEEP) and V_L is the volume above end-expiratory volume. When inspiratory and expiratory times are between zero and infinity, the shapes of the lung pressure and lung volume curves are defined by the τ. By plotting these curves over time in units of τ, clinically useful principles emerge (Fig. 3). Irrespective of the specific values of resistance and compliance, after one τ 63% of lung inflation or deflation occurs, 95% after 3τ, and, for all practical purposes, complete equilibration after 5τ.

The equation of motion is a useful means to more closely examine the differences between constant flow volume-limited ventilation, and constant pressure ventilation with a decelerating inspiratory flow waveform. Peak airway pressures are higher for a constant flow pattern compared to the constant pressure pattern. However, peak alveolar pressures depend only on the compliance and tidal volume, thereby making peak lung pressures independent of the pattern of ventilation. Second, at any point in time, airway pressure is equal to the volume/compliance plus the resistance/flow. The pressure required to overcome flow resistance (shaded area in Fig. 2) is constant with fixed inspiratory flow while it decreases exponentially with the decelerating flow pattern. In the example depicted, the area is equal for both patterns, since tidal volume and inspiratory times are equal. Third, the more rapid approach to the pressure limit during constant pressure decelerating flow ventilation leads to a higher P_{aw} compared to constant flow ventilation. Since all shaded areas are equal, the total area under the airway curve is equal to the total area under the lung pressure curve for each pattern. Therefore, P_{aw} is equal to mean P_L, a finding that has been verified in animals.[4]

The final feature of pulmonary mechanics that must be appreciated is the sigmoidal shape of the static pressure-volume (compliance) relationship of the respiratory system (Fig. 4). The respiratory system is

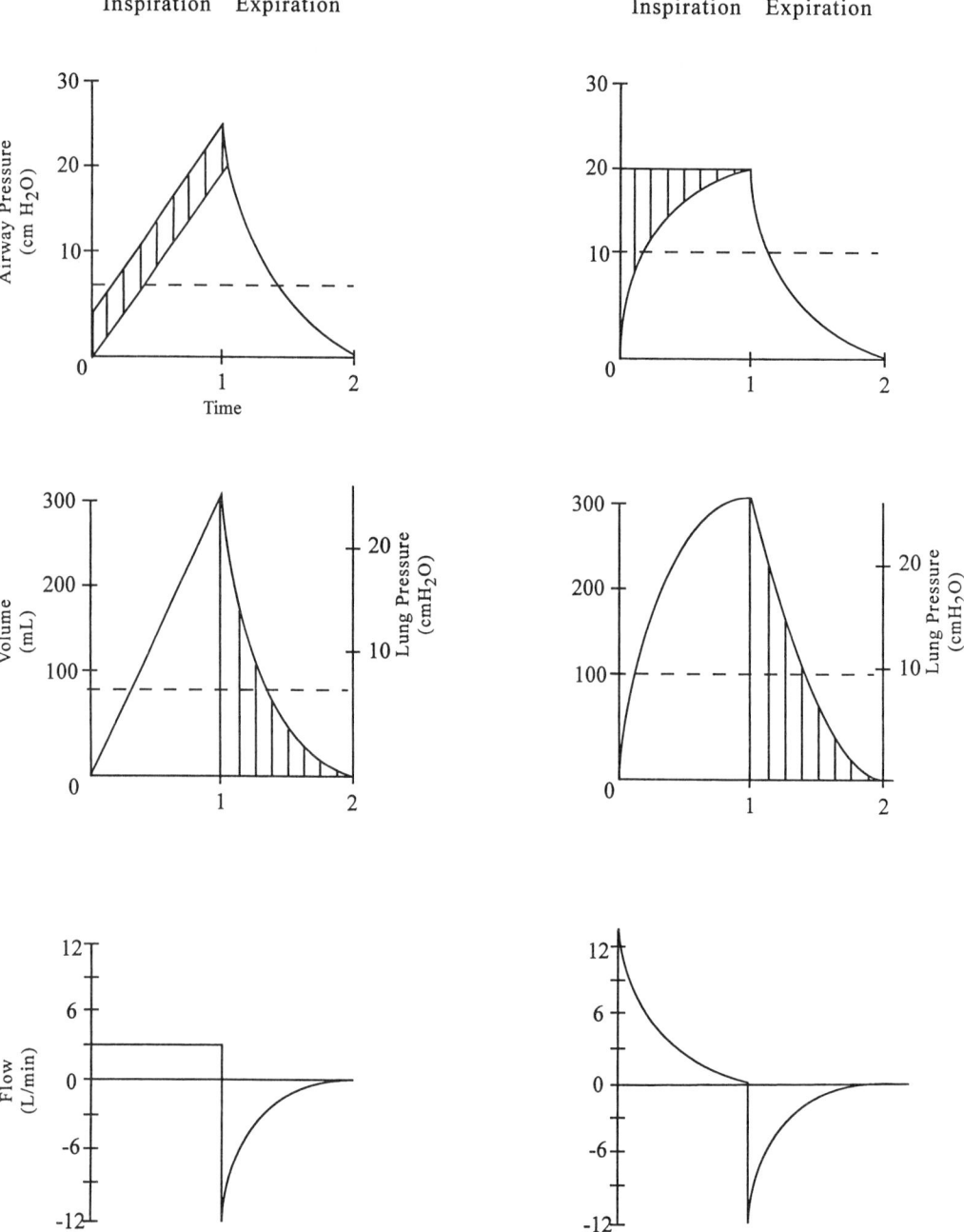

Figure 2. Graphic representation of the equation of motion for constant inspiratory flow (left) and constant inspiratory pressure (right) breaths. Pressure, volume, and flow are measured relative to their respective end-expiratory values. The shaded areas represent equal geometric areas proportional to the pressure required to overcome flow-resistance, while the unshaded areas correspond to the pressure required to overcome lung elastic recoil. The dotted line represents mean airway and lung pressures. Note the higher peak and lower mean airway pressures with the constant inspiratory flow breath (left) compared to the constant inspiratory pressure breath (right).

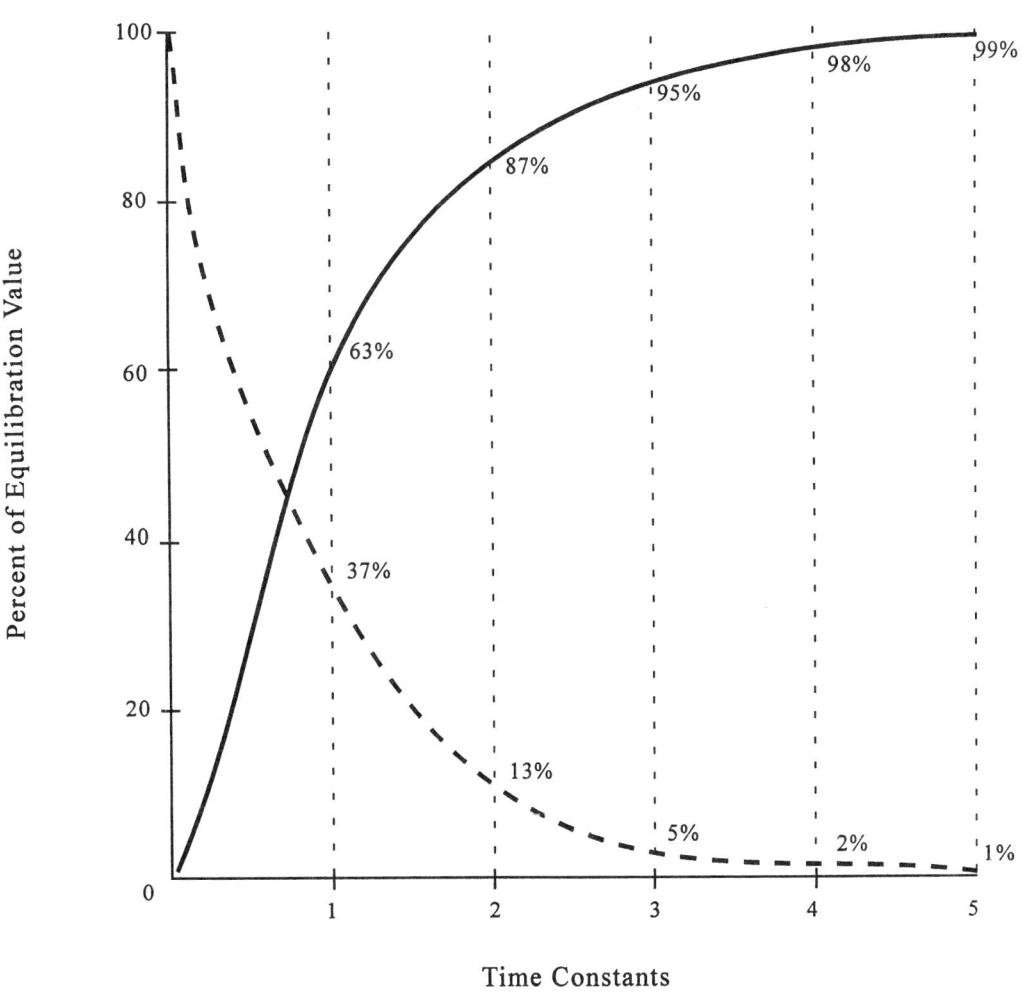

Figure 3. Exponential lung pressure or volume curves as a function of time constant during inspiration (solid line) and expiration (dotted line).

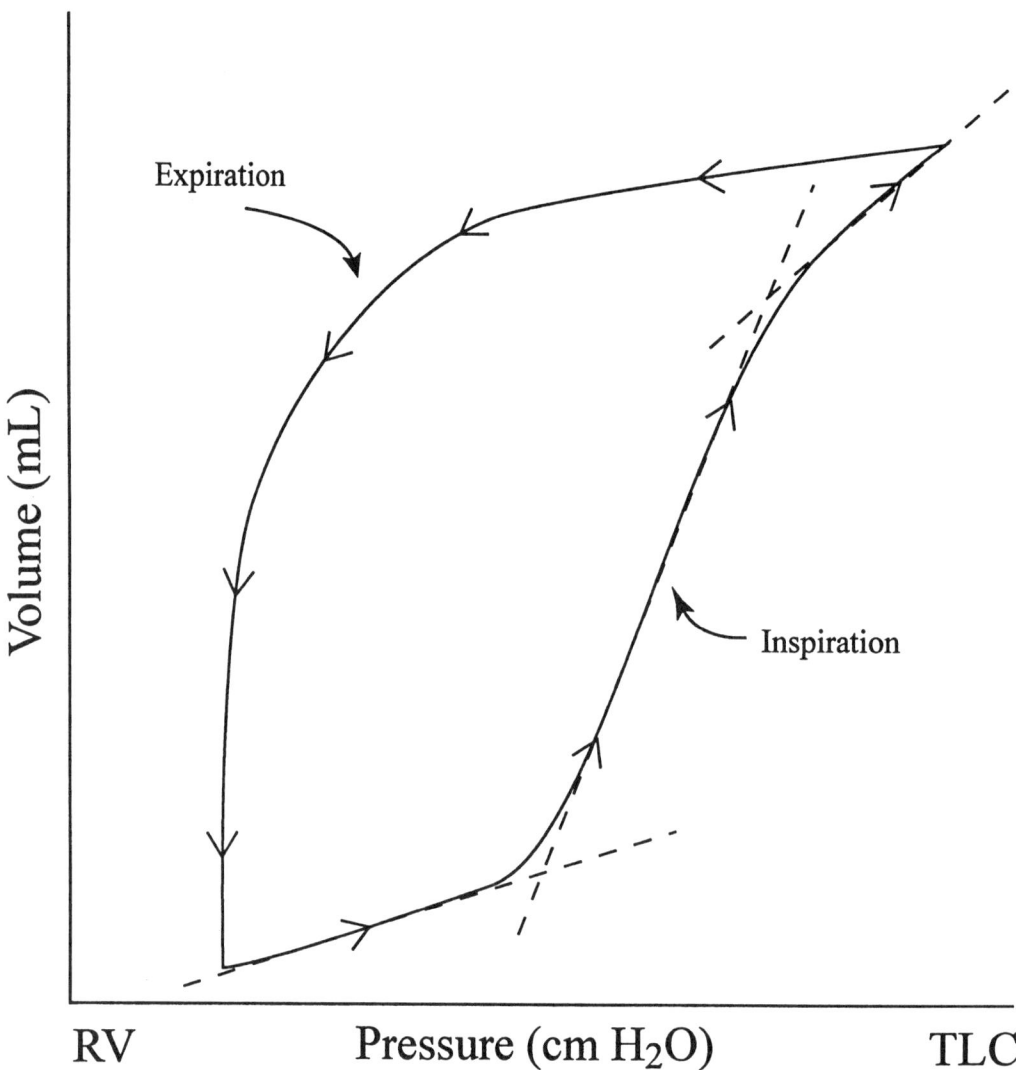

Figure 4. A hypothetical static pressure-volume curve of the respiratory system. Note the sigmoidal shape of the inspiratory limb with high compliance in the midvolume range and low compliance at either high or low lung volumes. Inflection points denote the change from low to high compliance regions.

most compliant in the midvolume range, becoming progressively less compliant at high (near total lung capacity) and low (approaching residual volume) volume extremes. Tidal ventilation near total lung capacity occurs under two conditions: 1) when total lung volume and/or vital capacity are decreased secondary to intrinsic lung disease, and 2) when end-expiratory volume is decreased. Conversely, ventilation near residual volume with a decrease in compliance also occurs under two conditions: 1) when obesity and/or abdominal distention increase residual volume and encroach on the lower range of vital capacity, and 2) when intrinsic lung disease results in airway or alveolar closure at end-expiratory volume.

The relationship between end-expiratory lung volume (ELV; the volume at which inspiration occurs), more commonly described as functional residual capacity (FRC), and closing capacity (the volume at which airway closure during expiration occurs) is critical. Conditions that decrease FRC below closing capacity or increase closing capacity above FRC result in a maldistribution of ventilation and perfusion, and adversely affect the mechanics of breathing (Table 3). In the school-aged child and in the adult, FRC is normally well above closing capacity. However, the relationship is more precarious in young infants, in whom studies suggest that closing capacity exceeds FRC.[7] A primary goal of mechanical ventilation is the restoration of the normal relationship between FRC and closing capacity. Conditions associated with a decrease in FRC (eg, pulmonary edema, pneumonitis, infant respiratory distress syndrome [IRDS] and acute respiratory distress syndrome [ARDS]) are treated with PEEP to increase FRC back to normal levels. Situations associated with increased closing capacity, such as bronchiolitis and reactive airway disease, are treated with bronchodilators and measures to control secretions in order to reduce closing capacity and maintain airway patency.

Table 3

Conditions Predisposing to Convergence of Closing and Functional Residual Capacities

Elevation of Closing Capacity
  Infancy
  Bronchiolitis
  Asthma
  Bronchopulmonary dysplasia
  Smoke inhalation (thermal airway injury)
  Cystic fibrosis
Reduction of Functional Residual Capacity
  Supine position
  Abdominal distention
  Thoracic or abdominal surgery/trauma
  Atelectasis
  Pulmonary edema
  Acute lung injury/acute respiratory distress syndrome
  Near drowning
  Diffuse pneumonitis
    aspiration pneumonitis
    idiopathic interstitial pneumonitis
    bacterial pneumonia
    viral pneumonitis
    opportunistic organism (ie *pneumocystis carinii*)
  radiation

Work of Breathing

The pressure-volume (compliance) and pressure-flow (resistance) characteristics of the respiratory system determine the work of breathing which, in reality, represents the afterload on the respiratory muscles.[8] The work of breathing overcomes two major sources of impedance: 1) elastic recoil of the lung and chest wall (Fig. 5, areas A, C, and D), and 2) the frictional resistance to gas flow in the airways (Fig. 5, areas A, B, and C). The total work of breathing (Fig. 5, areas A through D) is increased by a decrease in respiratory compliance and/or an increase in respiratory resistance properties. When total work of breathing against compliance and resistance is summated and plotted against respiratory frequency, an optimal respiratory frequency exists that minimizes the total work of breathing (Fig. 6). In patients with low lung compliance (restrictive lung diseases) such as pulmonary edema, IRDS, or ARDS, the optimal frequency is increased, leading to rapid, shallow breathing. In contrast, in obstructive lung diseases with increased resistance such as bronchiolitis or asthma, the optimal frequency is decreased with slow, deep breathing.

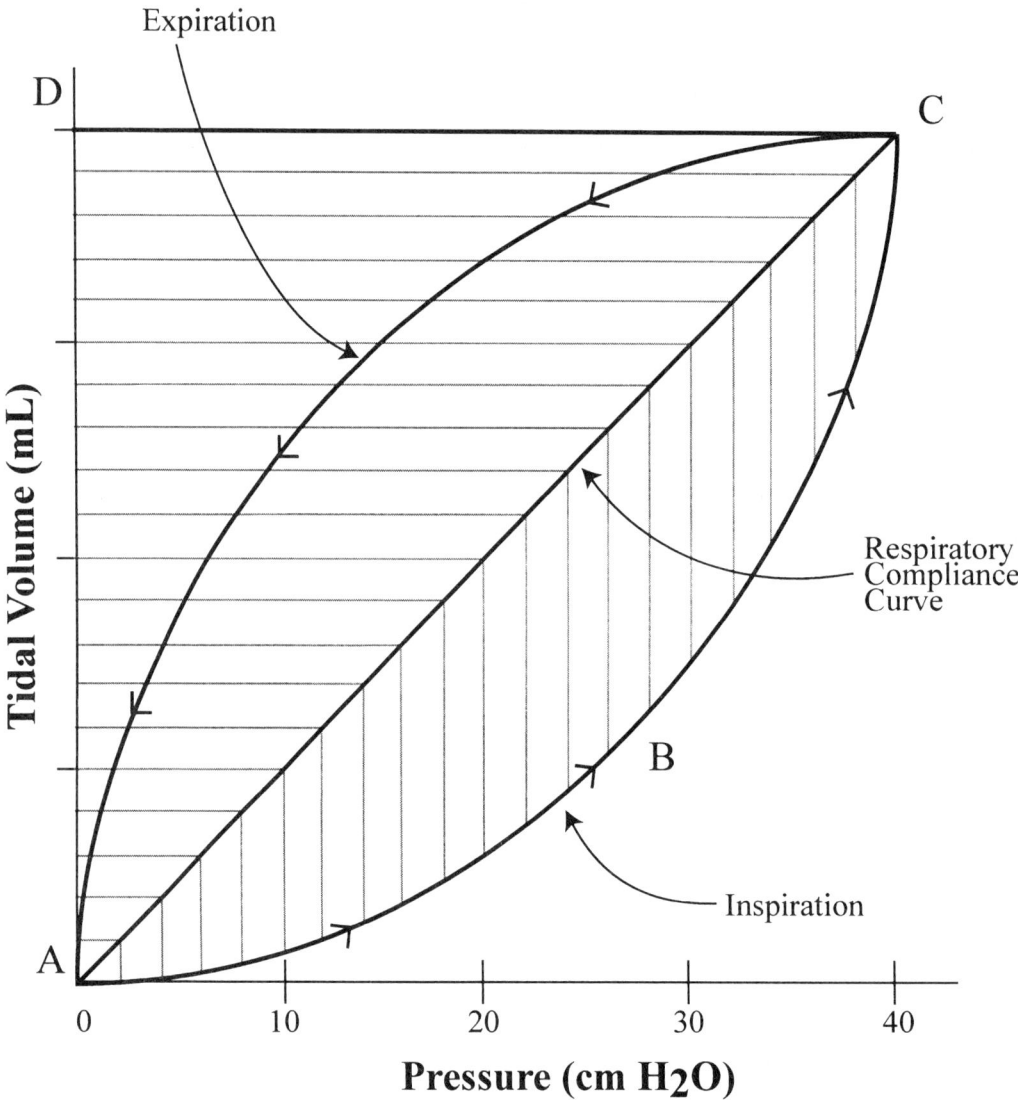

Figure 5. Inspiratory and expiratory pressure-volume curve recorded during a complete respiratory cycle. Total work of breathing (pressure × volume) is defined as the sum of resistive work (area defined by ABC) plus the elastic work (area defined by ACD). Total work (defined by area ABCD) is increased by either an increase in resistive properties of the respiratory system or by a decrease in compliance (slope of line between A and C).

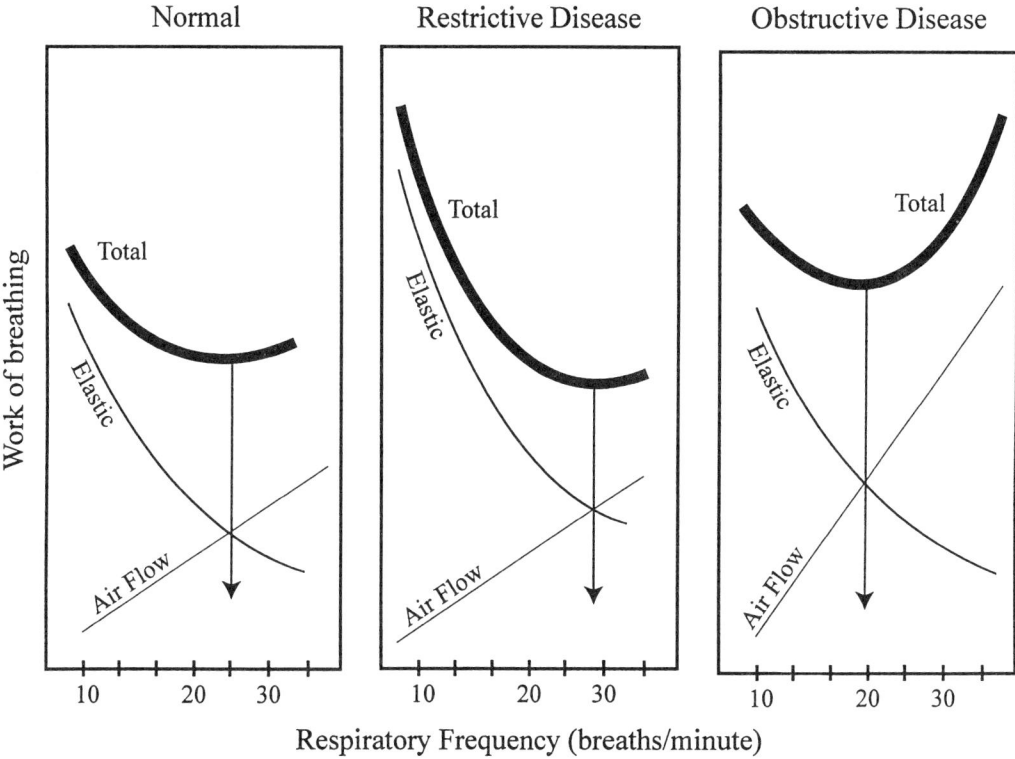

Figure 6. Hypothetical diagrams showing work done against elastic and resistance, separately, and summated to indicate total work at different respiratory frequencies. For a constant minute volume, minimum work is performed at higher frequencies with restrictive (low compliance) disease and at lower frequencies when airflow resistance is increased.

Developmental Aspects

A fundamental understanding of the developmental changes in static and dynamic components of respiratory mechanics is required in order to provide effective mechanical support of the respiratory system in pediatric patients. Age-related changes in respiratory rate, inspiratory time and flow, tidal volume, and other mechanical properties of the respiratory system (Table 4) determine the technical requirements of respiratory support equipment in children. Furthermore, these parameters limit the applicability of equipment and approaches designed primarily for the adult population.

Respiratory compliance and conductance (ie, reciprocal of resistance) define the mechanical forces required to inflate the lungs during positive pressure ventilation. Although the absolute values of compliance and conductance are much lower in the infant, when these parameters are expressed relative to size (lung volume, height, or weight), they are similar to values seen in adults. Therefore, comparable levels of positive inflating pressure are required in all age groups to deliver similar tidal volume. Because the absolute values of compliance and conductance are much lower in infants, pediatric ventilators must deliver low inspiratory tidal volumes and flows under pressures comparable to those used in adults. These conditions can lead to significant errors in tidal volume delivery to infants, due to the relatively large volume of the ventilator circuit. The distribu-

Table 4
Comparative Respiratory Physiology in the New Born and Adult

Parameters	Infant	Adult
Respiratory frequency (breaths/minute)	30–40	12–16
Inspiratory time (seconds)	0.4–0.5	1.2–1.5
Inspiratory/expiratory ratio	1:1.5–1:2	1:2–1:3
Tidal volume		
mL	20	500
mL/kg	6–8	6–8
Functional residual capacity (FRC)		
mL	100	2200
mL/kg	30	34
Vital capacity		
mL	120	3500
mL/kg	35	50
Total lung capacity		
mL	200	6000
mL/kg	63	86
Total respiratory system compliance		
mL/cm H_2O	2.5–5.0	100
mL/cm H_2O/mL FRC	0.04–0.06	0.04–0.07
Lung compliance		
mL/cm H_2O	4.8–6.2	170–200
mL/cm H_2O/mL FRC	0.04–0.07	0.04–0.07
Specific airway conductance (mL/sec · cm H_2O/mL FRC)	0.24	0.28

tion of volume delivered by a positive pressure ventilator between the ventilator circuit (ie, compressible volume) and the patient is determined by the relative compliance of the circuit and the patient. This relationship is expressed mathematically as: $V_T/V_S = 1/(1 + C_V/C_T)$, where V_T is tidal volume delivered to the patient, V_S is volume delivered by the ventilator, C_V is the compliance of the ventilator circuit, and C_T is total respiratory compliance. Modifications made to decrease compressible volume and circuit compliance enhance the efficacy of mechanical ventilators in infants and small children (Table 5).

Table 5
Measures to Decrease Ventilator System Compliance and Compressible Volume

Decrease circuit compliance
  small-diameter circuit tubing
  rigid, thick-walled, or reinforced circuit tubing
Decrease circuit volume
  short inspiratory circuit
  positioning of exhalation valve near the airway opening
Decrease humidifier volume
  decrease humidifier size
  maintaining humidifier fluid level

Classification of Mechanical Ventilators

Several generations of classification schemes for ventilators have been used in the past. As many of the systems are outdated, vague, or frankly contradictory, a new classification system has been proposed that is based on a theoretical framework that can be applied to all ventilators in a consistent manner with specific and appropriate detail.[9] This classification system is based on the physiologic principles of the equation of motion (pressure = volume/compliance + resistance × flow), and has five categories that form the framework for discussion (Table 6). The only two sources of power input used on commercial ventilators are electric and pneumatic (compressed gas). The original power input is converted to positive pressure gas that is delivered in a controlled manner via a power transmission drive mechanism. The ventilator's control scheme may be simple, as in most neonatal ventilators, or complex, as seen in microprocessor ventilators where the entire shape of the waveform is controlled during inspiration. Using mathematical terms, the ventilator can control only one variable (ie, the independent, or control, variable) while the resultant waveform is limited to only one dependent variable. The variable that becomes the dependent variable is determined by the selection of the independent or control variable. The ventilator-independent or control variable can be either pressure, volume, flow, or time.

Implicit in this classification system is the understanding that pressure, volume, and flow are functions of time. The pressure, volume, or flow is delivered over a specific interval of time. The ventilator controls the time intervals for inspiration and expiration. The ventilator cycle can be divided into four phases: 1) the change from expiratory to inspiratory phase; 2) the inspiratory phase; 3) the change from inspiratory to expiratory phase; and 4) the expiratory phase. The ventilator monitors pressure, volume, flow, or time (referred to as phase variables) and when a predetermined value is reached, the ventilator will switch from one phase to the next. The four phase variables can be more accurately defined as: 1) the trigger variable (the variable that initiates or triggers inspiration); 2) the limit variable (inspiratory pressure, volume, and flow increase above end-expiratory values to a preset limit but will not terminate inspiration); 3) the cycle variable (the specified variable that, when a predetermined value is reached, will result in termination of inspiration); and 4) the baseline variable (the variable that is controlled during expiration).

Consideration of whether the machine or the patient controls the phase variables provides a means for classifying mechanical ventilator breaths (Table 7). This system defines four possible breath types (controlled, assisted, supported, and spontaneous). Modern microprocessor ventilators combine the control and phase variables to de-

Table 6

Classification Scheme for Mechanical Ventilators

Power input
Power transmission
Control scheme
   control variable
   phase variable
   conditional variable
Output waveform
Alarms
   input power alarm
   control circuit alarm
   output alarms

Table 7

Classification of Mechanical Ventilator Breaths

Breath Type	Phase Variable		
	Trigger	Limit	Cycle
Mandatory	Machine	Machine	Machine
Assisted	Patient	Machine	Machine
Supported	Patient	Machine	Patient
Spontaneous	Patient	Patient	Patient

Modified, with permission, from Reference 11.

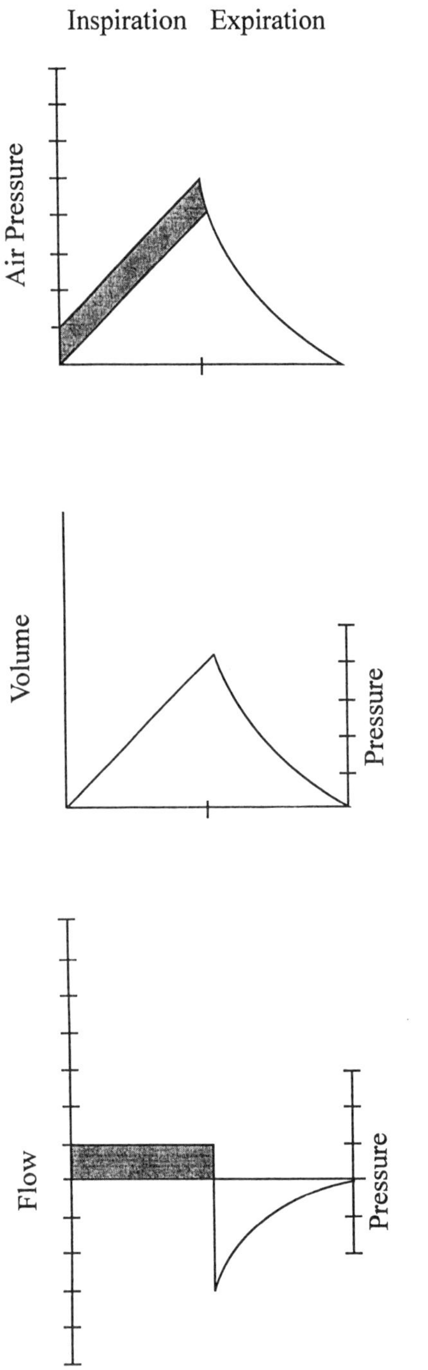

$$P_{total} = P_{elastic} + P_{resistance}$$

$$P_{total}$$

$$P_{elastic} = \frac{Volume}{Compliance}$$

$$P_{resistance} = Resistance \times Flow$$

Figure 7. Theoretical output waveforms for constant inspiratory flow presented as specified by the equation of motion (top-pressure, middle-volume, and bottom-flow). Note that the volume waveform is identical to the lung pressure waveform (ie, pressure is due to elastic recoil) and the flow waveform is the same shape as the airway pressure (ie, pressure is due to airway resistance). When all of the pressure scales are equal, the height of the airway pressure waveform at any point is the sum of the heights of the two waveforms indicated by the shaded and unshaded areas.

liver the predetermined waveform for each breath. The ventilator can either provide a constant pattern or a variable pattern (assisted and spontaneous breaths—synchronized intermittent mandatory ventilation [SIMV]; assisted and supported breaths—SIMV with pressure-support ventilation [PSV]; and all breaths assisted—assist control mode).

When considering assisted ventilation, two basic modes exist: assist control and SIMV. With assist control, the ventilator delivers the full support or breath (either pressure- or volume-limited) each time the patient initiates a breath. If the patient fails to breathe, the ventilator will deliver a fixed number of breaths per minute according to the preset rate. With SIMV, a set number of breaths per minute are synchronized (assisted) with the patient's respiratory effort. If the patient breathes above the preset number of breaths each minute, there will be additional minute ventilation but there will be no added support with these breaths if SIMV is used alone. As there is significant work of breathing during mechanical ventilation related to the resistance of the endotracheal tube, the circuit, and the ventilator, some form of support (eg, pressure support) may be added to augment the spontaneous breaths.

The ventilator must determine which pattern of control and phase variables to use for each breath, based on the value of the preset conditional variables. The study and understanding of ventilator operation is facilitated by the examination of the pressure, volume, and flow output waveform (Fig. 7).[10] Finally, nearly every aspect of the patient-ventilator respiratory pattern can be assessed, monitored, displayed, and alarmed. These alarms may be audible, visual, or both depending on the seriousness of the alarmed condition.

Modes of Mechanical Ventilation

Over the last two decades there has been a tremendous proliferation of different modes of mechanical ventilation, each with its loyal supporters and staunch critics. Perhaps the single greatest determinant of success for a mode of ventilation is the skill and experience of the clinician managing the ventilator. Because of the vast array of choices now available, common clinical descriptions and terminology for these modes of ventilation can easily confuse clinicians. Based on the previously described ventilator classification system, a categorizing scheme for the modes of ventilation has also been developed.[11] This system employs the same categories: control variables (pressure, volume, flow, and time), phase variables (trigger, limit, cycle), and conditional variables to describe all of the commonly used modes of ventilation (Table 8).

Controlled Ventilation

Controlled (or mandatory) ventilation is defined as a mode in which all breaths are triggered, limited, and cycled by the ventilator. The first generation of ventilators would deliver their mandatory breaths regardless of the patient's own ventilatory efforts, leading to patient-ventilator asynchrony and increased work of breathing. Modern microprocessor ventilators have overcome this inefficiency by their ability to sense a patient's inspiratory effort and synchronize ventilator breaths to meet all of the patient's inspiratory flow demands. Hence, all controlled modes of ventilation are in fact capable of assisting the patient's inspiratory efforts if they are present, and are best thought of as assisted modes of ventilation. Should the patient fail to make an inspiratory effort, the ventilator will deliver the mandatory mechanical breath.

Volume-Controlled Ventilation

Volume-controlled ventilation (VCV) is defined as ventilation with a preset tidal volume delivered over a set inspiratory time, with a set frequency and constant inspiratory flow (Figure 8). It can also be classified as assist control mode with volume-limited ventilation. The ventilator controls all timing parameters of the breath, although modern ventilators will respond to a patient's inspiratory efforts. Delivery of a

Table 8
Classification System for Common Modes of Positive Pressure Mechanical Ventilation

Modes*	Mandatory			Assisted			Spontaneous			Supported			Conditional Variable
	trigger	limit	cycle	trigger	limit	cycle	trigger	limit†	cycle†	trigger	limit	cycle	
VCV	time	flow	volume‡	patient§	flow	volume‡	—	—	—	—	—	—	—
PCV	time	pressure	time	patient§	pressure	time	—	—	—	—	—	—	—
PRVC	time	pressure	volume‡	patient§	pressure	time	—	—	—	—	—	—	minute volume
IMV													
volume	time	flow	volume‡	—	—	—	patient§	pressure	pressure	—	—	—	—
pressure	time	pressure	time	—	—	—	patient§	pressure	pressure	—	—	—	—
SIMV													
volume	time	flow	volume‡	patient§	flow	volume‡	patient§	pressure	pressure	—	—	—	pt. effort or time
pressure	time	pressure	time	patient§	pressure	time	patient§	pressure	pressure	—	—	—	pt. effort or time
PSV	—	—	—	—	—	—	—	—	—	patient§	pressure	flow‖	—
VSV	—	—	—	—	—	—	—	—	—	patient§	pressure	flow‖	minute volume
VAPS	—	—	—	—	—	—	—	—	—	patient§	pressure	flow‖	tidal volume
CPAP	—	—	—	—	—	—	patient	pressure	pressure	—	—	—	patient effort

Modified, with permission, from Reference 11.

*VCV = volume-controlled ventilation; PCV = pressure-controlled ventilation; PRVC = pressure-regulated volume control; IMV = intermittent mandatory ventilation; SIMV = synchronized intermittent mandatory ventilation; PSV = pressure support ventilation; VSV = volume support ventilation; VAPS = volume-assisted pressure support; CPAP = continuous positive airway pressure.

†Pressure-limited only on demand-valve systems in which the ventilator limits and cycles to maintain constant airway pressures (applies to all modes in this column).

‡Cycling can also be due to set inspiratory time in the setting of a fixed flow.

§May be either patient generated pressure or flow in the ventilator circuit.

‖Flow reflects the interaction of the patient's effort with the respiratory system impedance and ventilator flow rate.

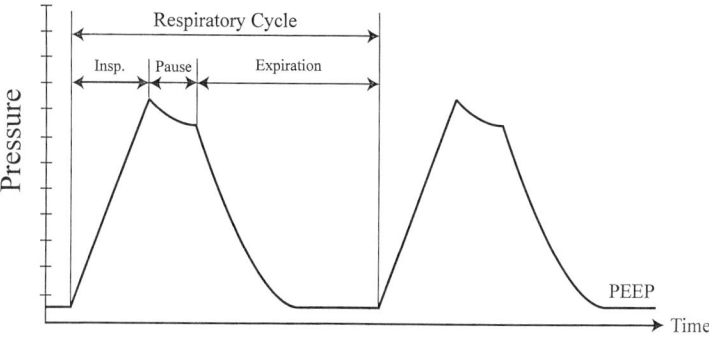

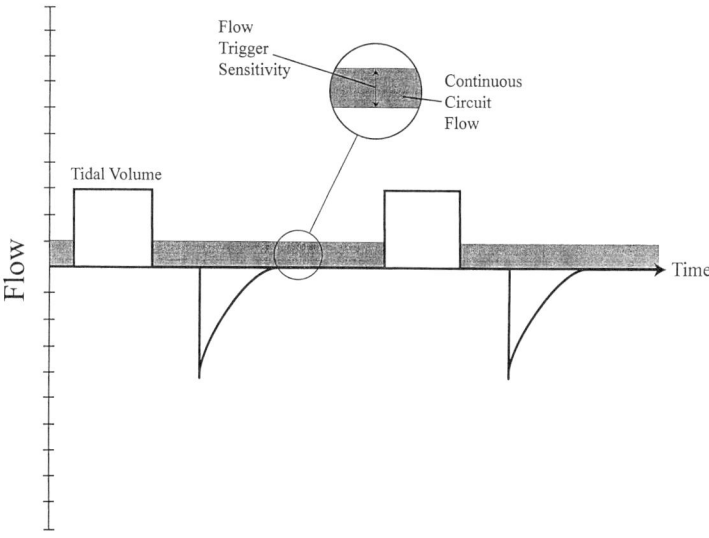

Figure 8. Pressure-time and flow-time diagrams during flow limited, time-cycled, volume-controlled ventilation. In this example, an inspiratory pause (hold) is used that results in both peak and plateau airway pressures. Note the constant inspiratory flow and increase in airway pressure. As seen in all subsequent modes of ventilation, mechanically limited breaths can be triggered by the patient via either a drop in circuit pressure (pressure-triggered) or by a decrease in continuous circuit flow (flow-triggered).

fixed inspiratory flow (limit variable) over a set inspiratory time results in the delivery of a constant tidal volume with changes in compliance and/or resistance reflected in changes in the peak airway pressure generated during the positive pressure breath. Each time the patient initiates a spontaneous breath, the full set volume is delivered. This mode is designed for patients with blunted ventilatory drive secondary to sedation/anesthesia, neuromuscular blockade, drug overdose, nervous system injury, or deliberate mechanical hyperventilation. A back-up rate is set so that if the patient does not initiate an adequate number of breaths per minute, the ventilator will deliver an adequate minute ventilation.

Pressure-Controlled Ventilation

Pressure-controlled ventilation (PCV) delivers positive pressure up to a preset limit above PEEP for a preselected inspiratory time (Fig. 9). The inspiratory flow depends

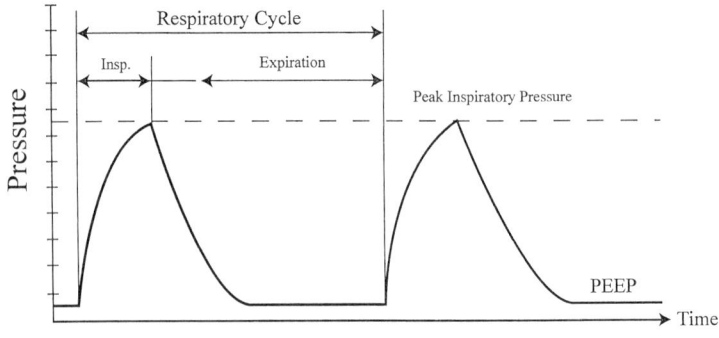

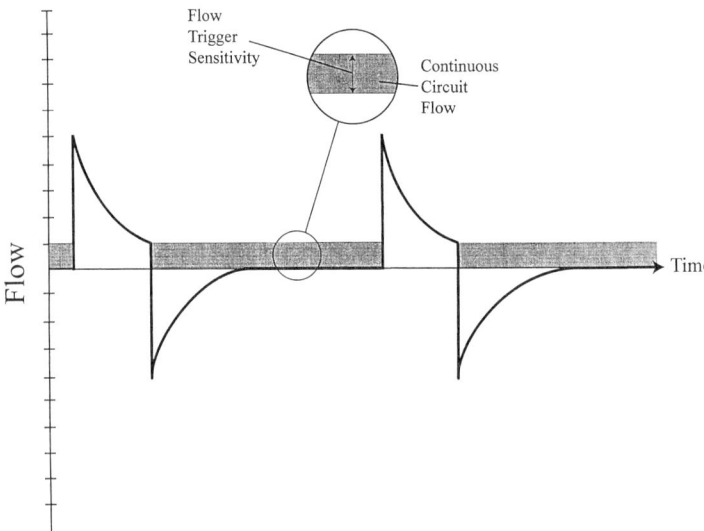

Figure 9. Pressure-time and flow-time diagrams during pressure-limited, time-cycled, pressure-controlled ventilation. Note the decelerating inspiratory flow and exponential increase in airway pressure up to the set peak inspiratory pressure.

on the airway pressure and respiratory system compliance, achieving high levels initially and decelerating toward zero near the end of inspiration. Because inspiratory pressure is the limiting variable, changes in respiratory system mechanics (ie, compliance and/or resistance) will result in changes in the delivered tidal volume and minute ventilation. With most ventilators, PCV is pressure-limited and time-cycled, so that when the preset level of pressure is achieved, it is held until a preset time is achieved, at which time exhalation begins. Like VCV, PCV is an assist control mode that is pressure-limited.

Each time the patient initiates a breath, the breath is assisted with the entire set pressure. A back-up rate is set so that a minimum minute ventilation is provided even if the patient does not initiate any respiratory effort. PCV is designed for patients with suppressed ventilatory drive secondary to sedation/anesthesia, neuromuscular blockade, drug overdose, nervous system injury, or for deliberate mechanical hyperventilation. Pressure-limited ventilation may be particularly beneficial in patients with decreased compliance related to high airway resistance or alveolar space disease such as pneumonia or ARDS. In these situations, pressure-limited ventilation may result in the provision of adequate tidal breaths while limiting the peak inspiratory pressure (see below).

Pressure-Regulated Volume-Controlled

Pressure-regulated volume-controlled (PRVC) is a new mode of ventilation, available on the newest generation of mechanical ventilators (eg, the Servo 300 [Siemens, Inc., Stockholm, Sweden]), that combines many of the features of both volume- and pressure-limited ventilation. This mode uses a decelerating inspiratory flow waveform to deliver a set tidal volume over a selected inspiratory time and frequency in a pressure-limited manner (Fig. 10). The ventilator monitors respiratory system compliance and resistance and uses a predetermined algorithm to deliver the preset tidal volume. The ventilator regulates the inspiratory pressure up or down by as much as 3 cm H_2O from the previous breath, to deliver the selected tidal volume. Thus, the ventilator is continuously

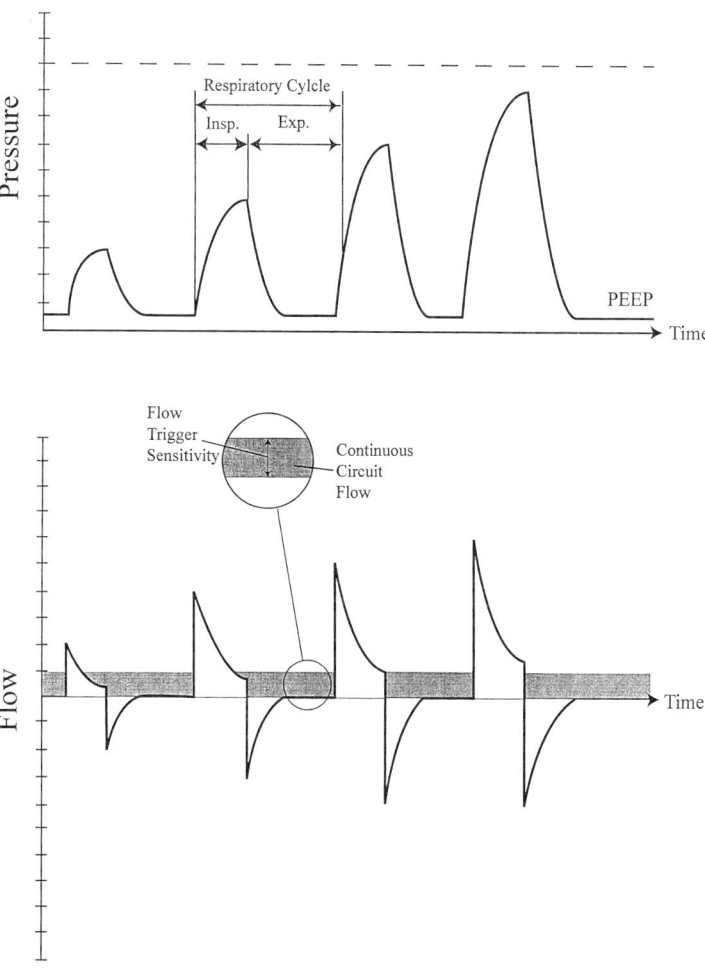

Figure 10. Pressure-time and flow-time diagrams during pressure-limited, time-cycled, pressure-regulated, volume-controlled ventilation. Note the decelerating inspiratory flow and exponential increase in airway pressure up to the set peak inspiratory pressure. The peak airway pressure is regulated up or down by as much as 3 cm H_2O each breath to deliver the desired tidal volume based on the volume-pressure relationship of the previous breath.

adapting the inspiratory pressure to changes in the volume/pressure relationship of the patient's respiratory system. As with both of the previous controlled modes of ventilation, with PRVC each of the patient's inspiratory efforts is sensed and responded to (assisted).

Intermittent Mandatory Ventilation

Intermittent mandatory ventilation (IMV) was introduced into clinical practice 25 years ago as a means for weaning patients from mechanical ventilation by allowing spontaneous, unsupported ventilation between mandatory mechanical breaths.[12] Theoretically, the gradual reduction in mechanical breaths and the concomitant increase in spontaneous breaths would allow a smooth transition from assisted to independent ventilation. Delivery of the mechanical breaths can be triggered at a predetermined time interval (asynchronous IMV) or in response to a patient's spontaneous inspiratory efforts (synchronized IMV or SIMV). In addition, as with assist control modes (PCV or VCV), either inspiratory volume (Fig. 11) or pressure (Fig. 12) can limit the mechanical breaths. For all practi-

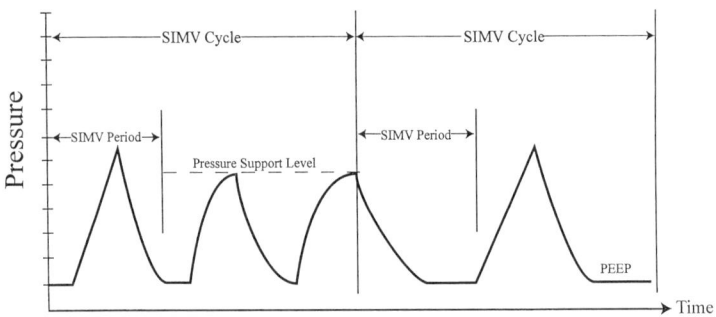

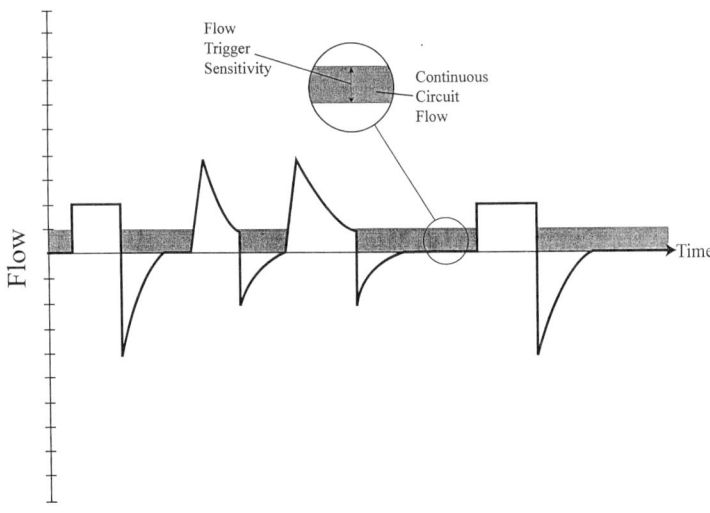

Figure 11. Pressure-time and flow-time diagrams during flow-limited, time-cycled, volume-controlled, synchronized intermittent mandatory ventilation (SIMV). Note the constant inspiratory flow and increase in airway pressure during the mandatory breaths. This diagram also shows pressure-limited, flow-cycled pressure-support ventilation breaths between the mandatory breaths. The mandatory breaths will be either the first triggered breath in each SIMV period or at the end of an SIMV period in which no spontaneously efforts triggered the ventilator.

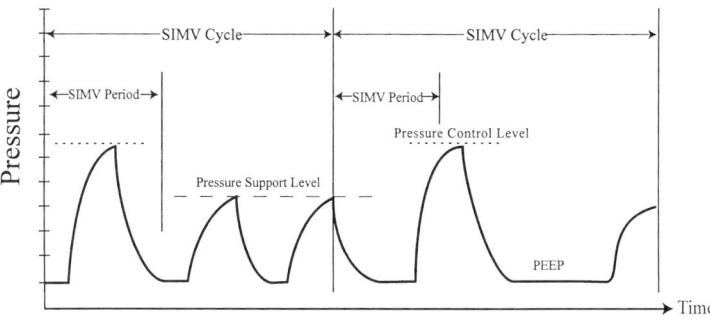

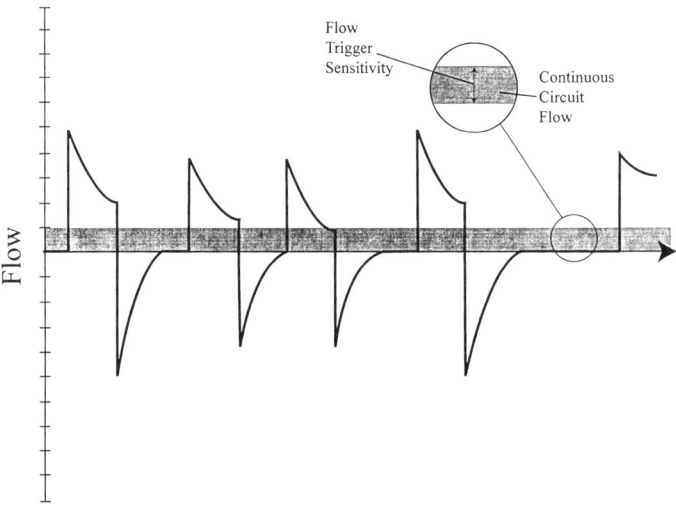

Figure 12. Pressure-time and flow-time diagrams during pressure-limited, time-cycled, pressure-controlled synchronized intermittent mandatory ventilation (SIMV). Note the decelerating inspiratory flow and exponential increase in airway pressure up to the set peak inspiratory pressure for the mandatory breaths. As in the previous diagram, pressure-limited, flow-cycled pressure-support ventilation breaths are seen between the mandatory breaths. The mandatory breaths will be either the first triggered breath in each SIMV period or at the end of an SIMV period in which no spontaneously efforts triggered the ventilator.

cal purposes, SIMV has become the standard mode of mechanical ventilation in most neonatal and pediatric centers worldwide. Despite the widespread use of SIMV, clear demonstration of the benefits of this mode of ventilation is lacking.

Supported Ventilation

Supported ventilation is defined as a breath that is triggered by the patient, limited by the ventilator (volume or pressure), and cycled by the patient. Ventilation is spontaneous in nature because the patient determines the ventilatory pattern (frequency, inspiratory, and expiratory times) by initiating and terminating each breath. Therefore, supported ventilation is only used in patients with intact ventilatory drives. With this form of ventilation, the patient provides the work to trigger the breath and then interacts with the ventilator to perform a variable amount of the remaining work with each breath.

PSV is a mode of ventilation in which the patient triggers the ventilator to deliver a flow of gas sufficient to meet inspiratory needs to a preset pressure level. The breath is terminated when inspiratory flow decreases to a percentage of its initial peak value, rather than by volume, pressure, or time. The exhalation valve closes to pressurize the circuit to the predetermined expiratory limit. Therefore, the patient retains control of the cycle length and flow characteristics while the patient's inspiratory efforts, the preset pressure limit, and respiratory system impedance determine the tidal volume (Fig. 13). PSV has been used to compensate for the inspiratory work of the endotracheal tube impedance and inspiratory demand valves. Inspiratory flow characteristics can significantly alter the efficiency of inspiration.[13,14] PSV has also been shown to abolish diaphragmatic fatigue in patients who failed to wean from conventional ventilation, possibly due to changes in the pressure-volume characteristics and enhanced endurance training of the diaphragm.[15-17]

Two different methods of weaning patients from mechanical ventilation by use of PSV have been advocated. One approach

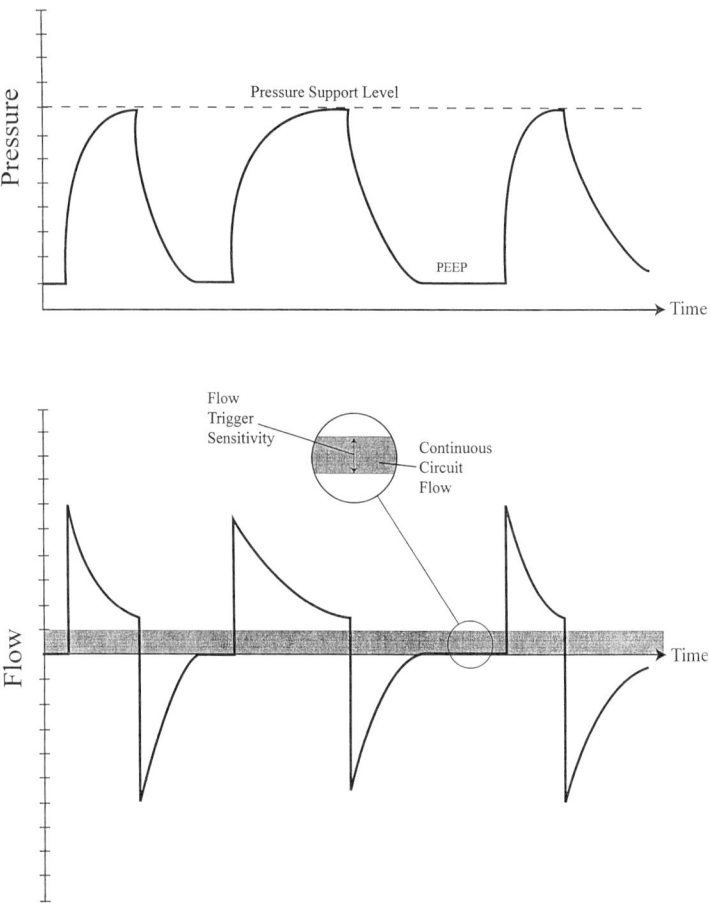

Figure 13. Pressure-time and flow-time diagrams during pressure-limited, flow-cycled pressure-support ventilation (PSV). Note that each breath is triggered (either flow- or pressure-triggered), terminated (flow-cycled) by the patient, and limited to a set pressure level. Thus, the patient determines the respiratory frequency as well as the inspiratory and expiratory times. No default mode of ventilation is available if the patient becomes apneic.

involves setting the pressure limit high enough to achieve delivery of the typical mechanical tidal volume (8 to 10 mL/kg) with no back-up SIMV rate and then gradually decreasing the pressure down to the minimum value needed to overcome the imposed work of the endotracheal tube and ventilator circuit before extubating. The second method involves the combined use of SIMV and PSV in which the pressure limit during PSV breaths is set to minimize the imposed work of the endotracheal tube and circuit only. The SIMV rate is gradually decreased until only PSV breaths are used, at which time the endotracheal tube is removed. Controlled studies have suggested that PSV weaning is more effective than SIMV weaning in adult patients who are difficult to liberate from mechanical ventilation.[18,19] Similar data in the pediatric population are not available.

Volume-support ventilation (VSV) is a new mode of ventilation in which supported breaths are volume-limited while using a decelerating inspiratory flow and flow-cycled mode with a conditional "if, then" variable (Fig. 14). With this mode of ventilation, the pressure assist is regulated

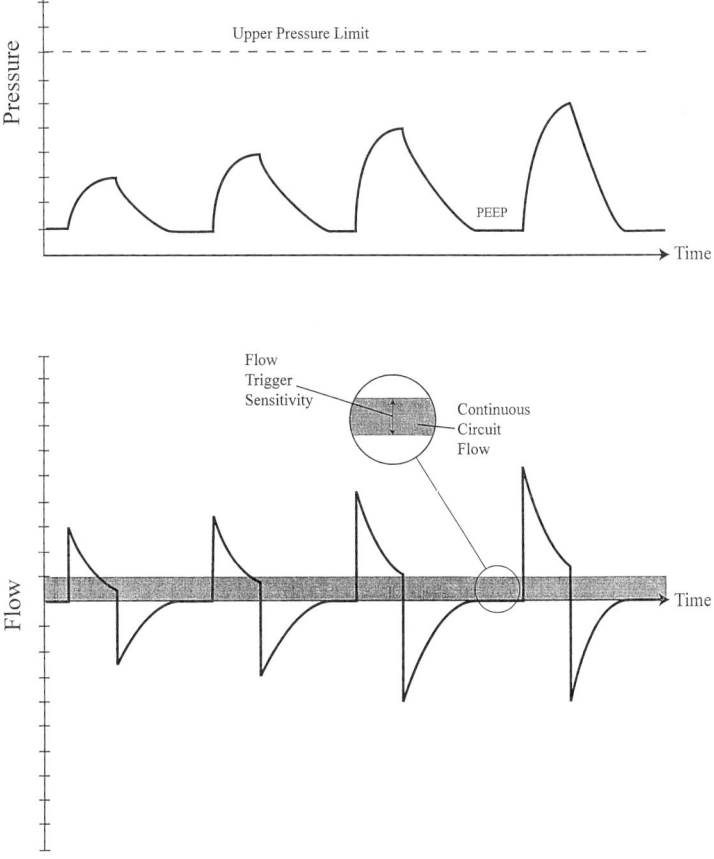

Figure 14. Pressure-time and flow-time diagrams during pressure-limited, flow-cycled, volume-support ventilation (VSV). Note the decelerating inspiratory flow and exponential increase in airway pressure up to the set peak inspiratory pressure. The peak airway pressure is regulated up or down by as much as 3 cm H_2O each breath, to deliver the desired tidal volume based on the volume-pressure relationship of the previous breath. When breathing frequency drops below the apneic threshold, the ventilator will automatically switch to pressure-regulated volume-controlled (PRVC).

to deliver the preset volume, provided a maximum pressure limit is not exceeded, with each supported breath. This mode has all of the theoretical benefits of PSV (the patient controls the inspiratory flow, time, and frequency) with the unique capability of providing a guaranteed minimum minute volume. Unlike PSV, this mode also can provide back-up mandatory breaths should the patient become apneic. Published clinical experience in children and in adults is limited to a single case series demonstrating the potential utility and problems associated with this mode of ventilation.[20]

Spontaneous Ventilation

Spontaneous ventilation is a mode of ventilation in which the patient triggers, limits, and cycles the "breaths" from the ventilator. In this mode (CPAP), the clinician selects a level of positive pressure that is maintained in the ventilator circuit while the patient breathes spontaneously (Fig. 15). Care must be exercised to avoid confusing CPAP and PEEP. This is best accomplished by thinking of CPAP as a mode of ventilation while PEEP represents simply the control of the baseline (expiratory) pressure during mechanical ventilation. In common

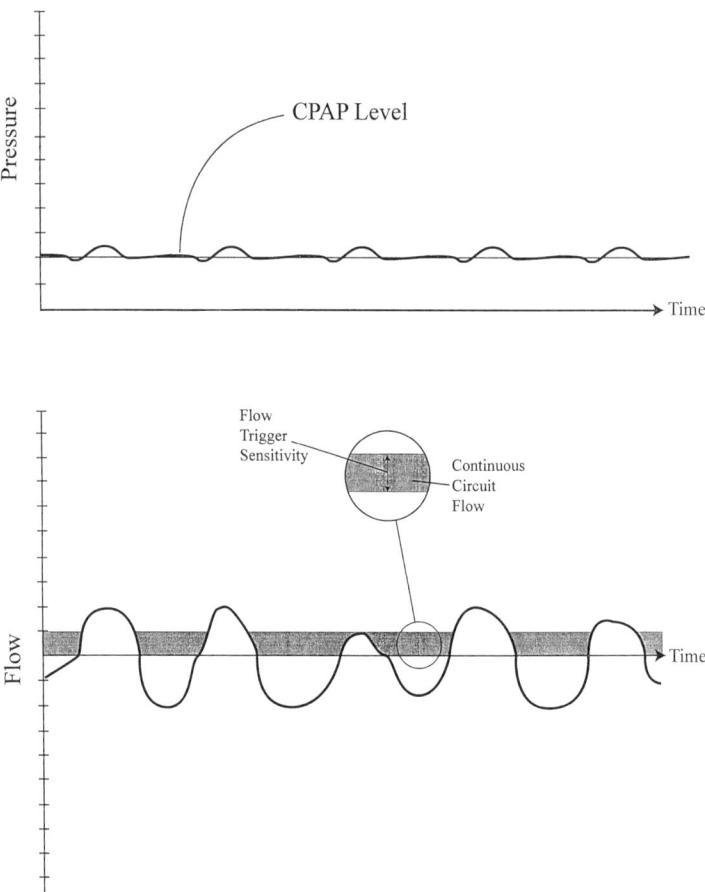

Figure 15. Pressure-time and flow-time diagrams during pressure-limited, flow-cycled, continuous positive airway pressure (CPAP). This mode allows the patient to breathe spontaneously at an elevated positive pressure baseline level while he or she determines the inspiratory flow, tidal volume, respiratory frequency, inspiratory time and expiratory time.

clinical practice, CPAP is used to describe the baseline pressure from which spontaneous or supported ventilation is initiated, while PEEP is used to describe the baseline pressure during assisted or controlled ventilation. Introduced in clinical practice for the management of acute respiratory failure in adults with ARDS[21] and in neonates with IRDS,[22] CPAP or PEEP has become a mainstay of modern mechanical ventilation as a means to increase ELV and improve the pressure-volume relationship of the lung (Fig. 4). Technically, CPAP or PEEP is provided by expiratory valves that function as either threshold resistors that allow unimpeded expiration until the preset end-expiratory pressure limit is reached or as expiratory flow resistors that impede flow throughout expiration until the initiation of the next breath, without achieving atmospheric pressure. Flow resistors have several undesirable characteristics (eg, increased mean airway pressure and dead space ventilation with potential for circulatory compromise) that make them less desirable in most clinical settings.[23]

Applications of Mechanical Ventilation

Physicians involved in the ventilatory management of patients with respiratory failure should base their decisions on a thorough understanding of physiologic principles of normal respiratory function, the pathophysiologic alterations induced by the patient's underlying disease process, ventilator technology, and patient-ventilator interactions.

Indications for Mechanical Ventilation

Because the desired endpoints of ventilatory support define the criteria for its use, indications for mechanical ventilatory support vary according to the clinician's goals. The most obvious indication is overt respiratory failure defined as inadequate alveolar ventilation and/or failure of arterial oxygenation (Table 9). However, there are many situations, besides in patients with apparent respiratory failure, in which mechanical ventilatory support may prove beneficial. For example, decreases in lactic acid production and redirection of blood flow from respiratory muscles to vital organs associated with the application of mechanical ventilation have been demonstrated in laboratory models of circulatory shock.[2,24] In addition, withdrawal of mechanical ventilatory support in newborn animals with acute respiratory failure has been associated with marked alterations in cardiac output attributable to the increase in the work of breathing.[25] Under these circumstances, standard criteria for initiation of mechanical support based on blood gas indices of gas exchange may be lacking. This is particularly true in the actively growing infant and child, who must channel considerable metabolic expenditures toward growth and development. Regardless of the possible indications, it is necessary to consider the clinical assessment of respiratory fatigue and failure, the anticipated course of the disease process at hand,

Table 9

Indications for Initiating Positive Pressure Mechanical Ventilation

Absolute
  Inadequate arterial oxygenation
    Cyanosis with $FiO_2 > 0.6$
    $PaO_2/FiO_2 < 200$
    Alveolar to arterial oxygen gradient
      $(AaDO_2) > 300$ mm Hg with $FiO_2 = 1.0$
    Intrapulmonary shunt $(Q_S/Q_T) > 15\%$
  Insufficient alveolar ventilation
    Respiratory failure
      apnea
      $PaCO_2 > 60$ mm Hg (in the absence of chronic hypercapnia)
    Impending hypoventilation/respiratory failure
      rising $PaCO_2$
      vital capacity < 15 mL/kg
      dead space/tidal volume $(V_D/V_T) > 0.6$
Relative
  Control of ventilatory pattern and or function
    pulmonary hypertension
    circulatory insufficiency
  Decrease metabolic cost of breathing
    chronic respiratory failure
    circulatory insufficiency

and its expected response to conservative interventions, before deciding to proceed with mechanical ventilation.

When the decision has been made to initiate mechanical ventilation, two further basic decisions must be made regarding the mode of ventilation (SIMV or assist control) and the limit variable, or the variable that is not exceeded during inspiration and that controls the tidal breath (pressure or volume). Oxygenation is controlled by manipulation of the inspired oxygen concentration and the mean airway pressure, the latter being controlled by the limit variable, the inspiratory time, and PEEP. Carbon dioxide removal is regulated by controlling minute ventilation, respiratory rate multiplied by tidal breath.

Once a decision has been made to initiate mechanical ventilatory support, a systematic approach to its application based on the patient's respiratory physiology is recommended. This should take into account both the developmental aspects (Table 10) and disease-associated changes in respiratory physiology (Table 11). In the absence of intrinsic lung disease (alterations in resistance or compliance), most patients do well with volume-limited ventilation. In this setting, the peak airway pressures required to deliver the tidal volume of 8 to 12 mL/kg are generally 18 to 22 cm H_2O. When initiating volume-limited ventilation, the peak airway pressure should be monitored. High pressures require immediate investigation including a check for kinking of the circuit or endotracheal tube, obstruction to the endotracheal tube or major airways by mucus, bronchospasm, increasing alveolar space disease (pneumonia or ARDS), or external

Table 10

Application of Normal Developmental Respiratory Physiology During Mechanical Ventilation

Parameter	Infant	Child	Adolescent
Inspired O_2 concentration (FiO_2)	<0.6	<0.6	<0.6
Tidal volume (mL/kg)	10	10	10
Peak inspiratory pressure (cm H_2O)	20	20	20
Positive end-expiratory pressure (cm H_2O)	3–5	2–4	0–3
Ventilator rate (breaths/minute)	30–40	20–30	12–20
Inspiratory time (seconds)	0.4–0.6	0.6–1.0	1.0–1.5

Table 11

Application of Altered (Disease-Related) Respiratory Physiology During Mechanical Ventilation*

Parameter	Normal Child	Restrictive Disease	Obstructive Disease
Inspired O_2 concentration (FiO_2)	<0.6	<0.6	<0.6
Tidal volume (mL/kg)	10	6–8	10
Peak inspiratory pressure (cm H_2O)[†]	20	<35–40	<35–40
Positive end-expiratory pressure (cm H_2O)	2–4	10–15[‡]	0–2[§]
Ventilator rate (breaths/minute)	20–30	30–40	15–20
Inspiratory time (seconds)	0.6–1.0	0.6–1.0	0.6–1.0

*For this example, a child is used for normal as well as restrictive and obstructive disease states.
[†]Plateau airway pressures should be used for volume-limited modes of ventilation.
[‡]PEEP may be higher or lower based on closing pressure determination during a PEEP trial.
[§]PEEP may need to be set equal to intrinsic or autoPEEP if pressure-trigger assisted/supported ventilation is used.
PEEP = positive end-expiratory pressure.

factors impeding respiratory excursion (pneumothorax, restrictive diseases of the thorax, abdominal distention). Lengthening the inspiratory time may allow the delivery of the tidal volume while lowering the peak airway pressure to an acceptable value. However, the longer inspiratory times (approaching inspiratory:expiratory (I:E) ratios of 1:2 or 1:1 with inspiratory times of greater than 0.5 to 0.7 seconds) may be relatively uncomfortable for the patient because the normal I:E ratio is 1:3 or 1:4. The latter is important, because with SIMV or assist control modes (assisted breaths), the ventilator determines the inspiratory time. If the peak airway pressure is unacceptably high or if the patient has underlying intrinsic lung disease with increases in resistance or decreases in compliance, the pressure-limited mode may be chosen. The latter may also be more practical in neonates, in whom the delivery of smaller tidal volumes may be somewhat inaccurate based on the working parameters of the ventilator. A discrepancy of 10 to 20 mL in the delivered tidal volume is not an issue when the set tidal volume is 500 mL, but can be a significant issue when the set tidal volume is 30 to 40 mL.

The same approach is used when initiating pressure-limited ventilation, except the tidal breath is controlled by the change in pressure from PEEP (the ΔP). The latter can be set depending on the ventilator by adjusting the PEEP and the peak inflating pressure (PIP) or by adjusting the pressure above PEEP. Under the former circumstances, it should be recognized that adjusting the PEEP will affect the pressure above PEEP and, hence, the tidal breath. The pressure above PEEP is adjusted to deliver the desired exhaled tidal volume. One advantage of pressure-limited ventilation is that a decelerating flow pattern is used to deliver the tidal breath. The decelerating flow pattern may help in the recruitment of alveoli with long time constants (high resistance and low compliance) and, thereby over time, improve compliance. As with volume-limited ventilation, an inspiratory time is set. Since most ventilators end the inspiratory cycle by a time signal, increasing the inspiratory time will increase the mean airway pressure and, hence, the exhaled tidal volume. During pressure-limited ventilation, the exhaled tidal volume should be monitored. A decrease in the exhaled tidal volume should prompt a thorough investigation into its cause that includes the same steps outlined above for investigating an increase in peak airway pressure during volume-limited ventilation.

Subtleties in the adjustment of inspiratory time vary from ventilator to ventilator. The inspiratory time may be set as a fixed time, by adjusting the inspiratory flow rate, as an I:E ratio, or as a percentage of the respiratory cycle. In the latter two cases, adjusting the rate will affect the actual inspiratory time in seconds. For example, if the respiratory rate is set at 15 breaths per minute with an inspiratory time of 25%, this results in an inspiratory time of 1 second. Changing the rate to 20 breaths per minute with an inspiratory time of 25% now results in an inspiratory time of 0.75 seconds. Such changes can result in changes in the peak airway pressure during volume-limited ventilation or in the tidal volume during pressure-limited ventilation.

Mechanical ventilation in patients with normal respiratory mechanics should attempt, when possible, to duplicate the normal physiologic state. Physiologic standards based on the developmental changes in respiratory mechanics should be employed (Table 10). This applies particularly to respiratory frequency as well as inspiratory and expiratory times. Selection of inspiratory mechanical tidal volumes must make allowances for: 1) compressible volume of the ventilator circuit and losses around uncuffed endotracheal tubes in younger patients; 2) associated increases in physiologic dead space as a result of the application of positive pressure; and 3) increased carbon dioxide production that may accompany acute respiratory failure. Consequently, the preset tidal volume (8 to 12 mL/kg) required for normal carbon dioxide clearance is often greater than that found during spontaneous breathing (4 to 6 mL/kg). As a first approximation, normal levels of $PaCO_2$ are generally achieved with preset, inspiratory tidal volumes of 8 to 12 mL/kg. Although absolute compliance and resistance vary greatly from the newborn to the adult, when they are indexed (ie, divided by lung volume, body height or weight) there is very little change with growth. Thus, delivery of physiologic tidal volumes will be associated with the generation of similar airway pressures (approximately 20 cm H_2O) across all ages in patients without pathologic conditions known to alter the compliance or resistance of the respiratory system. This constant relationship makes selection of peak airway pressure in pressure-limited modes of ventilation relatively straightforward without the need to alter pressure based on the patient's age and weight. In patients who do not have pathologic conditions that lead to alterations in respiratory resistance or compliance, adequate tidal volumes are generally provided with peak airway pressures of 18 to 22 cm H_2O.

The relatively compliant chest wall, the decreased elastic content of neonatal lungs, and the increased airway resistance all significantly alter the normal relationship between FRC, ELV, and closing volume (CV). In normal adults, FRC (the volume at which lung recoil inward is balanced by chest wall recoil outward) and ELV (the volume at which inspiration begins) are equal and exceed CV (the volume at which airway closure/atelectasis in the lungs occurs). Thus, healthy adolescents and adults require little or no PEEP to prevent atelectasis and its associated hypoxemia from occurring. In contrast, newborns with their highly compliant chest wall, will have an FRC that approaches and, in some cases, may be less than CV under passive (ie, sedated and/or paralyzed) conditions, thereby leading to the concept of physiologic PEEP (typically 3 to 5 cm H_2O) to avoid ventilation-perfusion inequalities. This mechanical inefficiency is avoided under dynamic (spontaneously breathing) conditions because ELV is greater than FRC secondary to: 1) rapid respiratory rate with short expiratory times (ie, there is insufficient time for expiratory flows to reach zero; therefore, intrinsic or auto PEEP is present); 2) laryngeal muscle contraction during expiration impedes expiratory airflow (this is absent when patients have endotracheal tubes in place); and 3) increased intercostal muscle tone which stabilizes the chest wall and increases elastic recoil outward. Thus, sedated infants will routinely require delivery of physiologic levels of PEEP to overcome the loss of these dynamic compensatory mechanisms. Higher levels of PEEP may be required in patients with alveolar space disease, increased abdominal distention, and other pathologic conditions that increase closing capacity and decrease FRC. Several different methods of determining the optimal PEEP have been suggested, including: 1) chest x-ray examination with an evaluation of the expansion of the lung fields; 2) increasing the PEEP to allow for an FiO_2 of less than 0.6; 3) performance of pressure-volume curves with increasing tidal breaths; and 4) measurement of shunt fraction using flow-directed pulmonary artery catheters.

Postoperative Patients

Although the vast majority of postoperative patients will not require mechanical ventilation, a small subset of postsurgical patients will require mechanical support: 1) secondary to residual anesthetics and/or neuromuscular blocking agents; 2) secondary to maintenance of airway patency (craniofacial or tracheal reconstructive surgery); 3) for therapeutic hyperventilation (intracranial or pulmonary hypertension); 4) due to underlying cardiorespiratory instability; or 5) for the provision of adequate pulmonary toilet. In the absence of significant pulmonary pathology, ventilatory needs are usually easily met. In this group, maintenance of ventilation and oxygenation can be provided by SIMV, volume-limited ventilation providing physiologic tidal volumes (8 to 12 mL/kg) at physiologic respiratory rates based on the patient's age, with minimal amounts of supplemental oxygen and small amounts of pressure support to overcome the work of breathing imposed by the ventilator and endotracheal tube. However, many patients who receive mechanical ventilation postoperatively do so because of actual or suspected alterations in respiratory mechanics. Therefore, the method and means of mechanical support should be adjusted based on these variations in respiratory mechanics as outlined in the section that follows.

Respiratory Pump Failure

Patients with respiratory pump failure generally fall into one of two categories: those with acute pump failure (eg, spinal cord trauma, Guillain-Barré syndrome, botulism, etc.) or those with chronic pump failure (eg, muscular dystrophies, myasthenia gravis, polio, etc.). These patients typically have normal ventilatory drives and pulmonary mechanics, but suffer from respiratory muscle weakness that promotes the development of atelectasis and pneumonia. The maintenance of a patent airway and normal lung volume are of primary importance for this population of patients.

Circulatory Pump Failure

The provision of airway patency and mechanical support of respiration is one of the primary therapeutic interventions for circulatory compromise regardless of its etiology. Although the increase in intrathoracic pressure during positive pressure mechanical ventilation has been commonly associated with a decrease in venous return and cardiac output in the normal state, the large negative intrathoracic pressures seen in patients with elevated respiratory work due to either compensatory hyperventilation for metabolic acid production or impaired pulmonary mechanics, leads to increased left ventricular transmural pressure, wall stress, and afterload with subsequent deleterious effects on myocardial function.[26,27] Reduction in the metabolic expenditures and the decreased requirements for blood flow to the respiratory muscles with the initiation of mechanical ventilation may help abate further ischemic injury to vital organs.[2] The decision to institute mechanical respiratory support must be tempered by the potential hemodynamic consequences associated with many of the medications used to facilitate airway management (see also chapter 1 for a full discussion of airway management and endotracheal intubation) and the physiologic alterations seen when transforming from a largely negative to a positive intrathoracic pressure environment.

Neurologic Injury

The maintenance of a patent airway and adequate minute ventilation continues to be one of the mainstays of therapy for acute neurologic injury. Hypercapnia and hypoxia are potent stimuli for cerebral vasodilation; consequently, one of the most effective means of acutely decreasing intracranial hypertension is to artificially lower $PaCO_2$ via hyperventilation. Short-term hyperventilation to decrease intracranial hypertension and allow time for other therapeutic measures (eg, diuretics, sedatives, barbiturates) to take effect is accepted practice; however, long-term hyperventilation in head-injured patients who do not have intracranial hypertension has been shown to be detrimental to ultimate neurologic outcome.[28] Thus, to prevent acute intracranial hypertension, stable head-injured patients should receive mechanical ventilation sufficient to achieve normocapnia, while hypoxemia should be prevented and care exercised to gradually return to a normocapnic state.

Abnormal Respiratory Mechanics and Physiology

The vast majority of children who require mechanical ventilation do so because of alterations in their respiratory mechanics that lead to clinically significant changes in PaO_2 and $PaCO_2$. Mechanical ventilation should be tailored to compensate for or correct the underlying pulmonary pathophysiology. The changes in respiratory mechanics can be roughly divided into two broad categories: 1) restrictive disease involving alveoli (alveolar space disease), and 2) obstructive disease involving the airways. Historically, lung disease has been thought of as relatively homogeneous (uniform); however, over the last decade it has become apparent that in most instances the lung disease is heterogeneous (regional) in nature with areas of abnormal airways and/or alveoli intermixed with areas of relatively normal airway and alveolar function. Despite this revelation, it is useful from a clinical perspective to categorize the disease process based on the predominate pathophysiology to guide delivery of mechanical ventilation.

Restrictive pulmonary disease is characterized by a decrease in lung volume and compliance, with a proportionate reduction in airflow. This constellation of changes results in an increase in the respiratory time constant, lower FRC/ELV relative to CV, increased V/Q mismatch with intrapulmonary shunting, and elevated work of breathing. These changes ultimately lead to the hallmark clinical finding for this category of diseases, namely hypoxemia. The etiology of hypoxemia can be divided into five broad categories: 1) a low FiO_2; 2) hypoventilation, characterized by associated hypercarbia; 3) true shunt as seen in patients with cyanotic cardiac lesions; 4) ventilation-perfusion mismatch or intrapulmonary shunt whereby some of the alveoli are adequately perfused and yet inadequately ventilated due to the presence of pathologic processes in the alveoli; and 5) diffusion abnormalities.

Restrictive diseases may be due to abnormalities in either thoracic (obesity, abdominal distention, scoliosis) or lung (alveolar filling or fibrosis) mechanics. For discussion purposes, ARDS will be used as the model for this category of diseases (see also chapter 6 for a full discussion of the etiology, pathogenesis, and treatment of patients with ARDS). The traditional approach to mechanical ventilation of patients with ARDS throughout the 1970s and 1980s was to fully compensate for abnormalities in lung function (ie, to normalize arterial blood gas values) without toxic inspired oxygen concentrations, barotrauma, or cardiovascular compromise. This was achieved principally through the recruitment of collapsed alveoli and improvement in oxygenation with the use of increased P_{aw}. The latter was achieved primarily through the use of tidal volumes of 10 to 12 mL/kg, resulting in high peak airway pressures. Under passive conditions, P_{aw} has been shown to correlate closely with forces that hold lungs distended, and is associated with the level of oxygenation.[4,29] In clinical practice, P_{aw} can be manipulated through changes in inspiratory pressure. Inspiratory pressure can be altered by changing the pressure in pressure-limited modes, the volume in the volume-limited modes, expiratory pressure (CPAP or PEEP), inspiratory time, and inspiratory flow waveform. With restrictive lung disease, there is a decrease in lung volumes to the lower, flat portion of the pressure-volume curve that results in the need to use large pressures to maintain the same tidal volumes.

In most instances, changing the PEEP, thereby moving to the steep portion of the pressure-volume curve and restoring normal compliance of the respiratory system, is the first method used for regulating P_{aw} in patients with restrictive disease. The application of PEEP prevents airway pressure from dropping below critical closing pressure (maintaining airway patency and alveolar volume throughout the ventilatory cycle), redistributes pulmonary edema fluid from alveoli to the interstitium, maintains alveolar surfactant activity, and improves ventilation to low V/Q lung units.[30,31] The latter effects result in an improvement in respiratory compliance. Excessive levels of PEEP can be counterproductive in patients with ARDS because they increase dead space ventilation, depress cardiovascular function, and decrease alveolar compliance via excessive distention. Various methods have been described to physiologically define "optimal PEEP." Examples include PEEP titrated to: maximal lung compliance, maximal oxygen delivery, and more recently, changes in respiratory mechanics as determined by the static pressure-volume curve of the respiratory system.[32,33] These methods are limited in the clinical setting due to their requirement of invasive monitoring (pulmonary artery catheter) or complicated respiratory mechanics measurements (static pressure-volume curve generation). For these reasons, a systematic evaluation of respiratory mechanics based on easily obtained clinical markers in an organized "PEEP trial" is recommended. During a PEEP trial, PEEP is incrementally altered while monitoring oxygenation (PaO_2, pulse oximetry [SpO_2], PaO_2/FiO_2, alveolar to arterial oxygen gradient [$AaDO_2$], and/or oxygenation index [OI = $FiO_2 \times P_{aw} \times 100/PaO_2$]), ventilation ($PaCO_2$, $PaCO_2$ −

$P_{et}CO_2$, V_D/V_T), compliance ($C_{dynamic}$ = VT/PIP − PEEP, C_{static} = VT/$P_{plateau}$ − PEEP), and cardiovascular function (perfusion, urine output, and occasionally cardiac index, oxygen delivery, and oxygen consumption) while keeping all ventilator and patient variables constant (Table 12). Historically, most clinicians have instituted PEEP trials at a low level of PEEP and increased in 2- to 5-cm H_2O increments approximately every 15 minutes; however, there are several reasons to suggest that the opposite approach (starting with a high level of PEEP and slowly decreasing it) may be preferable. First, injured lungs with decreased compliance will much more rapidly collapse with withdrawal of positive pressure than they will be recruited with application of increased levels of positive pressure. Hence, a PEEP trial with decreasing levels of PEEP can be completed much more rapidly and with a much greater likelihood of achieving steady state conditions than would an escalating PEEP trial. Second, a decreasing (derecruitment) PEEP trial defines the desired physiologic variable (ie, approximate critical closing pressure) versus an escalating (recruitment) PEEP trial that determines the critical opening pressure. Thus, the latter may lead to the selection of a PEEP slightly higher than actually necessary to achieve the goal of maintaining airway pressure slightly above critical closing pressure.

Recent insight regarding the role of alveolar overdistention in the pathogenesis of ARDS, defined by many as volutrauma, has led to a significant change in the approach to mechanical ventilation for the population of patients with this disorder.[34] Multiple experimental models have demonstrated that alveolar overdistention with high airway pressures produces insidious physiologic and morphologic injury in the previously healthy lungs, that ultimately leads to a clinical picture consistent with ARDS with progressive multiorgan injury and death.[34,35] To avoid this complication, the clinician uses either smaller V_T (in volume-limited modes of ventilation) or lower peak airway pressures (in pressure-limited modes of ventilation). Unfortunately, these are very little data to help the bedside clinician determine what is a safe V_T or peak airway pressure in patients with lung injury. One method suggests that alveolar pressure in excess of those obtained at total lung capacity ($P_{plateau}$ ≥35 to 40 cm H_2O) represents a reasonable upper limit. Regardless of the limit set, this scheme of limiting inspiratory pressure/volume lowers minute and alveolar ventilation, thereby resulting in an increase in $PaCO_2$. The term "permissive hypercapnia" has been coined to describe this overall strategy of small tidal ventilation with adequate P_{aw} to achieve satisfactory oxygenation without toxic inspired oxygen concentrations while allowing $PaCO_2$ to rise if necessary.[29,35,36] The application of permissive hypercapnia is not without adverse physiologic effects. Although generally well tolerated, these may include: 1) intracellular

Table 12

Hypothetical PEEP Trial During Pressure-Limited Mechanical Ventilation

PEEP (cm H_2O)	PIP (cm H_2O)	V_T (mL/kg)	C_{dyn} (mL/cm H_2O)	$PaCO_2$ (mm Hg)	PaO_2 (mm Hg)	SaO_2 (%)	CI (L/min/m²)	DO_2 (mL/min/m²)
24	44	8.0	0.40	52	280	1.0	3.5	742
20	40	8.8	0.44	45	260	1.0	3.7	784
16	36	9.0	0.45	44	240	1.0	3.8	802
12	32	8.5	0.43	45	120	0.99	3.9	803
8	28	8.2	0.41	45	60	0.90	4.0	744
4	24	7.8	0.39	46	50	0.80	4.0	660

PEEP = positive end-expiratory pressure; PIP = peak inspiratory pressure; V_T = exhaled tidal volume; C_{dyn} = dynamic compliance; $PaCO_2$ = partial pressure arterial carbon dioxide; PaO_2 = partial pressure arterial oxygen; SaO_2 = oxygen saturation of arterial hemoglobin; CI = cardiac index; DO_2 = oxygen delivery.

acidosis, which can alter cellular oxidative metabolism, ionic conductance, excitation-contraction coupling, and cell division; 2) increased sympathoadrenergic tone (elevated heart rate, stroke volume, cardiac output, and lower systemic vascular resistance); 3) cerebral vasodilation (intracranial hypertension); and 4) an increased incidence of arrhythmias.[37] Recently, a small prospective, controlled trial in adults and preliminary data from a large pediatric trial have suggested that this lung protective strategy of ventilation is associated with a decrease in the mortality rate of ARDS.[38,39] However, conflicting results from other controlled trials have been seen.[40,41]

Obstructive lung disease is characterized by a reduction in airflow (FEV_1) in excess of the reduction in forced vital capacity (FVC). The predominant change in respiratory mechanics is the increase in airway resistance. As the increase in airway resistance progresses, expiratory air trapping and an increase in residual volume (RV) occurs until the elevation in RV begins to encroach on vital capacity, a process called dynamic hyperinflation. The increase in RV and dynamic hyperinflation results in tidal ventilation occurring on the upper flat portion of the pressure-volume curve of the respiratory system, leading to a decrease in compliance and an increase in the work of breathing. Asthma is used as the prototypical obstructive disease for the purposes of this discussion.

Patients with severe asthma develop acute respiratory failure secondary to bronchoconstriction, airway edema, and mucous production. This triad produces an increase in airway resistance (expiratory > inspiratory) which can ultimately lead to expiratory airflow obstruction and dynamic hyperinflation. These patients will benefit from mechanical ventilatory strategies designed to maximize expiratory time, thereby decreasing ELV, intrinsic PEEP, and the risk of cardiovascular compromise.[42] A higher ELV when using the same tidal volume will produce a higher end-inspiratory lung volume, thus increasing the risk of excessive alveolar volume lung injury (volutrauma).[43] The employment of higher inspiratory flow rates will, in general, minimize ELV, intrinsic PEEP, and dynamic hyperinflation; however, this may be counterbalanced by the effects of turbulence, noncompliant airways, and/or bronchoconstriction, which can cause a flow-dependent increase in inspiratory resistance.[44] This approach will result in higher inspiratory airway pressures and a greater chance of volutrauma. The percentage of central airway pressure that is transmitted to the alveoli (the genuine risk factor for volutrauma) is difficult to determine. End-inspiratory plateau pressures best approximate alveolar pressures and should be used when selecting inspiratory flow rates and tidal volumes during mechanical ventilation. The latter can be estimated by using an end-inspiratory hold during a mechanical breath and allowing the pressure within the respiratory system to equilibrate.

A second method to limit dynamic hyperinflation involves using the lowest minute ventilation to achieve acceptable (not normal) gas exchange. This strategy of deliberate or controlled hypoventilation for patients with status asthmaticus was first described nearly 15 years ago and has become the standard approach for this patient population.[45] To minimize minute ventilation while providing as long an expiratory time as possible, most clinicians will use physiologic tidal volumes delivered at a low frequency. The low minute ventilation and increased dead space ventilation will invariably result in hypercapnia. This approach has been associated with a decrease in morbidity and mortality in children with asthma.[46,47] The method of ventilation is limited by its requirement for large amounts of sedation and sometimes administration of neuromuscular blocking agents, which, in combination with the high dose of corticosteroid, can produce prolonged myopathy.[48] Some investigators suggest that measurement of dynamic hyperinflation, defined as the failure of the lung volume to return to passive FRC prior to the onset of inspiration, may identify patients ventilated for status asthmaticus who are at risk for significant morbidity and/or mortality.[43,49] This risk for morbidity and/or mortality is assessed by using the end-expiratory hold mode on the ventilator and ensuring that the airway pressure returns to near zero. If airway pressure does not reach zero, there is significant air trapping, resulting in the generation of auto-PEEP and the risk of dynamic hyperinflation (Fig. 16). In such patients, alterations in the inspiratory time, inspiratory flow rate, or PEEP may be required to limit the dynamic hyperinflation.

In order to avoid the potential morbidity associated with neuromuscular blocking agent administration and/or hypercapnia, other investigators have advocated the use of supported modes of ventilation for the patient population.[50] Supported modes of ventilation allow the patient to determine the ventilatory pattern (ie, respiratory frequency and inspiratory and expiratory times). In addition, the patient's inspiratory muscles are partially supported to prevent fatigue while active exhalation by the patient permits ventilation on the lower, more compliant portion of the pressure-volume curve of the respiratory system. The initial yet limited clinical experience with this method shows great potential, as it has been associated with dramatic decreases in $PaCO_2$ levels while avoiding the use of neuromuscular blocking agents.[50]

Although rarely encountered, a patient with unilateral lung disease resulting in

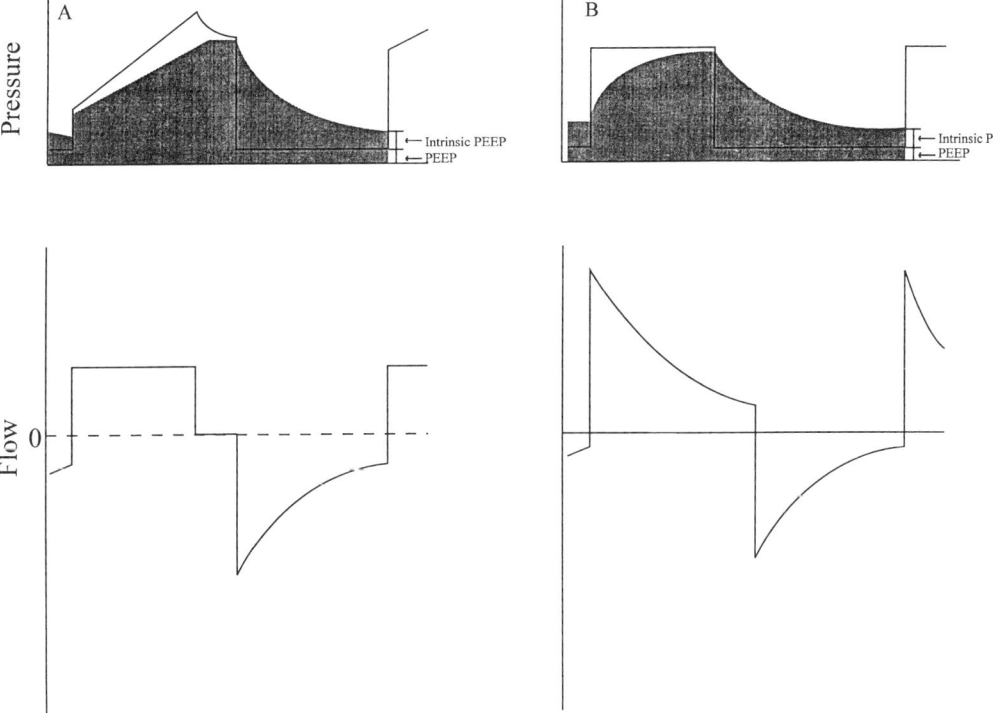

Figure 16. Pressure-time and flow-time diagrams during volume-controlled ventilation (VCV) (A) and pressure-controlled ventilation (PCV) (B). Note in both diagrams the discrepancy between alveolar (shaded) and airway pressures and persistent expiratory flows (auto-PEEP). During flow-limited, time-cycled VCV, there is a constant increase in airway pressure and difference in peak and plateau pressures (reflecting the resistive component of airway pressure). Mean airway pressure during VCV is increased by increased tidal volume, increased end-expiratory pressure, increased inspiratory time, and/or shortened expiratory time by either increasing frequency or decreased inspiratory flow. During pressure-limited, time-cycled PCV, there is a decelerating inspiratory flow that results in a square pressure waveform and both alveolar volume and pressure increase and decrease exponentially. Mean airway pressure during PCV is increased by increased peak and/or end-expiratory pressure, lengthened inspiratory time, or increased respiratory frequency (shortened expiratory time).

respiratory failure and the need for mechanical ventilatory assistance presents the ICU physician with a significant clinical dilemma. In almost every instance, the indication for mechanical ventilation in patients with focal disease is hypoxemia, similar to patients with restrictive lung disease. Unfortunately, measures designed to improve oxygenation in restrictive lung disease (increase mean P_{aw}) are applied uniformly throughout the lungs. This likely will result in excessive distention of the normally compliant areas of the lung, placing them at risk for volutrauma. Therapeutic efforts should be directed toward alterations to improve overall lung function, such as changes in inspiratory flow rates to equalize distribution of ventilation. Should this fail, a trial of ventilation with the normal lung in the dependent (down) position in older patients[51] and the diseased lung in the superior (up) position in infants[52] is indicated. When this is not sufficient, other methods to improve lung function, such as flexible fiber optic bronchoscopy for clearing of airway plugs, intubation with double-lumen endotracheal tubes for independent lung ventilation, or other experimental methods (high-frequency ventilation, extracorporeal life support) can be tried.

Controversies of Mechanical Ventilation

Pressure-Limited versus Volume-Limited Ventilation

While the provision of mechanical ventilatory support for patients with little or no alteration in respiratory mechanics is relatively straightforward, the best means of mechanical assistance in situations of severe changes in pulmonary function remains an area of controversy for clinicians. One of these controversial areas is the relative merits and risks of volume-limited versus pressure-limited ventilation (Table 13). During flow-limited, volume-cycled ventilation, the inspiratory flow and tidal volume (and thus the minute ventilation) are set by the clinician (Fig. 16, part A). This method of

Table 13

Comparison of Volume-Limited and Pressure-Limited Mechanical Ventilation

Volume-Limited	Pressure-Limited
Advantages	
Guaranteed tidal volume/minute ventilation	Precise control of end-inspiratory alveolar pressure
Precise control of inspiratory flow pattern	Decelerating inspiratory flow pattern reported to:
Easy detection of changed respiratory impedance	improve distribution of ventilation
Clinician familiarity	decrease dead space ventilation
	increase mean airway pressure
	decrease peak inspiratory pressure
	more easily match patient inspiratory demands
Disadvantages	
Peak airway/alveolar pressure/volume vary	Variable tidal volume/minute ventilation
Inspiratory flow may not match patient needs	Changes in respiratory impedance not easily detected
	Minute ventilation complex function of:
	peak and end-expiratory pressure
	respiratory system impedance
	respiratory frequency

ventilation facilitates the control of alveolar ventilation (and thus PaCO$_2$) by providing a constant tidal volume with each mechanical breath while allowing breath-to-breath monitoring of respiratory system impedance (ie, changes in peak airway pressure will be associated with alterations in respiratory system compliance and/or resistance). Disadvantages of volume-limited ventilation are related to variable end-inspiratory alveolar volume and pressure (with its associated risk of "volutrauma") and the constant inspiratory flow, which can be set too low to meet the patient's spontaneous inspiratory needs (flow dyssynchrony and imposed work of breathing). During pressure-limited, time-cycled ventilation, a decelerating inspiratory flow pattern is used to achieve a predetermined peak pressure early in the inspiratory cycle and then to maintain that pressure for a set time interval (Fig. 16, part B). By the nature of this design, the limitation in airway pressure also limits end-inspiratory alveolar pressure and, in theory, the associated risk of "volutrauma" while providing a higher mean P$_{aw}$ for the peak airway pressure than that achieved with comparable pressures with volume-limited ventilation. Treatment of severe restrictive lung disease requires recruitment of collapsed distal airways and alveoli using inspiratory pressures in excess of the critical opening pressure, for sustained periods of time. This situation is perhaps best treated with pressure-limited ventilation and its associated higher mean P$_{aw}$. Decelerating inspiratory flow also has been associated with a better, more homogenous distribution of ventilation and a decrease in dead space ventilation in patients with lung injury.[29,53] Unfortunately, the limitation of inspiratory pressure is associated with several disadvantages. Changes in respiratory system impedance are not apparent with changes in airway pressure (but are with alteration in exhaled tidal volume). The fluid nature of the tidal volume is evidence that minute ventilation is also changing. During pressure-limited ventilation, minute ventilation will not increase linearly with respiratory frequency, but will change in response to the change in applied pressure and respiratory system compliance and resistance. Thus, the control of alveolar ventilation and PaCO$_2$ are more variable during pressure-limited ventilation.[54] Randomized clinical trials comparing volume-limited and pressure-limited modes of mechanical ventilation in adults with ARDS have yielded conflicting results while no data specific to the pediatric population are available.[34]

When pressure-limited modes of ventilation are chosen, constant monitoring of the exhaled tidal volume is suggested. However, with volume-limited ventilation, the peak airway pressure is monitored. Decreases in the exhaled tidal volume or increases in peak airway pressure should prompt a thorough investigation into their etiology, starting with a check of the ventilator and circuit for disconnects or small leaks that may account for the loss of tidal volume. The investigation should the continue with the passing of a suction catheter down the endotracheal tube to ensure that secretions have not blocked the endotracheal tube or major airways. Auscultation ensures bilateral breath sounds, ruling out a mainstem intubation, bronchospasm, or pneumothorax. A chest x-ray may be indicated to rule out progressive alveolar space disease (worsening pneumonia or ARDS) or extrapleural problems (pneumothorax) that lead to the decreased tidal volume. Finally, extrapneumonic sources of altered compliance, such as increasing abdominal girth, are sought.

Weaning from Mechanical Ventilation

For the vast majority of patients requiring mechanical ventilatory assistance, weaning from this support is relatively simple and straightforward; however, a small but significant percentage of patients require ventilatory assistance for prolonged periods of time and represent a population of patients that are frequently difficult to wean from positive-pressure ventilation. The success of weaning a patient from ventilatory support is dependent upon the careful consideration of the patient's general status, the presence of adequate ventilatory reserve, and the attainment of favorable respiratory mechanics. A greater understanding of respiratory muscle performance in infants and children may improve the decision-making process for weaning them from mechanical ventilation.[55]

The determinants of the ability to resume and sustain spontaneous ventilation are the converse of the indications for mechanical ventilation and can be divided into hypoxemic failure and hypoventilation. Hypoxemia during a weaning trial may be the result of hypoventilation, impaired pulmonary gas exchange (typically lung volume loss), or decreased mixed venous oxygen content. Neurologic injury and/or suppression can occasionally be the reason for the decrease in ventilatory capacity and for the failure to wean from mechanical ventilation. The presence of an increased $AaDO_2$ is indicative of alterations in gas exchange and not of hypoventilation. When hypoxemia is encountered during a weaning trial, weaning must be stopped until the etiology is identified and corrected. Hypoventilation secondary to respiratory muscle failure is the most common reason for an inability to successfully wean from mechanical ventilation. The etiology of respiratory muscle failure can be divided into two categories: decreased ventilatory capacity and increased respiratory muscle load (Table 14).

Several other diverse conditions may affect the performance of the respiratory muscles. Examples include lung hyperinflation with impaired diaphragmatic performance,[56] malnutrition,[57] electrolyte imbalance (hypomagnesemia, hypophosphatemia, hypocalcemia, and hypokalemia),[55] shock with decreased substrate delivery to the respiratory musculature,[58-60] muscle fatigue,[61] and disuse atrophy.[62]

There are a vast array of factors that increase respiratory muscle load (the work the lungs must do) and lead to difficulty during attempts to wean from mechanical ventilation. A variety of both physiologic (eg, pain, agitation, fever, surgical stress) and pathologic (eg, seizures, sepsis, excessive carbohydrate intake, malignant hyperthermia) causes of increased carbon dioxide production lead to the need to increase minute ventilation to maintain normal $PaCO_2$ levels. Diseases that increase the dead space to tidal volume ratio (eg, asthma, bronchiolitis, and bronchopulmonary dysplasia) also cause a need for an increase in minute ventilation and respiratory muscle load. Excessive respiratory drive from neurologic lesions, psychologic stress, or pulmonary irritant receptors can cause inappropriate hyperventilation and an increase in respiratory muscle workload. Finally, respiratory work (ie, transpulmonary pressure times the tidal volume per minute) is increased and efficiency diminished by alterations in respiratory system compliance and/or resistance secondary to disease or developmental (ie, compliant chest wall, rapid breathing) changes.

Clinicians working in ICUs have attempted for many years to define objective measures that can be used to predict the success or failure of discontinuation of

Table 14

Potential Etiologies of Respiratory Pump Failure

Decreased Ventilatory Capacity	Increased Respiratory Muscle Load
Neurologic	Increased ventilatory requirements
Decreased respiratory center output	Increased carbon dioxide production
Cervical spinal cord injury	Increased dead space ventilation
Phrenic nerve dysfunction	Inappropriately elevated ventilatory drive
Respiratory Muscle	Decreased efficiency of breathing
Hyperinflation	Increased chest wall compliance
Malnutrition	Respiratory pattern
Metabolic derangements	Increased work of breathing
Decreased oxygen supply/fatigue	
Disuse atrophy	
Abdominal wall defects	

mechanical ventilation and extubation of the trachea in patients undergoing positive pressure ventilation (Table 15). The criteria are typically directed at ensuring adequate gas exchange (oxygenation) and the presence of sufficient ventilatory reserve (ventilatory pump function) to maintain acid-base homeostasis. Oxygenation criteria include: 1) $PaO_2 \geq 60$ mm Hg, with an $FiO_2 \leq 0.4$ and physiologic levels of PEEP; 2) $AaDO_2$ less than 350 mm Hg; and 3) PaO_2/FiO_2 greater than 200 and Q_S/Q_T less than 15%. Examples of ventilatory pump criteria include: 1) vital capacity greater than 10 to 15 mL/kg; 2) maximum negative inspiratory pressure greater than -30 cm H_2O; 3) maximum minute ventilation greater than 10 L/min; 4) respiratory frequency less than 25 breaths/min; 5) spontaneous V_T greater than 6 mL/kg; and 6) V_D/V_T less than 0.6. Unfortunately the majority of data are from adults with respiratory failure. Furthermore, many of the criteria used have been shown to have high false-positive and/or false-negative rates. Integration of several physiologic variables such as respiratory frequency/tidal volume, also known as the rapid, shallow breathing index (RSBI), has recently shown promise as a more accurate predictor of success for the weaning of adults from ventilation.[63] This was not shown in one study in the pediatric population in which integrated indices could not predict success or failure; however, other bedside measures of respiratory function (FiO_2, oxygenation index, PIP, mean P_{aw}, fraction of total minute ventilation provided by ventilator, dynamic compliance, mean inspiratory flow) were able to define low- and high-risk categories.[64] With a lack of reproducible predictive criteria, the bedside clinician will be left with somewhat subjective guidelines on which to base his or her decision to attempt withdrawal of ventilation and extubation (Table 15). A major problem that remains is that many of the criteria are based on an instantaneous measurement when, in fact, many patients fail extubation due to increasing respiratory muscle fatigue related to increased respiratory workload.

Many different methods of weaning patients from mechanical ventilation have been developed over the years. These methods include periods of T-tube weaning as well as decreases in SIMV and/or PSV. Despite the wealth of clinical experience with each of these weaning techniques, there are no controlled clinical trials that clearly demonstrate a superiority of one method over another.[18,19]

In defiance of these conclusive data, SIMV has emerged as the standard method for weaning from mechanical ventilatory support in the pediatric setting. This mode of ventilation allows for a gradual decrease in the fraction of minute ventilation delivered by the ventilator at a pace tailored to the capabilities of the patient. In general, the frequency of positive pressure breaths is decreased in 2 to 5 breath per minute increments followed by patient assessment for signs of distress with or without blood gas determination for hypoxemia and/or hypercapnia. As the rate is weaned, the level of

Table 15

Guidelines for Discontinuation of Mechanical Ventilatory Support (CALMS)

Central nervous system
   Adequate ventilatory drive
   Mental status sufficient to protect airway
Airway
   Lack of nasopharyngeal airway edema/obstruction
   Lack of subglottic edema (ie, air leak < 30 cm H_2O with cuff deflated or around uncuffed endotracheal tube)
Lungs
   Adequate oxygenation:
     PaO_2 >70 with $FiO_2 \leq 0.4$ (PaO_2/FiO_2 >200) and PEEP≤5
     $Q_S Q_T$<15%
   Sufficient ventilatory reserve:
     vital capacity>10–15 mL/kg
     spontaneous tidal volume>6mL/kg
     rapid shallow breathing index (RSBI)≤8
Muscles
   Negative inspiratory force (NIF)<−30–45 cm H_2O
   Recovery of neuromuscular junction function:
     sustained tetanus at 50 or 100 Hz for >4 seconds
     sustained head or leg lift
Secretions
   Quality/quantity
   Frequency of suctioning

pressure support is weaned to levels that are thought to provide only enough support to overcome the work of breathing imposed by the endotracheal tube, the circuit, and the ventilator. No formal studies exist to demonstrate the exact level of pressure support required to achieve this goal; however, it is generally accepted that levels of 6 to 10 cm H_2O provide minimal extra support. Higher levels may provide additional support, suggesting that the patient can be removed from mechanical ventilation, when in fact there is still a significant amount of support provided by the ventilator. When the patient has reached some arbitrary minimum SIMV rate (SIMV = 0 to 2 in children, SIMV = 4 in toddlers, and SIMV = 4 to 8 in infants), they are deemed ready for extubation. Regardless of the weaning method selected, the clinician must continuously monitor for signs of increased work of breathing, and halt weaning to avoid respiratory muscle fatigue. If the assist control mode is chosen, then both the rate and the level of support (volume or pressure) must be weaned. As each breath is assisted, the support provided for each breath (either volume or pressure) should be decreased. The assist control mode may be beneficial in neonates and infants who have difficulty triggering the pressure-support mode of some ventilators. The baseline amount of support that is acceptable prior to attempted extubation should be an amount estimated to provide only enough support to overcome the work of breathing imposed by the endotracheal tube and ventilator.

Complications of Mechanical Ventilation

While frequently life-saving, mechanical ventilation is also associated with numerous real and potential complications, some of which are themselves life-threatening. These complications include diverse problems from patient discomfort to unnecessary prolongation of mechanical ventilation with excessive use of limited health resources. These complications are generally related to positive pressure or inspired oxygen concentration.

Typical mechanical ventilation is linked to the application of positive intrathoracic pressure that may alter respiratory mechanics and that has the potential to alter the function of intra- and extrathoracic organs (Table 16). Most commonly, this includes a decrease in preload with decreased cardiac output in patients who have diminished myocardial contractility or who are hypovolemic. Alternatively, excessive levels of PEEP may increase pulmonary vascular resistance and right ventricular afterload, leading to decreases in left-sided filling pressures. The alterations in organ function are more accurately described as side effects rather than complications of the positive intrathoracic pressure.

Evidence has accumulated over the last decade, in many different mammalian species, that excessive alveolar distension

Table 16

Side Effects of Positive Pressure Mechanical Ventilation

Pulmonary Effects
  Increased physiologic dead space ventilation
  Alveolar-capillary membrane injury (i.e., acute lung injury - volutrauma)
  Alveolar membrane disruption (i.e., barotrauma):
    pulmonary interstitial/subcutaneous emphysema
    pneumomediastinium
    pneumothorax
    pneumopericardium
    pneumoperitoneum
    venous gas emboli
Cardiovascular
  Decreased systemic venous return
  Decreased left ventricular performance:
    decreased myocardial blood flow
    neural and/or humoral depression
    intraventricular septal displacement impeding ventricular filling
  Increased pulmonary vascular resistance
Other Organ Function
  Decreased cerebral perfusion secondary to ↑ intracranial pressure and/or ↓ systemic arterial pressure
  Decreased/redistributed renal blood flow
  Decreased sodium excretion and free water/creatinine clearance
  Decreased hepatic/intestinal blood flow

with high inflating pressures produces disruption of the alveolar-capillary membrane with resultant development of severe alterations in membrane filtration and permeability (high-volume lung injury). This injury to the alveolar-capillary membrane leads to interstitial and alveolar pulmonary edema and diffuse alveolar damage.[65-67] If left unchecked, these injuries progress to multiple organ failure and death.[29] Further studies with negative pressure ventilators and thoracoabdominal binding have clearly shown that this injury is not due to high positive airway pressure per se, but to excessive end-inspiratory alveolar volumes.[68,69] These experiments prompted the evolution of the concept that the mechanisms of high-pressure lung injury were from "pressure-related" injury (ie, barotrauma) to that of "volume-related" injury (ie, volutrauma).[70] Although these studies suggest that excessive end-inspiratory alveolar volumes are the primary determinant of volutrauma, it remains uncertain whether there is a volume threshold below which mechanical ventilation will not cause lung injury. It is clear, however, that multiple factors, including duration of inflation,[71] previous lung injury,[72-74] and age,[75] are involved in the complex process.

Other investigators have focused on the effects of mechanical ventilation at low lung volumes. Initial studies showed that lung injury can occur from purely mechanical factors when ventilation results in repeated small airway closure and opening with each respiratory cycle.[76] They further demonstrated that the use of PEEP to open airways and alveoli at end-expiration will change the site and severity of lung injury. The heterogeneous nature of lung injury associated with the uniform application of positive pressure during mechanical ventilation leads to the delivery of the bulk of ventilation to the more normal, compliant regions of the lungs. Traction exerted on the normally compliant parenchyma surrounding atelectatic areas also causes injury.[77] These works have led to the hypothesis that stretch caused by repetitive collapse and reopening of terminal lung units directly damages or worsens previously injured lung (low-volume lung injury).[78] Hence, it is apparent that clinicians have a narrow therapeutic window for delivery of mechanical ventilation to prevent iatrogenic lung injury.

When end-inspiratory alveolar volumes exceed a certain threshold, disruption occurs at the border of the alveolar base and the bronchovascular sheath. This allows access of gas under positive pressure into the interstitium (pulmonary interstitial emphysema) that is then free to dissect toward the hilum, up and down the mediastinum (pneumomediastinum), and into the subcutaneous tissue (subcutaneous emphysema), pleural (pneumothorax), pericardial (pneumopericardium), and peritoneal spaces (pneumoperitoneum). These pathologic collections of gas have been categorized under the all-inclusive term of barotrauma. Their clinical significance ranges from mild patient discomfort to severe life-threatening collapse of the lung and shift of mediastinal structures. The occurrence rate of barotrauma in some form varies between 3% and 65% in patients treated with continuous positive pressure ventilation.[79] Although many factors have been associated with an increased risk of pulmonary barotrauma (Table 17), the consensus is that excessive alveolar volumes (end-inspiratory alveolar volumes) are the primary offending factor.[80]

Alterations in extravascular lung water have been associated with the use of mechanical ventilation. For example, rapid re-expansion of a collapsed lung from a pneumothorax causes a dramatic increase in negative interstitial pressure and frank alveolar edema fluid accumulation.[81] Extravascular lung water has been reported to increase,[82] decrease,[68,83] or remain unchanged[84] in response to the application of CPAP/PEEP. The variable response in extravascular lung water is due to changes in transmural pressure across the pulmonary vasculature and vessel type,[85] to lymphatic flow,[86] and to alterations in alveolar epithelial and pulmonary endothelial permeability.[87,88] The clinical significance of the change in extravascular lung water in response to mechanical ventilation is not known.

Administration of continuous positive pressure has frequently been associated with alterations in cardiovascular function.

Table 17

Factors Associated with Pulmonary Barotrauma

Impedance to exhalation
  Small artificial airway
  Intrathoracic airway obstruction
    retained secretions
    disease (ie bronchiolitis)
  Positive pressure mechanical ventilation
    insufficient expiratory time
    mechanical expiratory retardation (ie PEEP valve)
Excessive alveolar volume/pressure
  Decreased respiratory compliance
  Positive pressure mechanical ventilation
    high inspiratory pressure
    prolonged inspiratory time
    inspiratory pause
    high end-expiratory pressure
    patient-ventilator dyssynchrony
Regional disparities in ventilation distribution
  Focal lung disease (ie, inhomogeneity of regional compliance and/or resistance)
  Endobronchial intubation

PEEP = positive end-expiratory pressure.

Decreased systemic venous return[89] and ventricular preload,[90] increased pulmonary vascular resistance and right ventricular afterload,[91] and leftward intraventricular septal displacement and impedance to left ventricular diastolic filling[92] have been suggested to contribute to the compromise in cardiac output during mechanical ventilation. Studies in open-chested animals free of mechanical heart-lung interactions have also demonstrated depressed cardiac output, suggesting that reflex neurohumoral factors contribute to ventricular dysfunction.[93] In general, depression of cardiovascular function associated with high levels of positive pressure ventilation can be reversed with expansion of intravascular volume or a low-dose dopamine infusion. It has been suggested that some of the adverse cardiovascular side effects can be minimized by some degree of spontaneous ventilation (eg, SIMV with PEEP) versus controlled positive pressure ventilation.

Continuous positive pressure ventilation is also associated with a variety of changes in peripheral organ function that are likely related to changes in cardiac output and end-organ perfusion. Decreases in urine output, creatinine clearance, and renal sodium excretion have been commonly seen with the use of PEEP.[94] These effects are related to changes in cortical-medullary distribution of kidney perfusion, decreased renal blood flow, and increased antidiuretic hormone secretion.[95] Other studies have shown decreased hepatic, portal venous, and mesenteric blood flow with continuous positive pressure ventilation.[95,96] Positive intrathoracic pressure has also been associated with decreased cerebral venous drainage and elevations in cerebral blood volume and intracranial pressure in head trauma victims.[97]

It is ironic that the very existence of humans is fully dependent on a gas that, in excess quantities, is toxic and lethal. Despite the fact that supplemental oxygen administration is the mainstay of our clinical inventory for hypoxemia, exposure to high concentrations of oxygen will cause pulmonary injury. Although the onset of oxygen toxicity varies from patient to patient, the contributing factors have been identified as: 1) the partial pressure of inspired oxygen; 2) the duration of exposure; and 3) the patient's underlying lung disease.[98] It should be noted that the partial pressure of inspired oxygen, and not the fraction of inspired oxygen, is related to pulmonary oxygen toxicity. This can be illustrated by comparing prolonged periods of exposure to 100% inspired oxygen under hypobaric conditions without ill effects, to the fact that brief exposures to 21% oxygen under hyperbaric conditions may cause significant injury. The exact level of partial pressure of oxygen that produces lung injury in humans has not been established; however, exposure to FiO_2 less than 0.5 at sea level has been tolerated for prolonged periods without overt effects on the lungs.[99] Oxygen radicals (superoxide, hydrogen peroxide, hydroxyl free radical, and singlet oxygen) that are normal metabolic byproducts are the major cause of pulmonary oxygen toxicity.[100] Increased production of cyclo-oxygenase and lipoxygenase pathway products has also been implicated with hyperoxic lung injury.[101] Pathologic changes in animals' lungs resulting from oxygen therapy have been divided into three phases: 1) the latent phase with no pathologic changes, 2) the inflammatory phase associated with atelectasis, alveolar edema, and hemorrhage, and 3) the destructive phase marked by hyaline membrane deposition and proliferation of type II alveolar pneumocytes. Capillary endothelial cell injury appears to occur earlier than alveolar epithelial cell damage. The rapidity of disease progression varies by species but is clearly hastened by increased partial pressure of inspired oxygen.

Respiratory Monitoring

Methods of monitoring the respiratory system have changed dramatically, from a reliance on physical assessment and direct observation to continuous electronic surveillance of multiple physiologic parameters. Noninvasive techniques to assess gas exchange and pulmonary mechanics supplement physical assessment and provide continuous data with alarm capabilities to identify changes in patient status and to alert care providers. Appropriate integration and interpretation of these data is essential for high-quality, cost-effective care in the modern ICU setting. However, the role for physical assessment continues today. Only by examination can the bedside care provider differentiate between monitor error and a true change in patient status.

Monitoring has several proposes: 1) to measure intermittently or continuously key physiologic variables that aid in diagnosis and guide management; 2) to provide alarms that notify the care providers that important changes in the patient's clinical condition have occurred; and 3) to create and evaluate trends that might assist with the assessment of treatment and prognosis.[102] Monitoring systems must provide pertinent, accurate, and reproducible data that are interpretable by the bedside care providers. The technology should be practical to use, easy to attach to the patient, should function independently, and should occupy little space. Finally, the monitoring system must achieve these goals with patient safety as the primary goal. Since the respiratory system is responsible for providing oxygen for transport to the tissues and removal of carbon dioxide produced by metabolic pathways, this discussion revolves around monitoring systems that quantify and evaluate these two functions.

Pulse Oximetry

One of the most important technological advances of modern medicine was the development of SpO_2 to noninvasively measure the percent oxygen saturation of hemoglobin. This technology had existed since the 1930s, but required the development of microprocessors and advancements in light-emitting diodes, plethysmography, and spectrophotometry in the 1970s before its application in a variety of clinical settings in the 1980s. This technology uses the different absorption characteristics of oxyhemoglobin and reduced hemoglobin at two separate wavelengths (660 nm-red and 940 nm-infrared). A miniature light source is applied to an area of the body that is narrow enough to allow light to transverse a pulsating capillary bed and be sensed by a photo detector (optical plethysmography). A microprocessor programmed with empirically derived data calculates the amounts of oxyhemoglobin and reduced hemoglobin (thus, the oxygen saturation) by comparing absorbencies at baseline (BA) and during the peak (PA) of transmitted pulse at 660 nm (red) and 940 nm (infrared): red absorbance (R)/infrared absorbance (IR) = $(PA_{660}/BA_{660})/(PA_{940}/BA_{940})$. The R/IR ratio determines the "functional" oxygen saturation. Functional saturation is the ratio of oxyhemoglobin to the sum of all functional hemoglobins (ie, hemoglobin capable of carrying oxygen): functional $SpO_2 = HbO_2/(HbO_2 + Hb)$, where HbO_2 is oxygenated hemoglobin and Hb is nonoxygenated hemoglobin. Functional SpO_2 differs from "fractional" SaO_2 measured by co-oximetry on most blood gas machines. Fractional SaO_2 gives the ratio of oxygenated hemoglobin to the sum of all other hemoglobin types, including carboxyhemoglobin (HbCO) and methemoglobin

(Hbmet), which do not carry oxygen: fractional $SaO_2 = HbO_2/(HbO_2 + Hb + HbCO + Hbmet)$. The disadvantage of functional saturation is that other possibly clinically pertinent hemoglobin species will be missed. For example, carbon monoxide poisoning with elevated levels of HbCO will lead to an overestimation of the true HbO_2 that will lead to falsely elevated SpO_2 values.[103] HbCO absorbs light in the red wavelength and is therefore interpreted by the pulse oximeter as oxygenated hemoglobin. As the partial pressure of oxygen is not altered by the presence of abnormal hemoglobin species, if HbCO or other abnormal hemoglobin components are suspected, the blood gas must be analyzed using co-oximetry.

Similarly, increased Hbmet levels will cause SpO_2 values to be inaccurate and plateau at 85% due to the absorption characteristics of Hbmet (absorbing at a wavelength between oxygenated and unoxygenated hemoglobin) and to the algorithm used by the pulse oximeter.[104] It has been clearly demonstrated that oxygen saturation of normal hemoglobin determined by the pulse oximeter correlates very closely with the oxygen saturation determined by the co-oximeter ($R = 0.98$) when the saturation is between 70% and 100%.[105]

Pulse oximetry, like most other technologies, has several limitations, most of which are predictable and understandable given a firm grasp of the basic operating principles of the instrument. As mentioned previously, abnormal hemoglobin species (ie, HbCO and Hbmet), due to their similar absorbencies at 660 nm to oxyhemoglobin and reduced hemoglobin, respectively, can lead to false estimates of oxyhemoglobin. Dyes like methylene blue and indocyanine green will cause brief false decreases in SpO_2 due to absorbance of light in the infrared range.[106] Because pulse oximetry depends on a pulsatile change in arterial blood (optical plethysmography), abnormalities in propagation of the pulse to the extremities can result in inaccuracy of SpO_2 values. Shock states, vasopressors, severe edema, and peripheral vascular disease challenge the oximeter to distinguish the true signal from background. External light sources can also adversely affect the performance of SpO_2 devices.[107] Variation in light transmission and reception due to excessive motion can produce false arterial pulse waveforms that the oximeter may not be able to differentiate from the true arterial waveforms, hence, producing spurious SpO_2 values. Pulse oximetry is clearly most valuable when used as a continuous monitor, and may decrease the need for frequent blood gas analysis. However, it must be remembered that these probes use infrared light (heat) and can alter perfusion; therefore, probe sites should changed periodically to prevent damage to tissues.

Carbon Dioxide Monitoring

Capnography is defined as the graphic waveform produced by variations in carbon dioxide concentration throughout the respiratory cycle as a function of time.[108] The two most common methods of capnography measurement are infrared spectroscopy and mass spectroscopy. Infrared spectroscopy (wavelengths >1 μ) uses the unique absorption characteristics of gases to quantify the amount (partial pressure) of a particular gas. This technology requires an infrared light source, a gas chamber, and a detector. Respiratory gases are either aspirated into the gas chamber (sidestream monitoring) or enter the gas chamber that is attached in-line at the endotracheal tube (mainstream monitoring).

Capnography has many potential uses in the ICU setting (Table 18). Perhaps the most common use is the determination of $P_{et}CO_2$ concentration, which is defined as the peak carbon dioxide value during the expiratory phase of respiration. The normal $P_{et}CO_2$ in healthy subjects is less than 5 mm Hg lower than the $PaCO_2$ because of the small amount of dead space ventilation. In the absence of significant lung disease, the $P_{et}CO_2$ will correlate with the arterial carbon dioxide and can be used as a means of adjusting minute ventilation without the need for repeated arterial blood gas determinations.

Numerous clinical conditions have been associated with changes in $P_{et}CO_2$ (Table 19). Uses of $P_{et}CO_2$ monitoring in

Table 18
Potential Clinical Uses of Capnography
Tracheal placement of endotracheal tube (ie, presence of exhaled carbon dioxide)
Quantify the partial pressure of exhaled (end-tidal) carbon dioxide ($P_{ET}CO_2$)
Determination of dead space ventilation (ie, V_T/V_D)
Approximation of arterial partial pressure of carbon dioxide (when dead space ventilation in minimal)
Evaluation of respiratory pattern
Rate and rhythm
Patient-ventilator synchrony
Mechanical ventilator failure alarm

Table 19	
Conditions Associated with Alterations in Partial Pressure of End-Tidal Carbon Dioxide	
Increases in $ETCO_2$	
Sudden	Increase in cardiac output
	Release of a tourniquet
	Administration of sodium bicarbonate
Gradual	Hypoventilation
	Increase carbon dioxide production
Decreases in $ETCO_2$	
Sudden	Sudden hyperventilation
	Decrease in cardiac output
	Pulmonary embolism
	Air embolism
	Endotracheal tube obstruction
Gradual	Hyperventilation
	Decrease oxygen consumption
	Increase in dead space ventilation
Absent $ETCO_2$	Esophageal intubation
	Ventilator disconnect
	Accidental extubation

the ICU include monitoring adequacy of alveolar ventilation during mechanical ventilation, respiratory monitoring in spontaneously breathing patients, patient-ventilator system function, and endotracheal tube patency. $P_{et}CO_2$ monitoring is used as a standard of care in the operating room to document correct placement of an endotracheal tube in the trachea. The graphic display of the capnography waveforms provides useful information in the mechanically ventilated patient. Mechanical failures, adequacy of ventilation, differentiation of mechanical versus spontaneous breaths, and patient-ventilator synchrony can be assessed with this technology. The amount of dead space (V_D/V_T) can be estimated using a variant of the Bohr equation: $V_D/V_T = (PaCO_2 - ETCO_2)/PaCO_2$ or $1 - (ETCO_2/PaCO_2)$, where $ETCO_2$ is mean expired carbon dioxide concentration. Conditions that significantly alter V_D/V_T will be easily detected by changes in $ETCO_2$.[109] Coronary perfusion pressure and the success rate of resuscitation during cardiopulmonary arrest have been found to correlate with $P_{et}CO_2$.[110,111]

Transcutaneous technology offers an additional option for the continuous estimation and monitoring of $PaCO_2$. The device heats the skin, producing local vasodilation that leads to arterialization of the capillary bed. While several technological and patient issues can interfere with the accuracy of these devices, recent studies have suggested their accuracy in monitoring carbon dioxide in the PICU population.[112] Variations in skin thickness, tissue edema, the administration of vasoconstricting agents, and tissue hypoperfusion can interfere with the accuracy of these devices. However, their accuracy has been demonstrated even in patients with respiratory failure and significant alterations in ventilation-perfusion patterns in whom $P_{et}CO_2$ is inaccurate.[112]

Respiratory Mechanics Monitoring

Recent technological advances now permit continuous respiratory mechanics monitoring, including graphic display of gas flow, tidal volume, and airway pressure. Output waveforms are useful tools with which to study the characteristics of

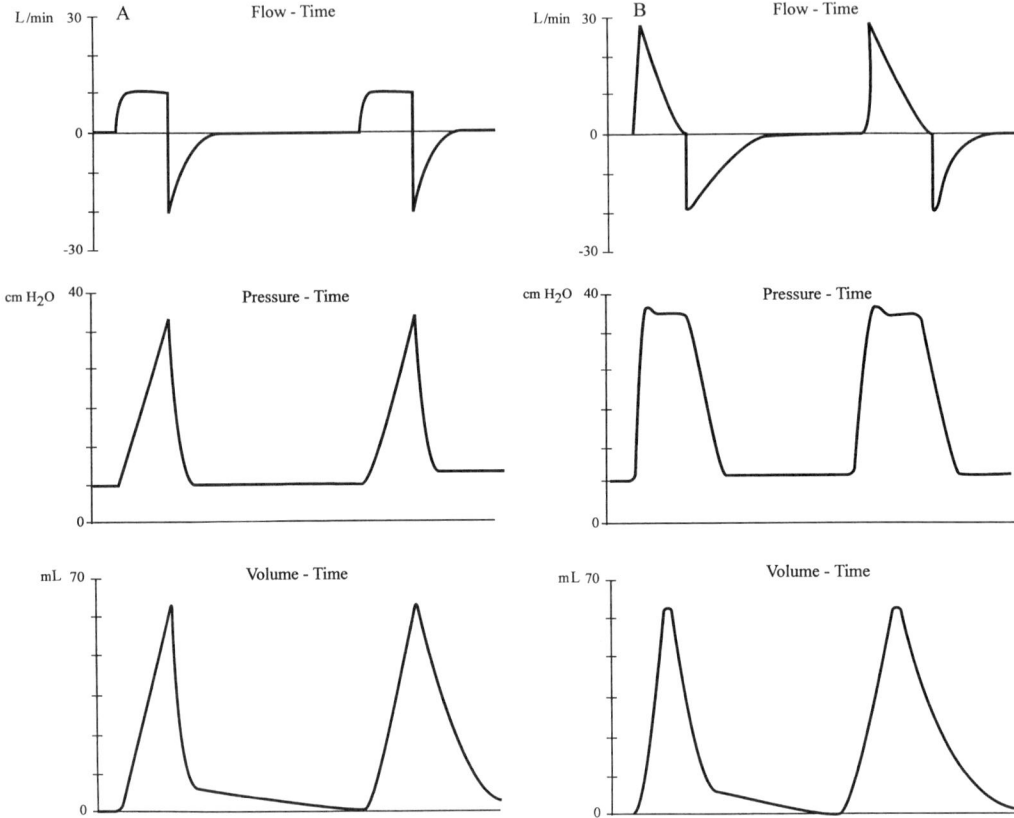

Figure 17. Examples of flow-time (top), pressure-time (middle), volume-time (bottom) curves during flow-limited, time-cycled ventilation (diagram A) and pressure-limited, time-cycled ventilation (diagram B). These diagrams are helpful for detecting problems such as patient-ventilator dyssynchrony, insufficient inspiratory time, or continued expiratory flow and pressure (auto-PEEP).

ventilator operation and provide a graphic display of the various modes of ventilation. Waveform analysis can be used to optimize mechanical ventilatory support and to analyze ventilator incidents and alarm conditions. It is also possible to alter ventilatory support to improve patient-ventilator synchrony, reduce work of breathing, and calculate a variety of physiologic parameters related to respiratory mechanics.

Respiratory mechanics monitoring can be accomplished using flow- and pressure-sensing devices internally in individual ventilators or by placement of a flow/pressure sensor between the endotracheal tube and ventilator circuit. Volume is generally measured by integrating the flow signal over time. The most common display is waveforms of flow, pressure, and volume (y axis) plotted against time (x axis) with inspiration positive values and expiration negative values (Fig. 17). The timing sequence of various respiratory events and patient-ventilator dyssynchrony can be determined by the graphs. In addition, flow, pressure, and volume can be plotted against each other (Fig. 18). Pressure-volume and flow-volume loops are particularly helpful in assessing alterations in resistance, compliance, work of breathing, overdistention of the lung, and premature termination of exhalation (auto-PEEP).

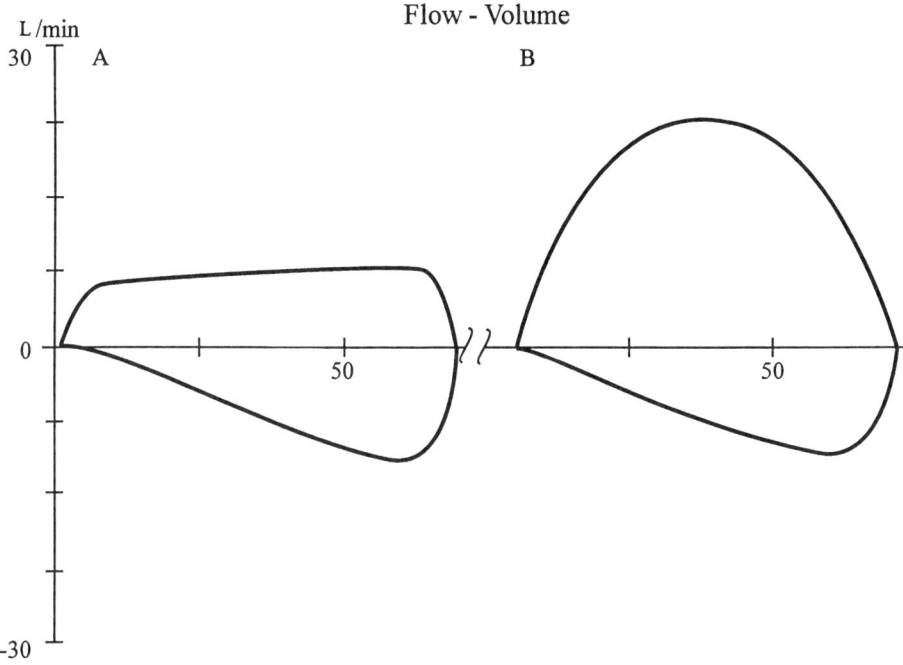
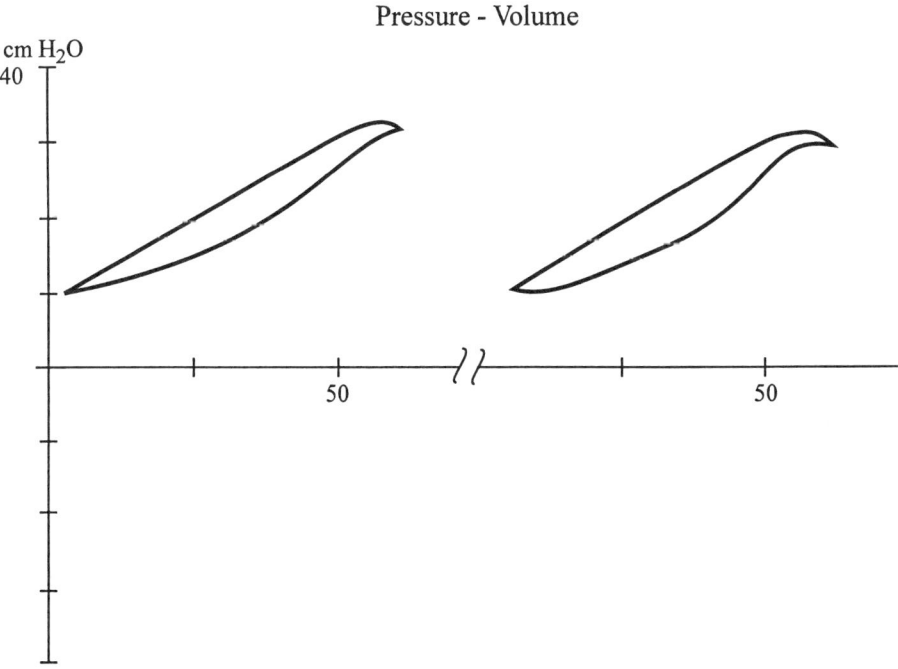

Figure 18. Examples of flow-volume and pressure-volume loops during flow-limited, time-cycled ventilation (diagram A) and pressure-limited, time-cycled ventilation (diagram B). These diagrams are helpful for detecting problems such as inspiratory or expiratory airflow obstruction, excessive tidal volumes, or changes in compliance.

Summary

During the last 20 years, tremendous technological advances in mechanical ventilation and respiratory monitoring have occurred. Regardless of the means, the primary goal of mechanical ventilation and respiratory monitoring remains cost-effective optimization of patient care and minimization of morbidity and mortality. However, it must be emphasized that the effectiveness of any device will be limited by the understanding of the pathophysiology of the disease process by the bedside care providers and by their ability to integrate this knowledge into therapeutic applications of the technology to slow or reverse the pathologic process. The reader is referred to chapter 5 for a full discussion of other means of respiratory support for those patients who fail standard mechanical ventilation.

References

1. Schreiner MS, Downes JJ, Kettrick RG, et al. Chronic respiratory failure in infants with prolonged ventilator dependency. *JAMA* 1987;258:3398–3404.
2. Viires N, Sillye G, Aubier M, et al. Regional blood flow distribution in dog during induced hypotension and low cardiac output: Spontaneous breathing versus artificial ventilation. *J Clin Invest* 1983;72:935–947.
3. Dantzker DR, Brook CJ, Dehart P, et al. Ventilation-perfusion distributions in the adult respiratory distress syndrome. *Am Rev Respir Dis* 1979;120:1039–1052.
4. Marini JJ, Ravenscraft SA. Mean airway pressure: Physiologic determinants and clinical importance-parts 1 & 2. *Crit Care Med* 1992;20:1604–1616.
5. Boros SJ, Matalon SV, Ewald R, et al. The effect of independent variations in inspiratory-expiratory ratio and end-expiratory pressure during mechanical ventilation in hyaline membrane disease: The significance of mean airway pressure. *J Pediatr* 1977;91:794–798.
6. Weisman IM, Rinaldo JE, Rogers RM, Sanders MH. Intermittent mandatory ventilation. *Am Rev Respir Dis* 1983;127:641–647.
7. Mansell A, Bryan C, Levison H. Airway closure in children. *J Appl Physiol* 1972;33:711–714.
8. Banner MJ, Jaegar MJ, Kirby RR. Components of the work of breathing and implications for monitoring ventilator-dependent patients. *Crit Care Med* 1994;22:515–523.
9. Chatburn RL. Classification of mechanical ventilators. *Respir Care* 1992;37:1009–1026.
10. Tobin MJ. Monitoring of pressure, flow and volume during mechanical ventilation. *Respir Care* 1992;37:1081–1093.
11. Branson RD, Chatburn RL. Technical description and classification of modes of ventilator operation. *Respir Care* 1992;37:1026–1034.
12. Downs JB, Klein EF Jr, Desaults D, et al. Intermittent mandatory ventilation: A new approach to weaning patients from mechanical ventilation. *Chest* 1973;64:331–335.
13. Banner MJ, Kirby RR, Blanch PB, Layton AJ. Decreasing imposed work of breathing apparatus to zero using pressure-support ventilation. *Crit Care Med* 1993;21:1333–1338.
14. Cohen IL, Bilen Z, Krishnamurthy S. The effects of ventilator working pressure during pressure support ventilation. *Chest* 1993;103:588–592.
15. Brochard L, Harf A, Lorino H, Lemaire F. Inspiratory pressure support prevents diaphragmatic fatigue during weaning from mechanical ventilation. *Am Rev Respir Dis* 1989;139:513–521.
16. MacIntyre NR, Leatherman NE. Mechanical loads on the ventilatory muscles: A theoretical analysis. *Am Rev Respir Dis* 1989;139:968–973.
17. Leith DE, Bradley M. Ventilatory muscle strength and endurance training. *J Appl Physiol* 1976;41:508–516.
18. Esteban A, Frutos F, Tobin MJ, et al. A comparison of four methods of weaning from mechanical ventilation. Spanish lung failure collaborative group. *N Engl J Med* 1995;332:345–350.
19. Brochard L, Rauss A, Benito S, et al. Comparison of three methods of gradual withdrawal from ventilatory support during weaning from mechanical ventilation. *Am J Respir Crit Care Med* 1994;150:896–903.
20. Keenan HT, Martin LD. Volume support ventilation in infants and children: Analysis of a case series. *Respir Care* 1997;42:281–287.
21. Ashbaugh DG, Bigelow DB, Petty TL, Levine BE. Acute respiratory distress in adults. *Lancet* 1967;2:319–323.
22. Gregory GA, Kitterman JA, Phibbs RH, et al. Treatment of the idiopathic respiratory-distress syndrome with continuous positive airway pressure. *N Engl J Med* 1971;284:1333–1340.
23. Link J. Increase of expiratory resistance by the PEEP-valve of the servoventilator. *Intensive Care Med* 1983;9:137–138.

24. Aubier M, Viires N, Syllie G, et al. Respiratory muscle contribution to lactic acidosis in low cardiac output. *Am Rev Respir Dis* 1982;126:648–652.
25. Shepard FM, Arango LA, Simmons JG, Berry FA. Hemodynamic effects of mechanical ventilation in normal and distressed newborn lambs: A comparison of negative pressure and positive pressure respirators. *Biol Neonate* 1971;19:83–100.
26. Buda AJ, Pinsky MR, Ingels NB Jr, et al. Effect of intrathoracic pressure on left ventricular performance. *N Engl J Med* 1979;301:453–459.
27. Mathru M, Rao TL, el-Etr AA, Pifarre R. Hemodynamic response to changes in ventilatory patterns in patients with normal and poor left ventricular reserve. *Crit Care Med* 1982;10:423–426.
28. Muizelaar JP, Marmarou A, Ward JD, et al. Adverse effects of prolonged hyperventilation in patients with severe head injury: A randomized clinical trial. *J Neurosurg* 1991;75:731–739.
29. Marini JJ. New options for the ventilatory management of acute lung injury. *New Horizons* 1993;1:489–503.
30. Wyszogrodski I, Kyei-Aboagye K, Taeusch HW Jr, Avery ME. Surfactant inactivation by hyperventilation: Conservation by end-expiratory pressure. *J Appl Physiol* 1975;38:461–466.
31. Hammon JW Jr, Wolfe WG, Moran JF, et al. The effect of positive end-expiratory pressure on regional ventilation and perfusion in the normal and injured primate lung. *J Thorac Cardiovasc Surg* 1976;72:680–689.
32. Suter PM, Fairley HB, Isenberg MD. Optimum end expiratory airway pressure in patients with acute pulmonary failure. *N Engl J Med* 1975;292:284–289.
33. Matamis D, Lemaire F, Harf A, et al. Total respiratory pressure-volume curves in the adult respiratory distress syndrome. *Chest* 1984;86:58–64.
34. Martin LD. New approaches to mechanical ventilation in infants and children. *Curr Opin Pediatr* 1995;7:250–261.
35. Tuxen DV. Permissive hypercapnic ventilation. *Am J Respir Crit Care Med* 1994;150:870–874.
36. Bidani A, Tzouanakis AE, Cardenas VJ Jr, Zwischenberger JB. Permissive hypercapnia in acute respiratory failure. *JAMA* 1994;272:957–962.
37. Feihl F, Perret C. Permissive hypercapnia. How permissive should we be? *Am J Respir Crit Care Med* 1994;150:1722–1737.
38. Amato MB, Barbas CS, Medeiros DM, et al. Effect of a protective-ventilation strategy on mortality in the acute respiratory distress syndrome. *N Engl J Med* 1998;338:347–354.
39. Fackler J, Bohn D, Green T, et al. ECMO for ARDS: Stopping a randomized clinical trial. *Am J Respir Crit Care Med* 1997;155:A504.
40. Stewart TE, Meade MO, Cook DJ, et al. Evaluation of a ventilation strategy to prevent barotrauma in patients at high risk for acute respiratory distress syndrome. Pressure- and Volume-Limited Ventilation Strategy Group. *N Engl J Med* 1998;338:355–361.
41. Weg JG, Anzueto A, Balk RA, et al. The relation of pneumothorax and other air leaks to mortality in the acute respiratory distress syndrome. *N Engl J Med* 1998;338:341–346.
42. Pepe PE, Marini JJ. Occult positive end-expiratory pressure in mechanically ventilated patients with airflow obstruction. *Am Rev Respir Dis* 1982;126:166–170.
43. Williams TJ, Tuxen DV, Scheinkestel CD, et al. Risk factors for morbidity in mechanically ventilated patients with acute severe asthma. *Am Rev Respir Dis* 1992;146:607–615.
44. Prezant DJ, Aldrich TK, Karpel JP, Park SS. Inspiratory flow dynamics during mechanical ventilation in patients with respiratory failure. *Am Rev Respir Dis* 1990;142:1284–1287.
45. Darioli R, Perret C. Mechanical controlled hypoventilation in status asthmaticus. *Am Rev Respir Dis* 1984;129:385–387.
46. Dworkin G, Kattan M. Mechanical ventilation for status asthmaticus in children. *J Pediatr* 1989;114:545–549.
47. Shugg AW, Kerr S, Butt WW. Mechanical ventilation of paediatric patients with asthma: Short and long term outcome. *J Paediatr Child Health* 1990;26:343–346.
48. Leatherman JW, Fluegel WL, David WS, et al. Muscle weakness in mechanically ventilated patients with severe asthma. *Am J Respir Crit Care Med* 1996;153:1686–1690.
49. Tuxen DV, Williams TJ, Schienkestel CD, et al. Use of a measurement of pulmonary hyperinflation to control the level of mechanical ventilation in patients with severe asthma. *Am Rev Respir Dis* 1992;146:1136–1142.
50. Wetzel RC. Pressure-support ventilation in children with severe asthma. *Crit Care Med* 1996;24:1603–1605.
51. Remolina C, Kahn AU, Santigo TV, Edekman NH. Positional hypoxemia in unilateral lung disease. *N Engl J Med* 1981;304:523–525.
52. Heaf DP, Helms P, Gordon I, Turner HM. Postural effects on gas exchange in infants. *N Engl J Med* 1983;308:1505–1508.

53. Al-Saady N, Bennett ED. Decelerating inspiratory flow waveform improves lung mechanics and gas exchange in patients on intermittent positive-pressure ventilation. *Intensive Care Med* 1985;11:68–75.
54. Marini JJ, Crooke PS III, Truwit JD. Determinants and limits of positive pressure-preset ventilation: A mathematical model of pressure control. *J Appl Physiol* 1989;67:1081–1092.
55. Nichols DG. Respiratory muscle performance in infants and children. *J Pediatr* 1991;118:493–502.
56. Weiner P, Suo J, Fernandez E, Cherniack R. The effect of hyperinflation on respiratory muscle strength and efficiency in healthy subjects and patients with asthma. *Am Rev Respir Dis* 1990;141:1501–1505.
57. Arora NS, Rochester DF. Respiratory muscle strength and maximal voluntary ventilation in undernourished patients. *Am Rev Respir Dis* 1982;126:5–8.
58. Aubier M, Trippenbach T, Roussos C. Respiratory muscle fatigue during cardiogenic shock. *J Appl Physiol* 1981;51:499–508.
59. Watchko JF, LaFramboise WA, Standaert TA, Woodrum DE. Diaphragmatic function during hypoxemia: Neonatal and developmental aspects. *J Appl Physiol* 1986;60:1599–1604.
60. Watchko JF, Standaert TA, Woodrum DE. Diaphragmatic function during hypercapnia: Neonatal and developmental aspects. *J Appl Physiol* 1987;62:768–775.
61. Keens TG, Bryan AC, Levison H, Ionize CD. Developmental patterns of muscle fiber types in human ventilatory muscles. *J Appl Physiol* 1978;44:909–913.
62. Knisely AS, Leal SM, Singer DB. Abnormalities of diaphragmatic muscle in neonates with ventilated lungs. *J Pediatr* 1988;113:1074–1077.
63. Yang KL, Tobin MJ. A prospective study of indexes predicting the outcome of trials of weaning from mechanical ventilation. *N Engl J Med* 1991;324:1445–1450.
64. Khan N, Brown A, Venkataraman ST. Predictors of extubation success and failure in mechanically ventilated infants and children. *Crit Care Med* 1996; 24:1568–1579.
65. Webb HH, Tierney DF. Experimental pulmonary edema due to intermittent positive pressure ventilation with high inflation pressures. Protection by positive end-expiratory pressure. *Am Rev Respir Dis* 1974;110:556–565.
66. Dreyfuss D, Basset G, Soler P, Saumon G. Intermittent positive-pressure hyperventilation with high inflation pressures produces pulmonary microvascular injury in rats. *Am Rev Respir Dis* 1985;132:880–884.
67. Parker JC, Hernandez LA, Longnecker GL, et al. Lung edema caused by high peak inspiratory pressures in dogs. Role of increased microvascular filtration pressure and permeability. *Am Rev Respir Dis* 1990;142:321–328.
68. Dreyfuss D, Soler P, Basset G, Saumon G. High inflation pressure pulmonary edema. Respective effects of high airway pressure, high tidal volume, and positive end-expiratory pressure. *Am Rev Respir Dis* 1988;137:1159–1164.
69. Hernandez LA, Peevy KJ, Moise AA, Parker JC. Chest wall restriction limits high airway pressure-induced lung injury in young rabbits. *J Appl Physiol* 1989;66:2364–2368.
70. Dreyfuss D, Soler P, Saumon G. Spontaneous resolution of pulmonary edema caused by short periods of cyclic overinflation. *J Appl Physiol* 1992;72:2081–2089.
71. Tsuno K, Prato P, Kolobow T. Acute lung injury from mechanical ventilation at moderately high airway pressures. *J Appl Physiol* 1990;69:956–961.
72. Hernandez LA, Coker PJ, May S, et al. Mechanical ventilation increases microvascular permeability in oleic acid-injured lungs. *J Appl Physiol* 1990;69:2057–2061.
73. Corbridge TC, Wood LD, Crawford GP, et al. Adverse effects of large tidal volume and low PEEP in canine acid aspiration. *Am Rev Respir Dis* 1990;142:311–315.
74. Coker PJ, Hernandez LA, Peevy KJ, et al. Increased sensitivity to mechanical ventilation after surfactant inactivation in young rabbit lungs. *Crit Care Med* 1992;20:635–640.
75. Adkins WK, Hernandez LA, Coker PJ, et al. Age affects susceptibility to pulmonary barotrauma in rabbits. *Crit Care Med* 1991;19:390–393.
76. Muscedere JG, Mullen JBM, Slutsky AS. Tidal ventilation at low airway pressures can augment lung injury. *Am J Respir Crit Care Med* 1994;149:1327–1334.
77. Mead J, Takisima T, Leith D. Stress distribution in lungs: A model of pulmonary elasticity. *J Appl Physiol* 1970;28:596–608.
78. Lachmann B. Open the lung and keep the lung open (editorial). *Intensive Care Med* 1992;18:319–321.
79. Haake R, Schlichtig R, Ulstad DR, Henschen RR. Barotrauma: Pathophysiology, risk factors, and prevention. *Chest* 1987;91:608–613.
80. Pierson DJ. Alveolar rupture during mechanical ventilation: Role of PEEP, peak airway pressure, and distending volume. *Respir Care* 1988;33:472–479.

81. Trapnell DH, Thurston G. Unilateral pulmonary oedema after pleural aspiration. *Lancet* 1970;1:1367–1369.
82. Demling RH, Staub NC, Edmunds LH Jr. Effects of end-expiratory airway pressure on accumulation of extravascular lung water. *J Appl Physiol* 1975;38:907–912.
83. Bshouty Z, Ali J, Younes M. Effect of tidal volume and PEEP on rate of edema formation in in situ perfused canine lobes. *J Appl Physiol* 1988;64:1900–1907.
84. Nolop KB, Braude S, Taylor KM, Royston D. Epithelial and endothelial flux after bypass in dogs: Effect of positive end-expiratory pressure. *J Appl Physiol* 1987;62:1244–1249.
85. Albert RK. Non-respiratory effects of positive end-expiratory pressure. *Respir Care* 1988;33:464–469.
86. van der Zee H, Cooper JA, Hakim TS, Malik AB. Alteration in pulmonary fluid balance induced by positive end-expiratory pressure. *Respir Physiol* 1986;64:125–133.
87. Egan EA. Response of alveolar epithelial solute permeability to changes in lung inflation. *J Appl Physiol* 1980;49:1032–1036.
88. Egan EA. Lung inflation, lung solute permeability, and alveolar edema. *J Appl Physiol* 1982;53:121–125.
89. Qvist J, Pontoppidan H, Wilson RS, et al. Hemodynamic responses to mechanical ventilation with PEEP. *Anesthesiology* 1975;42:45–55.
90. Fewell JE, Abendschein DR, Carlson CJ, et al. Continuous positive-pressure ventilation decreases right and left ventricular end-diastolic volumes in the dog. *Circ Res* 1980;46:125–132.
91. Scharf SM, Caldini P, Ingram RH Jr. Cardiovascular effects of increasing airway pressure in the dog. *Am J Physiol* 1977;232:H35-H43.
92. Jardin F, Farcot JC, Boisante L, et al. Influence of positive end-expiratory pressure on left ventricular performance. *N Engl J Med* 1981;304:387–392.
93. Liebman PR, Patton MT, Manny J, et al. The mechanism of depressed cardiac output of positive end-expiratory pressure (PEEP). *Surgery* 1978;83:594–598.
94. Hall SV, Johnson EE, Hedley-White J. Renal hemodynamics and function with continuous positive-pressure ventilation in dogs. *Anesthesiology* 1974;41:452–461.
95. Manny J, Justice R, Hechtman HB. Abnormalities in organ blood flow and its distribution during positive end-expiratory pressure. *Surgery* 1979;85:425–432.
96. Brienza N, Revelly JP, Ayuse T, Robotham JL. Effects of PEEP on arterial and venous blood flows. *Am J Respir Crit Care Med* 1995;152:504–510.
97. Shapiro HM, Marshall LF. Intracranial pressure responses to PEEP in head-injured patients. *J Trauma* 1978;18:254–256.
98. Lodato RF. Oxygen toxicity. *Crit Care Clin* 1990;6:749–765.
99. Clark JM, Lambertsen CJ. Pulmonary oxygen toxicity: A review. *Pharmacol Rev* 1971;23:37–133.
100. Halliwell B. Superoxide and superoxide dependent formation of hydroxyl radicals are important in oxygen toxicity. *Trends Biochem Sci* 1982;7:270–274.
101. Klein J. Normobaric pulmonary oxygen toxicity. *Anesth Analg* 1990;70:195–207.
102. Tobin MJ. Respiratory monitoring in the intensive care unit. *Am Rev Respir Dis* 1988;138:1625–1642.
103. Barker SJ, Tremper KK. The effect of carbon monoxide inhalation on pulse oximetry and transcutaneous PO_2. *Anesthesiology* 1987;66:677–679.
104. Barker SJ, Tremper KK, Hyatt J. Effects of methemoglobinemia on pulse oximetry and mixed-venous oximetry. *Anesthesiology* 1989;70:112–117.
105. Yelderman M, New W. Evaluation of pulse oximetry. *Anesthesiology* 1983;59:349–352.
106. Scheller MS, Unger RJ, Kelner MJ. Effects of intravenously administered dyes on pulse oximetry readings. *Anesthesiology* 1986;65:550–552.
107. Hanowell L. Ambient light affects pulse oximeters. *Anesthesiology* 1987;67:864–865.
108. Swedlow D, Irving S. Monitoring and patient safety. In Blitt C (ed): *Monitoring in Anesthesia and Critical Care Medicine*. New York: Churchill Livingstone; 1990:50.
109. Snyder J, Elliot L, Grevnik A. Capnography. In Spence A (ed): *Clinics of Critical Care Medicine*. Edinburgh: Churchill Livingstone; 1982:100.
110. Gudipati CV, Weil MH, Bisera J, et al. Expired carbon dioxide: A noninvasive monitor of cardiopulmonary resuscitation. *Circulation* 1988;77:234–239.
111. Trevino RP, Bisera J, Weil MH, et al. End-tidal CO_2 as a guide to successful cardiopulmonary resuscitation: A preliminary report. *Crit Care Med* 1985;13:910–911.
112. Tobias JD, Meyer DJ. Noninvasive monitoring of carbon dioxide during respiratory failure in toddlers and infants: End-tidal versus transcutaneous carbon dioxide. *Anesth Analg* 1997;85:55–58.

Chapter 5

Alternative Modes of Respiratory Support

Thomas V. Brogan, MD and Lynn D. Martin, MD

Introduction

The application of mechanical ventilation to critically ill patients has proven to be a life-saving advance for their care. However, it has also become evident that mechanical ventilation itself can cause pulmonary injury. This pulmonary injury includes alterations in lung fluid balance, increases in endothelial and epithelial permeability, changes in surfactant functions, and microscopic changes that do not differ considerably from the diffuse alveolar damage observed in the acute respiratory distress syndrome (ARDS). Initially, ventilator-induced lung injury (VILI) was believed to be due to the high pressures often employed to ventilate patients with acute lung injury or ARDS.[1] This pressure injury became known as barotrauma. More recently, animal model studies have demonstrated that damage is also produced by overdistention of normal respiratory units even with fairly low distending pressures.[2] This form of VILI is termed volutrauma.

The concept of VILI has spurred the search for alternative therapies that would limit pulmonary injury while providing or improving gas exchange. Consequently, nonconventional forms of mechanical ventilation such as high-frequency ventilation (HFV) and liquid ventilation using a conventional ventilator have been developed and employed at various levels. Alternatively, pharmacologic agents such as surfactant and nitric oxide (NO) have also become important adjuncts to mechanical ventilation, often decreasing the pressure and volume requirements of patients with severe pulmonary disease. When these measures fail, respiratory and cardiovascular function can be temporarily supported via the use of extracorporeal circulation of blood through an artificial lung. This chapter reviews the alternatives to conventional mechanical support for respiratory failure, and their recent advances.

High-Frequency Ventilation

HFV employs very small tidal volumes, often less than anatomic dead space, at supraphysiologic rates (up to 900 breaths/min). HFV attempts to limit damage to airways and alveoli by decreasing the large phasic swings of pressure and volume that are present with conventional mechanical ventilators.

HFV can be divided into four different categories (Table 1): 1) high-frequency positive pressure ventilation (HFPPV); 2) high-frequency oscillatory ventilation (HFOV); 3)

From: Tobias JD (ed): *Pediatric Critical Care: The Essentials*. ©Futura Publishing Co., Inc., Armonk, NY, 1999.

Table 1

Technical Features of the Methods of High-Frequency Ventilation

Feature	HFPPV	HFJV	HFOV	HFFI
Flow generator	high-pressure gas source	high-pressure gas source	piston pump or acoustic speaker	high-pressure gas source
Fresh gas delivery system	continuous or valved gas flow	jet catheter continuous bias flow	continuous gas flow	valved flow interrupter
Tidal volume	> dead space	> or < dead space	< dead space	> or < dead space
Expiratory phase	passive	passive	active	passive
Airway pressure waveform	variable	triangular	sine wave	triangular
Gas entrainment	none	possible	none	none
Frequency (cycles/min)	60–150	60–600	60–3600	300–1200

HFPPV = high-frequency positive pressure ventilation; HFJV = high-frequency jet ventilation; HFOV = high-frequency oscillatory ventilation; HFFI = high frequency flow interruptor.

Table 2

Characteristics of Available High-Frequency Ventilatory Devices

Ventilator	Classification*	Control mean P_{aw}†	Expiratory Phase	Frequency (Hz)	Inspiratory Time
Sensor Medics *3100A*	HFOV	direct	active	3–15	variable
Senko Med. Instr. *Humming II*	HFOV	direct	active	2–15	fixed
Bunnell *Life Pulse*	HFJV	indirect	passive	4–11	variable
Infrasonics *Infant Star HFV*	HFFI	indirect	active‡	2–22	fixed
Bird Space Tech. *PVDR-4*	HFFI	indirect	passive	2–22	variable

Modified with permission from Clark RH. High-frequency ventilation. *J Pediatr* 1994;124:661.
*HFOV = high-frequency oscillatory ventilator; HFJV = high-frequency jet ventilator; HFFI = high frequency flow interrupter.
†mean P_{aw} = mean airway pressure.
‡active exhalation with a venturi-type device attached.

high-frequency jet ventilation (HFJV); and 4) high-frequency flow interrupters (HFFI). The majority of data on HFV have involved the use of one of five high-frequency ventilators (Table 2). The principal differences between these devices relate to the control of mean airway pressure and expiration.

High-Frequency Positive Pressure Ventilation

Originally developed as a method to limit blood pressure fluctuations while maintaining gas exchange with positive pressure mechanical ventilation, HFPPV uses conventional mechanical ventilators with low-compliance circuit tubing to deliver small tidal volumes at nonconventional rates (>60 breaths/min).[3] This system uses a pneumatic valve to deliver compressed gas during inspiration while allowing passive exhalation. Tidal volumes are typically 3 to 4 mL/kg and respiratory frequency range from 60 to 150 breaths per minute with inspiratory-to-expiratory ratios of 0.3. Caution must be exercised when increasing frequency because tidal volume delivery may be compromised such that actual alveolar ventilation decreases despite an absolute increase in minute ventilation.[4] Some clinicians have used this form of HFV very effectively for children with ARDS, demonstrating survival rates of 89%.[5]

High-Frequency Oscillatory Ventilation

HFOV, developed by Lunkenheimer and colleagues,[6] uses a piston that generates small tidal volumes (1 to 3 mL/kg) at very high rates, usually greater than 5 Hz (300 breaths/min). Ventilation occurs through variable pressure oscillations around a set mean pressure with both active inspiration and expiration through movement of the piston. HFOV, when used with a high lung volume strategy, limits lung damage compared to conventional mechanical ventilation (CMV), including atelectasis, hyaline membrane formation, and interstitial and alveolar infiltrates.[7] HFOV also appears to decrease the level of inflammatory activation in the lungs that results from mechanical ventilation. Animal models of saline lavage, surfactant-depletion lung injury have shown decreased granulocytes, platelet-activating factor, thromboxane B_2, and tumor necrosis factor-α in the fluid from bronchoalveolar lavage.[7-10]

Initial clinical experience with HFOV occurred mainly in neonates.[11-13] The first large study of HFOV in 673 premature neonates with respiratory distress syndrome showed no decrease in the incidence of bronchopulmonary dysplasia in the infants who received HFOV.[11] Furthermore, those infants who were treated with HFOV demonstrated a significantly increased occurrence of pneumoperitoneum, intraventricular hemorrhage (IVH; grades 3 and 4), and periventricular leukomalacia. However, the study was criticized on the basis that adequate lung volumes were not achieved in the patients on HFOV, as the strategy attempted to minimize mean airway pressure and lung volume.[14]

The "high-volume" technique currently recommended for HFOV aims to recruit airways and alveoli by providing an adequate mean airway pressure (P_{aw}) when the patient is placed on the ventilator.[7] The initial P_{aw} is higher than the P_{aw} on CMV. The P_{aw} is then kept at levels to prevent atelectasis while simultaneously avoiding pulmonary overdistention as assessed by lung expansion on chest x-rays. This high lung volume strategy has been shown in animal studies to be less destructive to lung tissue while providing improved gas exchange.[7] Based on these findings, further studies using high lung volume strategies in neonates were performed and showed an improvement in oxygenation and a decrease in the incidence of chronic lung disease and airleak.[12,13]

Studies in the pediatric population have shown both the usefulness and difficulties of HFOV. Arnold et al[15] prospectively evaluated the application of the "high-volume" strategy of HFOV as a rescue therapy in seven pediatric patients with diffuse alveolar disease or pulmonary airleak syndrome. Six of the seven children responded and five survived to discharge. Four patients had hemodynamic measurements at the time of conversion to HFOV with no evidence of significant compromise. Rosenberg et al[16] then reported a post hoc analysis of data collected both retrospectively and prospectively on 12 children with acute lung injury unresponsive to CMV, who were treated with either HFOV or HFFI. They found that both methods of HFV improved gas exchange while survivors had more rapid and sustained improvements in oxygenation than nonsurvivors and a shorter duration of CMV prior to initiation of HFV. Six of seven patients treated with HFOV survived.

The first prospective, randomized, multicenter, controlled study comparing HFOV and CMV in pediatric patients with diffuse alveolar disease and/or airleak syndrome was published in 1994.[17] The study compared the strategy of "ideal" lung volume HFOV with low peak inflation pressures, best positive end-expiratory pressure CMV. Both strategies were designed to achieve optimal lung recruitment and to minimize VILI. HFOV was shown to improve oxygenation and ranked outcome (survival, survival with chronic lung disease) compared to CMV. Age and oxygenation index (OI) at 24 hours were both independent variables that predicted survival. Furthermore, an OI of greater than 42 at 24 hours of HFOV was suggested by the authors as a potential indicator of absence of response to HFOV, thus identifying patients who might benefit from alternative forms of therapy early in the course of their disease process when maximum benefit may still be derived.

More recently, Sarnaik and colleagues[18] treated 31 children with severe acute respiratory failure with either HFOV (20 patients) or HFJV (11 patients). Unlike previous studies, they started patients on HFOV at the same mean P_{aw} as CMV. The researchers found improvements in both ventilation and oxygenation associated with an increase in mean P_{aw} by 6 hours on HFV. They also found that an initial OI of ≤20 correlated with 100% survival. Patients who had an initial OI greater than 20 and who failed to show a decrease in OI by greater than 20% at 6 hours had an 88% mortality. A preliminary study of HFOV in adults has shown the efficacy of this modality in larger patients.[19]

Gas exchange during HFOV is believed to be a complex interplay of a number of different mechanisms.[20] A thorough discussion of this complex physiology is beyond the scope of this chapter but is well reviewed by Chang.[20] As a result of bulk convection, a certain percentage of alveoli may be reached by each tidal breath, producing direct ventilation of those alveoli. Differential time constants of various lung units may lead to asynchronous filling and emptying of lung units, known as Pendelluft. This inhomogeneity of time constants with differential filling is greatly exaggerated during HFOV, producing extensive Pendelluft in the lung. Another mechanism depends on asymmetric velocity profiles in the bifurcating system of airways in the lungs. Hence, after successive cycles of oscillatory flow, a gas particle is displaced through the lung. Taylor-type dispersion, also known as augmented diffusion, states that dispersion of material in a conduit results from the interaction of axial velocity profile and the radial concentration gradient. Finally molecular diffusion, resulting from random thermal oscillation of gas molecules, causes gas exchange across the alveolar-capillary membrane and contributes to the transport of oxygen and carbon dioxide in the gas phase near the membrane.

The use of HFOV is associated with certain risks. Concerns have been raised about hemodynamic compromise due to decreased venous return to the heart,[21] although reports of the use of HFOV show little hemodynamic deterioration.[15,17] Airleak[15] and gas trapping[22] have also been documented. Neuromuscular blockade is often required to prevent loss of lung volume with spontaneous respiration. Pulmonary compliance is difficult to assess with standard measures. Pulmonary toilet may also be problematic during HFOV because it may be accompanied by loss of lung volume. Extreme bradycardia of unknown etiology in patients on HFOV has also been reported.[23] Despite these concerns, HFOV appears to offer excellent respiratory support for ARDS, airleak syndrome, and other pulmonary diseases such as pulmonary hemorrhage.[24]

There remain no clear-cut criteria identifying those patients who should be placed on HFOV. Such decisions are based on the bedside clinician's experience and familiarity with various forms of ventilatory support. When switching from conventional to HFOV, the settings are quite different. It is generally recommended, based on the success of the "high volume" technique, to start with a P_{aw} of 4 to 8 cm H_2O greater than the value currently being generated by conventional ventilation. Optimal lung volume is reached once there is an increase in the oxygen saturation, thereby allowing weaning of the fraction of inspired oxygen (FiO_2) to 0.6 or less. A chest x-ray is obtained in 1 to 2 hours and the P_{aw} is adjusted to obtain an expansion of the lung fields to T_{8-9} in neonates and T_{9-10} in older patients. The frequency is set based on the patient's weight, and is generally not adjusted except when other maneuvers fail to lower the partial pressure of arterial carbon dioxide ($PaCO_2$). The recommended frequencies based on weight are provided in the information manual that accompanies the ventilator. The percent-inspiratory time is also generally held constant at 33%. As the inspiratory time is a percentage of the respiratory cycle, increasing the frequency (going from 7 to 8 Hz) will decrease the absolute inspiratory time, decrease the excursion of the diaphragm, and lead to an increase in the

PaCO$_2$. The other settings on the ventilator are the amplitude or ΔP. Increasing the power increases the ΔP. A power setting of 4 is recommended for pediatric patients, and 2 for neonates. Once the ventilator is connected to the patient, the power is adjusted to provide adequate movement of the chest. The chest should vibrate down to the level of the groin. The ΔP is increased in increments of 5 cm H$_2$O to achieve adequate carbon dioxide removal. If a point is reached where the ΔP is three times greater than the P$_{aw}$, the frequency is decreased by 1. As mentioned previously, when switching from conventional ventilation to HFOV, especially when using the high volume technique to recruit alveoli, careful attention must be paid to cardiovascular status. Due to the increase in P$_{aw}$ and the resultant increase in intrathoracic pressure, cardiovascular compromise may occur. If adequate cardiovascular function, manifested by appropriate urine output and peripheral perfusion, cannot be maintained with volume loading, invasive hemodynamic monitoring should be considered.

High-Frequency Jet Ventilation

The indications for the use of HFJV appear to be less well developed than those for HFOV. The use of HFJV also seems to vary considerably between institutions and practitioners. HFJV employs high-velocity jets of air that are injected into the patient's airway at rates of up to 600 breaths per minute. The devices currently used are listed in Table 2. Newer models of HFJ ventilators have been developed that no longer require specialized endotracheal tubes (ETTs), thereby eliminating the need to change an ETT in a critically ill patient. These ventilators can be used by replacing the 15-mm adaptor at the end of the ETT to allow for the measurement of P$_{aw}$ and adjustment of the ventilator parameters. As with HFOV, the P$_{aw}$ is adjusted to achieve the desired oxygen saturation and PaCO$_2$. Alterations of the inspiratory time and breath frequency are used only when the desired levels of oxygenation and ventilation cannot be achieved with adjustments of the P$_{aw}$.

Reports in neonates have demonstrated that persistent bronchopleural airleak is a commonly accepted indication for the use of HFJV.[25] Theoretically, HFJV might be beneficial with persistent airleak because it does not depend on mass gas flow for ventilation. However, studies have been divided on this point. In a multicenter trial of neonates with pulmonary interstitial emphysema, Keszler and colleagues[25] found that survival was significantly better with HFJV only when used in patients who failed CMV and crossed over to HFJV. There are both successful and unsuccessful reports of the use of HFJV for airleak syndrome in older children.[26–28] Clearly, definitive evidence of the effectiveness of HFJV in airleak syndrome is lacking.

HFJV has also been shown to support gas exchange in patients with severe lung disease.[29–32] There are few definitive comparisons of HFJV to CMV in the pediatric population. The aforementioned study by Sarnaik et al[18] utilized HFJV in 11 patients and HFOV in 20 others. The results were reported for both groups without breakdown of the device used. Again, ventilation and oxygenation improved by 6 hours of HFV for the entire group. OI ≤20 appeared to correlate with 100% survival, and failure to improve by 6 hours was suggestive of a poor outcome. Smith and colleagues[29] described 29 children treated with HFJV for progressive respiratory failure and volutrauma. HFJV resulted in a survival rate of 69%. Survivors in this study spent a shorter time on CMV prior to the initiation of HFJV. Other reports also suggest a role for HFJV in severe hypoxemic respiratory failure, but there is a lack of hard evidence with prospective randomized studies to demonstrate its potential superiority to other modes of ventilation for acute lung injury.[29-32]

HFJV has also been suggested to improve cardiovascular hemodynamics in patients who have undergone repairs of cardiac defects. Meliones et al[33] found that HFJV, by providing similar ventilation and oxygenation with a 50% lower mean airway pressure, actually improved cardiac function in children who had undergone the Fontan procedure. Yet other reports suggest that HFJV does not contribute to improved hemodynamics in children undergoing cardiac surgery.[34] Cardiac output does seem to be improved by adjusting P_{aw} by use of higher rates and lower tidal volumes.[35]

Like HFOV, HFJV may be subject to many or all of the complications of CMV, such as volutrauma. Additionally, a severe necrotizing tracheitis has been reported in association with HFJV.[36] This type of injury may have been most commonly associated with inadequate humidification of the gas flowing from the jet orifice.

High-Frequency Flow Interrupters

Although HFFI ventilators have been marketed, there are little clinical data available. Similar to HFJV, with HFFI small tidal volumes (2 to 5 mL/kg) are delivered at high frequency (300 to 1200 breaths/min) by interrupting flow or a high-pressure gas source.[37] As with HFJV, expiration is passive. No injector jet cannula or specialized ETT or gas entrainment is required during HFFI.

Nitric Oxide

NO was originally believed to be simply a component of air pollution, but over the past decade NO has proven to be a particularly versatile biologic messenger molecule, almost ubiquitous in its tissue distribution. NO is produced by the action of the enzyme nitric oxide synthase (NOS). L-arginine is oxidized to citrulline with the production of NO[38] (Fig. 1). There are three isoforms of NOS: endothelial NOS (eNOS), inducible NOS (iNOS), and neuronal (nNOS).[39] eNOS and nNOS are constitutive

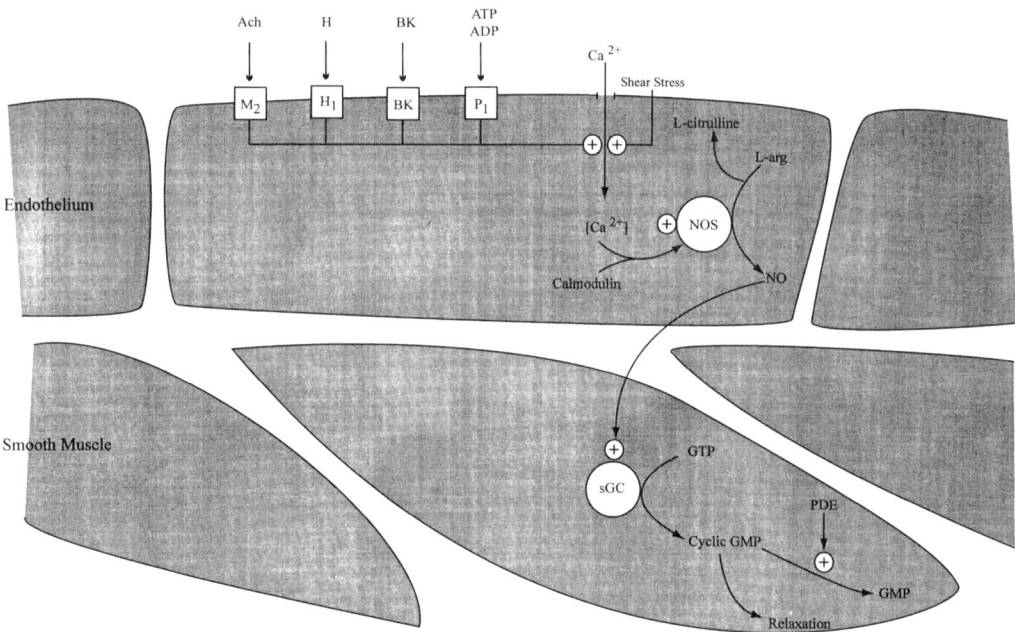

Figure 1. Cross-sectional diagram of a typical blood vessel. Note the endothelial surface receptors (muscarinic-M_2, histamine-H_1, bradykinin-BK, purinoreceptor-P_1) that, when stimulated, cause an increase of intracellular calcium concentration. The calcium stimulates the enzyme nitric oxide synthase (NOS) to produce nitric oxide (NO) from L-arginine (L-arg). The lipid-soluble NO diffuses into the vascular smooth muscle and binds to soluble guanylate cyclase (sGC), causing the production of cyclic guanosine monophosphate (cGMP). The cGMP activates a protein kinase that leads to vascular smooth muscle relaxation.

enzymes that consistently produce small amounts of NO, require calcium and calmodulin, and augment their production of NO in response to certain stimuli, including: 1) binding of effector molecules, like acetylcholine or bradykinin, to receptors; 2) increases in sheer stress; and 3) changes in pH. In contrast, iNOS is regulated at the level of gene transcription. Production of the enzyme is activated by stimuli such as endotoxin and certain cytokines (tissue necrosis factor-α). These stimuli result in upregulation of the enzyme itself, which produces NO in quantities several times higher than the constitutive enzyme.

In both the pulmonary and systemic vasculatures, NO is produced by endothelial cells and acts by stimulating smooth muscle guanylate cyclase with the resultant production of cyclic guanosine monophosphate (cGMP). This cGMP results in the relaxation of smooth muscle cells and in vasodilation.[38,40] Hemoglobin, however, rapidly and avidly binds NO, thereby inactivating it. Consequently, when NO is delivered by inhalation, it can act selectively at the level of the pulmonary vasculature because it becomes inactivated before it can produce systemic vasodilation such as hypotension. Thus, it has been seen as a potential therapy for conditions in which pulmonary hypertension plays an important role, such as persistent pulmonary hypertension of the newborn (PPHN), following certain congenital cardiac surgeries, and ARDS.

In a multicenter, randomized trial in 58 newborns with PPHN, iNO was found to improve systemic oxygenation.[41] The initial dose of iNO was 80 ppm. The improvement in oxygenation, as measured by the decrease in OI, was proportional to the degree of hypoxemia at baseline. This improvement in oxygenation was sustained in 75% of the infants during long-term administration of iNO. The duration of iNO therapy was less than 2 days in half the infants and the longest treatment was 8.5 days. The need for extracorporeal membrane oxygen (ECMO) was 40% in the iNO group compared to 71% in the control group. Other studies[42–44] have shown generally favorable responses to iNO in infants with PPHN: results include improved oxygenation and decreases in pulmonary artery pressure without decreases in systemic blood pressure; there does, however, appear to be a heterogeneity of responses.[45,46]

In a group of full-term and nearly full-term infants with respiratory failure, inhaled NO resulted in a significant decrease in the number of patients requiring ECMO.[47] The NO group also experienced a significant improvement in PaO_2 and OI, but there was no difference in mortality. Other studies of inhaled NO in respiratory failure have measured response to iNO in terms of gas exchange.[48,49] iNO appears to enhance pulmonary gas exchange, usually at doses of 20 ppm or less. Such studies have showed no advantage to higher doses of iNO (ie, 80 ppm). One study showed a positive correlation between early response to iNO and patient outcome.[48] The authors suggested that this might be due to the reversibility of the pulmonary pathophysiologic condition.

Inhaled NO has also been employed in the treatment of hypoxemic respiratory failure and ARDS. The results of a phase II trial of the use of iNO in adult patients with ARDS were recently reported.[50] Patients received 1.25, 5.0, 20.0, 40.0, or 80.0 ppm iNO. All treatment groups except those patients receiving 1.25 ppm had significantly improved oxygenation during the first 4 hours of iNO therapy compared to controls. There was also a statistically significant improvement in pulmonary artery pressure during this period. There continued to be improvement in oxygenation at 3 days of iNO therapy as measured by the OI, but not by the PaO_2/FiO_2. Patients receiving 5 ppm iNO had improved outcomes compared to all other treatment groups and to placebo controls as measured by mortality, the number of days alive and off mechanical ventilation, or the number of days alive after meeting oxygenation criteria for extubation. There were no differences in the other treatment groups and placebo controls in any of these outcome measures. There were also no differences in the number or type of adverse events.

NO has also been used in pediatric patients who suffer pulmonary hypertension following repair of congenital cardiac defects.[51–59] Studies have examined the effect of iNO on arterial oxygenation, pulmonary artery pressure, and pulmonary vascular resistance. Although there is a great deal of variety in the types of cardiac defects and measurements, iNO appears to decrease pulmonary artery pressure and to improve oxygenation. The reduction in pulmonary artery pressure often seems to be proportional to the extent of pulmonary hypertension. To date, there are no prospective, randomized, placebo-controlled trials of the use of iNO in these patients.

The complications of iNO are few. Methemoglobinemia and oxides of nitrogen (NO_x) are concerns, as iNO is readily oxidized and can also oxidize hemoglobin to methemoglobin. Nitrogen dioxide (NO_2) produces histologic changes to the lung at doses of 25 ppm and, in animals, doses of 500 ppm have produced pulmonary edema, hemorrhage, and death.[60] Clinical studies to date have shown this to be a relatively minor concern. However, levels of methemoglobin and NO_2 should be monitored when using iNO.

Another problem that has recently been appreciated is a resurgence of pulmonary artery pressures and resistance to weaning from or withdrawal of iNO in patients with persistent pulmonary hypertensive disorders.[61,62] If the underlying pulmonary hypertensive process has not resolved, then the tendency for an abrupt increase in pulmonary artery pressure may be hazardous if NO therapy must be withdrawn or interrupted.[63–65] Withdrawal of NO before resolution of the pathologic process may also result in hemodynamic instability. The reason(s) for this rebound in pulmonary artery pressure is unclear, but it may be due to suppression of endogenous production of NO from the pulmonary endothelium.[66] Negative feedback inhibition by iNO has been demonstrated for inducible[67] and endothelial[68] NOS. Alternatively, inhaled NO may modulate production of endogenous pulmonary vasoconstrictors or alter membrane receptor conformation in vascular smooth muscle, which could account for its withdrawal effects.

Despite the promising results and the overwhelming enthusiasm, NO remains an investigational drug and has yet to be approved by the Food and Drug Administration for any indication. Controlled clinical trials demonstrating clinical benefit are needed before initiation of its widespread clinical use.

Surfactant Replacement

Abnormalities of surfactant production in premature infants and the importance of replacement therapy have been appreciated for some time. Likewise, abnormalities of surfactant composition and function have been found in patients with ARDS, bacterial pneumonia, and viral pneumonitis.[69,70] Proteins such as albumin, hemoglobin, fibrinogen, and fibrin, which leak into the alveoli, interfere with the organization of the surfactant monolayer. Furthermore, many inflammatory mediators present in the lungs of patients with ARDS can directly damage surfactant.[71]

The findings of abnormal surfactant function and concentration were the basis for the application of surfactant therapy to patients with acute lung disease. In a prospective, multicenter, randomized, placebo-controlled trial involving 725 adults with sepsis-induced ARDS, there was no difference in survival at 30 days of aerosolized synthetic surfactant.[72] In several smaller studies in children, the results were more promising. One study of 19 children with ARDS showed that surfactant alone and surfactant in combination with iNO had positive outcomes.[73] In another multicenter study of 29 children with acute hypoxemic respiratory failure, after the first dose of surfactant, in 24 of the 29 patients there was immediate improvement in oxygenation and moderation of ventilator support.[74] The remaining doses had a modest effect, but the overall mortality was 14%. Definitive randomized controlled trials are lacking.

Liquid Ventilation

Liquids instilled into the lungs reduce the normal air-liquid surface tension found in the lungs. In addition, chemically inert perfluorocarbons have excellent oxygen and carbon dioxide solubilities. Based on these findings, the use of perfluorocarbons to fill alveoli of injured lungs and to assist with gas exchange has been investigated in the laboratory and in the clinical setting. Perflubron[R] (Alliance Pharmaceuticals, San Diego, CA) is the only perfluorocarbon specifically approved for medical use. Perflubron is not readily absorbed across the alveolar membrane. Since it readily evaporates, frequent reinstillation is required. Oxygenation and ventilation can be achieved by filling the lungs completely with the perfluorocarbon and ventilating with the liquid at slow rates using either gravity or a liquid ventilator (total liquid ventilation [TLV]). Another method, known as perfluorocarbon-associated gas exchange (PAGE), or partial liquid ventilation (PLV), fills the lungs to functional residual capacity with perfluorocarbon and then uses a standard mechanical ventilator for gas tidal ventilation.

With liquid ventilation, both infant and adult animal models of ARDS have shown improved oxygenation, ventilation, and lung compliance.[75–78] Histologically there is reduction of alveolar lung fluid accumulation, inflammatory infiltration, and disruption of the alveolar-capillary membrane.[75,79] In some studies, survival was also improved with liquid ventilation.

Clinical experience, however, remains limited. The initial clinical study was in moribund premature infants, and demonstrated only that liquid ventilation could be applied safely in the clinical arena.[80] In two follow-up studies,[81,82] children received PLV while on ECMO. Over the 96 hours after the initial dose, oxygenation improved and all children survived. Complications included pneumothoraces in two children. Several large, randomized, multicenter, controlled clinical trials of PLV have been started in infants, children, and adults with various forms of lung injury. Unfortunately, all of these studies were suspended (temporarily?) when preliminary data from the controlled pediatric trial revealed a lower than expected mortality rate in the control group.

Extracorporeal Life Support

Extracorporeal life support (ECLS) is a term used to describe prolonged but temporary provision of heart and/or lung function with the use of mechanical devices. This technology originated nearly 50 years ago with the development of the first mechanical heart-lung machine, by Gibbon and Kirklin, for operations on the heart.[83,84] While many investigators converged on the apparatus as a means to develop the field of cardiac surgery, others focused on modifying the device itself to allow prolonged partial support of heart and/or lung function. The 1960s and 1970s were periods of rapid progression and discovery of the use of prolonged ECLS that proceeded in three distinct phases. The first phase, in the 1960s, evolved around the use of ECLS as an alternative to the recently developed mechanical ventilator for treatment of respiratory failure in preterm and term infants.[85,86] These attempts failed, primarily based on a high incidence of intracranial hemorrhage. The second phase, in the early 1970s, was characterized by the use of this technology in adults with acute respiratory failure. This period was culminated by the National Institutes of Health sponsored, randomized clinical trial of ECLS that was terminated early secondary to a less than 10% survival rate in both control and ECLS groups.[87] Further investigations with the use of ECLS in adult and pediatric populations in the United States virtually ended with the publication of the study. The third phase, in the late 1970s, focused on the use of this developing technology in term neonates with reversible forms of respiratory failure and pulmonary hypertension.[88] The success of this work led to the widespread application of ECLS in this population, with an estimated mortality rate of greater than 80% and an overall survival rate of greater than 80%.[89] Today, there are more than 100 centers and over 15,000 patients around the world who have been successfully treated with these techniques. This success has led to a resurgence of interest in this technique as an alternative form of therapy for severe cardiac and/or respiratory failure in older children and adults.

Classification of ECLS

Most classification schemes for ECLS focus on the site of blood withdrawal and return. Three distinct options are available: 1) venoarterial (VA) ECLS, where blood is typically withdrawn from the right jugular vein and returned via the right carotid artery; 2) venovenous (VV) ECLS, in which blood is withdrawn from the jugular or femoral vein and returned to the jugular or femoral vein; and 3) arteriovenous (AV) ECLS in which blood is withdrawn from an artery and returned to a vein. For all practical purposes, AV ECLS remains an experimental tool and will not be considered further. Although VA ECLS remains the most popular method of ECLS, the use of VV ECLS is increasing, particularly in the pediatric and adult populations. Both VA and VV ECLS have unique technical and physiologic aspects (Table 3). VA ECLS is associated with higher levels of PaO_2, a significant amount of right and left ventricular support, and relatively low levels of ECLS flow. Unfortunately, these benefits are associated with significant risks that include ligation of a large artery (right common carotid), risk of arterial embolization, and decreased pulmonary arterial blood flow. In VV ECLS, in which blood is withdrawn and returned to the venous side of the circulation, systemic blood flow and oxygen delivery are dependent on intrinsic cardiac output. Because of various amounts of "recirculation," VV ECLS usually requires higher flow rates to maintain adequate oxygenation, if the pulmonary vascular bed is nonfunctional. Thus, VV ECLS eliminates the risks of arterial ligation and embolization while improving mixed venous oxygen saturation, but requires the function of the right and left ventricles in the face of pulmonary hyper-

Table 3

Comparison of Venoarterial (VA) and Venovenous (VV) Extracorporeal Life Support (ECLS)

Parameter	VA ECLS	VV ECLS
Cannulation site:		
Drainage	right jugular vein	right jugular or femoral vein
Return	right common carotid artery	right jugular or femoral vein
Typical ECLS flows	100–120 mL/kg/minute	125–150 mL/kg/minute
Gas exchange:		
PaO_2	60–150 mm Hg	45–80 mm Hg
$PaCO_2$	35–50 mm Hg (CO_2 added)	35–50 mm Hg (CO_2 added)
Ventilator requirements	allows complete lung rest	requires inflated lungs
Cardiac effects:		
Preload	decreased	no change
Afterload	increased	no change
Contractility	"cardiac stun syndrome"	no change or improved
Pulse pressure	decreased	no change
Coronary oxygen delivery	decreased (dependent on LV flow)	increased
Systemic oxygen delivery	high	moderate
Circulatory support	partial to complete	minimal (may improve cardiac output)
Vasopressor requirement	rarely	common in first several days
Pulmonary circulation:		
Total blood flow	decreased	no change
Pulm. arterial saturation	no change	increased
Right-to-left shunt	decreased SaO_2 in aorta	increased SaO_2 in aorta
Left-to-right shunt	may cause pulmonary congestion and/or systemic hypotension	may cause pulmonary congestion and/or systemic hypotension

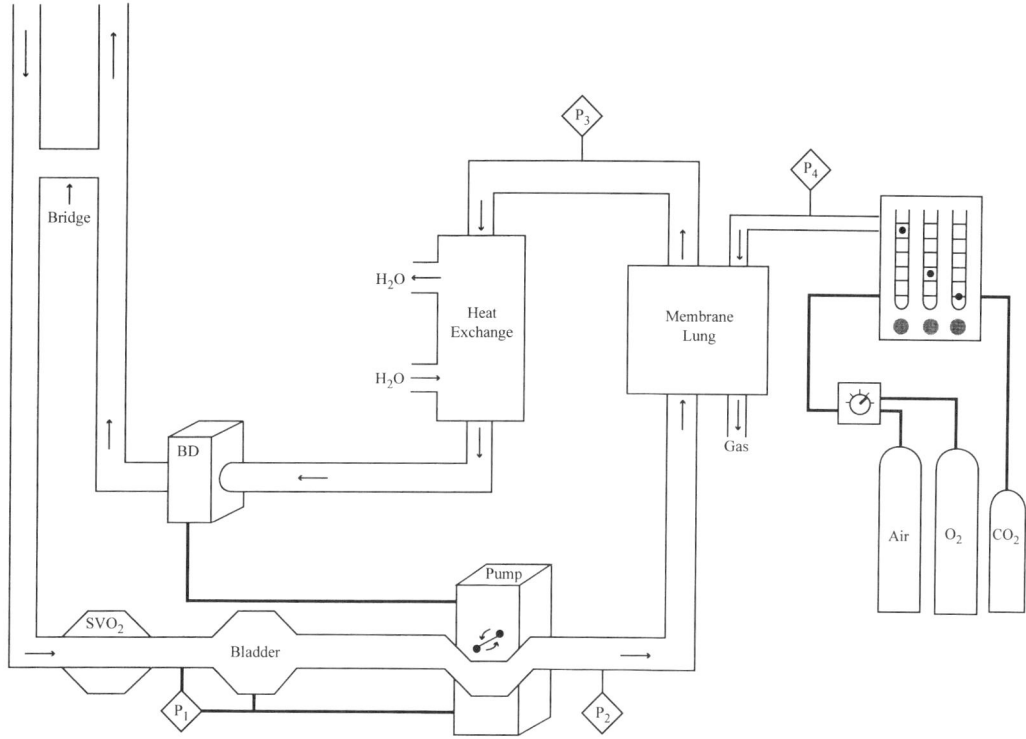

Figure 2. Schematic representation of a typical extracorporeal life support circuit. Blood drains from the venous cannula, through a venous saturation monitor (SVO_2), through the distensible bladder into the membrane lung via the roller head pump. Oxygenated blood exits the membrane and is warmed through the heat exchanger, passes through the bubble detector (BD) that is capable of servoregulating pump power, and back to the patient via the infusion cannula. Note the four possible locations of pressure monitors: P_1 = venous pressure monitor, which can be used to servoregulate the pump; P_2 = premembrane pressure; P_3 = postmembrane pressure; and P_4 = sweep gas pressure. Sweep gas flow is controlled by calibrated flow meters, gas concentration is controlled by blenders, and oxygen concentration is monitored with an in-line analyzer. Not included in the diagram are multiple ports throughout the circuit for sampling blood or injection of medications and/or blood products.

tension for systemic oxygen delivery. Regardless of the method selected, cannulation is typically extrathoracic. Although, initially the vessels used were ligated, the recent trend has been to attempt salvage and repair of at least the carotid artery at the time of decannulation.

Despite the variation in drainage and return sites, the equipment used to provide ECLS is remarkably similar. The standard ECLS circuit is composed of three main components: mechanical pump, artificial lung, and heat exchanger. There are also numerous other devices attached to the circuit as safety monitors (eg, pressure transducers, oximeters, bubble detectors, etc.). A typical ECLS circuit is schematically shown in Figure 2. Each component is discussed separately.

Cannulae

The size of the drainage cannula is the rate-limiting factor that determines the blood flow rate and, hence, the level of ECLS. The flow-pressure characteristics of a given cannula are determined by a number of geometric factors including length, internal diameter, and side hole placement.

A standardized means for comparing pressure-flow characteristics (M number) has been described.[90] To maximize blood flow capability, the largest possible cannula is inserted, typically into the right internal jugular vein, providing direct access to the right atrium. Drainage (venous) cannulae range in size from 8F to 40F and in length from 22 to 50 cm, to accommodate neonatal to adult patients. The size of the arterial cannula is less critical, although it must be large enough to tolerate the predicted blood flow rate without generating an excessive proximal circuit pressure (ie, premembrane pressure >350 mm Hg). Arterial cannulae also vary in size from 8F to 21F and in length from 12 to 37 cm, to accommodate all patients sizes. Arterial cannulae differ in construction from venous cannulae by their lack of side holes. Catheters, both arterial and venous, that can be percutaneously inserted, thereby avoiding the need for surgical incision, have recently been developed and released for use.

Pumps

The vast majority of ECLS programs use a roller pump for extracorporeal perfusion. Because application of high negative pressures to the drainage circuit can cause hemolysis, endothelial damage, and cavitation as air is drawn out of solution, a small (typically about 30 mL) distensible bladder is incorporated on the venous side of the circuit. This venous bladder provides a small reservoir of blood when pump flow exceeds blood flow draining from the venous cannula. The bladder also uses a spring-loaded switching device that interrupts power to the roller pump when the bladder collapses (ie, servoregulation of the mechanical pump) thereby decreasing the risk of entrainment of air and air embolism. An alternative method for roller pump servoregulation involves the use of a pressure monitor which signals reduction in venous circuit pressure and interrupts pump power. Complications related to roller pumps include pump malfunction (neonatal 2%, pediatric 4%, adult 7%), hemolysis (3% to 12%) frequently related to the occlusion pressure with which the roller heads compress the "raceway tubing," and "raceway rupture" (neonatal 1%, pediatric and adult 7%). To avoid this latter complication, most programs will advance or "walk the raceway" on a scheduled basis determined by the revolutions per minute of the roller heads.

A small number of ECLS programs use centrifugal pumps to generate flow via a spinning rotor that is magnetically coupled to a motor. Venous drainage is dependent on suction generated by the rotor (negative pressures as high as –200 to –700 mm Hg), which can produce cavitation and hemolysis. Centrifugal pumps have the advantage of not being able to generate high positive pressures with distal occlusion; this minimizes the likelihood of circuit rupture.

Artificial Lungs or Membrane Oxygenators

The success of ECLS is directly related to the design and performance of the artificial lung. The optimal design requirements for the artificial lung include: 1) maximal oxygen transfer capabilities due to minimal blood film thickness and membrane thickness with secondary flow for blood mixing; 2) large gas space to allow water condensation without compromising carbon dioxide elimination; 3) low compliance to maintain a constant blood volume; 4) large blood path cross-sectional area to minimize blood flow resistance and the translung circuit pressure drop; 5) small priming volume to minimize blood product exposure; 6) ease of debubbling the lung to allow rapid institution of ECLS; and 7) blood flow characteristics to minimize the development of thrombosis, hemolysis, and blood element activation.

There are currently three types of commercially available artificial lungs: bubble oxygenators, membrane lungs, and hollow fiber devices. Bubble oxygenators were the original gas exchange devices developed for short-term extracorporeal support for operative procedures. While they are easily primed and have low pressure-flow characteristics and cost, they are not useful for prolonged ECLS because of increased thrombogenicity, variable blood volume, and increased hemolysis and thrombocytopenia due to direct exposure of blood to gas. The standard gas exchange device used for prolonged ECLS remains the spiral wound silicone membrane lung developed by Kolobow in 1963.[91] This membrane lung is composed of two sheets of silicone sealed at the edges, which are wound up on a polycarbonate spool and have connector tubing at opposite ends. Blood enters and flows across one side of the silicone membrane while on the opposite side gas (oxygen and sometimes air and carbon dioxide) flows. Membrane lungs that are available range in size from 0.4 to 4.5 m^2 surface area and are approved for use for prolonged ECLS. In general, they meet most of the desirable design characteristics, although they require moderate systemic anticoagulation to minimize thrombosis and have relatively high pressure-flow (resistance) characteristics. Hollow fiber artificial lungs use a woven, microporous, capillary-sized hollow fiber through which gas is channeled while blood flows around and among the fibers as oxygen and carbon dioxide are exchanged. Although the gas exchange efficiency of the hollow fiber lungs is far superior to that of the membrane lung, their use is limited by the increased rate of water condensation in the gas phase and the frequent need for lung replacement due to the development of plasma leak. Artificial lung failures that require replacement occur more commonly in children and adult patients due to the increased duration of ECLS in those populations (neonatal 5%, pediatric 17%, and adult 23%).

Heat Exchangers

Because a significant amount of heat is lost through evaporation of water as blood flows through the artificial lung, it is frequently necessary to warm the patient on ECLS. This is typically accomplished by incorporation of a heat exchanger into the ECLS circuit after the artificial lung, to rewarm blood before it returns to the patient. This is particularly true for the maintenance of normothermia in the newborn requiring ECLS. The majority of programs use a narrow tubular device in which blood flows through the inside of stainless steel conduits while warm water flows in a countercurrent manner on the outside. Heat exchange failure is a rare complication of prolonged ECLS (neonatal 1%, pediatric 4%, and adult 7%).

Safety Devices

A number of devices that have become standard parts of the extracorporeal circuit are intended to provide safety and/or monitoring functions. The vast majority of ECLS programs monitor circuit pressure in up to four locations (prepump, premembrane lung, postmembrane lung, and sweep gas into the membrane lung). As discussed previously, the first site can be used to servoregulate the pump power to prevent large negative pressures and air entrainment. The pre- and postmembrane pressures are used to identify distal occlusion or membrane lung thrombosis (ie, increased transmembrane pressure drop). Many programs also use a bubble detector to halt pump flow when bubbles 0.3 to 1.0 mL in size and 0.002 to 0.1 mL in volume are detected. Fortunately, bubbles are rarely detected, perhaps because each circuit has three potential bubble traps incorporated into the design (the distensible bladder, the artificial lung, and the heat exchanger). The gas flow to the membrane lung is regulated by calibrated (low-flow) flow meters with a pressure pop-off valve (neonatal 50 mm Hg, pediatric and adult 100 mm Hg) to control gas composition and prevent the potentially disastrous complication of air embolus by keeping gas pressure less than the blood pressure in the membrane lung. Some programs also use an oximeter device on the venous (drainage) and the arterial (infusion) side of the circuit to estimate mixed venous and arterial hemoglobin saturation as well as to assist with oxygen delivery consumption estimation.

Clinical Application

Because of its invasive nature, potential for significant complications, and high cost, the use of ECLS is typically reserved for cases of severe cardiorespiratory failure that have failed optimal conventional management but are thought to be reversible if temporary support of cardiac and/or respiratory function is provided. The frequency of severe disease, the ability to define treatment failure, and the potential for reversibility are much greater in the neonatal population; hence, the widespread use of ECLS was initiated in this group. The clinical application, including eligibility criteria and typical management of ECLS, is reviewed separately for the neonatal and pediatric populations, followed by a review of its use for circulatory failure.

The majority of ECLS worldwide continues to be in the neonatal population; however, other forms of cardiorespiratory support such as surfactant replacement, HFOV, and inhaled NO, have resulted in a decrease in the use of ECLS in this population over the last 5 years (Fig. 3). The six most common primary diagnoses for the neonatal group and associated survival rate are shown in Figure 4 and the method used for ECLS is shown in Figure 5.

One of the more controversial topics related to ECLS has been the patient selection criteria. In general, each ECLS center will develop its own eligibility criteria based on a historical review of mortality rates for the common ECLS-related diagnoses. Despite minor variations, several criteria appear to be nearly uniformly accepted based primarily on historical experience, patient safety, and mechanical physics relative to the equipment required (Table 4). The need for systemic anticoagulation for ECLS with the associated risk for intracranial hemorrhage in premature infants limits its application to infants of greater than 33 weeks' complete

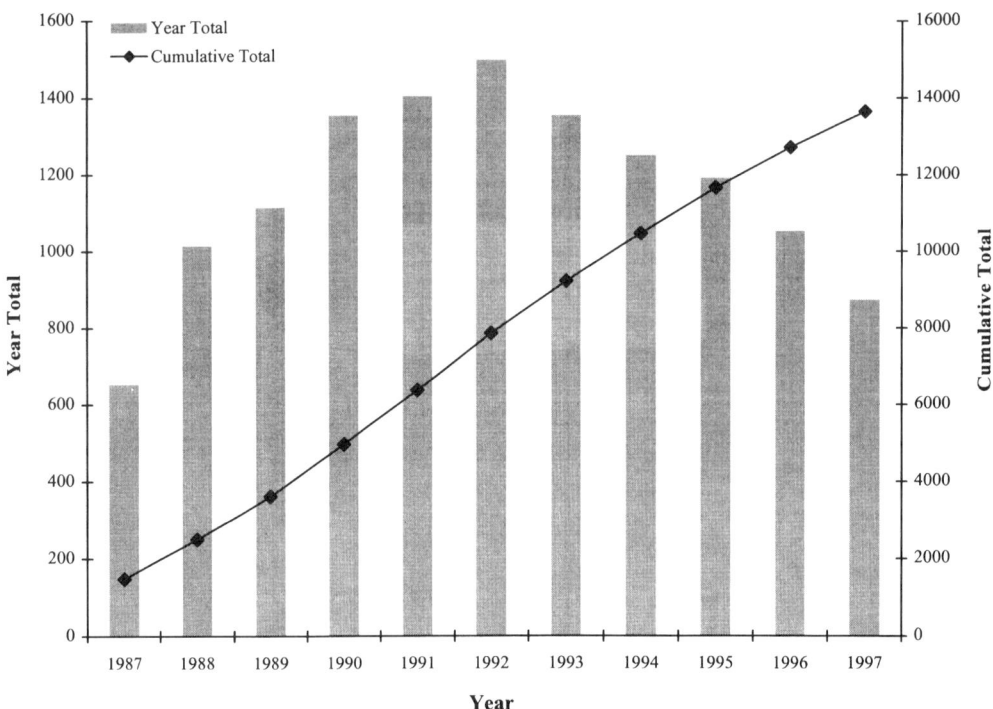

Figure 3. Graphic demonstration of the yearly totals (gray bar) and cumulative totals (solid line) of neonatal extracorporeal life support (ECLS) cases worldwide through 1997. Note the progressive decrease in yearly totals of neonatal ECLS cases over the last 5 years. Data obtained from the Registry Report of the Extracorporeal Life Support Organization (July 1998).

Neonatal ECLS

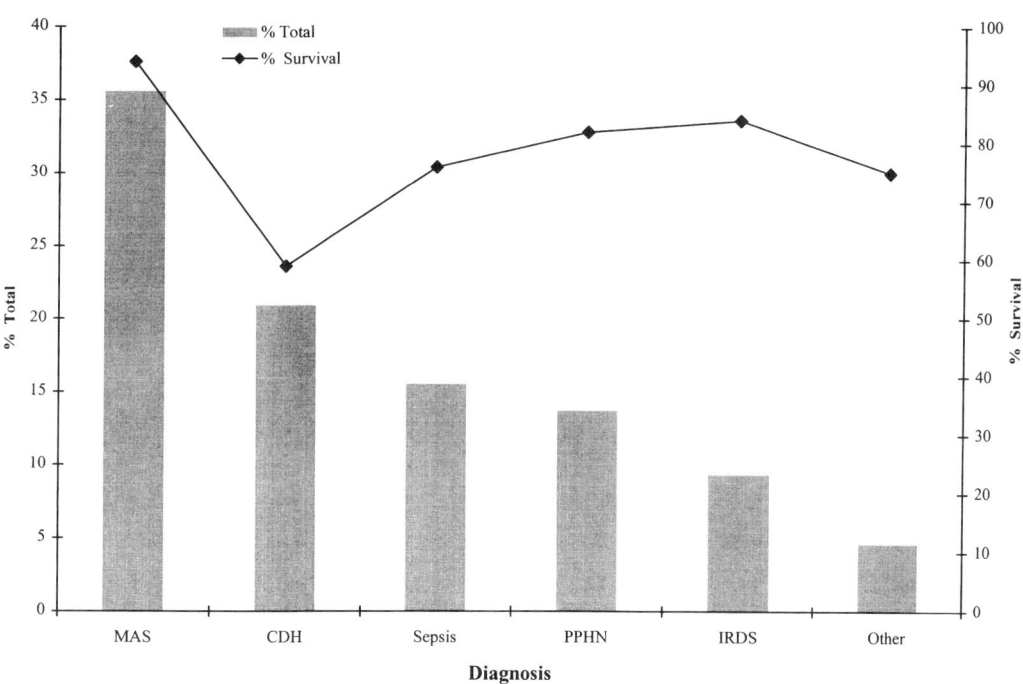

Figure 4. Graphic display of the total percentage for the top six diagnoses leading to the need for neonatal ECLS (gray bar) and their associated survival rates (solid line). Data obtained from the Registry Report of the Extracorporeal Life Support Organization (July 1998).

gestation. Similarly, patients with uncontrolled coagulopathy or preexisting interventricular hemorrhage are at high risk for further bleeding with significant morbidity or mortality. Due the technical difficulties associated with cannulation of small vessels, most programs have a lower size limit of approximately 2000 grams. Every effort should be made to identify the etiology of the cardiorespiratory failure before initiation of ECLS. Complete cardiologic evaluation, including cardiac ultrasound, should be completed prior to initiation of ECLS to rule out correctable congenital cardiac malformation as the cause for respiratory failure and/or PPHN. Furthermore, some conditions, such as pulmonary hypoplasia, alveolar capillary dysplasia, and congenital alveolar proteinosis, are nonsurvivable conditions in which the use of ECLS would only delay an inevitable death. Perhaps most difficult of all the selection criteria is the attempt to define failure of optimal (ie, the most favorable) therapy as opposed to maximal (ie, the greatest or highest possible) therapy. Failure is easily defined in terms of hypoxemia (increased alveolar to arterial oxygen gradient [$AaDO_2$], OI, and PaO_2) or inability to maintain acid-base status (acidosis) or blood pressure. The difficulty comes in determining optimal medical management. Each medical center has a subtly different approach to the care of the critically ill neonate; hence, each center must define its own selection criteria. Currently, optimal medical management in most centers includes conventional mechanical ventilation with sedatives/analgesics with or without neuromuscular blocking agents in addition to pharmacologic support with inotropic agents and/or vasoconstrictors/vasodilators. Many cen-

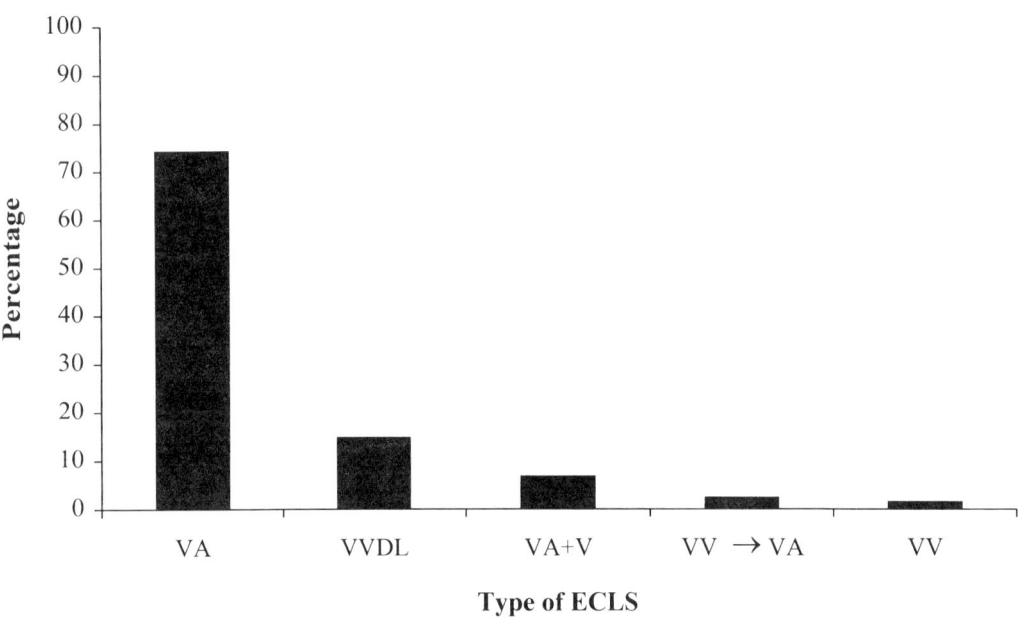

Figure 5. Bar graph representation of the method of neonatal extracorporeal life support. VA = venoarterial; VVDL = double-lumen venovenous; VA + V = venoarterial with additional venous drainage catheter; VV→VA = venovenous converted to venoarterial support; and VV = venovenous. Data obtained from the Registry Report of the Extracorporeal Life Support Organization (July 1998).

Table 4

Patient Selection Criteria for Neonatal ECLS

Gestational age > 33 weeks
Birthweight ≥ 2000 grams
No significant coagulopathy/uncontrolled bleeding
No major intracranial hemorrhage (IVH > grade I)
No major congenital cardiac malformations
No lethal congenital malformations
Severe cardiorespiratory failure unresponsive to <u>optimal</u> conventional medical management
    $AaDO_2$ = alveolar $O_2 - PaO_2 > 600$ mm Hg
    Oxygenation Index (OI) = mean airway pressure $\times$ FiO_2 $\times$ $100/PaO_2 > 40$
    Acute deterioration:
        $PaO_2 < 30$ mm Hg
        pH < 7.20
        intractable hypotension
Reversible cardiorespiratory pathophysiology (ie, limited duration of mechanical ventilation)

ECLS = extracorporeal life support.

ters will also try nonconventional mechanical ventilation (eg, HFPPV, HFJV, HFOV, HFFI, inverse inspiratory/expiratory ratio, etc.) and other pharmacologic interventions (eg, surfactant administration, inhaled NO) prior to considering ECLS. Unfortunately, the multiple choices can often delay initiation of ECLS and may be associated with an increase in chronic lung disease.[92] Hence, many programs attempt to identify the reversible nature of the primary disease process as well as the extent of lung injury as selection criteria.

Over the last two decades two distinct approaches to the application of ECLS for critically ill neonates have been developed, namely VA and VV ECLS. The former required cannulation and ligation of both the internal jugular vein for blood drainage and the common carotid artery for blood return. In an attempt to provide support without arterial ligation, a specialized flexible, thin-walled, double-lumen cannula with channels of unequal size was developed for insertion into the jugular vein for venovenous support (DLVV-ECLS). As routine management varies for each method, both are briefly reviewed.

Following priming of the ECLS circuit, systemic anticoagulation, and cannulation of the vessels, the circuit is connected to the cannula and flow is initiated at a low level (approximately 20 mL/kg/min) and increased as determined by the clinical condition of the patient over a period of minutes. Once the desired flow has been achieved (100 to 150 mL/kg/min), the ventilator should be slowly weaned to minimize further injury to the lungs. The nature of "ideal" pulmonary (ventilator) management during VA ECLS has been the subject of considerable study and debate.[93] Ventilator settings are generally reduced to levels that are believed to be noninjurious (FiO_2 <0.4, peak inspiratory pressure <30 cm H_2O, positive end-expiratory pressure 4 to 20 cm H_2O, and rate 4 to 20 breaths/min). The patient's oxygenation and ventilation are regulated by controlling the concentration of oxygen, nitrogen, and carbon dioxide gas through the artificial membrane (via sweep gas) and native lungs (via the ventilator), and controlling the percentage of cardiac output perfusing the membrane and native lungs (ie, ECLS flow). The rapid improvement in oxygenation and acid-base status commonly associated with the initiation of ECLS will allow the weaning from most or all inotropic and vasoactive medications.

The maintenance phase of ECLS is hopefully characterized by a slow resolution of the primary disease process responsible for the cardiorespiratory failure. Throughout this period, the lowest level of systemic anticoagulation is maintained via a continuous infusion of heparin that is titrated by hourly measurement of the activated clotting time. Thrombocytopenia due to consumption of platelets on the plastic surface of the circuit leads to the need for frequent platelet concentrate transfusions to maintain an arbitrarily defined minimum platelet count. During the first 24 to 72 hours of ECLS, the release of cytokines and other inflammatory mediators commonly causes a sustained capillary leak syndrome with an ongoing fluid administration requirement to maintain intravascular volume, followed by the subsequent development of generalized edema. Following this period, fluid intake is usually restricted to minimize further edema accumulation, with provision of nutrition via either the enteral or parenteral route. Resolution of this process is typically associated with a brisk diuresis that is frequently promoted by the administration of diuretics. Occasionally, persistent edema or progressive renal failure requires incorporation of a hemofiltration circuit into the ECLS circuit itself. Patients will generally require sedatives and/or analgesics to limit agitation and its associated risk for accidental dislodgment of essential equipment. Neuromuscular blocking agents are avoided to allow assessment of neurologic status as well as to promote movement and speed resolution of the edema fluid accumulation. Cranial ultrasounds are used to monitor for possible intracranial hemorrhage.

With resolution of the primary disease process, the amount of ventilator and extracorporeal support required to maintain oxygenation and ventilation decrease until a "trial-off" ECLS can be attempted. In a trial-off ECLS, the patient is placed on ventilator settings that are felt to be acceptable for the postbypass period. Then the venous and arterial lines are clamped while the bridge is opened to allow recirculation of the extracorporeal blood. The cannulae are "flashed" (briefly opened to allow passage of heparinized blood) and patient and circuit activated clotting times checked every 15 minutes to prevent development of thrombi. Vital signs and arterial blood gases are closely monitored throughout the trial-off, which may last up to several hours. Permanent removal from ECLS (decannulation) proceeds following either a successful trial-off, a severe complication preventing further ECLS (ie, IVH, uncontrollable bleeding), or a lack of resolution of the primary or secondary disease process. The decannulation process itself is a relatively straightforward, brief, sterile surgical procedure requiring sedation/analgesia and paralysis. Following discontinuation of ECLS, patients can experience slow ongoing hemolysis and thrombocytopenia for up to 48 hours.

In contrast to VA ECLS, the VV route does not bypass the circulation or provide direct support of ventricular function. Blood flow remains pulsatile in nature. Hence, VV ECLS does not decrease right ventricular preload, pulmonary blood flow, left atrial return, or left ventricular output.[94,95] Contraindications to VV ECLS include myocardial failure following recent cardiac surgery, recent cardiac arrest, or refractory rhythm disturbance associated with systemic hypotension. Despite the lack of direct myocardial support, VV ECLS may indirectly enhance cardiac performance by improving mixed venous oxygen content.[96] Thus, cardiac depression in critically ill neonates will frequently respond well to the institution of VV ECLS.

A second unique aspect of VV ECLS is recirculation. Recirculation fraction is defined as that portion of blood returning from the patient to the ECLS circuit that was just delivered to the patient's right atrium from the ECLS circuit, but returned to the catheter rather than going on to the pulmonary circulation. Factors that affect the recirculation fraction include: 1) pump flow (higher flows lead to higher recirculation fraction); 2) catheter position (proximity of the drainage and return ports increases recirculation fraction); 3) cardiac output (high cardiac output will more quickly remove returned blood, thereby decreasing recirculation fraction); and 4) right atrial size or intravascular volume (a small mixing chamber will lead to a larger recirculation fraction). For the purposes of this discussion, this overview is limited to DLVV ECLS in neonates.

The right jugular vein is cannulated with the 14F Kendall double-lumen cannula oriented such that the arterial side holes will be directed toward the tricuspid valve orifice (arterial arm directed up or anterior to the venous arm). This catheter is limited to flows of less than 600 mL/min, limiting it to patients who weigh less than 4 kg. Simultaneous drainage from a 10F or 12F cephalad-directed internal jugular catheter might extend the useful weight range to 4.5 kg. Circuit flow is initiated at 10 to 15 mL/kg/min and advanced over 10 to 15 minutes up to a maximum of 150 mL/kg/min. Flow is then slowly decreased to reduce the recirculation fraction, and optimal flow is determined by monitoring of patient oxygenation. Most other details of management for VV ECLS are not different than for VA ECLS. The ventilator settings are slowly reduced and inotropic medications weaned as tolerated. The "trial-off" is much more straightforward during VV ECLS as compared to VA ECLS. With the patient on ventilator settings that are acceptable, the gas flow to the membrane is simply "capped off" and serial arterial blood gases are obtained to demonstrate adequate pulmonary function. This form of trial-off can be continued for many hours to ascertain the stability of the pulmonary vascular tone and reactivity, with no additional risk to the patient.

As stated previously, the overall survival rate for neonates requiring ECLS remains close to 80% with an estimated mortality rate of 80%. Survival rates are, not surprisingly, highest with meconium aspiration syndrome (94%) and lowest with congenital diaphragmatic hernia (58%). Approximately 15% of infants treated with ECLS require supplemental oxygen at 28 days of life (the most common criteria defining chronic lung disease or bronchopulmonary dysplasia). Risk factors for the development of chronic lung disease include the primary diagnosis of congenital diaphragmatic hernia, lower birth weight, and age on initiation of ECLS.[92] The rate of sensorineural handicap among ECLS survivors ranges from 2% to 18% (mean 6%) and does not appear to differ significantly from that of other critically ill neonates.[97]

With the worldwide success of neonatal ECLS, the use of this technology has been, in recent years, extended to the pediatric population with increasing frequency (Fig. 6). Unlike the neonatal population, children with severe respiratory failure represent a largely heterogenous population. The most common primary diagnoses for the pediatric group, as well as associated survival rates, are shown in Figure 7. Similar to the neonatal population, the majority of children studied received VA ECLS (76%) while the remainder (24%) received VV ECLS.

Attempts at establishing objective criteria for pediatric ECLS have been problematic due to the diversity and difficulty in determining the primary disease process responsible for severe respiratory failure in children. Several studies from single institutions have served as predictors of mortality for pediatric respiratory failure.[98-101] These studies clearly demonstrate that mortality rates in pediatric patients were much higher for a given oxygenation parameter ($AaDO_2$, OI, etc.) when compared to the neonatal population. Retrospective review of the Extracorporeal Life Support Registry with stepwise, multivariate, logistic regression modeling has demonstrated that patient age and duration of mechanical ventilation prior to the start of ECLS correlated with survival.[102] A large multicenter, prospective study used physiologic data to develop a multivariable prediction tool to estimate mortality within 28 days of diagnosis.[103] De-

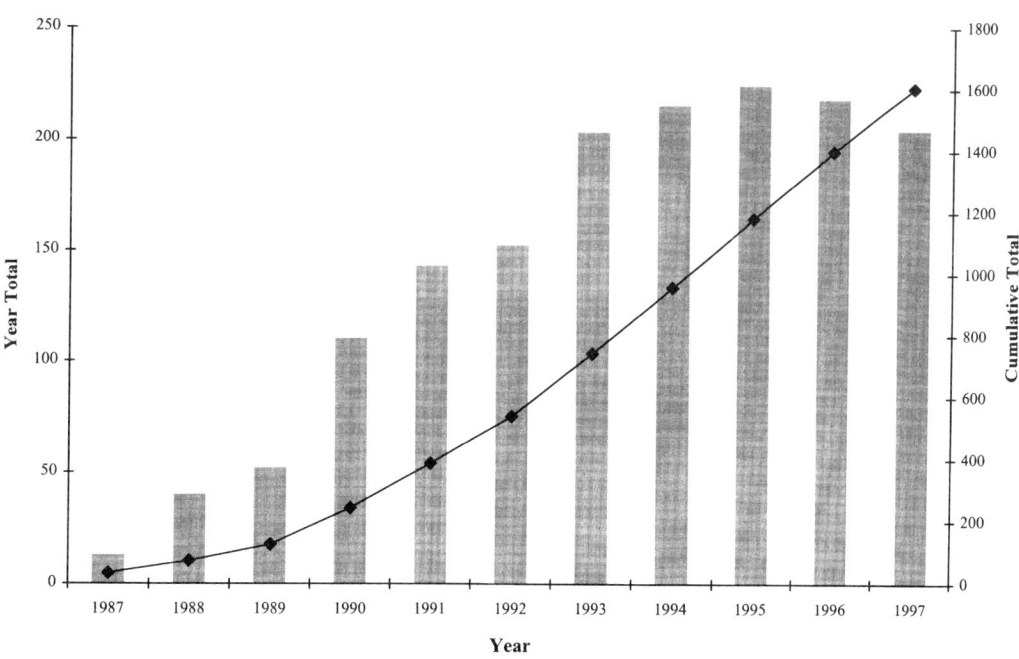

Figure 6. Graphic demonstration of the yearly totals (gray bar) and cumulative totals (solid line) of pediatric extracorporeal life support cases worldwide through 1997. Note that yearly totals have stabilized over the last 4 years. Data obtained from the Registry Report of the Extracorporeal Life Support Organization (July 1998).

Pediatric ECLS

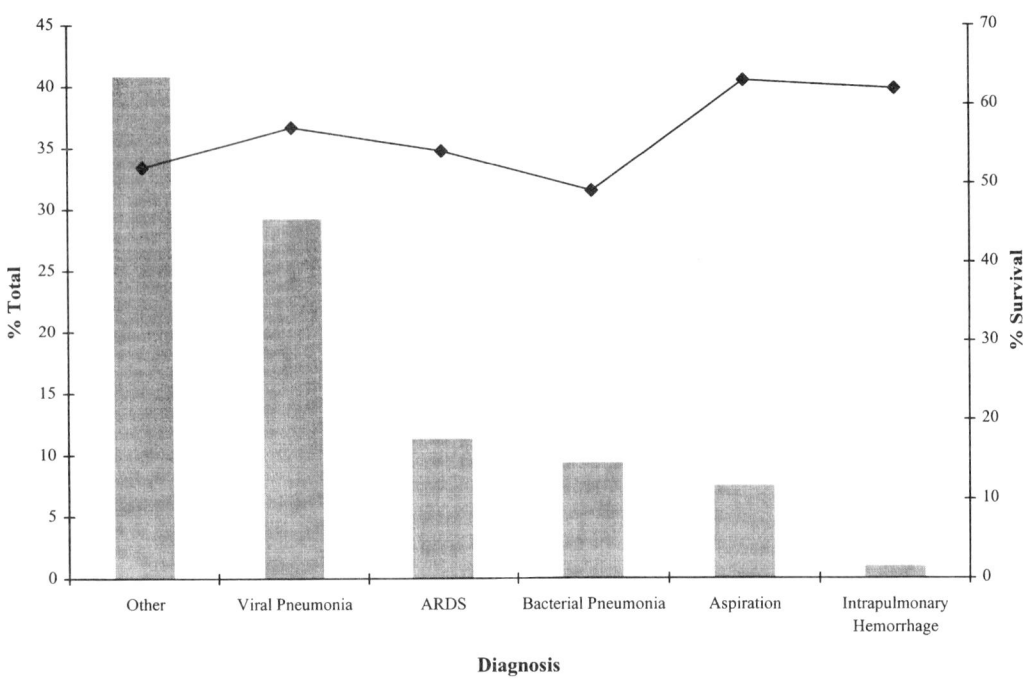

Figure 7. Graphic display of the total percentage for the top six diagnoses leading to the need for pediatric extracorporeal life support (gray bar) and their associated survival rates (solid line). Note that the most commonly listed diagnosis is other, likely representing that no definitive etiology for the respiratory failure was established. Data obtained from the Registry Report of the Extracorporeal Life Support Organization (July 1998).

spite these efforts, uniformly accepted criteria for ECLS in the pediatric population are lacking. Commonly reported criteria are listed in Table 5.

In general, the techniques of cannulation and provision of ECLS differ little from those described for the neonates. Cannula size, circuit size, and membrane surface area increase with the size of the patient. Attempts at VV ECLS will typically require cannulation of two veins. In most cases, the right internal jugular vein is used for drainage of blood that is returned via the right femoral vein into the inferior vena cava. Weaning and withdrawal from ECLS in children is similar to that described for neonates, although the duration of support is generally longer.

As of the end of December 1997, ECLS had been used in 1631 children (883 survivors, 54%), 2 weeks to 18 years of age, for respiratory failure. The yearly totals have been approximately 200 patients each of the last 4 years. The diagnosis leading to the need for ECLS was unknown in 41%, while viral pneumonia (29%) was the most common etiology identified. To date there are very little long-term data on the survivors of ECLS in the pediatric population.

Despite improvements in cardioplegia, cardiopulmonary bypass, surgical techniques, and postoperative intensive care unit care, children still expire from low cardiac output states after cardiac surgery. With the successful clinical application of ECLS for operative repair of congenital heart disease and the subsequent spread of neonatal ECLS worldwide, the use of this

Table 5

Patient Selection Criteria for Pediatric ECLS

No immunosuppression
No significant coagulopathy/uncontrolled bleeding
No acute neurologic injury
Reasonable medical certainty of quality of life
Severe cardiorespiratory failure unresponsive to <u>optimal</u> conventional medical management
   $PaO_2/FiO_2 < 150$
   $AaDO_2 > 450$ mm Hg
   Oxygenation Index (OI) = mean airway pressure $\times$ FiO_2 $\times$ $100/PaO_2 > 30$
   Acute deterioration:
      $PaO_2 < 30$ mm Hg
      pH < 7.28 with peak airway pressure > 40 cm H_2O or airleak syndrome
      intractable hypotension
Reversible cardiorespiratory pathophysiology:
   pulmonary fibrosis on lung biopsy or

Age	Duration of Ventilation
<2 years	≥10 days
2–8 years	≥8 days
>8 years	≥6 days

ECLS = extracorporeal life support.

technology has been logically extended to the pediatric population with primary myocardial dysfunction (Fig. 8). Similar to the pediatric respiratory failure population, children with severe cardiovascular failure represent a largely heterogeneous population. The most common primary diagnoses for the cardiac group, as well as associated survival rates, are shown in Figure 9. Due to the need for support of ventricular function, the vast majority (94%) of children studied received VA ECLS.

The unique response of failing ventricular function during cardiac ECLS must be considered. In the setting of myocardial depression, blood reinfused from the ECLS circuit into the aorta will increase left ventricular afterload, wall stress, myocardial work, and oxygen consumption.[104] Although the right ventricle is decompressed, some forward blood flow from the right ventricle into the pulmonary artery still occurs. This forward flow is frequently increased in the volume-overloaded state following cardiopulmonary bypass. The resultant pulmonary venous return in association with the left ventricular dysfunction and the increased afterload can cause an increase in left ventricular end-diastole pressure and volume and an increase in oxygen demand, and can lead to subendocardial ischemia. Animal studies have also shown that coronary perfusion occurs predominately from the left ventricular output (underscoring the importance of lung inflation and mixed venous saturation for oxygen delivery to the myocardium).[105] Attempts to decompress the left heart by increasing ECLS flow may paradoxically worsen myocardial ischemia in the failing heart by progressively increasing afterload and wall stress before augmenting coronary blood flow with oxygenated blood at high flow rates.[106] Therefore, the need to directly vent or decompress the left heart in the setting of severe left ventricular dysfunction when associated with ventricular dilatation and pulmonary edema is common.

Indications and uniformly accepted criteria for cardiac ECLS are not established. Each ECLS center must develop its own cardiac ECLS criteria. Commonly recognized criteria are listed in Table 6. In general, ECLS is considered for any patient who, despite optimal medical and surgical management, cannot be weaned from cardiopulmonary bypass in the operating room, or in whom a severe, refractory, low cardiac out-

Cardiac ECLS

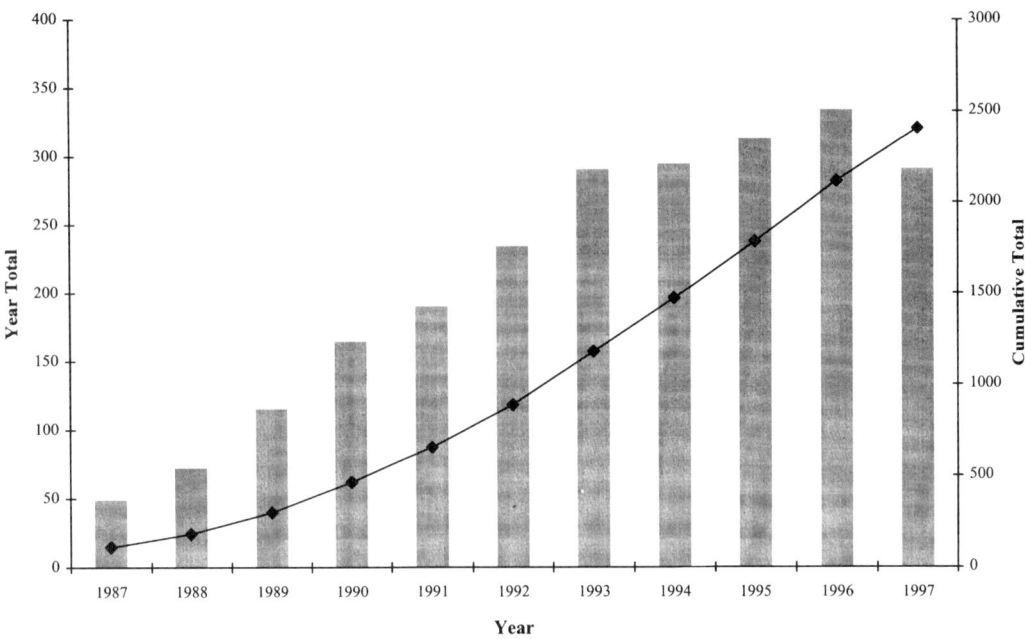

Figure 8. Graphic demonstration of the yearly totals (gray bar) and cumulative totals (solid line) of cardiac extracorporeal life support cases worldwide through 1997. The total number of cases each year has not changed over the last 4 years. Data obtained from the Registry Report of the Extracorporeal Life Support Organization (July 1998).

put syndrome develops in the immediate postoperative period. Other indications include progressive circulatory failure due to cardiomyopathy, myocarditis, or sepsis. Optimal medical management is defined as the provision of adequate ventricular filling pressures, correction of dysrhythmias, and use of inotropic and vasoactive medications to maximize systemic cardiac output and systemic oxygen delivery. Optimal surgical management is defined as the correction of any hemodynamically significant and correctable residual cardiac defect. Possible contraindications include acute neurologic injury, prematurity, irreversible organ injury, or the lack of a reasonable medical certainty of quality of life. While some programs exclude palliated hypoplastic left heart syndrome and shunt-dependent single ventricles,[107] others consider patients with these conditions poor candidates for ECLS, but do not absolutely exclude these patients.[108]

Because of the specific need to provide circulatory support for this population of patients, VA ECLS is used almost exclusively (94%). The majority of patients requiring ECLS for circulatory support are patients who have recently undergone surgical repair of congenital or acquired cardiac disease. Most of these patients are identified in the early postoperative period. Depending on the circumstances, cannulation can be via the standard approach (right internal jugular and common carotid artery) for the postoperative patients, or transthoracic with use of the intraoperative cannulae, if they fail to wean off bypass. The incidence of clinically significant bleeding is much higher in the latter setting. Because of the high risk of bleeding in this postoperative population, efforts are generally made to use the lowest

Cardiac ECLS

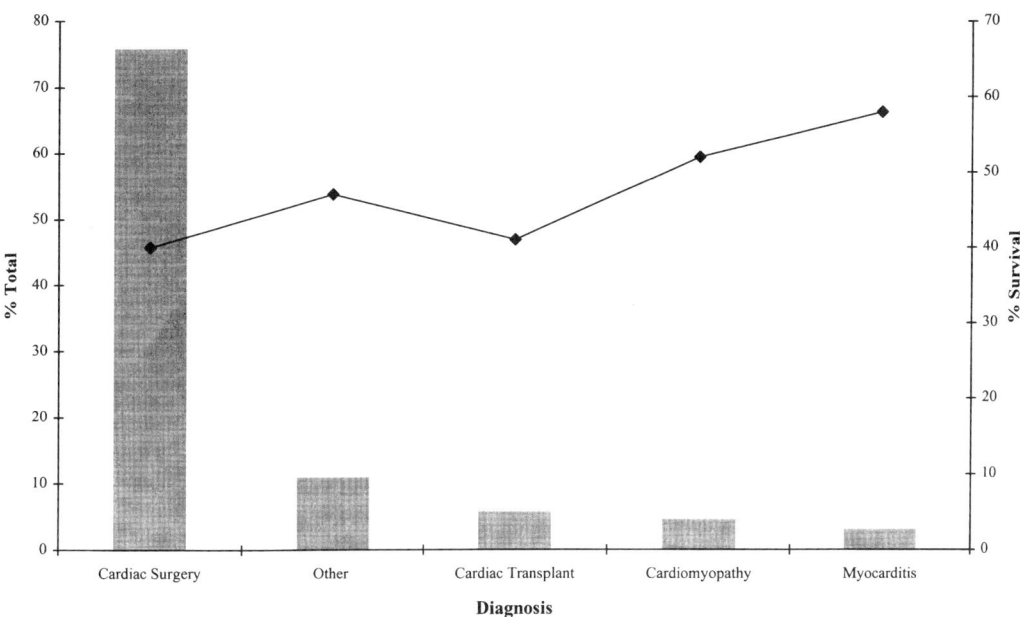

Figure 9. Graphic display of the total percentage for the top five diagnoses leading to the need for cardiac extracorporeal life support (gray bar) and their associated survival rates (solid line). The vast majority of patients had undergone cardiac surgery. Data obtained from the Registry Report of the Extracorporeal Life Support Organization (July 1998).

level of systemic anticoagulation and to very aggressively treat thrombocytopenia.

Regardless of the route of cannulation, several general principles are followed when using ECLS for circulatory support. First, a modest amount of ECLS flow is used to ensure sufficient systemic oxygen delivery, while excessive flows with their associated increase in left ventricular afterload are avoided. Maintenance of lung inflation, alveolar oxygenation, and thus higher mixed venous oxygenation via continued use of supplemental inspired oxygen and mechanical ventilation, are required to assure maximal myocardial oxygen delivery. Immediately following initiation of ECLS in patients with left ventricular failure, it is imperative to obtain an echocardiographic evaluation of left heart size. Evidence of massive ventricular dilatation or pulmonary edema/hemorrhage would be an indication for placement of a left heart drainage catheter or atrial septostomy.

Patients maintained on ECLS for circulatory failure usually undergo daily evaluation to assess return of myocardial function. Specifically, the ECLS flow is slowly decreased over a matter of minutes while monitoring of myocardial function and volume is continuously assessed via surface echocardiography. Should the patient successfully maintain adequate pulse pressure and perfusion with reasonable levels of pharmacologic support, a brief trial-off ECLS can be completed. When the patient is able to sustain sufficient oxygen delivery on acceptable levels of pharmacologic and mechanical ventilatory support during the trial-off, ECLS is discontinued. The duration of ECLS is generally shorter for postoperative circulatory failure (5 to 7 days) than it is for respiratory failure (10 to 21 days). This is likely due to the widely held belief that if myocardial function is recoverable, improvements and the ability to stop ECLS will be seen within 5 days. Use of this tech-

Table 6

Commonly Recognized Patient Selection Criteria for Cardiac ECLS

Gestational age >33 weeks
No acute neurologic injury or intracranial hemorrhage (IVH > grade I)
Reasonable medical certainty of quality of life
Severe cardiovascular failure unresponsive to optimal medical management:
  excessive or increasing ventricular filling pressures
  progressive or intractable hypotension
  oliguria (<0.5 mL/kg/h)/anuria
  elevated core temperature (>38° C) or core/peripheral temperature gradient >10° C
  mixed venous saturation <65%
  persistent or progressive metabolic acidosis
Acute, severe reversible obstructive pulmonary vascular disease unresponsive to optimal medical management
Reversible cardiorespiratory pathophysiology:
  limited duration of mechanical ventilation
  absence of significant correctable residual surgical defect

ECLS = extracorporeal life support.

nology is increasing as a means to provide temporary circulatory support until a suitable donor for cardiac transplantation can be obtained for patients who fail to recover ventricular function. The duration of ECLS for this purpose is obviously much longer, and is limited due to complications such as infections, bleeding, or end-organ failure.

Because of the inherent difficulty in the ability to predict the reversibility of primary cardiovascular dysfunction, the overall survival rate for cardiac ECLS (42%) is lower than that seen for pediatric (54%) or neonatal (80%) respiratory failure. Most investigators have found the major predictor of outcome to be severity of the underlying cardiac defect.[109,110] Reduced survival has also been associated with renal failure, sepsis, bleeding, and the duration of ECLS. More recent work has shown that survival rates with the use of ECLS intraoperatively following palliative procedures were limited (0%) while survival rates were highest for patients requiring ECLS postoperatively following complete repair of their underlying defect (56%). There are currently no data available regarding long-term complications associated with ECLS in the specific patient population.

Summary

Several options exist for the attempt to save the patient with progressive respiratory failure that is unresponsive to conventional mechanical ventilation. These techniques include HFV, NO, liquid ventilation, surfactant administration, and ECLS. One of the problems encountered in the evaluation of such salvage therapy is the lack of large, prospective studies to demonstrate the efficacy of these techniques. Another problem with these nonconventional means of respiratory support is the lack of clear-cut indications for their use, and limited information to demonstrate in which order these techniques should be attempted. Without information to identify those patients at the highest risk of mortality, the exact point at which to switch from conventional to nonconventional techniques remains unclear. Despite such problems, anyone who practices intensive care medicine will have personal anecdotes concerning patients who have survived against all odds with the use of these therapies. Future studies may help us to better use these nonconventional means of respiratory support.

References

1. Webb HH, Tierney DF. Experimental pulmonary edema due to intermittent positive pressure ventilation with high inflation pressures: Protection by positive end-expiratory pressure. *Am Rev Respir Dis* 1974; 110:556–565.
2. Dreyfuss D, Basset G, Soler P, Saumon G. High inflation pressure pulmonary edema: Respective effects of high airway pressures, high tidal volumes, and positive end-expiratory pressure. *Am Rev Respir Dis* 1988;137: 1159–1164.
3. Oberg PA, Sjostrand U. Studies of blood pressure regulation. I: Common carotid artery clamping in studies of the carotid-sinus baroreceptor control of the systemic blood pressure. *Acta Physiol Scand* 1969;75: 276–286.
4. Boros SJ, Bing DR, Mammel MC, et al. Us-

ing conventional infant ventilators at unconventional rates. *Pediatrics* 1984;74:487–497.
5. Paulson TE, Spear RM, Silva PD, Peterson BM. High-frequency pressure-control ventilation with high positive end-expiratory pressure in children with acute respiratory distress syndrome. *J Pediatr* 1996;129:566–575.
6. Lunkenheimer PP, Rafflenbeul W, Keller H, et al. Application of transtracheal pressure oscillations as a modification of "diffusion respiration". *Br J Anaesth* 1972;44:627–631.
7. Hamilton PP, Onayemi A, Smyth JA, et al. Comparison of conventional and high-frequency ventilation: Oxygenation and lung pathology. *J Appl Physiol* 1983;55:131–138.
8. Imai Y, Kawano T, Miyasaka K, et al. Inflammatory chemical mediators during CMV and during high frequency oscillatory ventilation. *Am J Respir Crit Care Med* 1994; 150:1550–1554.
9. Matsuoka T, Kawano T, Miyasaka K. Role of high frequency ventilation in surfactant-depleted lung injury as measured by granulocytes. *J Appl Physiol* 1994;76:539–544.
10. Takata M, Abe J, Tanaka H, et al. Intraalveolar expression of tumor necrosis factor-α gene during conventional and high-frequency ventilation. *Am J Respir Crit Care Med* 1997;156:272–279.
11. HIFI Study Group. High-frequency oscillatory ventilation compared with conventional mechanical ventilation in the treatment of respiratory failure in preterm infants. *N Engl J Med* 1989;320;88–93.
12. Clark RH, Gerstmann DR, Null DM Jr, de Lemos RA. Prospective randomized comparison of high frequency oscillatory and conventional ventilation in respiratory distress syndrome. *Pediatrics* 1992;89:5–12.
13. HiFO Study Group. Randomized study of high-frequency oscillatory ventilation in infants with severe respiratory distress syndrome. *J Pediatr* 1993;122:609–619.
14. Bryan AC, Froese AB. Reflections on the HIFI trial (editorial). *Pediatrics* 1991;87: 565–567.
15. Arnold JH, Truog RD, Thompson JE, Fackler JC. High-frequency oscillatory ventilation in pediatric respiratory failure. *Crit Care Med* 1993;21:272–278.
16. Rosenberg RB, Broner CW, Peters KJ, Anglin DL. High frequency ventilation for acute pediatric respiratory failure. *Chest* 1993;104:1216–1221.
17. Arnold JH, Hanson JH, Toro-Figuero LO, et al. Prospective randomized comparison of high-frequency oscillatory ventilation and conventional mechanical ventilation in pediatric respiratory failure. *Crit Care Med* 1994;22:1530–1539.
18. Sarnaik AP, Meert KL, Pappas MD, et al. Predicting outcome in children with severe acute respiratory failure treated with high-frequency ventilation. *Crit Care Med* 1996; 24:1396–1402.
19. Fort P, Farmer C, Westerman J, et al. High frequency oscillatory ventilation for adult respiratory distress syndrome-a pilot study. *Crit Care Med* 1997;25:37–47.
20. Chang HK. Mechanisms of gas transport during ventilation by high-frequency oscillation. *J Appl Physiol* 1984;56:553–563.
21. Gutierrez JA, Levin DL, Toro-Figuero LO. Hemodynamic effects of high-frequency oscillatory ventilation in severe pediatric respiratory failure. *Intensive Care Med* 1995; 21:505–510.
22. Bancalari A, Gerhardt T, Bancalari E, et al. Gas trapping with high-frequency ventilation: Jet versus oscillatory ventilation. *J Pediatr* 1987;110:617–622.
23. Mellema JD, Baden HP, Martin LD, Bratton SL. Severe paroxysmal sinus bradycardia associated with high-frequency oscillatory ventilation. *Chest* 1997;112:181–185.
24. Baden HP, Li CM, Hall D, et al. High frequency oscillatory ventilation in the management of infants with pulmonary hemorrhage after cardiac surgery. *J Cardiothorac Vasc Anesth* 1995;9:578–580.
25. Keszler M, Donn SM, Bucciarelli RL, et al. Multicenter controlled trial comparing high frequency jet ventilation and conventional mechanical in newborn infants with pulmonary interstitial emphysema. *J Pediatr* 1991;119:85–91.
26. Payne DK, Anderson WM, Romero MD, et al. Tracheosophageal fistula formation in intubated patients: Risk factors and treatment with high-frequency jet ventilation. *Chest* 1990;98:161–164.
27. Rubio JJ, Algora-Weber A, Dominguez de Villota E, et al. Prolonged high-frequency jet ventilation in a patients with bronchopleural fistula. An alternative mode of ventilation. *Intensive Care Med* 1986;12:161–163.
28. Roth MD, Wright JW, Bellamy PE. Gas flow through a bronchopleural fistula. Measuring the effects of high-frequency jet ventilation and chest-tube suction. *Chest* 1988; 93:210–213.
29. Smith DW, Frankel LR, Derish MT, et al. High-frequency jet ventilation in children

with the adult respiratory distress syndrome complicated by pulmonary volutrauma. *Pediatr Pulmonary* 1993;15:279–286.
30. Carlon GC, Howland WS, Ray C, et al. High-frequency jet ventilation: A prospective randomized evaluation. *Chest* 1983;84:551–559.
31. Jonson B, Lachmann B. Setting and monitoring of high-frequency jet ventilation in severe respiratory distress syndrome. *Crit Care Med* 1989;17:1020–1024.
32. Bysani GK, Rucoba RJ, Noah ZL. Treatment of hydrocarbon pneumonitis. High frequency jet ventilation as an alternative to extracorporeal membrane oxygenation. *Chest* 1994;106:300–303.
33. Meliones JN, Bove EL, Dekeon MK, et al. High-frequency jet ventilation improves cardiac function after the Fontan procedure. *Circulation* 1991;84:III364–III368.
34. Davis DA, Russo PA, Greenspan JS, et al. High frequency jet versus conventional ventilation in infants undergoing Blalock-Taussig shunts. *Ann Thorac Surg* 1994;57:846–849.
35. Traverse JH, Korvenranta H, Carlo WA. Effects of ventilatory strategy on cardiac output during high frequency jet ventilation. *Cardiovasc Res* 1991;25:309–313.
36. Boros SJ, Mammel MC, Lewallen PK, et al. Necrotizing tracheobronchitis: A complication of high-frequency ventilation. *J Pediatr* 1986;109:95–100.
37. Frantz ID III, Wertammer J, Stark AR. High-frequency ventilation in premature infants with lung disease: Adequate gas exchange at low tracheal pressures. *Pediatrics* 1983;71:483–488.
38. Palmer RMJ, Ferrige AG, Moncada S. Nitric oxide release accounts for the biological activity of endothelium-derived relaxing factor. *Nature* 1987;327:524–526.
39. Stuehr DJ, Griffith OM. Mammalian nitric oxide synthases. *Adv Enzymol Mol Relat Areas Biol* 1992;65:287–346.
40. Celermajer DS, Dollery C, Burch M, Deanfield JE. Role of endothelium in the maintenance of low pulmonary vascular tone in children. *Circulation* 1994;89:2041–2044.
41. Roberts JD, Fineman JR, Morin FC, et al. Inhaled nitric oxide and persistent pulmonary hypertension of the newborn. The Inhaled Nitric Oxide Study Group. *N Engl J Med* 1997;336:605–610.
42. Roberts JD, Polaner DM, Lang P, Zapol WM. Inhaled nitric oxide in persistent pulmonary hypertension of the newborn. *Lancet* 1992;340:818–819.
43. Kinsella JP, Neish SR, Shaffer E, Abman SH. Low-dose inhaled nitric oxide in persistent pulmonary hypertension of the newborn. *Lancet* 1992;340:819–820.
44. Wessel DL, Adatia I, Van Marter LJ, et al. Improved oxygenation in a randomized trial of inhaled nitric oxide for persistent pulmonary hypertension of the newborn. *Pediatrics* 1997;100:E7.
45. Finer NN, Etches PC, Kamstra B, et al. Inhaled nitric oxide in infants referred for extracorporeal membrane oxygenation: Dose response. *J Pediatr* 1994;124:302–308.
46. Turbow R, Waffarn F, Yang L, et al. Variable oxygenation response to inhaled nitric oxide in severe persistent pulmonary hypertension of the newborn. *Acta Paediatr* 1995;84:1305.
47. The Neonatal Inhaled Nitric Oxide Study Group. Inhaled nitric oxide in full-term and nearly full-term infants with hypoxic respiratory failure. *N Engl J Med* 1997;336:597–604.
48. Goldman AP, Tasker RC, Hosiasson S, et al. Early response to inhaled nitric oxide and its relationship to outcome in children with severe hypoxemic respiratory failure. *Chest* 1997;112:752–758.
49. Demirakca S, Dotsch J, Knothe C, et al. Inhaled nitric oxide in neonatal and pediatric acute respiratory distress syndrome: Dose response, prolonged inhalation, and weaning. *Crit Care Med* 1996;24:1913–1919.
50. Dellinger RP, Zimmerman JL, Taylor RW, et al. Effects of inhaled nitric oxide in patients with acute respiratory distress syndrome: Results of a randomized phase II trial. Inhaled Nitric Oxide in ARDS Study Group. *Crit Care Med* 1998;26:15–23.
51. Roberts JD Jr., Lang P, Bigatello LM, et al. Inhaled nitric oxide in congenital heart disease. *Circulation* 1993;87:447–453.
52. Curran RD, Mavroudis C, Backer C, et al. Inhaled nitric oxide for children with congenital heart disease and pulmonary hypertension. *Ann Thorac Surg* 1995;60:1765–1771.
53. Journois D, Pouard P, Mauriat P, et al. Inhaled nitric oxide as a therapy for pulmonary hypertension after operations for congenital heart defects. *J Thorac Cardiovasc Surg* 1994;107:1129–1135.
54. Yahagi N, Kumon N, Tanigami H, et al. Inhaled nitric oxide for the postoperative management of Fontan-type operations. *Ann Thorac Surg* 1994;57:1371–1373.
55. Miller OI, Celermejer DS, Deanfield JE, Macrae DJ. Very low-dose inhaled nitric ox-

ide: A selective pulmonary vasodilator after operations for congenital heart disease. *J Thorac Cardiovasc Surg* 1994;108:487–494.
56. Beghetti M, Habre W, Friedli B, Berner M. Continuous low dose inhaled nitric oxide for treatment of severe pulmonary hypertension after cardiac surgery in paediatric patients. *Br Heart J* 1995;73:65–68.
57. Morris GN, Lowson SM, Rich GF. Transient effects of inhaled nitric oxide for prolonged postoperative treatment of hypoxemia after surgical correction of total anomalous pulmonary venous return. *J Cardiothorac Vasc Anesth* 1995;9:713–716.
58. Goldman AP, Delius RE, Deanfeld JE, et al. Nitric oxide might reduce the need for extracorporeal support in children with critical postoperative pulmonary hypertension. *Ann Thorac Surg* 1996;62:750–755.
59. Luciani GB, Chang AC, Starnes VA. Surgical repair of transposition of the great arteries in neonates with persistent pulmonary hypertension. *Ann Thorac Surg* 1996;61: 800–805.
60. Greenbaum R, Bay J, Hargreaves MD, et al. Effects of higher oxides of nitrogen on the anaesthetized dog. *Br J Anaesth* 1967;39: 393–404.
61. Atz AM, Adatia I, Wessel DL. Rebound pulmonary hypertension after inhalation of nitric oxide. *Ann Thorac Surg* 1996;62:1759–1764.
62. Francoise M, Gouyon JB, Mercier JC. Hemodynamic and oxygenation changes induced by the discontinuation of low-dose inhalational nitric oxide in newborn infants. *Intensive Care Med* 1996;22:477–481.
63. Grover R Murdoch I, Smithies M, et al. Nitric oxide during hand ventilation in patient with acute respiratory failure (letter). *Lancet* 1992;340:1038–1309.
64. Miller OI, James I, Elliott MJ. Intraoperative use of inhaled low-dose nitric oxide (letter). *J Thorac Cardiovascular Surg* 1993;105:550–551.
65. Lavoie A, Hall JB, Olson D, Wylam ME. Life-threatening effects of discontinuing inhaled nitric oxide in severe respiratory failure. *Am J Respir Crit Care Med* 1996;153: 1985–1987.
66. Goldman AP, Haworth SG, Macrae DJ. Does inhaled nitric oxide suppress endogenous nitric oxide production? *J Thorac Cardiovasc Surg* 1996;112:541–542.
67. Assruey J, Cunha FQ, Liew FY, Moncada S. Feedback inhibition of nitric oxide synthase activity by nitric oxide. *Br J Pharmacol* 1993;108:833–837.
68. Ravichandran LV, Johns RA, Rengasamy A. Direct and reversible inhibition of endothelial nitric oxide synthase by nitric oxide. *Am J Physiol* 1991;268:H2216-H2223.
69. Gregory TJ, Longmore WJ, Moxley MA, et al. Surfactant chemical composition and biophysical activity in acute respiratory distress syndrome. *J Clin Invest* 1991;88: 1976–1981.
70. LeVine AM, Lotze A, Stanley S, et al. Surfactant content in children with inflammatory lung disease. *Crit Care Med* 1996; 24:1062–1067.
71. Seeger W, Gunther A, Walmrath HD, et al. Alveolar surfactant and adult respiratory distress syndrome: Pathogenic role and therapeutic prospects. *Clin Invest* 1993;71: 177–190.
72. Anzueto A, Baughmam RP, Guntupali KK, et al. Aerosolized surfactant in adults with sepsis induced acute respiratory distress syndrome. Exosurf Acute Respiratory Distress Syndrome Sepsis Study Group. *N Engl J Med* 1996;334:1417–1421.
73. Moller JC, Schaible TF, Reiss I, et al. Treatment of severe non-neonatal ARDS in children with surfactant and nitric oxide in a "pre-ECMO" situation. *Int J Artif Organs* 1995;18:598–602.
74. Willson DF, Jiao JH, Bauman LA, et al. Calf's lung surfactant extract in acute hypoxemic respiratory failure in children. *Crit Care Med* 1996;24:1316–1322.
75. Tutuncu AS, Faithfull NS, Lachman B. Intratracheal perfluorocarbon administration combined with mechanical ventilation in experimental respiratory distress syndrome: Dose-dependent improvement in gas exchange. *Crit Care Med* 1993;21:962–969.
76. Leach CL, Fuhrman BP, Morin FC, Rath MG. Perfluorocarbon-associated gas exchange (partial liquid ventilation) in respiratory distress syndrome: A prospective, randomized controlled study. *Crit Care Med* 1993;21:1270–1278.
77. Papo MC, Paczan PR, Fuhrman BP, et al. Perfluorocarbon associated gas exchange improves oxygenation, lung mechanics, and survival in a model of adult respiratory distress syndrome. *Crit Care Med* 1996; 24:466–474.
78. Hernan LJ, Fuhrman BP, Kaiser RE, et al. Perfluorocarbon associated gas exchange in normal and acid-injured large sheep. *Crit Care Med* 1996;24:475–481.
79. Hirschl RB, Tooley R, Parent A, et al. Evaluation of gas exchange, pulmonary compliance, and lung injury during total and par-

tial liquid ventilation in the acute respiratory distress syndrome. *Crit Care Med* 1996;24:1001–1008.
80. Greenspan JS, Wolfson MR, Rubenstein D, Shaffer TH. Liquid ventilation of human preterm neonates. *J Pediatr* 1990;117:106–111.
81. Hirschl RB, Pranikoff T, Gauger PG, et al. Liquid ventilation in adults, children, and full-term neonates. *Lancet* 1995;346:1201–1202.
82. Gauger PG, Pranikoff T, Schreiner RJ, et al. Initial experience with partial liquid ventilation with the acute respiratory distress syndrome. *Crit Care Med* 1996;24:16–22.
83. Hill JD. John H. Gibbon Jr: Part I. The development of the first successful heart-lung machine. *Ann Thorac Surg* 1982;34:337–341.
84. Kirklin JW, Donald DE, Harshburger HG, et al. Studies in extracorporeal circulation. Applicability of Gibbon-type pump-oxygenator to human intracardiac surgery: 40 cases. *Ann Surg* 1956;144:2–15.
85. Rashkind WJ, Freeman A, Klein D, Toft RW. Evaluation of a disposable plastic low volume pumpless oxygenator as a lung substitute. *J Pediatr* 1965;66:94–101.
86. White JJ, Andrews HG, Risenberg H, et al. Prolonged respiratory support in newborn infants with a membrane oxygenator. *Surgery* 1971;70:288–296.
87. Zapol WM, Snider MT, Hill JD, et al. Extracorporeal membrane oxygenation in severe acute respiratory failure. *JAMA* 1979;242:2193–2196.
88. Bartlett RH, Andrews AF, Toomasian JM, et al. Extracorporeal membrane oxygenation (ECMO) in neonatal respiratory failure: 45 cases. *Surgery* 1982;92:425–433.
89. Stolar CJ, Snedecor SS, Bartlett RH. Extracorporeal membrane oxygenation and neonatal respiratory failure: Experience from the extracorporeal life support organization. *J Pediatr Surg* 1991;26:563–571.
90. Montoya JP, Merz SI, Bartlett RH. A standardized system for description flow/pressure relationships in vascular access devices. *ASAIO Transactions* 1991;37:4–8.
91. Kolobow T, Boman RL. Construction and evaluation of an alveolar membrane artificial heart lung. *ASAIO Transactions* 1963;9:238–242.
92. Kornhauser MS, Cullen JA, Baumgart S, et al. Risk factors for bronchopulmonary dysplasia after extracorporeal membrane oxygenation. *Arch Pediatr Adolesc Med* 1994;148:820–825.
93. Keszler M, Subramanian KN, Smith YA, et al. Pulmonary management during extracorporeal membrane oxygenation. *Crit Care Med* 1989;17:495–500.
94. Kolobow T, Spragg RG, Pierce JE. Massive pulmonary infarction during total cardiopulmonary bypass in unanesthetized spontaneously breathing lambs. *Int J Artif Organs* 1981;4:76–81.
95. Martin GR, Short BL. Doppler echocardiographic evaluation of cardiac performance in infants on prolonged extracorporeal membrane oxygenation. *Am J Cardiol* 1988;62:929–934.
96. Strieper MJ, Sharma S, Dooley KJ, et al. Effects of venovenous extracorporeal membrane oxygenation on cardiac performance as determined by echocardiographic measurements. *J Pediatr* 1993;122:950–955.
97. Glass P, Wagner A, Papero P, et al. Neurodevelopmental status at age five years of neonates treated with extracorporeal membrane oxygenation. *J Pediatr* 1995;127:447–457.
98. Rivera RA, Butt W, Shann F. Predictors of mortality in children with respiratory failure: Possible indications for ECMO. *Anaesth Intensive Care* 1990;18:385–389.
99. Tamburro RF, Bugnitz MC, Stidham GL. Alveolar-arterial oxygen gradient as a predictor of outcome in patients non-neonatal pediatric respiratory failure. *J Pediatr* 1991;119:935–938.
100. Timmons OD, Dean JM, Vernon DD. Mortality rates and prognostic variables in children with adult respiratory distress syndrome. *J Pediatr* 1991;119:896–899.
101. Davis SL, Furman DP, Costarino AT Jr. Adult respiratory distress syndrome in children: Associated disease, clinical course, and predictors of death. *J Pediatr* 1993;123:35–45.
102. Moler FW, Palmisano JM, Custer JR. Extracorporeal life support for pediatric respiratory failure: Predictors of survival from 220 patients. *Crit Care Med* 1993;21:1604–1611.
103. Timmons OD, Havens PL, Fackler JC. Predicting death in pediatric patients with acute respiratory failure. Pediatric Critical Care Study Group. Extracorporeal Life Support Organization. *Chest* 1995;108:789–797.
104. Bavaria JE, Ratcliffe MB, Gupta KB, et al. Changes in left ventricular systolic wall stress during biventricular circulatory assistance. *Ann Thorac Surg* 1988;45:526–532.
105. Kinsella JP, Gerstman DR, Rosenberg AA. The effect of extracorporeal membrane oxygenation on coronary perfusion and regional blood flow distribution. *Pediatr Res* 1992;31:80–84.

106. Secker-Walker JS, Edmonds JF, Spraftt EH, Conn AW. The source of coronary perfusion during partial bypass for extracorporeal membrane oxygenation (ECMO). *Ann Thorac Surg* 1976;21:138–143.
107. Weinhaus L, Canter C, Noetzel M, et al. Extracorporeal membrane oxygenation for circulatory support after repair of congenital heart defects. *Ann Thorac Surg* 1989;48:206–212.
108. Dalton HJ, Siewer RD, Fuhrman BD, et al. Extracorporeal membrane oxygenation for cardiac rescue in children with severe myocardial dysfunction. *Crit Care Med* 1993;21:1020–1028.
109. Ziomek S, Harrell JE, Fascules JW, et al. Extracorporeal membrane oxygenation for cardiac failure after congenital heart operation. *Ann Thorac Surg* 1992;54:861–867.
110. Raithel SC, Pennington DG, Boegner E, et al. Extracorporeal membrane oxygenation in children after cardiac surgery. *Circulation* 1992;86:II305-II310.

Chapter 6

Acute Respiratory Distress Syndrome in Children

J. Steven Hata, MD

Introduction

The acute respiratory distress syndrome (ARDS) is a severe form of acute lung injury that is a major cause of morbidity and mortality in both pediatric and adult intensive care units (ICUs). Although originally described as the *adult* respiratory distress syndrome, it clearly affects the pediatric age group. This chapter reviews the fundamentals in the pathophysiology, diagnosis, and management of this syndrome, which can account for a significant proportion of pediatric ICU mortality.

Diagnostic Criteria

In the pediatric age group, the differential diagnosis of severe respiratory failure can be extensive. ARDS should be considered, particularly in any severely ill child with significant risk factors associated with severe direct or indirect lung injury (as defined below). To simplify establishment of the diagnosis, the American-European Consensus Conference on ARDS has recommended four major diagnostic criteria: 1) the period of onset; 2) severity of hypoxemia; 3) chest radiography; and 4) absence of left atrial hypertension (Table 1).[1] The latter distinguishes ARDS (noncardiogenic pulmonary edema) from cardiogenic pulmonary edema in patients with left ventricular dysfunction.

ARDS develops acutely after a temporally related risk factor (such as severe trauma, bacteremia, hypotension) and persists for days to weeks. Hypoxemia is severe, often refractory to oxygen therapy. The oxygenation index (PaO_2/FiO_2), a ratio of the oxygen tension from an arterial blood gas to the concentration of inspired oxygen, is typically less than 200 mm Hg. Other forms of acute lung injury can have presentations and radiographic findings that are similar to ARDS, but lack the severity of hypoxemia.

Physical examination findings are not specific in the child who is developing ARDS, and include dyspnea, tachypnea, cyanosis, rales, and, frequently, hypotension with accompanying septic shock. The initial evaluation should assess the need for mechanical ventilation and hemodynamic support, and potential sources of infection. In addition, urgent diagnostic evaluation is required, with concomitant, supportive critical care. A deliberate diagnostic approach is outlined in Table 2. Arterial blood gas analysis assesses the severity of hypoxemia and identifies the development of respiratory and/or metabolic acidosis. Pulmonary function at the

From: Tobias JD (ed): *Pediatric Critical Care: The Essentials.* ©Futura Publishing Co., Inc., Armonk, NY, 1999.

Table 1

Diagnostic Criteria for ARDS

History of illness	Acute onset
PaO$_2$/FiO$_2$ ratio	<200 mm Hg regardless of PEEP level
Chest x-ray	Diffuse, bilateral infiltrates
Pulmonary capillary wedge pressure	<18 mm Hg or no evidence of left atrial hypertension

ARDS = acute respiratory distress syndrome.
Adapted from The American-European Consensus Conference on ARDS. *Am J Respir Crit Care Med* 1994;149:818–824.

Table 2

Diagnostic Evaluation of the Patient with Suspected ARDS

Medical history	Chest x-ray
Arterial blood gases	Blood cultures
Continuous pulse oximetry	Urine cultures
Urinalysis	Leukocyte differential
Complete blood count	Sputum culture
Sputum Gram's stain	Blood lactate level
Liver and renal function	Echocardiography
Bronchoscopy*	
Physical exam	

ARDS = acute respiratory distress syndrome.
*Bronchoscopy may be particularly relevant to the immunocompromised patient at risk for opportunistic infection, as well as the child at risk for noscomial pneumonia.

onset of ARDS is significantly impaired with a marked increase in the P(A/a)O$_2$ gradient, a decreased PaO$_2$/FiO$_2$ ratio, and reduced dynamic lung compliance. Formal pulmonary function studies are not indicated with the usual severity of illness. ARDS can be associated with increased airway resistance, restrictive indices, and impairment of diffusion capacity. There is a significant overlap of pulmonary dysfunction and hypoxemia between survivors and nonsurvivors early in the course of ARDS, thus limiting their predictive prognostic value. The severity of pulmonary function does not appear to be related to the mechanism of disease.

Similar to that of adults with ARDS, the chest x-ray of pediatric ARDS shows bilateral alveolar infiltrates, consistent with pulmonary edema.[2] The diffuse roentgenographic pattern can lag behind the clinical presentation of respiratory failure, but patchy, ill-defined opacities consolidate progressively over time, affecting all lung zones (Fig. 1). Localized forms of ARDS, although infrequent, can occur and have been reported in 10% of one autopsy series.[3] The cardiac silhouette is generally not enlarged, and pleural effusions are not common. The degree of consolidation on chest x-ray can be significantly affected by the level of positive end-expiratory pressure (PEEP). Computed tomography scan of the lung in ARDS shows opacities that distribute throughout the lung, with a predisposition for dependent areas.[4]

The pulmonary artery catheter aids in the diagnosis of ARDS, excluding left atrial hypertension contributing to hydrostatic pulmonary edema (eg, pulmonary artery occlusion pressure >18 mm Hg). In the initial assessment of ARDS, echocardiography has significant potential as a noninvasive method to determine causes of hypotension and left atrial hypertension, and to evaluate left ventricular preload and cardiac output. Its widespread use awaits supportive clinical studies.

Multiple laboratory tests on plasma and bronchoalveolar lavage (BAL) fluid analysis have been linked with ARDS (Table 3).[5] These factors reflect activation of pulmonary and systemic inflammatory cascades as well as the increased permeability of endothelial and epithelial lung barriers that define this syndrome. To date, however, there is not a sensitive or specific plasma or cellular laboratory marker to confirm the diagnosis of ARDS. The major role of BAL and bronchoscopically obtained samples is to diagnose pulmonary infection (see below). Laboratory abnormalities indicative of kidney and liver dysfunction are common and can be associated with the multiple organ dysfunction syndrome ([MODS] as discussed in a following section). Elevation in blood lactate level is an ominous finding, associated with an increased risk for mortality in the patient presenting with shock.[6]

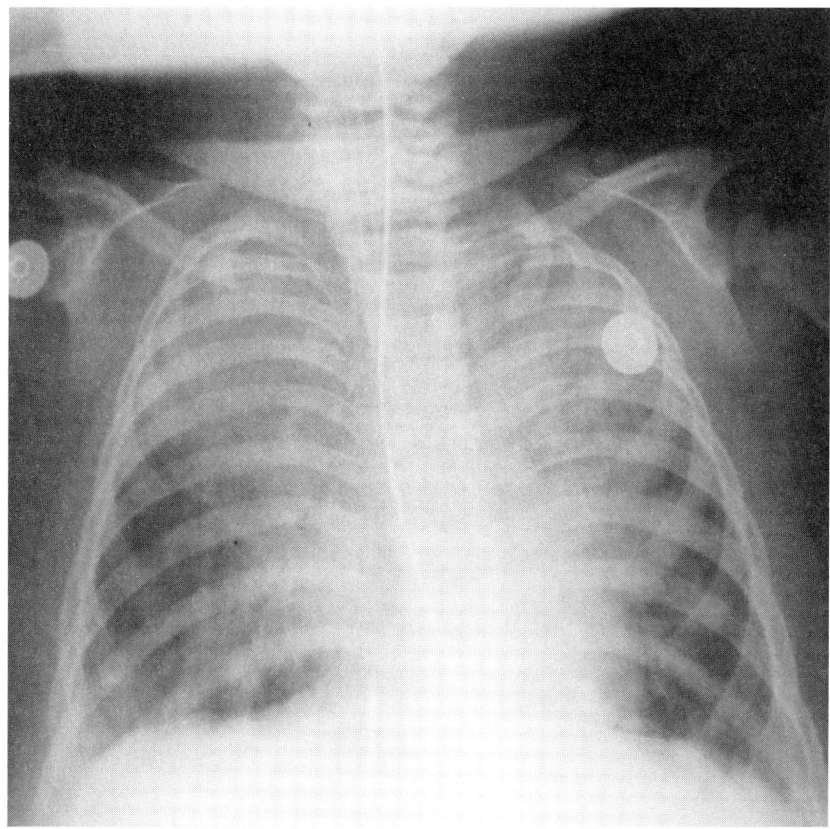

Figure 1. Chest x-ray of an immunocompromised 3-year-old child with acute respiratory distress syndrome, presenting with septic shock. The chest x-ray shows bilateral alveolar infiltrates in all lung zones.

Table 3

Biological Markers Associated with ARDS

Plasma elastase	Plasma TNF-α
Plasma LTB$_4$	Plasma IL-8
Plasma L-selectin	Plasma Von Willebrand
Plasma catalase	factor antigen
BAL L-1β	Plasma CD$_{11b}$/CD$_{18}$
Pulmonary edema/	leukocyte ratio
plasma protein ratio	BAL C3a
Neutrophil percentage	
in bronchoalveolar	
lavage	

ARDS = acute respiratory distress syndrome. Adapted from Reference 5.

Risk Factors for ARDS

In both pediatric and adult populations, ARDS can develop after a myriad of insults including both direct and indirect injury to the lung. Direct injury to the lungs can initiate ARDS. Pneumonia, aspiration of gastric contents, smoke inhalation, near drowning, and traumatic lung contusion are common causes that present rapidly after the insult. Indirect pulmonary damage also occurs, a manifestation of the body's systemic inflammatory response. Clinical examples of indirect injury include the sepsis syndrome, massive blood transfusions, pancreatitis, long bone fractures, postcardiopulmonary resuscitation, cardiopulmonary bypass, hypotension, drug overdose, and disseminated intravascular coagulation. ARDS in the pediatric age group is frequently associated with underlying illness. In one large pediatric series[7] the sepsis syndrome preceded ARDS in 37% of patients; isolated abdominal or blood infections were the most frequent sources. Pneumonia is an important etiology of ARDS that develops with viral, bacterial, or fungal infections. The respiratory syncytial virus, cytomegalovirus, influenza virus, and measles are important causative viral pathogens of ARDS.

Severity of ARDS

The prognosis of ARDS is dependent on factors including the underlying patient diagnoses, severity of illness, etiology of ARDS, physiologic reserve, chronologic age, and immune status. There appears to be a modest improvement in survival of ARDS since its original description in 1967.[8-10] This observation withstanding, mortality from ARDS remains significant, estimated between 40% and 70%.

A clinical scale has been proposed for ARDS, in order to assign a numerical number to estimate the severity of illness (Table 4).[11] This information has relevance to research and it aids in the communication among clinicians and clinical trials. To date, reviews of studies that use lung injury scores have shown a poor correlation with mortality (r = 0.23).[11] That is, this scoring system does not predict survival by the initial severity of lung injury. In contrast, mortality from ARDS has been better assessed with scoring systems of nonpulmonary organ system dysfunction, chronic liver disease, and sepsis at time of ICU admission.[12]

Table 4
Lung Severity Score

		Value
1. Chest roentgenogram score		
No alveolar consolidation		0
Alveolar consolidation confined to 1 quadrant		1
Alveolar consolidation confined to 2 quadrants		2
Alveolar consolidation confined to 3 quadrants		3
Alveolar consolidation in all 4 quadrants		4
2. Hypoxemia score		
PaO_2/FiO_2	>300	0
PaO_2/FiO_2	225–299	1
PaO_2/FiO_2	175–224	2
PaO_2/FiO_2	100–174	3
PaO_2/FiO_2	<100	4
3. PEEP score		
PEEP	>5 cm H_2O	0
PEEP	6–8 cm H_2O	1
PEEP	9–11 cm H_2O	2
PEEP	12–14 cm H_2O	3
PEEP	>15 cm H_2O	4
4. Respiratory system compliance score		
Compliance	>80 mL/cm H_2O	0
Compliance	60–79 mL/cm H_2O	1
Compliance	40–59 mL/cm H_2O	2
Compliance	20–39 mL/cm H_2O	3
Compliance	<19 mL/cm H_2O	4

The sum of each group divided by the number of components defines the lung injury score: No lung injury = 0; mild to moderate injury = 0.1–2.5, severe lung injury >2.5.
PEEP = positive and expiratory pressure.
Adapted from Doyle RL et al. *Am J Resp Crit Care Med* 1995;152:1818–1824.

Clinical Course

After ARDS is diagnosed, a prolonged, intensive period of medical support is required. The duration of hospitalization in pediatric ARDS patients has been reported at 28±20 days (median 20 days) in survivors, versus 9±9 days (median 7 days) in nonsurvivors.[7] Mechanical ventilation is necessary for a duration of 22±18 days (median 18 days). Death within the first 72 hours relates to the original presenting illness or injury (eg, refractory circulatory failure from sepsis or severe neurologic injury).[13] Similar to adult ARDS, the causes of death occurring in the later phases of ARDS in the pediatric age group is related MODS. With the current standards of mechanical ventilatory support, refractory hypoxemia is an uncommon cause of mortality. Sepsis, a contributing factor to MODS, remains a major cause of morbidity and mortality in ARDS. Therefore, most patients with ARDS do not die from respiratory failure, but rather from progressive dysfunction in other organ systems related to the MODS.

Differential Diagnosis of ARDS

The pattern of the chest x-ray is a major supportive factor for the diagnosis of ARDS. The differential diagnosis of the radiographic pattern of bilateral alveolar infiltrates (also known as an acinar pattern) on chest x-ray in the patient presenting with acute dyspnea and marked hypoxemia, can be extensive (Table 5). These disease processes should be ruled out prior to establishing the diagnosis of ARDS. Many of the diseases listed can meet the diagnostic criteria for ARDS when accompanied by other supportive clinical data as listed in Table 1.

Pathology of ARDS

Lung specimens from surgical biopsy and autopsy show the diffuse alveolar damage that is prerequisite for pathologic diagnosis of ARDS. Despite diversity of clinical predisposing events, the lung lesion of ARDS evolves through a similar pattern of presentation. The temporal evolution of ARDS can be divided into three phases: 1) an exudative phase of lung edema and hemorrhage; 2) a proliferative phase of lung organization and repair; and 3) a fibrotic phase of end-stage fibrosis.[14] The exudative phase occurs during the first week of illness. Morphologically, the lungs of dying patients are heavy, edematous, and airless in consistency. Microscopically, edema develops in the pulmonary interstitium and in the intra-alveolar and septal areas. Microthrombi lodge in the pulmonary arterioles and capillaries, contributing to the severity of hypoxemia. Hyaline membranes, composed of plasma proteins including fibrinogen, complement, and other

Table 5

Differential Diagnosis of Diffuse Alveolar Infiltrates on Chest X-Ray

Infectious	Bacterial, viral, and fungal pneumonias; ascaris lumbricoides
Immunologic	Goodpasture's syndrome, idiopathic pulmonary hemorrhage, leukocytoclastic vasculitis
Neoplastic	Hematogenous metastases
Thromboembolic	Fat embolism, amniotic pulmonary embolism
Cardiovascular	Pulmonary edema: hydrostatic or permeability (ARDS)
Inhalational	Near drowning, acute berylliosis, acute silicoproteinosis
Poisoning	Aspirin overdose, heroin, contrast media, fluorocarbon/hydrocarbon ingestion, paraquat ingestion, inhaled toxic gases (nitrogen dioxide, sulfur dioxide, hydrogen sulfide, ammonia, chlorine, phosgene, cadmium, burns)
Metabolic	Alveolar proteinosis
Idiopathic	Sarcoidosis

ARDS = acute respiratory distress syndrome.

cellular debris, are deposited along the walls of alveolar ducts and alveoli.[15] Type I pneumocytes show extensive degenerative changes within alveoli. In the subsequent, proliferative phase of ARDS, widespread fibrosis begins in the intra-alveolar spaces and interstitium. Type II pneumocytes proliferate and become hyperplastic in appearance. Patients who survive the initial weeks of ARDS can develop a fibrotic phase, characterized by extensive remodeling of lung tissue, interspersed with microcystic air spaces and widespread scarring. During this phase, lung collagen progressively increases, correlating with the degree of lung fibrosis.

Major abnormalities in the pulmonary vasculature associated with ARDS (Table 6) contribute to pulmonary hypertension, a common and often severe finding during the course of ARDS.[16] Early in the course of illness, microthrombi and large pulmonary emboli have been identified on autopsy. These events contribute to the severity of hypoxemia. Pulmonary emboli can be systemic in origin or they can form in situ in the pulmonary vasculature. Postmortem examinations have identified thromboemboli in 95% of ARDS patients. Hypoxic vasoconstriction and interstitial edema promote increased pulmonary artery pressures. In the later phases of ARDS the muscular layers of the pulmonary arteries and arterioles hypertrophy. Theories explaining this "muscularization" of the pulmonary vasculature include the effects of chronic hypoxemia, sustained pulmonary hypertension, and oxygen toxicity.

Table 6

Pulmonary Vasculature Abnormalities Associated with ARDS

Microthrombi	Pulmonary vasoconstriction
Arterial muscularization	
Pulmonary infarction	Venous and lymphatic obstruction
Pulmonary hypertension	
Pulmonary emboli	
Vascular bed remodeling	

ARDS = acute respiratory distress syndrome.

Mechanisms of ARDS

Over the past two decades, much has been learned about the immune pathophysiology promoting ARDS. After a severe clinical insult (eg, microbial invasion), the body initiates an inflammatory cascade to limit the extent of injury. Conversely, this acute inflammatory response can create substantial host injury (ie, the development of diffuse alveolar damage). Mechanistically, the systemic inflammatory response encompasses a complex, interlocking pathophysiology of molecular, cellular, and organ networks.[17] On a molecular level, cytokines are low molecular weight proteins that stimulate, amplify, and control the degree of the inflammatory response. Released from pulmonary macrophages as well as from endothelial cells, epithelial cells, and fibroblasts, cytokines recruit neutrophils and monocytes to the lung. Two early response cytokines, tumor necrosis factor-alpha (TNF-α) and interleukin 1-B (IL-1B), stimulate other cells, amplifying the immune response with resulting cellular chemoattraction, release of growth factors, and adhesion molecules. Neutrophils, which are multifunctional cells that are essential for microbial defense, aggregate within the lungs releasing reactive oxygen species and proteases. In the setting of ARDS, these factors can damage both lung vasculature and parenchyma. Platelet aggregation occurs in the pulmonary circulation, releasing factors that contribute to pulmonary vasoconstriction and thrombosis.

The inability to balance the immune system in its role of host defense against its potential organ-damaging properties is an intense area of study in the development of ARDS. For example, other cytokines, such as IL-10 or interleukin-1 receptor-antagonist protein (IL-1RA), promote an anti-inflammatory response and limit damage by proinflammatory cytokines. The uncontrolled inflammatory response, whether the etiology of ARDS is direct or indirect, damages both endothelium and epithelium in the lung. Bypassing normal homeostatic controls, vascular fluid and protein move readily into the lung interstitium. The end result of this cascade of inflammation contributes to lung injury in ARDS.

Hypoxemia is a major criterion for the diagnosis of ARDS. As described previously, autopsy lung sections show significant and often nonhomogeneous alveolar collapse. This can result in increased intrapulmonary shunt, a significant cause of hypoxemia in ARDS.[18] The intrapulmonary shunt can be magnified with pathologic or iatrogenic increases in cardiac output.[19] Increased shunt can create higher capillary filtration pressures and subsequent pulmonary edema or an increase in the blood-capillary transit time, both of which contribute to the severity of hypoxemia. Hypoxic vasoconstriction normally serves a protective function by limiting blood flow to impaired alveoli. In ARDS, high cardiac output and the resulting increased pulmonary blood flow can reduce hypoxic vasoconstriction, resulting in increased intrapulmonary shunt.[20] With sophisticated multiple inert gas methodology, studies of ARDS patients show areas of low ventilation to perfusion (V/Q) contributing to severity of hypoxemia.[21] Dead space ventilation is increased, requiring a high minute ventilation to preserve normal arterial oxygen and carbon dioxide partial pressures. Lung mechanics in the setting of ARDS show significant reduction in lung compliance, related to the histopathologic findings of pulmonary edema. Airway resistance usually increases, particularly with mechanical ventilation at high levels of PEEP.[22] Respiratory failure, occurring with ARDS, can be categorized as lung failure, characterized by gas exchange abnormalities and hypoxemia, or pump failure, in which abnormalities of ventilation result in hypercarbia and respiratory acidosis.[23] Pump failure can result from respiratory muscle fatigue or from depression of the central respiratory drive. Factors that increase energy demand or decrease energy supply to the respiratory muscles clearly contribute to respiratory muscle fatigue. Increased work of breathing associated with high minute ventilation, increased airway resistance, high respiratory rates, malnutrition, sepsis, neuromuscular disorders, and abnormal mechanical properties of the chest wall or lungs contributes to high energy demand. Low cardiac output associated with septic shock, hypoxemia, anemia, and malnutrition results in inadequate energy supply to respiratory muscles. In the face of these clinical conditions, the dichotomy of high energy demand and low energy supply can lead to respiratory failure.

Diagnosis of Pneumonia in the Child with ARDS

Pneumonia and pneumonia-associated sepsis are important risk factors for the development of ARDS. The diagnosis of pneumonia, particularly with the wide host of potential pathogens, can be problematic. As shown in Table 5, multiple illnesses can mimic the chest x-ray of pneumonia and ARDS. Common diagnostic criteria for pneumonia, such as new pulmonary infiltrates, hypoxemia, leukocytosis or leukopenia, fever, and pathogenic bacteria in sputum, are associated with a significant rate of misdiagnosis when compared with postmortem histologic studies.[24] Fiber optic bronchoscopy can improve the accuracy in diagnosis of pneumonia and aid in the selection of antibiotic therapy. In the diagnosis of bacterial pneumonia, airway colonization by potentially pathogenic bacteria confounds pneumonia diagnosis and can contribute to unnecessary and ill-advised use of antibiotics. Bronchoscopic methods using protected specimen brush (PSB) catheters or BAL to avoid bacterial contamination of upper airways may facilitate distal lung parenchymal sampling. These bronchoscopic methods combined with quantitative bacterial cultures can limit false-positive results. Studies to date, when performed in the absence of antibiotic therapy in the involved bronchopulmonary segment, suggest that the quantitative thresholds of $\geq 10^3$ colony-forming units (CFU)/mL for PSB and $\geq 10^4$ CFU/mL for BAL support the diagnosis of bacterial pneumonia. For the PSB technique, supportive statistics from the medical literature are variable with sensitivities reported between 65% and 100% with specificities of 80% to 100%.[25] In a combination of several studies, BAL has a reported sensitivity of 77% and specificity of 69%.[26] A major source of false-positive results in both of these

Table 7
Diagnostic Utility of Bronchoalveolar Lavage

Infectious organisms diagnosed by BAL isolation
    Mycobacterium tuberculosis
    Legionella pneumophila
    Pneumocystis carinii
    Toxoplasmosis gondii
    Mycoplasma
    Influenza virus
    Respiratory syncytial virus
    Stronglyoides

Infectious organisms isolated by BAL requiring supportive clinical criteria for diagnosis
    Bacteria
    Aspergillus
    Cryptococcus
    Atypical mycobacterium
    Herpes simplex
    Cytomegalovirus

BAL = bronchalveolar lavage.

methods is contamination from the upper airway. False-negative studies can result from prior antibiotic therapy, improper processing of specimens, and failure to evaluate the involved bronchopulmonary segment. The isolation of certain pathogens by culture or by special stains is diagnostic (Table 7). Importantly, certain pathogens can colonize the airways and not be associated with active infection. In this group, supporting clinical criteria are required for diagnoses.[27]

Multiple Organ Dysfunction Syndrome

MODS is a significant cause of death in patients with ARDS. Examples of organ dysfunction in MODS are shown in Table 8. MODS can develop from inadequate resuscitation from shock, from persisting infection, and from persistent inflammation in the absence of infection. Importantly, in the ARDS patient who fails to improve, occult clinically unrecognized infection should be a major concern. In one postmortem series of ARDS patients with associated multiple system pathology, 98% of autopsied patients had evidence of bacterial infection.[28] Common causes of occult infection include pneumonia, intravenous catheter-related sepsis, cholecystitis, sinusitis, endocarditis, infected decubitus ulcers, and fungal infections. Other reports support MODS development in absence of infection in the presence of ongoing systemic inflammatory response syndrome. No infectious etiology can be isolated in 30% to 60% of patients who meet the American College of Chest Physicians/Society of Critical Care Medicine definition of sepsis or severe sepsis. MODS has been described in a variety of pathologic states including trauma, burns, pancreatitis, shock, and sickle cell crises. Quantitative scoring systems of MODS that predict mortality are described.[12]

MODS is classified as primary or secondary in origin. Primary MODS develops from a well defined insult such as microcirculatory hypoperfusion, bacteremia/sepsis, or direct tissue injury, and results in clinically measurable organ dysfunction. Sec-

Table 8
Evaluation for the Multiple Organ Dysfunction Syndrome (MODS)

System	Variable
Respiratory	PaO_2/FiO_2 ratio, respiratory compliance
Cardiovascular	Mean arterial pressure, cardiac output
Renal	Serum creatinine, glomerular filtration rate
Hepatic	Serum bilirubin, hepatic enzymes, coagulation profile
Hematologic	Platelet count, white blood cell count
Gastrointestinal	Upper gastrointestinal bleeding
Neurologic	Glasgow coma scale

ondary MODS, occurring days after initial presentation, can be a manifestation of persisting inflammation, such as ongoing nosocomial infection or injured tissue. Organ function can deteriorate with the ongoing or progressive release of cytokines, oxygen free radicals, and other inflammatory mediators. In ARDS patients with progressive MODS the clinician must evaluate for potential treatable causes, such as occult infection or necrotic tissue, which contribute to the ongoing inflammatory state.

Therapy for ARDS

The intensive care of the child with ARDS requires significant support over an extended period from the medical, nursing, and respiratory therapy staff. Because of the potential for rapid deterioration, the multisystem nature of the illness, and the requirement of frequent clinical assessment, early admission to a critical care unit seems essential in order to limit morbidity and mortality. The following sections summarize aspects of supportive care of the ARDS patient.

Mechanical Ventilation

Mechanical ventilation is an essential component of ICU support of the ARDS patient, to provide adequate oxygenation, carbon dioxide clearance, and decreased work of breathing. An international consensus conference on mechanical ventilation[29] suggested the following guidelines in the support of patients with ARDS: 1) a mode of ventilation should be capable of adequate oxygenation and ventilation of the patient, together with appropriate physician familiarity; 2) an acceptable arterial oxygen saturation (SaO_2) should be achieved; 3) plateau pressures ≤ 35 cm H_2O should be targeted to minimize the risk of barotrauma; 4) permissive hypercapnia is acceptable and can lessen the need for large tidal volumes or high airway pressures; 5) PEEP with appropriate use can improve oxygenation; and 6) the FiO_2 should be minimized if the SaO_2 allows, to avoid pathologic oxygen toxicity.

It is increasingly evident that clinical management of mechanical ventilation can cause pathologic lesions that mimick diffuse alveolar injury of ARDS,[30,31] and are currently termed ventilator-induced lung injury. A common theme in ventilator-induced lung injury associates iatrogenic overdistention of the lung with the pathophysiology of lung injury. High airway pressures accompanying mechanical ventilation lead to pulmonary edema in human and animal models (ie, barotrauma). Furthermore, large ventilator tidal volumes can produce acute lung injury in animal models, even in the absence of increased airway pressure, and can exacerbate pathologic microvascular permeability (ie, volutrauma). PEEP can similarly be detrimental if it produces significant alveolar overdistention. Lungs that are injured by a variety of clinical insults (eg, trauma, aspiration, pneumonia) may be more susceptible to ventilator-induced lung injury. In contrast, excessively low tidal volumes can be similarly injurious. Low tidal volumes may fail to keep the lungs "open," with resulting atelectasis and decreased compliance. The injured lung units are then subjected to stress injury related to repeated opening and collapse, furthering diffuse alveolar damage. This, in turn, can stimulate the inflammatory cascade, augmenting the lung injury (Fig. 2).

Since the description of ARDS by Ashbaugh and colleagues,[8] PEEP has been used to treat hypoxemia and to lower FiO_2 requirements. Theories to explain PEEP's effectiveness in ARDS involve its reexpansion of collapsed alveoli as well as its ability to shift perfusion from nonventilated to ventilated lung regions.[21] Additionally, it may preserve surfactant function and limit microvascular fluid filtration into alveoli. Of emphasis, PEEP does not seem to open alveoli in a linear manner. Rather, increasing PEEP to a critical airway pressure abruptly opens alveoli in recruitable areas, improving oxygenation as shown in Figure 3.[32] PEEP seems to have limited effect on severely diseased alveoli. Excessive PEEP can contribute to injury in healthy lung parenchyma when accompanied by hyperinflation, potentially because of stress failure of the involved alveolar epithelial membrane. Increasing PEEP

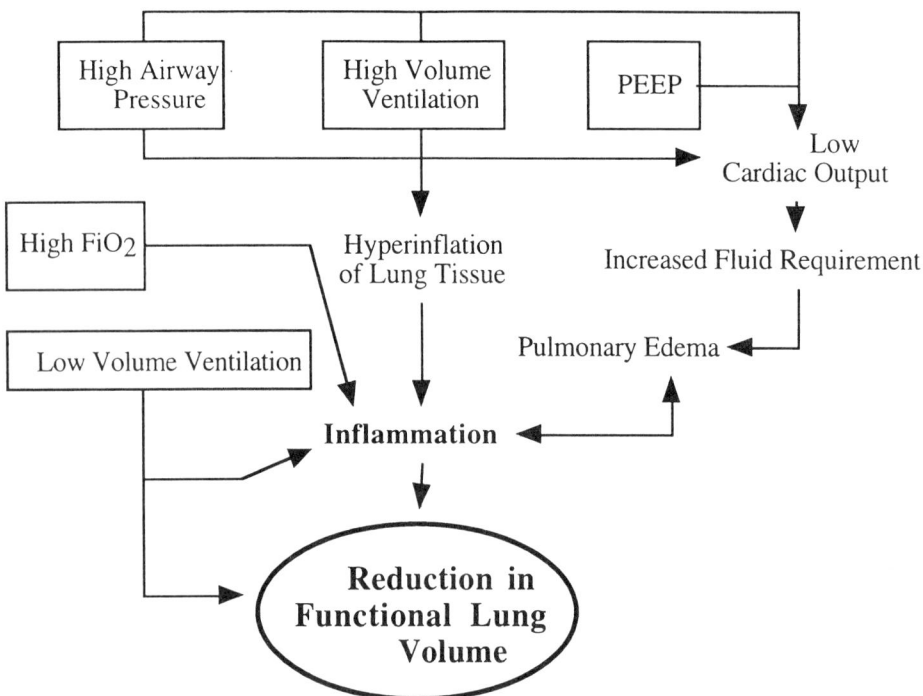

Figure 2. Flow diagram showing factors contributing to ventilator-induced lung injury. Ventilator management can lead to excessive hyperinflation of the lung, augmenting the inflammatory cascade of ARDS and creating hemodynamic instability. Conversely, excessively low tidal volumes can fail to keep the lung "open" and potentially exacerbate stress injury to the lung. Excessive FiO_2 can cause oxygen toxicity, worsening lung injury.

can improve oxygenation, but its potential to decrease cardiac output and oxygen delivery is well founded. The increased intrathoracic pressure with increased PEEP can impede venous return and increase right ventricular afterload. After PEEP level is changed, the effect on cardiac output is generally seen within 15 minutes.[33] The goals of PEEP titration are to provide effective oxygenation with nontoxic FiO_2, to maintain effective cardiac output, and to avoid hyperinflation (overdistention) of alveoli. Different methods of PEEP titration are listed in Table 9. Regardless of the method chosen to determine the optimal PEEP, invasive hemodynamic monitoring with placement of a pulmonary artery catheter may be indicated in patients with ARDS to provide an accurate measurement of the cardiac output, the intrapulmonary shunt fraction, and tissue oxygen delivery/consumption, as well as a direct measurement of pulmonary artery pressure. The reader is referred to chapter 2 for a full discussion of invasive hemodynamic monitoring.

Bedside determination of pressure-volume curves has been used to prescribe optimal PEEP (Fig. 3) and to limit overdistention of the alveoli. As shown in Figure 3, the inflection point (P_{flex}) represents the pressure at which alveoli or airways open, corresponding to closing volume. Setting PEEP at a pressure above P_{flex} has been suggested as a means to guide PEEP therapy and limit ventilator-induced lung injury secondary to hyperinflation. PEEP does not prophylactically prevent pulmonary edema or prevent ARDS. Other ventilator manipulations may be useful to improve oxygenation. For the patient with refractory hypoxemia, "bedside" empiric ventilator changes such as prolongation of inspiratory to expiratory time (ie, I:E ratio) and the addition of an inspiratory pauses can be beneficial. The ra-

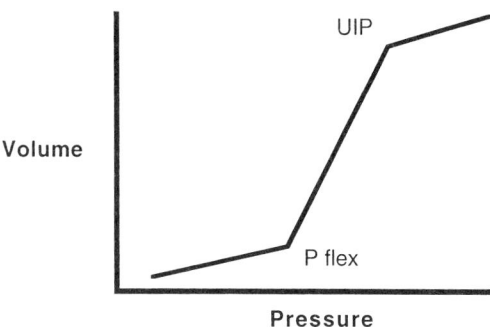

Figure 3. Pressure-volume curve of the respiratory system in ARDS. This stylized schema shows the lower inflection point (P_{flex}) and upper inflection point (UIP). P_{flex} represents the pressure at which there is massive opening of collapsed lung units. UIP represents lung volume at which there is progressive overdistention. Maintenance of positive end-expiratory pressure above P_{flex} can result in improved oxygenation in select patients. Reducing the prescribed tidal volume or peak inflating pressure to a point on the curve below UIP has been proposed as a method to limit ventilator-associated lung injury.

tionale for these changes is to maintain "open" alveoli.

Intravenous sedation and, in specific cases, the addition of neuromuscular blockade can alleviate dyssynchrony between the patient and the ventilator, limit marked alterations in tidal volume, decrease oxygen consumption and, potentially, minimize ventilator-induced lung injury. The role of appropriate fluid management and the use of diuretics are discussed in another section. Other methods to enhance systemic oxygenation and improve carbon dioxide clearance, include extracorporeal membrane oxygenation (ECMO), extracorporeal carbon dioxide removal, high-frequency jet ventilation, high-frequency oscillation, intravenous oxygenator, and tracheal gas insufflation to reduce dead space ventilation. These methods have been proposed as methods to provide "lung rest" by limiting excessive airway pressure and high tidal volumes, and by decreasing respiratory acidosis. Each of the described methods has been reported to be effective for respiratory failure in selected patients, but the improvement in overall survival in ARDS requires further clinical supportive evidence. For example, in a large multicenter trial, ECMO showed an improvement in oxygenation but no overall improvement in survival.[34] For a full discussion of conventional and nonconventional means of support of oxygenation and ventilation, the reader is referred to chapters 4 and 5.

Permissive Hypercapnia

Permissive hypercapnia is a strategy of ventilator management for ARDS that limits ventilator inflation pressure and allows for a significant increase in arterial $PaCO_2$. Its purpose is to prevent or limit ventilator-associated lung injury associated with high peak airway pressures or large tidal volumes, as well as hemodynamic impairment associated with hyperinflation of the lung.[35] Limiting ventilator peak pressures to less than 40 cm H_2O has been associated with lower than predicted mortality in a series of ARDS patients. This is in face of marked elevation of $PaCO_2$ levels, even to greater than 120 mm Hg.[36] Significant arterial carbon dioxide accumulation and associated respiratory acidosis appear to be well tolerated in selected critically ill patients, as long as concomitant hypoxia is avoided. Detrimental host effects of permissive hypercapnia include impairment of left ventricular contractility, coronary artery vasodilation, pulmonary artery hypertension, a rightward shift of the oxygen-hemoglobin dissociated curve, and increased intracranial pressure. The cardiac depressant effect of hypercarbia is offset by carbon dioxide's stimulatory effects on the central and auto-

Table 9

Methods to Determine Optimal PEEP

Pressure volume curve analysis (P_{flex})
Best SaO_2
Best SvO_2
Best oxygen delivery
Lowest Q_s/Q_t
Maximum tidal volume
Lowest deadspace (V_d/V_t)

PEEP = positive end-expiratory pressure.

nomic nervous system. Permissive hypercapnea is contraindicated in patients prone to increased intracranial pressure. This is a result of hypercapnea-associated increases in cerebral blood flow, resulting from arterial hypertension and cerebral vasodilation.

With time, the ensuing respiratory acidosis is buffered by renal reabsorption of bicarbonate, and systemic acidosis is thereby limited. Generally, an arterial pH of ≥7.20 is hemodynamically well tolerated. Intravenous sedation and occasionally neuromuscular blockade are required to facilitate patient comfort, limit dyspnea, and allow for tolerance of mechanical ventilation.

Liquid Ventilation

Liquid ventilation is a novel form of ventilatory support that holds promise, but whose value remains unclear. The introduction of oxygen-carrying perfluorocarbons into the lungs potentially offers a reduction in ventilator-induced barotrauma as compared with standard ventilation. Clearance of the alveolar exudate that occurs in ARDS by the perfluorocarbon has been observed, potentially reducing the level of inflammation.[37] Results of large controlled trials that show benefit over standard therapy are not yet available.

Nitric Oxide

Inhaled nitric oxide (NO) has gained significant interest for the patient with ARDS who is difficult to oxygenate. NO, formerly known as endothelial-dependent relaxing factor, acts through the cyclic guanosine monophosphate system, resulting in vasodilation. As it is immediately inactivated following interaction with hemoglobin, it acts preferentially on the pulmonary endothelium. Mechanistically, as an inhaled gas through the ventilator circuit, NO distributes to functional (ie, ventilated) alveoli. As a direct pulmonary vasodilator, it augments blood flow to these alveoli, enhancing ventilation and perfusion matching. Thus, NO improves arterial oxygenation by reducing intrapulmonary right-to-left shunt. Pulmonary artery pressure and pulmonary vascular resistance can be reduced without significant reduction of system blood pressure because of the rapid metabolism of NO. Although theoretically attractive in the treatment of ARDS, the use of NO remains controversial and awaits evidenced-based support. Clinical trials to date have not shown that inhaled NO offers a significant decrease in ARDS-related mortality. Its promoters, however, suggest that modest improvements in oxygenation may simplify ventilator management and ventilator-induced lung injury.[38] In an important, placebo-controlled, multicenter trial for adults with ARDS,[39] NO showed no significant improvement over placebo in terms of mortality, days of mechanical ventilation, clinically significant reduction in mean pulmonary artery pressure, or indices of oxygenation. Methemoglobinemia is a potential toxicity, but appears infrequent in carefully monitored clinical trials. Furthermore, production of nitrogen dioxide (NO_2), a byproduct of oxygen and NO metabolism, can cause primary lung injury at high levels in animal models. In clinical trials using NO at ≤40 ppm, NO_2 toxicity has not been significant. In two major pediatric studies using NO,[40,41] its use reduced the requirements for ECMO therapy.

Oxygen Therapy and Toxicity

Oxygen, although fundamental for the support of the patient with ARDS, has the potential to contribute to the toxicity of the underlying lung lesion. It is well known that the biochemical byproducts of oxygen metabolism include water, hydrogen peroxide, superoxide radicals, and hydroxyl radicals; the latter three all have direct potential for cellular toxicity. Pathologic changes of oxygen toxicity include atelectasis, alveolar capillary leak, airway and alveolar inflammation, alveolar hemorrhage, fibrin deposition, and hyaline membranes.[42,43] The normal host has natural defenses against these reactive oxygen species including superoxide dismutase, catalases, glutathione, and peroxidases. In the ICU patient, antioxidant defenses can be depleted, predisposing the patient to oxygen toxicity. On a clinical basis, it is difficult to separate the primary pathologic changes that occur during ARDS from those occurring with oxygen toxicity. Based on this dichotomy, it is generally recommended that the lowest tolerable FiO_2, preferably below 0.60, be used.

Prone Positioning

Placing the patient with ARDS in the prone position can provide significant improvements in oxygenation. Thoracic computed-tomography scans have shown that during the course of ARDS, consolidation develops in dependent areas of the lungs. Multiple clinical series have shown that the change from the supine to prone position can create a marked improvement in the PaO_2/FiO_2 ratio and reduced intrapulmonary shunt, occurring within 30 minutes of position change.[44] These improvements are sustained over time while the patient is prone and revert back with resumption of the supine position.[45] The mechanisms of improved oxygenation with the prone position have been attributed to redistribution of ventilation to areas of atelectasis or redistribution of blood flow to areas of effective ventilation and perfusion. The position change is generally well tolerated without cardiovascular compromise and with no significant changes in pulmonary compliance. Contraindications to the prone position have included uncontrolled cerebral hypertension as well unstable cervical spine injuries. Regardless of the scenario, the prone position does impose some difficulties with providing nursing care, etc. Despite improvements in oxygenation, further studies are needed to demonstrate improvements in mortality.

Fluid Management

Fluid management in the patient with ARDS is controversial. The Starling equation for the formation of pulmonary edema suggests that an increase in hydrostatic pressure can increase lung water in acute lung injury. Based on this, several clinical studies support the hypothesis that modifying iatrogenic fluid therapy can improve overall outcome. In a prospective, observational study of adult ARDS patients, mortality was increased in those patients with cumulative fluid excess (quantified by daily fluid input greater than output measurements) and progressive weight gain.[46] There was no evidence of increasing renal failure in the patients with decreased fluid accumulation. A subsequent study analyzed the benefits of the therapeutic reduction of pulmonary capillary wedge pressures using diuretics, fluid restriction, phlebotomy, dialysis, or ultrafiltration.[47] The patients were divided into two groups: group I had greater than 25% reduction in the pulmonary capillary wedge pressure while group II did not achieve this goal. The group with the reduced pulmonary capillary wedge pressure showed significant improvement in overall survival (75% versus 29%) and decreased length of stay in the ICU. The downside to this approach to care is that excessive reduction in preload could result in impairment of cardiac output and oxygen delivery. Based on these studies, a fluid management trial with the lowest pulmonary capillary wedge pressure that allows an acceptable blood pressure and cardiac output is an appropriate goal, especially during the first days of ARDS.

Antibiotic Therapy

The initial choice of antibiotic therapy can be critical for the survival of patients with ARDS. Previous studies have shown that survival from nosocomial pneumonia and sepsis is dependent on the correct choice of the initial empiric antibiotic(s). Despite aggressive means for diagnosis of infection, identification of pathogens will be delayed in most centers for 24 to 48 hours. Thus, antibiotic selection initially must be empirically based on the epidemiology of potential infections and the patient's risk factors for infection. In the deteriorating patient with high risk for infection and no known pathogen, broad-spectrum antibiotic therapy should be instituted promptly.

Surfactant

Produced by type II alveolar cells, surfactant lines the alveolar cell surface, reducing surface tension and thus limiting atelectasis. Surfactant is composed primarily of phospholipids, as well as neutral lipids, and at least three different surfactant specific proteins (eg, SP-A, SP-B, SP-C). In the setting of ARDS surfactant shows both quantitative and qualitative abnormalities.[48-51] Furthermore, pulmonary factors associated with ARDS can inactivate surfactant function. With the known response of surfactant in neonatal respiratory distress syndrome—a condition associated with surfactant deficiency—there has been a theoretical appeal for use of nebulized surfactant to improve respiratory function in acute lung injury. Thus far, its use in ARDS is controversial. A prospective, multicenter, double-blind, randomized, placebo-controlled trial of 725 sepsis-induced ARDS patients failed to improve 30-day survival, length of stay in the ICU, duration of mechanical ventilation, or physiologic lung function.[52] In contrast, smaller trials have suggested improvements in oxygenation and mortality.[53] Details such as the appropriate dose, the method of delivery, and the chemical characteristics of the surfactant require further definition.

Sedation and Analgesia

Sedation and analgesia are essential considerations in the supportive ICU care of the pediatric patient with ARDS.[54] With the prolonged course of ARDS, sedative and analgesic therapy can provide the child with pain relief, sleep, amnesia, and adaptation to mechanical ventilation. Effective use of sedative and analgesic drugs, either alone or in combination, can limit the requirement for neuromuscular blocking agents and their associated problems (prolonged neuromuscular toxicity). In selecting the appropriate drug or combination of drugs, a goal-oriented approach can be used as directed by the need for sedation, pain relief, and amnesia (see Table 10). The opioid class, including morphine or fentanyl, is the mainstay of analgesic therapy. The appropriate use of opioids will limit pain and the physiologic response associated with pain (eg, tachycardia and increased oxygen consumption). The benzodiazepine class (midazolam, diazepam, lorazepam) combines the benefits of amnesia with sedation. In contrast to the opioid class, benzodiazepines do not provide effective analgesia. Propofol is an intravenous general anesthetic which can provide sedation and amnesia. After discontinuation of infusion, propofol is rapidly cleared, allowing for early patient assessment. For a full discussion of sedation and analgesia, the reader is referred to chapter 11.

Corticosteroids

In the treatment of ARDS, the use of high-dose corticosteroids has been appealing, to temper the well described, intense inflammatory state. At this point, corticosteroids early in the clinical course of ARDS do not appear beneficial. A prospective, randomized, double-blind, placebo-controlled,

Table 10

Characteristics of Sedatives for the ARDS Patient

Class of Drug	Sedation	Analgesia	Amnesia
Opioid:			
Morphine	+	+	−
Fentanyl	+	+	−
Benzodiazepine:			
Midazolam	+	−	+
Diazepam	+	−	+
Lorazepam	+	−	+
Miscellaneous:			
Propofol	+	−	+

ARDS = acute respiratory distress syndrome.

multicenter trial of methylprednisolone for ARDS in adults showed that early use of corticosteroids did not improve overall outcome in terms of mortality or reversal of ARDS.[55] A subsequent report has suggested that corticosteroids used late in the clinical course may limit the fibroproliferative stage of ARDS,[56] but this observation requires further substantiation.

Failed Pharmacologic Trials for ARDS

Because of well supported data that emphasize inflammation in the pathogenesis of ARDS, several trials have targeted essential points of this inflammatory cascade to limit the development and progression of ARDS. Other pharmacologic therapies that have not shown significant benefit or that lack large clinical supporting trials in the treatment of ARDS include acetylcysteine, ibuprofen, prostaglandin E_1, pentoxifylline, antiendotoxin, and cytokine immunotherapies.

Enhancement of Oxygen Delivery

It has been proposed that multiple system organ dysfunction in critical illness may be a result of inadequate oxygen delivery. There is little disagreement that patients with ARDS and associated hemodynamic compromise (oliguria, low perfusion pressure) require resuscitation including intravenous fluids to correct hypovolemia, intropic support of low cardiac output, judicious use of vasopressors to enhance compromised perfusion pressure, and blood for severe anemia. Some investigators have proposed that increasing cardiac output to supranormal levels with use of drugs such as dobutamine is beneficial in surgical patients and critical illness.[57] Importantly, two large multicenter trials question this "supranormal" oxygen delivery approach to ICU support. In a prospective, randomized, controlled study of patients with the sepsis syndrome or septic shock,[58] specific hemodynamic goals were targeted (a cardiac index of ≥ 4.5 L/min/m^2, oxygen delivery >600 mL/min/m^2, and an oxygen consumption >170 mL/min/m^2). In the treatment groups, catecholamines, including dobutamine and norepinephrine, were used to achieve the desired hemodynamic goals. Increased oxygen delivery did not result in decreased mortality, decrease in days of ICU care, or decreased MODS. Similarly, another multicenter study of a general population of critically ill patients[59] randomized patients to one of three groups including supranormal cardiac indices, high mixed venous oxygen saturations, and a control group. No differences were seen in mortality, PaO_2/FiO_2 ratio, days of mechanical ventilation, length of stay in ICU, or organ dysfunction. Based on the results of these two large clinical trials, routine hemodynamic pursuit of supranormal physiology in ARDS patients is not recommended.

Long-Term Outcome of Pulmonary Function after ARDS

ARDS patients who survive the acute illness have the potential for functional recovery and improvement in measured pulmonary parameters.[60] This fact is based on long-term follow-up of adult ARDS patients in addition to similar, albeit less extensive, studies in the pediatric literature. During the recovery phase of ARDS after discontinuation of mechanical ventilation, pulmonary function typically shows restrictive physiology with reduction in forced vital capacity (FVC) and total lung capacity. In contrast, a smaller subset of ARDS survivors shows obstructive physiology with reduction of the forced expiratory volume in 1 second (FEV_1)/FVC ratio. The carbon monoxide diffusion capacity, also known as transfer factor, is reduced in the majority of ARDS patients (75% to 100%). Significant improvement in pulmonary function occurs during the first 3 months after tracheal extubation and, to a lesser degree, over 6 months to 1 year. In a study of 41 patients with ARDS, only 28% of patients showed moderate to severe reduction in measurements of pulmonary function during their recovery period.[61] The severity of the subsequent pulmonary abnormality correlates with the degree of lung injury during the acute phase of illness.[62] There does not ap-

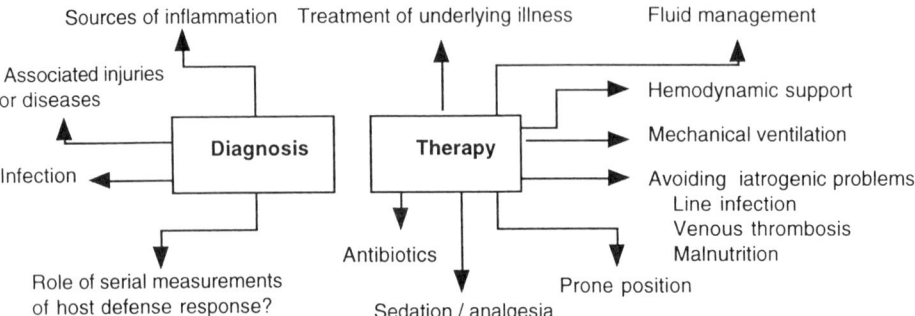

Figure 4. Essentials of the management of acute respiratory distress syndrome.

pear to be a significant relationship between the causative factor for ARDS and the severity of pulmonary sequelae.

Frequent symptoms during the recovery phases of ARDS include cough, sputum production, and shortness of breath, but these usually do not limit lifestyle.[63] In the follow-up of patients after resolution of ARDS, other causes of dyspnea developing after discontinuation of mechanical ventilation can include laryngeotracheostenosis and vocal cord dysfunction associated with prolonged endotracheal intubation.

Summary

Aggressive management of ARDS in the pediatric patient should include a broad-spectrum approach, in terms of both diagnosis and therapeutic support, as reviewed and summarized in Figure 4. Because of the risk of uncontrolled inflammation with inadequately treated infection, a thorough analysis for potential sources of infection is suggested. Supportive therapy with meticulous fluid management, treatment of shock, attention to methods of ventilatory support, effective selection of antibiotics, and avoidance of common iatrogenic complications may limit the damage of this challenging condition. Although pharmacologic modifications of the basic inflammatory event have been, to date, less than optimistic, the understanding of basic mechanisms of ARDS has significantly advanced over the past three decades. With the current level of mortality associated with ARDS, there exists significant need for further investigation in both the basic pathophysiology and clinical support of this patient population.

References

1. Bernard GR, Artigas A, Brigham KL, et al. The American-European Consensus Conference on ARDS: Definitions, mechanisms, relevant outcomes, and clinical trial coordination. *Am J Respir Crit Care Med* 1994; 149:818–824.
2. Effmann EL, Merten DF, Kirks DR, et al. Adult respiratory distress syndrome in children. *Radiology* 1985;157:69–74.
3. Yazdy AM, Tomashefski JF Jr, Yagan R, Kleinerman J. Regional alveolar damage (RAD): A localized counterpart of diffuse alveolar damage. *Am J Clin Pathol* 1989;92:10–15.
4. Gattinoni L, Pesenti A, Bombino M, et al. Relationships between lung computed tonometry, gas exchange, and PEEP in acute respiratory failure. *Anesthesiology* 1988;69:824–827.
5. Pittet JF, Mackersie RC, Martin TR, Matthay MA. Biological markers of acute lung injury: Prognostic and pathogenetic significance. *Am J Respir Crit Care Med* 1997; 155:1187–1205.
6. Bakker J, Coffernils M, Leon M, et al. Blood lactate levels are superior to oxygen-derived variables in predicting outcome in septic shock. *Chest* 1991;99:956–962.
7. Davis SL, Furman DP, Costarino AT Jr. Adult respiratory distress syndrome in children: Associated disease, clinical course, and predictors of death. *J Pediatr* 1993;123: 35–45.

8. Ashbaugh DG, Bigelow DB, Petty TL, et al. Acute respiratory distress syndrome in adults. *Lancet* 1967;ii:3319-3323.
9. Miller JA, Davis DR, Steinberg KPO, Hudson LD. Improved survival of patients with acute respiratory distress syndrome (ARDS): 1983-1993. *JAMA* 1995;273:306-309.
10. Paulson TE, Spear RM, Peterson BM. New concepts in the treatment of children with acute respiratory distress syndrome. *J Pediatr* 1995;127:163-175.
11. Murray JF, Matthay MA, Luce JM, Flick MR. An expanded definition of the adult respiratory distress syndrome. *Am Rev Respir Dis* 1988;138:720-723.
12. Marshall JC, Cook DJ, Christous NV, et al. Multiple organ dysfunction score: A reliable descriptor of a complex clinical outcome. *Crit Care Med* 1995;23:1638-1652.
13. Montgomery AB, Stager MA, Carrico J, Hudson LD. Causes of mortality in patients with the adult respiratory distress syndrome. *Am Rev Respir Dis* 1985;132:485-489.
14. Tomashefski JF Jr. Pulmonary pathology in the adult respiratory distress syndrome. *Clin Chest Med* 1990;11:593-619.
15. Royall JA, Levin DL. Adult respiratory distress syndrome in pediatric patients (I): Clinical aspects, pathophysiology, pathology, and mechanisms of lung injury. *J Pediatr* 1988;112:169-179.
16. Tomashefski JF, Davies P, Boggis C, et al. The pulmonary vascular lesions of the adult respiratory distress syndrome. *Am J Pathol* 1983;112:112-126.
17. Rinaldo JE, Christman JW. Mechanisms and mediators of the adult respiratory distress syndrome. *Clin Chest Med* 1990;11:621-632.
18. Lemaire F. Hypoxaemia in adult respiratory distress syndrome. In Artigas A, Lemaire F, Suter PM, Zapol WM (eds): *Adult Respiratory Distress Syndrome*. New York: Churchill Livingstone; 1992:329-339.
19. Lynch JP, Mhyre JG, Dantzker DR. Influence of cardiac output on intrapulmonary shunt. *J Appl Physiol* 1979;321:315-321.
20. Benumof JL, Wahrenbrock EA. Blunted hypoxic pulmonary vasoconstriction by increased lung vascular pressure. *J Appl Physiol* 1975;38:846-850.
21. Dantzker DR, Brook LJ, Dehart P, et al. Ventilation-perfusion distributions in the ARDS. *Am Rev Respir Dis* 1979;120:1039-1052.
22. Pesenti A, Pelosi P, Rossi N, et al. The effects of positive end-expiratory pressure on respiratory resistance in patients with the adult respiratory distress syndrome and in normal anesthetized subjects. *Am Rev Respir Dis* 1991;144:101-107.
23. Roussos C, Macklem PT. The respiratory muscles. *N Engl J Med* 1982;307:786-797.
24. Andrews CP, Coalson JJ, Smith JD, Johanson WG Jr. Diagnosis of nosocomial bacterial pneumonia in acute, diffuse lung injury. *Chest* 1981;80:254-258.
25. Goldstein RA, Rohatgi PK, Bergofsky EH, et al. Clinical role of bronchoalveolar lavage in adults with pulmonary disease. *Am Rev Respir Dis* 1990;142:481-486.
26. Meduri GU, Chastre J. The standardization of bronchoscopic techniques for ventilator-associated pneumonia. *Chest* 1992;102:557S-564S.
27. Hata JS, Schenk DA, Dellinger RP. Fiberoptic bronchoscopy. In Civetta JM, Taylor RW, Kirby RR (eds): *Critical Care*. Philadelphia: Lippincott-Raven Publishers; 1997:683-702.
28. Bell RC, Coalson KK, Smith JD, et al. Multiple organ system failure and infection in adult respiratory distress syndrome. *Ann Intern Med* 1983;84:1045-1049.
29. Slutsky AS. ACCP Consensus Conference: Mechanical ventilation. *Chest* 1993;104:1833-1859.
30. Dreyfuss D, Saumon G. Ventilator-induced lung injury: Lessons learned from experimental studies. *Am J Respir Crit Care Med* 1998;157:294-323.
31. Hickling KG. Ventilatory management of ARDS: Can it affect outcome. *Intensive Care Med* 1990;16:219-226.
32. Matamis D, Lemaire F, Harf A, et al. Total respiratory P-V curves in ARDS. *Chest* 1984;86:58-66.
33. Patel M, Singer M. The optimal time for measuring the cardiorespiratory effects of positive end-expiratory pressure. *Chest* 1993;104:139-142.
34. Zapol WM, Snider MT, Hill JD, et al. Extracorporeal membrane lung oxygenation in severe acute respiratory failure. *JAMA* 1979;242:2193-2196.
35. Tuxen DV. Permissive hypercapnic ventilation. *Am J Respir Crit Care Med* 1994;150:870-874.
36. Hickling KG, Henderson SJ, Jackson R. Low mortality associated with low volume pressure limited ventilation with permissive hypercapnia in severe adult respiratory distress syndrome. *Intensive Care Med* 1990;16:372-377.
37. Hirschl RB, Parent A, Tooley R, et al. Liquid

ventilation improves pulmonary function, gas exchange, and lung injury in a model of respiratory failure. *Ann Surg* 1995;221:79–88.
38. Rossaint R, Falke KJ, Lopez F, et al. Inhaled nitric oxide for the adult respiratory distress syndrome. *N Engl J Med* 1993;328:399–405.
39. Dellinger RP, Zimmerman JL, Taylor RW, and the Inhaled Nitric Oxide in ARDS Study Group. Effects of inhaled nitric oxide in patients with acute respiratory distress syndrome: Results of a randomized phase II trial. *Crit Care Med* 1998;26:15–23.
40. Roberts JD, Fineman JR, Morin FC, et al. Inhaled nitric oxide and persistent pulmonary hypertension of the newborn. *N Engl J Med* 1997;326:605–610.
41. The Neonatal Inhaled Nitric Oxide Study Group. Inhaled nitric oxide in full-term and nearly full-term infants with hypoxic respiratory failure. *N Engl J Med* 1997;336:597–604.
42. Deneke SM, Fanburg BL. Normobaric oxygen toxicity and the lung. *N Engl J Med* 1980;303:76–86.
43. Davis WB, Rennard SI, Bitterman PB, Crystal RG. Early reversible changes in human alveolar structures induced by hyperoxia. *N Engl J Med* 1983;309:878–883.
44. Pappert D, Rossaint R, Slama K, et al. Influence of positioning on ventilation-perfusion relationships in severe adult respiratory distress syndrome. *Chest* 1994;106:1511–1516.
45. Fridrich P, Krafft P, Hochleuthner H, Mauritz W. The effects of long term prone positioning in patients with trauma-induced adult respiratory distress syndrome. *Anesth Analg* 1996;83:1206–1211.
46. Simmons RS, Berdine GG, Seidenfeld JJ, et al. Fluid balance and the adult respiratory distress syndrome. *Am Rev Respir Dis* 1987;135:924–929.
47. Humphrey H, Hall J, Sznajder I, et al. Improved survival in ARDS patients associated with a reduction in pulmonary capillary wedge pressure. *Chest* 1990;97:1176–1180.
48. Lewis JF, Jobe AH. State of the art: Surfactant and the adult respiratory distress syndrome. *Am Rev Respir Dis* 1993;147:218–233.
49. Pison U, Seeger W, Buchhorn R, et al. Surfactant abnormalities in patients with respiratory failure after multiple trauma. *Am Rev Respir Dis* 1989;140:1033–1039.
50. Weg JG, Balk RA, Tharratt RS, et al. Safety and potential efficacy of an aerosolized surfactant in human sepsis-induce adult respiratory distress syndrome. *JAMA* 1994;272:1433–1438.
51. Gregory TJ, Gadek JE, Weiland JE, et al. Survanta supplementation in patients with acute respiratory distress syndrome (ARDS). *Am J Respir Crit Care Med* 1994;149:A567.
52. Anzueto A, Baughman RP, Guntupalli KK, et al. Aerosolized surfactant in adults with sepsis-induced acute respiratory distress syndrome. *N Engl J Med* 1996;334:1417–1421.
53. Gregory TJ, Steinberg KP, Spragg R, et al. Bovine surfactant therapy for patients with acute respiratory distress syndrome. *Am J Respir Crit Care Med* 1997;155:1309–1315.
54. Shapiro BA, Warren J, Egol AB, et al. Practice parameters for intravenous analgesia and sedation for adult patients in the intensive care unit: An executive summary. *Crit Care Med* 1995;23:1596–1600.
55. Bernard GR, Luce JM, Sprung CL, et al. High dose corticosteroids in patients with acute respiratory distress syndrome. *N Engl J Med* 1987;317:1565–1570.
56. Meduri GU, Chinn AJ, Leeper KV, et al. Corticosteroids rescue treatment in late ARDS: Patterns of response and predictors of outcome. *Chest* 1994;105:1516–1527.
57. Shoemaker WC, Appel PL, Kram HB, et al. Prospective trial of supranormal values of survivors as therapeutic goals in high-risk surgical patients. *Chest* 1988;94:1176–1186.
58. Hayes MA, Timmins AC, Yau EHS, et al. Elevation of systemic oxygen delivery in the treatment of critically ill patients. *N Engl J Med* 1994;330:1717–1722.
59. Gattinoni L, Brazzi L, Pelosi P, et al. A trial of goal-oriented hemodynamic therapy in critically ill patients. *N Engl J Med* 1995;333:1025–1032.
60. Hart R, Albert RK. Sequelae of the adult respiratory distress syndrome. *Thorax* 1994;49:8–13.
61. Ghio AJ, Elliott G, Crapo RO, et al. Impairment after adult respiratory distress syndrome: An evaluation based on American Thoracic Society Recommendations. *Am Rev Respir Dis* 1989;139:1158–1162.
62. McHugh LG, Milberg JA, Whitcomb ME, et al. Recovery of function in survivors of the acute respiratory distress syndrome. *Am J Respir Crit Care Med* 1994;150:90–94.
63. Peters JI, Bell RC, Prihoda TJ, et al. Clinical determinants of abnormalities in pulmonary functions in survivors of the adult respiratory distress syndrome. *Am Rev Respir Dis* 1989;139:1163–1168.

Chapter 7

Congenital Heart Diseases/Arrhythmias

Marcus S. Schamberger, MD

Introduction

The frequency of congenital heart disease in the newborn population is 0.8% to 1%. The majority of affected children have minor cardiac lesions and require little or no treatment. Patients who have more serious heart defects may become symptomatic during the newborn period, or their problem may be detected on routine examination, due to the presence of a murmur. Symptoms are frequently nonspecific, especially in the newborn period, and include respiratory distress, poor feeding, excessive sweating, hepatomegaly, cyanosis, poor perfusion, and shock.[1] Findings on cardiac auscultation can be variable, but tachycardia and gallops are frequent findings in ill patients. The chest x-ray typically shows cardiomegaly (Table 1). Pulmonary blood flow may be increased, decreased, or normal, depending on the cardiac defect. The classification of pulmonary blood flow based on review of the initial chest x-ray may guide the clinician in arriving at the correct diagnosis.

Cardiac defects can also be classified into acyanotic lesions (left-to-right shunts), left-sided obstructive lesions, and cyanotic lesions (right-to-left shunts). The lesions with large left-to-right shunts include ventricular septal defect, atrioventricular (AV) canal, large patent ductus arteriosus (PDA), and aortopulmonary window. These defects have the potential to develop into congestive heart failure, but are otherwise relatively well tolerated. The other two classes of defects are discussed below.

Left-Sided Obstructive Heart Disease

Critical aortic stenosis of the newborn, severe neonatal coarctation of the aorta, and hypoplastic left heart syndrome (HLHS) are characterized by obstruction to systemic blood flow from the left side of the heart. Systemic blood flow is therefore partially or totally dependent on the presence of a PDA allowing for right-to-left shunting of blood from the pulmonary artery to the aorta. Although this is deoxygenated blood, at least there is blood flow. The saturation of 70% to 75% in deoxygenated blood is sufficient to support systemic metabolic needs.

Hypoplastic Left Heart Syndrome

In HLHS, the left ventricle is extremely underdeveloped. In addition, the mitral and aortic valves are too small to allow adequate left-sided blood flow. These changes are caused by obstruction to blood flow during

From: Tobias JD (ed): *Pediatric Critical Care: The Essentials.* ©Futura Publishing Co., Inc., Armonk, NY, 1999.

Table 1

Differential Diagnosis of Cardiomegaly on Chest X-Ray

Congenital heart disease
Acquired heart disease
  myocarditis
  dilated cardiomyopathy
  prolonged arrhythmias
  ischemic heart disease
Pericardial effusion
Acute fluid overload
Artifact (expiratory film, portable CXR)
Noncardiac lesions
  thymus
  anterior mediastinal mass

---

fetal development. Since there is very little or no flow through the aortic valve, the ascending aorta does not develop appropriately and remains small, often measuring only 2 or 3 mm in diameter. All systemic blood flow is maintained through the right side of the heart and the PDA. To allow sufficient right-to-left shunting at the ductal level, the systolic pulmonary artery pressures must be at least equal to the systemic pressures. The perfusion to the innominate, carotid, and the coronary arteries is retrograde through the aortic arch, also provided by blood flow from the PDA. The pulmonary venous blood enters the left atrium and has to cross though an atrial septal defect or foramen ovale, since the flow through the mitral valve is minimal (Fig. 1).

With the availability of prenatal ultrasound screening, more and more patients with HLHS are diagnosed prior to delivery. If undiagnosed, the newborn babies can remain asymptomatic for several days. When the PDA starts to close or when the pulmonary vascular resistance decreases, systemic perfusion becomes compromised. Patients will develop symptoms of shock, including pallor, poor capillary refill, hypotension, decreased urine output, and metabolic acidosis. Because less blood is pumped to the body, the pulmonary blood flow dramatically increases. The pulmonary artery saturation is higher than normal, often up to 100%, and the little amount of blood that reaches the systemic circulation is normally saturated. This explains why normal systemic oxygen saturation on pulse oximetry or blood gas analysis is often noted (in combination with metabolic acidosis). The increased pulmonary blood flow also leads to pulmonary vascular congestion, which may result in "wet lungs" and pulmonary edema. An enlarged liver may be palpable. On auscultation, a murmur may not necessarily be present; a gallop is frequently heard and there is always a single second heart sound. The chest x-ray usually shows increased pulmonary vasculature and cardiomegaly. It may be very hard to differentiate the clinical findings of decompensating HLHS from those of sepsis. And in fact, many patients who have HLHS are misdiagnosed initially and treated as if they were in septic shock. The latter may necessitate many of the same treatments necessary for HLHS including endotracheal intubation, controlled ventilation, and correction of metabolic disturbances. In HLHS, the administration of prostaglandin E is also necessary to stop the process and allow for the return of systemic blood flow.

Treatment of HLHS is aimed toward reestablishing sufficient systemic circulation. To assure the patency of the PDA, prostaglandin E_1 is started as a continuous infusion at 0.1 μg/kg/min. If present, metabolic acidosis is corrected with sodium bicarbonate. Attempts to limit pulmonary overcirculation and to increase pulmonary artery pressures are undertaken by increasing pulmonary vascular resistance. As the blood leaves the single ventricle, it may travel through the pulmonary circulation or across the PDA to the systemic circulation. The ratio of pulmonary blood flow to systemic blood flow (Q_p/Q_s) is determined by the difference in the vascular resistance of the two beds (pulmonary versus systemic). Since oxygen is a potent pulmonary vascular dilator, the FiO_2 is reduced to room air (21%)[2] or as low as possible as long as the systemic oxygen saturation is 70% to 80%.

The ventilatory management includes the use of positive end-expiratory pressure (PEEP) and appropriate tidal volumes. Avoidance of overventilation, by acceptance of $PaCO_2$ values in the 40 mm Hg to 50 mm Hg range, is essential.[3] Lower levels of $PaCO_2$

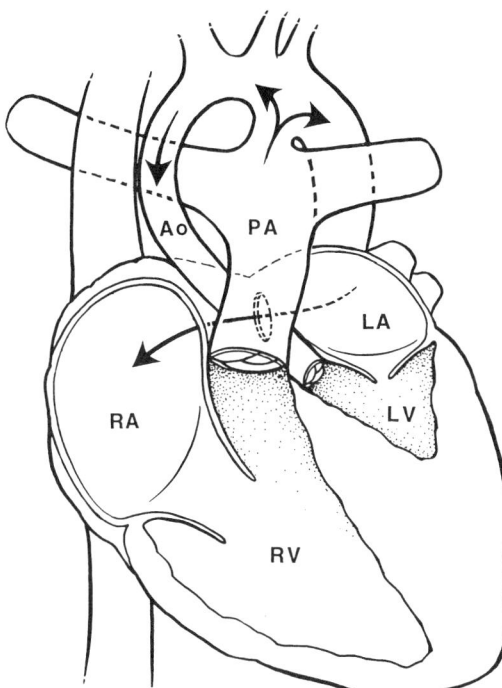

Figure 1. Diagram demonstrating the anatomy of hypoplastic left heart syndrome. See text for details. Ao = aorta; LA = left atrium; LV = left ventricle; PA = pulmonary artery; RA = right atrium; RV = right ventricle.

will lower pulmonary vascular resistance. Occasionally, the addition of 1% to 4% CO_2 to the inspired air may help to increase pulmonary vascular resistance.[4,5] Use of inotropic agents is often helpful; especially dobutamine in doses of 5 to 15 μg/kg/min to increase cardiac contractility without increasing the already elevated systemic vascular resistance. Dopamine, although known to increase systemic vascular resistance, may also increase pulmonary vascular resistance and is not generally contraindicated. Systemic arterial saturations between 75% and 80% represent an acceptable balance between pulmonary and systemic circulations.

After the patient is stabilized, the prostaglandin E_1 may be weaned to 0.01 to 0.05 μg/kg/min. The ultimate treatment for the HLHS is surgical. Surgical options include cardiac transplantation or Norwood surgery (see chapter 8) in the newborn period. Once the patient's cardiovascular status has been resuscitated and metabolic abnormalities corrected, it is often possible to wean and discontinue mechanical ventilatory support. In such cases, in an attempt to increase pulmonary vascular resistance and decrease pulmonary blood flow, some centers use concentrations of oxygen of less than 21% as long as the systemic saturation is greater than or equal to 75%. While waiting for either surgery, nutritional support should be maximized. Enteral feedings should be started as soon as the patient is considered stable. If enteral feedings are not possible, parenteral nutrition may be used.

Critical Aortic Stenosis

In the setting of critical aortic stenosis in the newborn, only a little systemic flow is maintained through the aortic valve. Prenatally, the left ventricle fails in an attempt to pump against the left ventricular outflow obstruction and eventually the left ventricle dilates. Like in HLHS, systemic perfusion depends on the patency of the PDA, which shunts right to left.[6] Findings on physical examination and clinical management are identical to that of HLHS. After initial stabilization, an aortic valvotomy is performed. This can be done in the cardiac catheterization laboratory with a balloon catheter or during an open procedure in the operating room. Even after valvotomy, patients remain critically ill and may require continuation of prostaglandin E_1 infusion, until the left ventricular function improves. Secondary problems may arise due to a poorly developed left ventricle, associated mitral valve anomalies, or an extremely dysplastic or small aortic annulus which is difficult to correct even during an open cardiac procedure.

Severe Coarctation of the Aorta/Interrupted Aortic Arch

In severe coarctation of the aorta in the newborn period, the left-sided obstruction is located just proximal to the PDA. Perfusion of the brachiocephalic vessels is antegrade through the ascending aorta and perfusion of the lower body takes place through the PDA, with right-to-left shunting (Fig. 2). As long as the PDA is widely open, patients may be asymptomatic. Once the PDA begins to close, the blood supply to the lower body becomes restricted. In addition, the coarctation may become more severe, since the aorta often contains some periductal tissue. This tissue constricts with the PDA, thereby further narrowing the aortic lumen.[7]

An extreme form of this lesion is the interrupted aortic arch, which may be associated with DiGeorge syndrome. Therefore, patients who have interrupted aortic arch should have their calcium and phosphorus levels monitored frequently. Chromosomal analysis for microdeletion on chromosome 22 should be performed. If positive, T cell count and T cell function will eventually need to be checked. It is imperative to irradiate all blood products in these patients, because the administration of immunocompetent T cells can result in a fatal form of graft-versus-host disease.

When the PDA begins to constrict, the lower body perfusion becomes compromised. This may present clinically as a difference in perfusion and color between upper and lower body. Pulses in the lower extremities are weak or absent. There is frequently a difference between preductal and postductal oxygen saturation, with a saturation in the legs 5% to 10% lower than in the right arm. There are signs of congestive heart failure, such as tachypnea and hepatomegaly. Often no murmur is auscultated, but due to the frequent association with a bicuspid aortic valve, a systolic ejection click may be heard. A gallop is also frequently found.

Treatment is aimed toward opening the PDA with prostaglandin E_1. As in HLHS and critical aortic stenosis, the body perfusion depends on the pulmonary artery pressure and resistance. Medical management is essentially identical to that of these two lesions, as discussed above. The use of preductal and postductal pulse oximeters is often helpful in the initial management. The oxygen saturation in the lower body depends on the severity of the coarctation, as well as the mixture of blood from the ascending aorta and PDA. In addition to routine methods, progress of treatment may be monitored by assessing pulses in the lower extremities as well as urine output. Final treatment consists of surgical repair of the stenosis with simultaneous PDA ligation. More recently, balloon coarctation angioplasty has been successful in some patients and may be an alternative to surgery. Surgical repair may include resection of the coarctation and an end-to-end anastomosis. With this repair, there may be progressive narrowing later on from progressive scar formation that may require reoperation or balloon dilation. The other option for treatment of patients younger than 6 to 12 months of age is to use a segment of the left subclavian artery and incorporate it into the repair thereby decreasing the incidence of subsequent narrowing (subclavian flap). Perfusion to the left upper extremity is provided by collateral circulation. It is our practice to avoid this extremity as a site for future placement of venous or arterial cannulae.

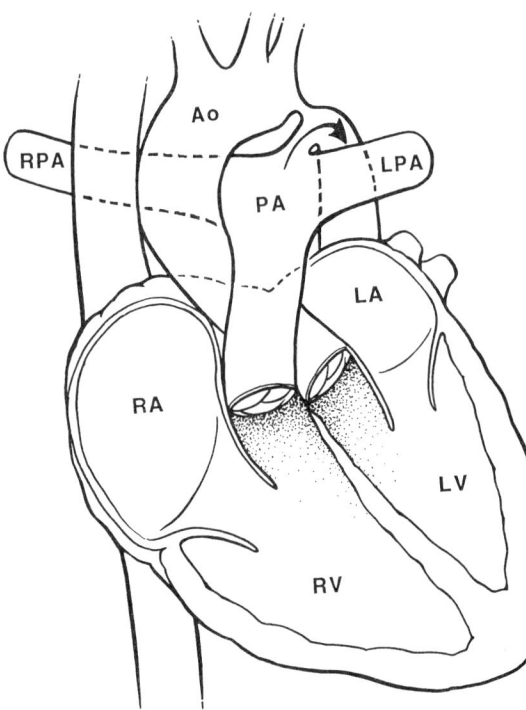

Figure 2. Diagram demonstrating the anatomy of coarctation of the aorta. See text for details. Ao = aorta; LA = left atrium; LPA = left pulmonary artery; LV = left ventricle; PA = pulmonary artery; RA = right atrium; RPA = right pulmonary artery; RV = right ventricle.

Cyanotic Heart Disease

Cyanosis is visible when the amount of reduced (unoxygenated) hemoglobin is at least 5 mg/dL. This means that patients with high hemoglobin levels are more likely to appear cyanotic than are anemic patients. The term cyanotic heart disease is relative, since some of the lesions grouped in this category may not demonstrate visible cyanosis until later in life. Specifically, the term is used for cardiac lesions that have a predominant right-to-left shunt, which results in some degree of desaturated systemic arterial blood.

The degree of cyanosis also depends on the amount of shunting and the oxygen saturation of the blood before mixing. Many lesions require a PDA for pulmonary perfusion and are considered PDA-dependent. In these lesions, the flow across the PDA is left to right from the aorta to the pulmonary artery. If there is a suspicion that a PDA-dependent congenital heart lesion is present, prostaglandin E_1 should always be started, until a definitive diagnosis can be made.[8]

Transposition of the Great Arteries

In transposition of the great arteries, the origins of the aorta and pulmonary artery are switched. The aorta (including the coronary arteries) originates from the right ventricle and the pulmonary artery from the left ventricle so that the pulmonary and systemic circuits are parallel, rather than in series. Oxygenated blood is then pumped back to the lungs and unsaturated blood is pumped to the body. The right ventricle empties into the aorta, which delivers blood to the systemic circulation, which returns to the right atrium, to the right ventricle, and to the aorta again. The left ventricle pumps blood to the pulmonary artery, which carries it to the lungs; the blood returns to the left atrium, to the left ventricle, and to the pulmonary artery again.

When the PDA begins to close, patients may become visibly cyanotic. Preductal (right arm) blood gas analysis shows a low systemic arterial saturation and possibly metabolic acidosis. Depending on additional cardiac defects (ventricular septal defect, atrial septal defect), the PDA may be the main source of mixing between systemic and pulmonary blood. Since vascular resistance and pressures are usually higher on the systemic side compared to the pulmonary side, the PDA will have left-to-right shunting (Fig. 3). If the pulmonary artery systolic pressures are at least equal to systemic pressures, bidirectional shunting across the PDA is seen. In this case, the preductal oxygen saturation may be significantly lower than the postductal saturation (place pulse oximeters on right arm and either leg).

Patients will present with varying degrees of cyanosis. There may be signs of respiratory distress due to increased pulmonary blood flow. On auscultation a murmur is not necessarily present, but the second heart sound is single. The chest x-ray shows cardiomegaly, possibly a narrow mediastinum (caused by the unusual position

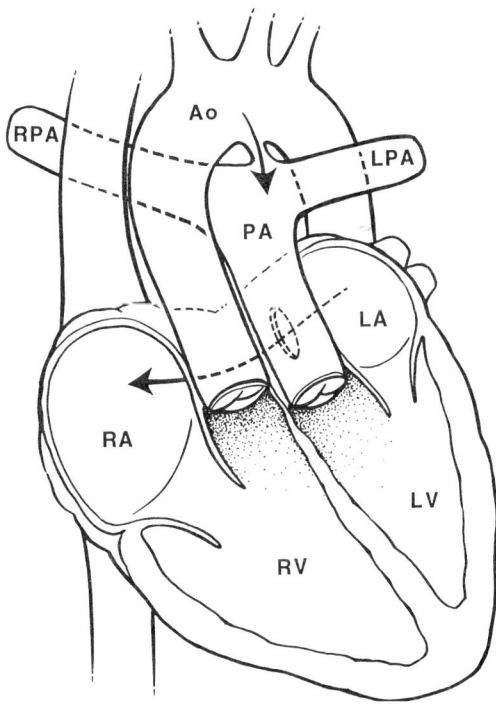

Figure 3. Diagram demonstrating transposition of the great arteries, in which the origins of the aorta and pulmonary artery are switched. See text for details. Ao = aorta; LA = left atrium; LPA = left pulmonary artery; LV = left ventricle; PA = pulmonary artery; RA = right atrium; RPA = right pulmonary artery; RV = right ventricle.

of aorta and pulmonary artery) and *increased vascularity*. Prostaglandin E_1 should be started at 0.1 µg/kg/min as a continuous infusion, to maintain the patency of the PDA. Administration of oxygen may improve the systemic saturation. A foramen ovale with left-to-right shunting is always present, allowing oxygenated blood to cross to the right side of the heart and to be pumped to the body. Shunting across the patent foramen ovale is the major site of mixing in these patients. While some mixing occurs across the PDA, the major effect of the patent PDA is to increase shunting of blood in a unidirectional manner and to subsequently increase atrial pressure and thereby increase shunting at the atrial level. If the foramen ovale is restrictive to flow, the amount of atrial shunting may not be sufficient to maintain adequate systemic oxygenation (in spite of a widely open PDA). Affected patients are deeply cyanotic and require emergency balloon atrial septostomy. This procedure enlarges the foramen ovale and creates an artificial atrial septal defect, thereby improving systemic oxygenation. Postprocedure improvement is usually immediate.

Definitive treatment for transposition of the great arteries is the arterial switch operation. In this surgery, the aorta and pulmonary artery are switched and the coronary arteries are reimplanted. Atrial septal defects and ventricular septal defects are closed during the same surgery. If this surgery cannot be performed within the first few days, an elective balloon atrial septostomy will assure adequate mixing of the circulations. Prostaglandin E_1 may then be discontinued, if shunting at the atrial level is adequate.

Tricuspid Valve Atresia and Pulmonary Valve Atresia

In tricuspid valve atresia, the systemic venous blood has to cross from the right atrium via the foramen ovale or an atrial septal defect to the left atrium. Pulmonary blood flow is provided from the left ventricle via a ventricular septal defect to a hypoplastic right ventricle and to the pulmonary artery. If the ventricular septal defect is large, patients will develop signs of congestive heart failure as the pulmonary vascular resistance decreases. Under these circumstances, a PDA is no longer beneficial for pulmonary blood flow. If the ventricular septal defect is very restrictive, or if the pulmonary valve is stenotic, pulmonary blood flow is decreased. In this setting, similar to pulmonary valve atresia, a PDA may be necessary to provide blood flow to the lungs (Fig. 4). Patients who depend on the PDA will develop severe cyanosis as the PDA begins to constrict. As long as oxygen saturations are sufficient, the patients may otherwise show little sign of distress. A chest x-ray will show *decreased pulmonary blood flow* and varying degrees of cardiomegaly. An electrocardiogram (ECG) is very helpful,

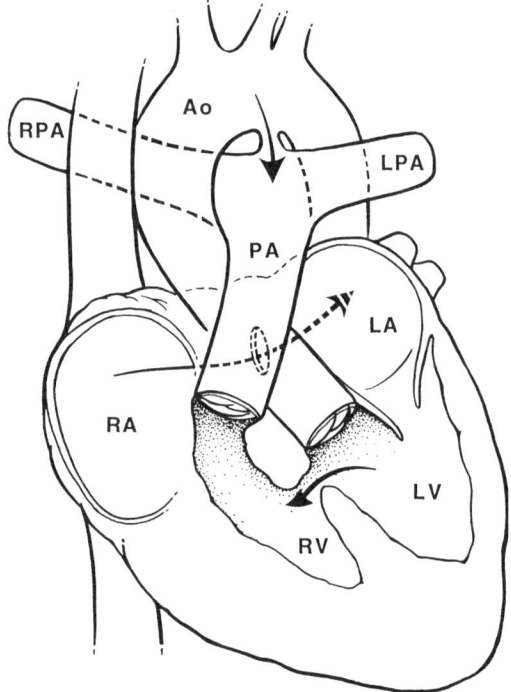

Figure 4. Diagram demonstrating tricuspid valve atresia, in which the systemic venous blood has to cross from the right atrium via the foramen ovale or an atrial septal defect to the left atrium. See text for details. Ao = aorta; LA = left atrium; LPA = left pulmonary artery; LV = left ventricle; PA = pulmonary artery; RA = right atrium; RPA = right pulmonary artery; RV = right ventricle.

as it often shows left ventricular hypertrophy for age and always shows extreme left axis deviation (negative QRS axis). Tricuspid atresia is the only cyanotic congenital heart defect with these easily recognizable ECG findings. Pulmonary valve atresia has a similar presentation, but without the left axis changes on ECG. In pulmonary valve atresia, the PDA is essential for providing pulmonary blood flow.

Administration of oxygen may improve the systemic oxygen saturation somewhat, but prostaglandin E_1 must be started as a continuous infusion to assure adequate pulmonary perfusion. In either of these lesions, atrial right-to-left shunting can be seen. Especially in tricuspid valve atresia, a restrictive atrial septal defect must be enlarged, by atrial balloon septostomy, in the cardiac catheterization laboratory. Eventually a shunt from the subclavian artery to the pulmonary artery (Blalock-Taussig shunt) is surgically placed in most patients. In tricuspid valve atresia, the eventual surgical repair is the Fontan procedure, to achieve an acyanotic state. In pulmonary valve atresia, further surgeries depend on the ventricular morphology. If the right ventricular size is adequate, a valved conduit can be placed from the right ventricle to the remnant of the main pulmonary artery to maintain a two-ventricular system. If the right ventricle is rudimentary, a Fontan procedure is performed.

Ebstein's Anomaly of the Tricuspid Valve

In Ebstein's anomaly, the septal leaflet of the tricuspid valve is displaced apically. This leads to severe tricuspid valve regurgitation and a smaller than normal right ventricle. Often this lesion is associated with varying degrees of pulmonary stenosis. Patients may be symptomatic shortly after birth with severe degrees of cyanosis, respiratory distress, and signs of heart failure with hepatomegaly. On chest x-ray, *decreased pulmonary blood flow* is noted in combination with massive cardiomegaly. The severe cardiomegaly is caused by the enlarged right atrium, due to the tricuspid valve regurgitation. Auscultation often reveals a loud holosystolic tricuspid regurgitation murmur and several additional heart sounds or clicks caused by the abnormal tricuspid valve. If the displacement of the tricuspid valve is severe and there is pulmonary valve stenosis, very little blood reaches the lungs. Affected patients require a PDA with left-to-right shunt for adequate pulmonary perfusion. If patients are clinically cyanotic, prostaglandin E_1 should be started.[9] As pulmonary vascular resistance and pressure decrease, it becomes easier for the right ventricle to pump to the lungs. The pulmonary blood flow may therefore improve during the first days of life in patients who have less severe pulmonary stenosis. Oxygen is a potent pulmonary vasodilator which decreases the pulmonary vascular resistance, and should therefore be used liberally in this lesion.

Ebstein's anomaly is associated with an increased frequency of supraventricular tachycardia (SVT). The SVT is treated as in all other patients, while keeping in mind that patients with Ebstein's anomaly of the tricuspid valve are hemodynamically less stable and may not tolerate SVT for a prolonged time.

Tetralogy of Fallot

The cardiac defects that characterize tetralogy of Fallot (TOF) include a large ventricular septal defect, an overriding aorta, right ventricular hypertrophy, and infundibular/valvular pulmonary stenosis. The magnitude of the right-to-left shunt and the amount of cyanosis depend on the severity of the right ventricular outflow tract obstruction. The infundibular component of the pulmonary stenosis frequently increases over the first few months of life, leading to more cyanosis (Fig. 5). If the right ventricular outflow tract obstruction is already severe in the newborn period, patients may develop significant cyanosis with the closure of the PDA. In this case, prostaglandin E_1 should be started, to reestablish adequate pulmonary perfusion. Oxygen may help to improve systemic saturations. On clinical examination, a loud systolic ejection murmur at the left sternal border radiating to the back, and a single

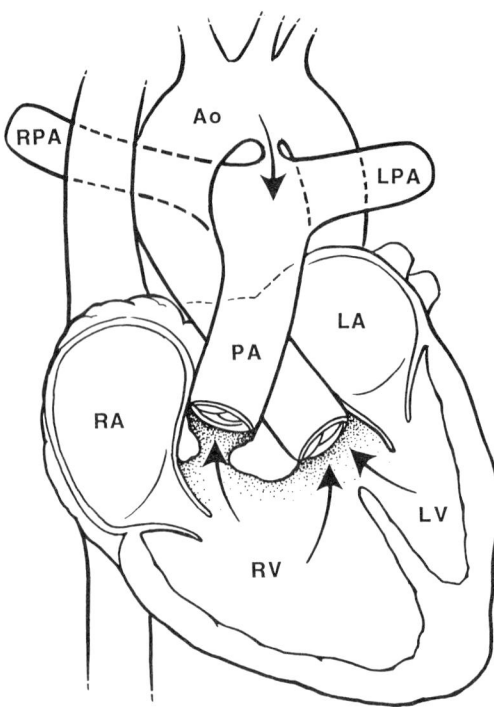

Figure 5. Diagram demonstrating the anatomic findings of tetralogy of Fallot, including a ventricular septal defect, overriding aorta, right ventricular hypertrophy, and obstruction to pulmonary blood flow (either pulmonary valve or infundibular stenosis). See text for details. Ao = aorta; LA = left atrium; LPA = left pulmonary artery; LV = left ventricle; PA = pulmonary artery; RA = right atrium; RPA = right pulmonary artery; RV = right ventricle.

second heart sound (no pulmonary component) are typical findings. The chest x-ray shows *decreased pulmonary vascularity* and, frequently, a boot-shaped heart (*cor en sabot*), due to elevation of the ventricular apex caused by the right ventricular hypertrophy. Due to the decreased pulmonary blood flow, congestive heart failure is very uncommon in patients who have TOF.

The infundibular pulmonary stenosis can change in severity, as the infundibulum is part of the right ventricular myocardium. Acute constriction of the infundibulum, resulting in increased right-to-left shunt and decreased pulmonary perfusion, causes a hypercyanotic episode, also known as a hypoxemic spell or "Tet spell." These episodes may occur in almost any patient with unoperated TOF, even if the patient is only mildly cyanotic at baseline. They can be caused by any event that increases cardiac contractility, such as the release of endogenous catecholamines during painful procedures (blood draws, intravenous starts) or the use of inotropic agents. They can also occur after only minor stimulation (normal crying, etc). Besides the obvious increase in cyanosis, the patient appears agitated and restless. Older patients often assume a squatting, knee-to-chest position. This position increases the systemic vascular resistance and, since blood flow follows the path of least resistance, more blood is pumped to the lungs. The usual, loud systolic ejection murmur may be barely audible during a hypoxic spell, because less blood crosses the narrowed right ventricular outflow tract. Many of the Tet spells are self-limited. Comforting of the patient in the parent's arms and avoidance of further stimulation, may be all that is required. Administration of 100% oxygen is suggested. Pressing the patient's knees against his or her chest while consoling the patient increases the systemic vascular resistance and increases pulmonary blood flow. Morphine, as an anxiolytic agent, should be given in a dose of 0.05 to 0.2 mg/kg by the intravenous or subcutaneous route, if conservative management fails. More specific medical management requires intravenous access. β-Adrenergic antagonists such as propranolol or esmolol relax the subpulmonary infundibulum. Most experience exists with the use of intravenous propranolol in doses of 0.01 to 0.1 mg/kg. The advantage of esmolol lies in its more rapid onset of action and the shorter half-life time. Therefore, possible hemodynamic side effects are shorter in duration. Often a single intravenous bolus of 0.5 mg/kg of esmolol is sufficient to end a hypoxic spell. If needed, a continuous esmolol infusion (0.1 to 0.3 mg/kg/min) may be started. Phenylephrine, a selective α-adrenergic agonist, increases the systemic vascular resistance (similar to knee-chest maneuver). It is administered intravenously in bolus doses of 2 to 5 μg/kg and a continuous infusion of 0.1 to 5.0 μg/kg/min, if needed. One or two 10 mL/kg boluses of isotonic fluid may be helpful by increasing right ventricular preload. Rarely, a hypoxic episode may be severe enough to require intubation. In this event, heavy sedation with opioids is necessary to avoid protracted spells due to patient agitation and discomfort. Emergent surgical placement of a systemic-to-pulmonary shunt has been necessary in rare situations that were refractory to medical management. The occurrence of hypoxic spells in patients with TOF is always an indication for surgical intervention in the near future (complete repair or placement of an aorta-to-pulmonary-artery shunt). Although oral propranolol has no place in the short-term treatment of a hypoxic episode, it is helpful as a baseline medication for prevention of episodes. Every patient with TOF and a history of hypoxic spells should be started on maintenance propranolol therapy while awaiting surgery.

Cardiac inotropic medications should be used cautiously in patients with unoperated TOF, as these medications (including digoxin) have the potential to increase the contractility of the infundibular muscle bundle and may cause a hypoxic episode. Inotropic agents that decrease the systemic vascular resistance (dobutamine, amrinone, milrinone, isoproterenol) may increase right-to-left shunting and should be avoided in most instances. Diuretics are usually avoided since they may decrease right ventricular preload, which may lead to increased narrowing at the subpulmonary infundibulum.

Truncus Arteriosus

In patients with truncus arteriosus, the pulmonary artery and aorta failed to separate during embryologic development. As a result, there is a single large artery originating from both ventricles, over a large ventricular septal defect. Unless there is additional coarctation of the aorta, a PDA does not develop in the embryologic period (Fig. 6). Patients are typically minimally symptomatic in the first few days of life. As the pulmonary vascular resistance begins to drop, most patients develop signs of pulmonary congestion and congestive heart failure. On physical examination, a murmur may be absent, but the second heart sound is always

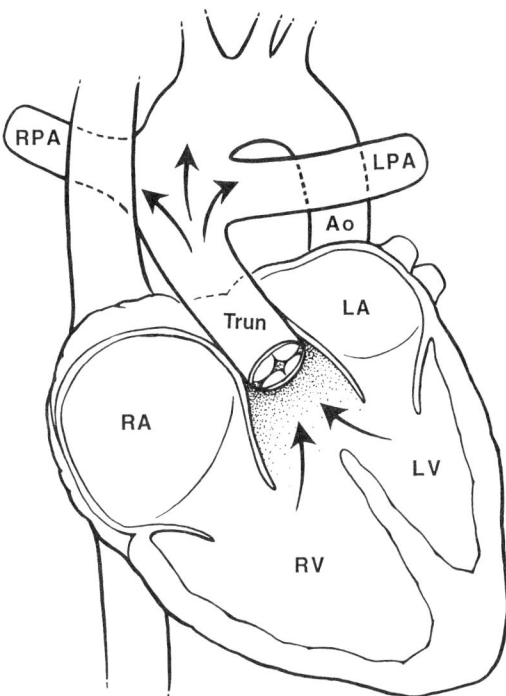

Figure 6. Diagram demonstrating truncus arteriosus, which involves a single vessel with a single valve arising from both ventricles. This vessel bifurcates into the aorta and the pulmonary arteries. Congestive heart failure develops early on due to increased pulmonary blood flow and a left-to-right shunt. Treatment involves closing the ventricular septal defect and using the single great vessel as the aorta. Pulmonary flow is provided by a valved conduit from the right ventricle to the right and left pulmonary arteries, which are divided and removed from the single great vessel. Ao = aorta; LA = left atrium; LPA = left pulmonary artery; LV = left ventricle; PA = pulmonary artery; RA = right atrium; RPA = right pulmonary artery; RV = right ventricle; Trun = truncus arteriosus.

single. Hepatomegaly depends on the severity of heart failure. Depending on the amount of pulmonary blood flow, systemic artery saturations vary between 80% and 100%. The chest x-ray shows *increased pulmonary vascularity* and varying degrees of cardiomegaly. A thymus may be absent, due to the frequent association with DiGeorge syndrome.

The clinical management of truncus arteriosus is aimed toward control of the heart failure. Use of diuretics, such as furosemide, decreases pulmonary edema. Inotropic agents may help to limit the effects of the volume overload on the heart. Oxygen, a potent pulmonary vasodilator, should be used only if absolutely necessary. The desired balance between systemic and pulmonary blood flow is present with systemic oxygen saturations in the 75% to 80% range. Although this may be the ideal goal, often the pulmonary blood flow cannot be controlled well and saturations are in the high 90% range even with an FiO_2 of 0.21. If heart failure cannot be controlled with medications alone, endotracheal intubation and ventilation with liberal use of PEEP may allow limitation of pulmonary blood flow. Unless additional coarctation of the aorta or an interrupted aortic arch are present, prostaglandin E_1 is of no use for treatment of truncus arteriosus.

All patients with truncus arteriosus should undergo a work-up for DiGeorge syndrome. Specific gene probes for chromosome 22 are available, but are not currently highly specific and do not correlate with the severity of the syndrome. Frequent monitoring of calcium and phosphorus levels is indicated. If the gene probe is positive, T-lymphocyte count and function should be assessed at some later point. All patients with truncus arteriosus should receive only irradiated blood products until DiGeorge syndrome is ruled out (risk of graft-versus-host syndrome). The definitive management of truncus arteriosus is surgical repair. During this surgery, the ventricular septal defect is patched so that the truncal vessel originates completely from the left ventricle. The truncal vessel is used as the aorta to supply systemic circulation. A conduit is placed from the right ventricle to the pulmonary arteries, which are separated from the truncal vessel.

Total Anomalous Pulmonary Venous Return

Total anomalous pulmonary venous return (TAPVR) is the fifth of the five T's (transposition of the great arteries, tricuspid atresia, TOF, truncus arteriosus, and TAPVR) that cause cyanosis in the newborn. Embryologically, the pulmonary veins develop independently from the heart and drain into a separate chamber, which eventually fuses with the left atrium. If this connection does not take place, the pulmonary veins will drain abnormally. TAPVR is classified according to location of this drainage. There is a "supracardiac type," characterized by drainage into the innominate vein or the superior vena cava. In the "cardiac type," the pulmonary veins are connected to the coronary sinus or directly to the right atrium. In the "infradiaphragmatic form" of TAPVR, the pulmonary veins drain into the portal vein and via the ductus venosus to the inferior vena cava. The latter type frequently has a significant degree of pulmonary venous congestion, as the drainage is frequently stenotic or obstructed. A combination of any of the three types is also possible. As a result of the TAPVR, patients have a large left-to-right shunt. Unless there is an associated cardiac lesion, an atrial septal defect with right-to-left shunting must be present to provide blood flow to the left-sided cardiac chambers (Fig. 7). The age and severity of clinical presentation depend on the form of TAPVR. Patients in which the drainage of the pulmonary veins is obstructed (95% of infradiaphragmatic and up to 50% of supracardiac) typically present in the immediate newborn period. They are severely ill and there is pulmonary hypertension and venous congestion, which mimics the picture of persistent pulmonary hypertension of the newborn. The chest x-ray is characterized by "white lungs" and a normal heart size. In TAPVR below the diaphragm, a blood gas sample from an umbilical venous line positioned high in the inferior vena cava will have a high oxygen saturation and is almost diagnostic of the disease. Prostaglandin E_1 infusion may be helpful for those patients in whom the pulmonary venous obstruction is at the level of the ductus venosus, as prostaglandin is believed to have a dilating effect on this tissue. Otherwise, aggressive cardiorespiratory support and early surgical repair are the appropriate interventions.

Patients who do not have initial obstruction during the newborn period are only minimally symptomatic. Over time, signs of heart failure develop and the systemic oxy-

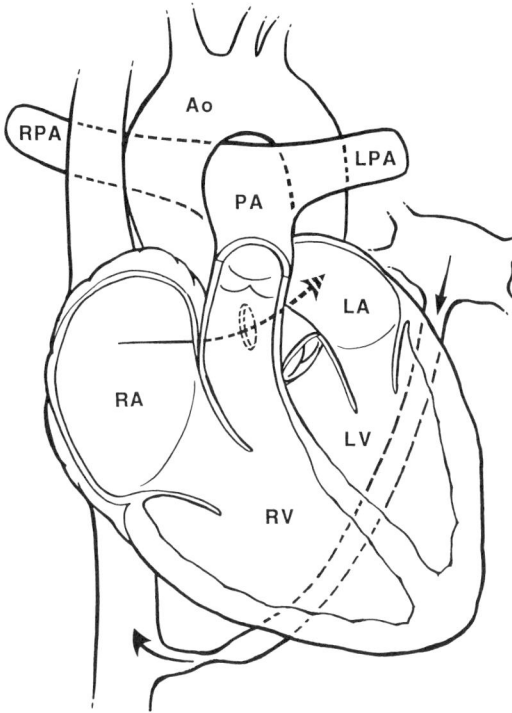

Figure 7. Diagram demonstrating total anomalous pulmonary venous return, which is classified according to location of the anomalous drainage. The infradiaphragmatic form consists of drainage of the pulmonary veins into the portal vein and via the ductus venosus to the inferior vena cava. A significant degree of pulmonary venous congestion is usually present because the drainage is frequently stenotic or obstructed. An associated atrial septal defect is frequently present and allows blood to flow from the right atrium to the left atrium.

gen saturations are mildly decreased due to the atrial level right-to-left shunt. As long as heart failure can be controlled with medications (furosemide and digoxin), and no obstruction of the pulmonary veins develops, patients may be followed conservatively. In these patients, surgical correction of the TAPVR can be performed electively at 2 to 6 months of age.

Patients who have complex congenital heart disease in combination with TAPVR have an increased frequency of polysplenia and asplenia. If the presence of a spleen is uncertain, a radionuclide scan for spleen tissue should be performed or a peripheral smear examined for Howell-Jolly bodies. The latter are nuclear remnants in red blood cells that are normally removed by splenic tissue.

Congestive Heart Failure

Congestive heart failure is not a diagnosis, but rather should be considered the symptom of an underlying disease process (Table 2). Although short-term management may be similar for many of the etiologies, specific treatment may be required.[10]

Myocarditis/Cardiomyopathy

Myocarditis is characterized by an inflammation of the heart muscle. Frequently, the inflammatory process is not limited to the myocardium, but also involves the pericardium (pericarditis) and, less frequently, the endocardium (endocarditis). There is a wide range in severity of the disease from the asymptomatic to the critically ill patient in cardiogenic shock. Many patients have a few-day history of an upper respiratory infection, but have been otherwise healthy. Newborns and infants often have a rapid onset and presentation of the disease. Frequently the myocarditis/pericarditis is of viral origin, with adenoviruses, coxsackie B, coxsackie A, and echovirus being most common. Almost any virus has the potential to cause myocarditis (including the HIV virus).[11] Bacterial myocarditis (including mycobacterium tuberculosis) is less common. Rickettsiae, mycoplasma, fungi, and protozoa can all cause myocarditis. Chagas disease (Trypanosoma cruzi) may involve the heart and is endemic

Table 2

Differential Diagnosis of Congestive Heart Failure

Congenital and acquired heart disease
Cardiomyopathy
Myocarditis
Pericardial effusion
Arrhythmias
Cardiac ischemia
High-output cardiac failure (anemia, AV fistula)

AV = arteriovenous.

in Central and South America. Rheumatic fever, other rheumatic diseases, and medications should be included in the differential diagnosis of myocarditis and pericarditis (Table 3). Travel and medication history may occasionally be helpful in determining a cause for the disease. A positive family history and abnormal neurologic examination may be suggestive of metabolic/genetic causes of the cardiomyopathy.

On cardiac auscultation, findings such as tachycardia, a gallop, and possibly a valvular insufficiency murmur (due to dilation of the valve annulus) may be present. Right-sided heart failure may lead to jugular venous distention, hepatomegaly, and edema in dependent body parts (ankles and feet in older children, sacral edema in infants). Left-sided heart failure presents as pulmonary venous congestion with rales, rhonchi, respiratory distress, and symptoms of decreased systemic output. With decreased systemic output, peripheral extremities are cool, capillary refill is prolonged, and urine output is frequently diminished. In an attempt to compensate for the diminished stroke volume, the heart rate is increased. A decreased blood pressure is an alarming sign, and is due to the inability to maintain systemic vascular resistance due to poor vasomotor control. Most patients maintain an adequate blood pressure by increasing systemic vascular resistance in response to the decreased cardiac output. All forms of arrhythmia are possible and may further compromise the already low cardiac output.

The chest x-ray in myocarditis or cardiomyopathy shows varying degrees of cardiomegaly and pulmonary edema. ECG changes may include low voltage (especially in the limb leads), flattened T waves, prolonged QT interval, AV block, and other arrhythmias. The echocardiogram is characterized by a decrease in left ventricular contractility indices, frequently with dilatation of the ventricles. A pericardial effusion may be present. Intracardiac thrombi in the dilated heart chambers may be seen in long-standing disease states. In infants, an aberrant origin of the left coronary artery from the pulmonary artery must be excluded by the echocardiographic examination.

Laboratory work should include serum electrolytes, calcium, magnesium, blood urea nitrogen, creatinine, arterial blood gas, a complete blood count, sedimentation rate, blood cultures, and viral cultures from the nasopharynx and stool. Serum troponin I level,[12] creatine phosphokinase, transaminases, and lactate dehydrogenase may be useful. Calculation of the anion gap should be performed and, if abnormal, lactate, pyruvate, and ammonia levels should be measured. Serum carnitine and acyl carnitine levels are always obtained in younger children, since a metabolic cause for the cardiomyopathy is possible.[13] Urine metabolic screening should be routine in newborns and infants with cardiomyopathy. Biopsies of skeletal muscle and skin can identify mitochondrial-related causes and other disorders.[14] An endomyocardial biopsy may be diagnostic for myocarditis and may show typical inflammatory changes. However, myocardial biopsy, even with immunohistochemical staining, has a sensitivity of less than 60%, and carries a significant risk. For this reason, it is rarely indicated in the acute phase of the disease. The differential diagnosis of cardiomyopathy includes myocarditis, as well as all other causes for cardiac dilatation and decreased contractility (Table 4).

The initial management of myocarditis or cardiomyopathy is aimed toward stabilization of the ill patient. See also chapter 1 for a full discussion of airway management and chapter 2 for a full discussion of cardiovascular physiology, invasive hemodynamic monitoring, and the administration of inotropic agents. In addition to the pulmonary congestion, decreased perfusion of

Table 3

Etiologic Agents for Myocarditis

Viral
Bacterial (including mycobacterium tuberculosis)
Rickettsial
Protozoal (Trypanosoma cruzi)
Fungal
Rheumatic/immunologic
Kawasaki disease
Medications
Idiopathic

Table 4

Differential Diagnosis of Dilated Cardiomyopathy

Medications
Myocarditis
Familial cardiomyopathy
Chronic hypertension
Congenital or acquired structural heart disease
Prolonged arrhythmia (supraventricular tachycardia)
Ischemia, hypoxia
Myocarditis
Metabolic/genetic disorders
Aberrant left coronary artery

the diaphragm (caused by the low cardiac output) may lead to deterioration in respiratory status. Oxygen is administered via face mask to improve tissue oxygenation. To allow for more effective ventilation and to decrease the work of breathing, endotracheal intubation should be used early on in the critically ill patient. Endotracheal intubation also permits effective sedation of agitated patients and thereby further reduces the workload on the heart. For the same reason, fever should be treated aggressively. Metabolic acidosis is corrected with sodium bicarbonate.

Frequent electrolyte monitoring is required, as electrolyte abnormalities may precipitate arrhythmias. Hypomagnesemia should be treated with 50 mg/kg (maximum: 2 grams) of magnesium sulfate administered intravenously over 30 minutes. Hypocalcemia is corrected with either 0.3 mL/kg of calcium gluconate or 0.1 mL/kg of 10% calcium chloride administered intravenously over 30 minutes, preferably via a central venous catheter. Both hyperkalemia and hypokalemia may cause arrhythmias, with the former being more serious. Due to the risk of hyperkalemia, especially in the presence of impaired renal function, extreme caution must be used in the correction of hypokalemia. Hypokalemia is treated carefully in increments of 0.25 mEq/kg (maximum 20 mEq) of potassium chloride administered intravenously over 60 minutes or, if tolerated, 0.25 to 1.0 mEq/kg (maximum 40 mEq) of potassium chloride

by mouth or via a nasogastric tube. The goal is to achieve values in the low normal range and to avoid overcorrection. Arrhythmias must be treated effectively, as cardiac output in patients with myocarditis is very dependent on rhythm and heart rate. Cardiac compensation by increasing the stroke volume is not possible in patients with myocarditis or cardiomyopathy.

In severely ill patients, placement of an arterial line for blood pressure and blood gas monitoring is very helpful. Urine output is monitored with a Foley catheter. A central venous line connected to a pressure transducer is valuable for assessing the intravascular fluid status and right-sided preload. Decreasing oxygen saturations on serial central venous blood gases may allow early detection of dropping cardiac output. Placement of a Swan-Ganz catheter may be indicated in patients who have progressive cardiac failure and high central venous pressure values with a low urine output. The placement of a pulmonary artery catheter carries a significant risk of precipitating arrhythmias in the patient with a dilated cardiomyopathy. Additionally, successful placement, without the aid of fluoroscopy, may be difficult due to the dilated right ventricle. With these considerations in mind, a risk-benefit ratio must be made when considering the use of a pulmonary artery catheter.

Essentially, all patients show fluid retention. For this reason, total fluid intake is restricted, and intravenous furosemide in doses of 0.5 to 1.0 mg/kg/dose is frequently helpful for decreasing left ventricular end-diastolic pressures (LVEDPs) and alleviating pulmonary congestion. A small subset of patients may show relative intravascular fluid depletion and, in these patients, one careful fluid bolus of 5 to 10 mL/kg of isotonic fluid may improve cardiac output by increasing preload. Long-term fluid management is guided by serial measurements of central venous pressure, urine output, and weight.

Cardiac inotropes (see chapter 2) may be useful for improving myocardial contractility.[15] Medications that possess a mild vasodilatory effect are especially useful in that they additionally decrease afterload. Dobutamine, in doses of 5 to 20 μg/kg/min, is well established in this role. It is frequently combined with dopamine, in renal doses (2 to 5 μg/kg/min) or inotropic doses (5 to 20 μg/kg/min), in patients with a low mean arterial pressure.[16] Either of the above agents can cause arrhythmias in patients with a dilated, irritable myocardium. The use of more vasoconstrictive inotropic agents (epinephrine, norepinephrine) is avoided whenever possible, since these agents increase afterload and thus increase cardiac workload, thereby decreasing cardiac output. In patients who have stable or even mildly elevated blood pressure, additional careful afterload reduction appears useful. Nitroprusside may be started at low doses (0.25 μg/kg/min). If well tolerated, it is slowly increased over the next several hours up to 2 to 3 μg/kg/min (monitor cyanide and thiocyanate levels especially in renal failure). Phosphodiesterase inhibitors (amrinone and milrinone) also have vasodilator properties and may be used instead of or in addition to dobutamine. After the initial loading doses, amrinone is administered in doses of 5 to 20 μg/kg/min and milrinone in doses of 0.5 to 1.0 μg/kg/min. Since digoxin has a long half-life and may cause severe arrhythmias in patients who have myocarditis, it is used with extreme caution. It is usually not started until several days after stabilization of the patient. Due to the increased myocardial irritability, the digoxin dose is lowered to about two thirds of the usual dosage. Angiotensin-converting enzyme inhibitors (captopril and enalapril) are potent vasodilators and can lead to severe hypotension. They should only be started at very low doses (captopril 0.05 mg/kg/dose) after hemodynamic stability is established. Their main role lies in preparation for discontinuation of intravenous vasodilators and in long-term oral afterload reduction. If tolerated initially, the dose may be increased slowly over several days.

If intracardiac thrombi are seen on echocardiogram, anticoagulation with heparin or coumadin is recommended. If no thrombi are present, low-dose aspirin may be started to counteract the increased risk of thrombus formation. Intravenous γ-globulin for myocarditis remains controversial. If used, a total dose of 2 g/kg is administered intravenously.[17] To minimize fluid overload, it may be helpful to give this amount in divided doses over several days.[18] High-dose corticosteroids (methylprednisolone or dexamethasone) are believed by some experts to be of benefit to patients who have myocarditis.[19] Since the potential benefit of steroids lies in their anti-inflammatory properties, treatment is frequently continued throughout the entire acute phase of the disease. After several days, tapering to lower doses appears reasonable. A decision for eventual discontinuation may be guided by the results of an endomyocardial biopsy. Other anti-inflammatory agents (azathioprine or cyclosporine) have been used, but no formal, prospective, randomized studies are available to determine their efficacy.[20] If metabolic etiologies for a dilated cardiomyopathy are being considered (especially in infants), carnitine should be administered orally or intravenously after drawing blood for carnitine and acylcarnitine levels.[14]

Patients who fail to respond to the above measures may develop progressive cardiac failure. Mechanical assist devices (intra-aortic balloon pump, ventricular assist device, extracorporeal membrane oxygenation) may be indicated to support the patient until there is return of myocardial function or as a bridge to cardiac transplantation.[21] Results of cardiac transplantation in the acute phase of myocarditis have been discouraging. In spite of aggressive medical immunosuppression, the transplanted graft frequently develops myocarditis.[22]

Long-term management in the intensive care unit is mainly supportive. Special attention should be paid to the nutritional status of the patient. Enteral or parenteral nutrition is started as soon as the fluid management permits.

Aberrant Origin of the Left Coronary Artery

The origin of the left coronary artery from the pulmonary artery is a rare anomaly. Nevertheless, it must be ruled out in every pediatric patient with a dilated cardiomyopathy or with cardiac failure. Patients with this condition are typically asymptomatic in the newborn period. Over time, when the pulmonary vascular resistance falls, the pulmonary artery pressure is not sufficient to provide forward flow in the left coronary artery. With this anomaly, the lower saturation of blood from the pulmonary artery is not the problem, but rather the problem is its low driving pressure. Flow reversal in the left coronary artery develops, with "stealing" of blood flow from left and right coronary arteries into the pulmonary artery. The typical age of presentation is from 1 to 4 months (occasionally later, even after the first year of life).

Review of the patient's recent history often reveals general irritability, increased sweating, and poor feeding. At the time of presentation, patients typically have dilation of the left ventricle with cardiomegaly and pulmonary edema on chest x-ray. Signs of left-sided ischemia on ECG include prominent Q waves and ST-T wave changes in leads I, II, aVL, and V_4 through V_6. Clinical signs of heart failure are similar to those described in myocarditis. Poor perfusion with cold extremities, tachycardia, tachypnea, wheezes, rales, and hepatomegaly are frequent in the patient with aberrant origin of the left coronary artery.

The diagnosis of aberrant left coronary artery is typically made by echocardiography, the clinical history, and the ECG. The left ventricle is dilated, with poor function. Most of the focus is on identification of the left coronary orifice, which is often positioned just opposite of the aortic sinuses at the main pulmonary artery. If the diagnosis of an aberrant origin of the left coronary artery cannot be made or ruled out by echocardiography, cardiac catheterization is indicated.

Medical management is limited to stabilization of the patient. Supportive measures include administration of oxygen. Endotracheal intubation is performed based on the patient's clinical status, but may be helpful in decreasing the myocardial oxygen demands as well as allowing the aggressive use of opioids to control pain related to myocardial ischemia. The judicious use of inotropic agents (low-dose dobutamine) may be indicated, as long as oxygen demand on the heart is not increased. Careful attention is directed toward the myocardial oxygen delivery-demand ratio. Delivery is determined by the diastolic time (related to heart rate) and the coronary perfusion pressure: diastolic blood pressure minus the LVEDP. In aberrant origin of the left coronary artery, the coronary perfusion pressure is decreased, as the pulmonary arterial diastolic pressure is much lower than the systemic diastolic blood pressure. Oxygen consumption is determined by heart rate, myocardial contractility, LVEDP, and afterload. The prime determinant in both delivery and consumption is heart rate. Vasoconstrictive inotropic agents are avoided. Afterload reduction with low-dose nitroprusside or nitroglycerin infusion may be helpful. Diuretics are used to reduce retained fluid. Definitive therapy requires surgical correction of the coronary anomaly as soon as possible.

Arrhythmias

The diagnosis and management of arrhythmias requires a systematic approach. Electrolyte abnormalities (K^+, Ca^{++}, Mg^{++}) must be excluded. The reader is also referred to chapter 13. Hyperkalemia presents with widening of the QRS complex and tall, peaked T waves. With the further rise of the serum potassium, the P wave becomes widened and the PR interval is prolonged. Eventually the QRS complex enlarges so much that the ECG shows a typical "sine wave pattern," which may progress to ventricular fibrillation and asystole. Changes in the ECG associated with hypokalemia include the appearance of a U wave and flattening of the T wave. This may be "misread" as a long QT interval. Additional changes may include ST depression and prolongation of the PR interval. Low levels of magnesium may also predispose to ventricular ectopy, bigeminy, or ventricular tachycardia especially following cardiac surgery.

Low serum levels of calcium and/or magnesium lead to prolongation of the ST segment, which results in a long QT interval. These changes reverse with correction of the electrolytes. High serum levels of calcium and/or magnesium result in shortening of the ST segment. This is visible mainly in the form of a short QT interval.

Almost all antiarrhythmic medications

have the potential to cause arrhythmias and may interact with other medications (quinidine increases digoxin levels). A one-lead rhythm strip may be sufficient to handle acute emergencies, but for the diagnosis of more complex arrhythmias, a 12-lead ECG should be obtained.

Sinus Tachycardia

Sinus tachycardia is characterized by a fast heart rate that originates from the sinus node. On the ECG, all QRS complexes are narrow and preceded by a p wave. The p waves have a normal axis (positive in lead I and II, negative in aVR). The heart rate varies with changing activity or agitation. Newborns and young children can have sinus tachycardia with heart rates in excess of 200 beats per minute. The sinus tachycardia may be a symptom of underlying heart disease (myocarditis or congenital heart disease). More frequently, it is caused by noncardiac problems including dehydration, anemia, shock, fever, pain, hyperthyroidism, and agitation. Sinus tachycardia may also be an effect of medications (cardiac inotropic agents, nasal decongestants, nebulized albuterol, atropine, methylxanthines) or of abnormally high levels of endogenous catecholamines. Treatment is aimed at correction of the underlying problem. Only in the rare case of unexplainable inappropriate sinus tachycardia, should the use of β-adrenergic antagonists be considered.

Some forms of SVT originate high in the right atrium (sinus node reentry tachycardia, ectopic high right atrial tachycardia). These tachycardias have a normal p wave axis and are difficult to distinguish from sinus tachycardia by surface ECG. Permanent junctional reciprocating tachycardia (PJRT) may also look similar to sinus tachycardia on a one-lead rhythm strip. Differentiation from a sinus tachycardia may require placement of esophageal electrodes and more invasive forms of ECG monitoring.

Atrial Flutter/Fibrillation

Atrial flutter is caused by a single atrial reentry circuit. The rate of atrial flutter depends on the size of this circuit and varies markedly between patients. Older children and adolescents with large atria (eg, after Fontan surgery) may have atrial flutter rates of less than 150 beats per minute. This makes it difficult to recognize the flutter waves on ECG. Typically, a sawtooth pattern is seen on the ECG with varying ventricular conduction (1:1, 2:1, 3:1, etc) (Fig. 8). Vagal maneuvers (eg, Valsalva) may change AV conduction and allow recognition of this sawtooth pattern. Intravenous injection of adenosine does not convert atrial flutter to sinus rhythm, but causes a short, complete AV block and reveals the atrial flutter waves. If the physician is in doubt about the rhythm, this may be a useful diagnostic maneuver.

Atrial fibrillation is caused by multiple small reentry circuits, which lead to high-rate atrial excitation without coordinated contraction. The atrial fibrillation spikes are usually visible on the ECG (exclude baseline artifact!). The QRS complexes demonstrate a randomly irregular R-R interval due to variable AV nodal conduction. Usual ventricular rates vary between 70 and 160 beats per minute, with rapid ventricular response being rare. In the otherwise healthy child, hyperthyroidism as a cause of atrial fibrillation should be ruled out.

Some patients with poor baseline cardiac function require AV synchrony for the maintenance of a sufficient cardiac output (eg, status post-Fontan procedure). These patients may acutely decompensate with the onset of atrial flutter or fibrillation. Even otherwise healthy patients in atrial flutter with 1:1 AV conduction may not tolerate the high ventricular rates. If the patient is acutely unstable, immediate synchronized electric cardioversion with 0.5 to 2.0 J/kg is the treatment of choice. As this is acutely painful, it is preferable to perform it under adequate anesthesia, if the situation allows.

In stable patients, atrial flutter and fibrillation are typically treated with intravenous digoxin, procainamide, esmolol, or propranolol. Other potentially useful medications include amiodarone, flecainide, quinidine, and disopyramide. Nevertheless, conventional pharmacologic conversion of atrial flutter and fibrillation is unsuccessful in many patients.

Atrial Flutter:

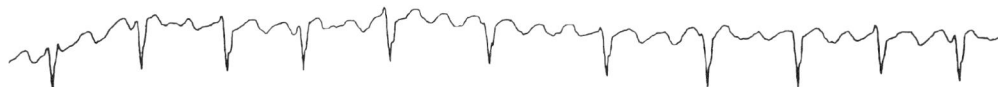

Supraventricular Tachycardia:

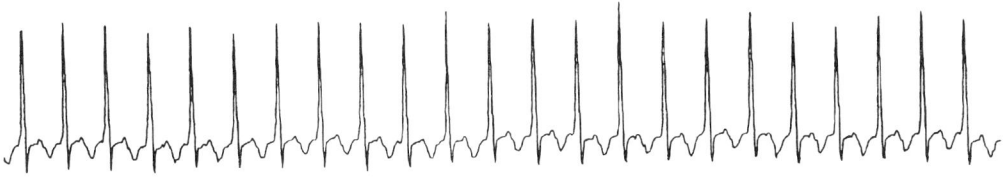

Ventricular Tachycardia:

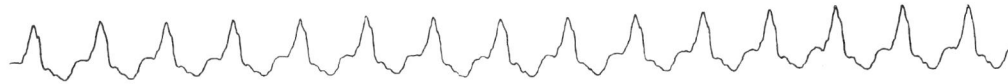

3rd Degree AV-Block:

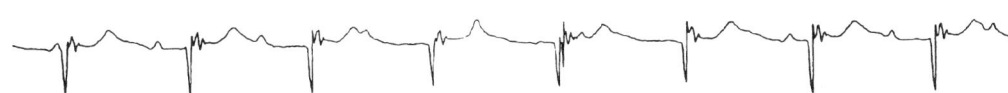

Figure 8. ECG rhythm strips demonstrating the classic pattern of various arrhythmias that can occur in the pediatric population. See text for a thorough description of the morphology, etiology, and treatment of these arrhythmias.

Ibutilide is a new antiarrhythmic medication with success rates of up to 50% for conversion of recent-onset atrial flutter and fibrillation to sinus rhythm.[23] It is administered as a continuous intravenous infusion and discontinued when conversion to sinus rhythm occurs.[24] Prolongation of the QT interval during infusion is typical. The major side effect is sustained polymorphic ventricular tachycardia (torsades de pointes), which requires electrical cardioversion. Monitoring of the patient for 4 hours after completion of the infusion is recommended.[25] Currently, little information on the use of this new drug in children is available.

Esophageal or intracardiac overdrive pacing are often successful in stable patients with atrial flutter. Overdrive pacing is not possible in atrial fibrillation. Synchronized electrical cardioversion is the most frequently used treatment for patients in sustained atrial fibrillation or refractory atrial flutter. Appropriate anesthesia or analgesia are mandatory prior to elective cardioversion. Since there is an increased risk of atrial thrombus formation with atrial fibrillation or atrial flutter, anticoagulation with coumadin or heparin, for at least 1 week prior to elective cardioversion, is typically indicated, unless formation of a thrombus can be excluded on transthoracic or transesophageal echocardiogram. Anticoagulation is especially important if the time of onset of the atrial arrhythmia is unknown or if it has been present for more than 2 days.

Supraventricular Tachycardia

All forms of reentry or increased automaticity tachycardias that have their origin above the level of the ventricles are called SVT. SVT is typically characterized by a narrow QRS complex (Fig. 8). Most SVTs are of the reentry type and their onset and termination is very abrupt. Heart rates depend on the size of the reentry circuit. A feature that distinguishes SVT from sinus tachycardia is that in SVT there is generally only minimal variation of the heart rate from baseline. In neonates and infants, the heart rates are often in excess of 220 to 300 beats per minute. Older patients complain about palpitations, chest pain, or dizziness, while SVT can remain undetected for hours or even days in infants. Irritability, poor feeding, and eventually congestive heart failure may be the only clinical signs. If the patient is unstable, synchronized electric cardioversion with 0.5 to 2.0 J/kg is the treatment of choice. If intravenous access and adenosine are immediately available, an attempt to break the arrhythmia with a rapid injection of 100 to 250 μg/kg of adenosine may be indicated even in the presence of hemodynamic instability. Adenosine breaks reentry SVT by causing temporary, complete AV block. The effect of adenosine is limited by its short half-life of only a few seconds. For this reason the injection is performed as a rapid intravenous bolus, followed by an immediate saline flush.[26] If the initial dose of 100 μg/kg (maximum dose: 6 mg) is ineffective, a second dose of 200 μg/kg (maximum dose: 12 mg) can be given immediately. Adverse effects include temporary, complete AV block, bronchospasm, and chest pain. Doses may need to be increased in patients receiving methylxanthines because these agents are adenosine antagonists.

In stable patients, vagal maneuvers may be attempted first to break the SVT. Coughing or eliciting the gag reflex or the diving reflex may be attempted. The diving reflex is easily provoked by filling a rubber examination glove with ice water and placing it over the patient's face and forehead, thereby obstructing the nose and mouth for about 5 to 10 seconds (apnea is part of the diving reflex!). If conversion to sinus rhythm does not occur, adenosine should be used. It is important to realize that return to sinus rhythm, for even a few beats, means successful conversion. If the patient fails to maintain the sinus rhythm, a longer lasting, baseline antiarrhythmic medication (usually digoxin or procainamide) must be started before multiple repeated attempts to convert the SVT are undertaken. Another fairly successful treatment option is esophageal overdrive pacing. Verapamil is frequently effective in breaking SVT and has a long half-life to limit its recurrence. Verapamil, however, is contraindicated in infants and young children (<6 to 12 months of age), because of the risk of myocardial depression and sudden death! Other pharmacologic agents used for conversion of SVT include α-adrenergic agonists (phenylephrine), which act to increase systemic vascular resistance and thereby cause a reflex slowing of the heart rate and anticholinesterase inhibitors (edrophonium). The latter agent inhibits acetylcholinesterase thereby increasing the concentration of acetylcholine at the sinoatrial (SA), AV node.

A baseline antiarrhythmic medication is almost always started at the time a diagnosis of SVT is made. In newborns and infants, digoxin is the drug of choice. If necessary, a Class I antiarrhythmic (procainamide, flecainide) or a β-blocker (propranolol, atenolol) may be added to or may replace the digoxin. In refractory cases, amiodarone is sometimes used. In older patients or patients who have Wolf-Parkinson-White syndrome, digoxin is not recommended. In these patients, β-blockers, Class I antiarrhythmic medications, calcium antagonists, or amiodarone (for refractory cases) are used. If the patient is already being treated, medication levels should be obtained (usually predose levels) to assess the adequacy of the dose.

SVT in the form of ectopic atrial tachycardia is characterized by a wider variation of the heart rate during tachycardia. It rarely breaks with adenosine, but often responds to the above medications, at least by a slowing of the heart rate. If the arrhythmia has been present for a long time, infants may present with chronic ventricular dysfunction and a clinical picture similar to that of myocarditis with cardiomyopathy.

Other forms of SVT include junctional ectopic tachycardia (JET) (see below) and PJRT. PJRT is a reentry tachycardia characterized by a slower heart rate (as low as 150 beats per minute) and relative wide variations of heart rates, depending on the sympathetic and vagal tone. On a one-lead rhythm strip, it can easily be confused with sinus tachycardia, because it has a short PR interval. Atrial excitation is retrograde, which results in an abnormal P wave axis (negative in lead II), as can be seen on the 12-lead ECG. The tachycardia may start and stop frequently, alternating with sinus rhythm. Even though PJRT may be hard to control medically, acute heart failure is less common in this condition compared to other tachycardias due to the lower heart rates.

JET is seen mostly in the first few days after open heart surgery. It is a narrow, complex SVT caused by increased automaticity in the His bundle or the AV node. In the setting of JET there is complete AV dissociation, and the ventricular rate is always higher than the atrial rate. Occasional atrial beats may be conducted to the ventricles, when the atrial impulse is timed correctly.[27] Hemodynamic compromise depends primarily on the heart rate and the tolerance of AV dissociation. As long as heart rates are only mildly accelerated and cardiac output is appropriate, no treatment for JET is required. Due to the potential for high morbidity and mortality, however, extremely close monitoring of heart rate and cardiac output is indicated. If the heart rate increases, attempts to control the rate and to establish AV synchrony are indicated. Inotropic agents should be reduced to a minimum, since their chronotropic effect further increases heart rate and outweighs the benefit of increased contractility. Digoxin loading doses are administered intravenously (unless contraindicated for other reasons) to rapidly achieve adequate levels. Procainamide or esmolol, as continuous infusions, may be added in an attempt to further slow the rate of JET. In this or any other form of arrhythmia, the use of β-adrenergic antagonists such as esmolol or propranolol can cause significant decreases in myocardial contractility, and their use is contraindicated in patients who have poor ventricular function. Intravenous amiodarone has recently been suggested as an effective alternative for the control of the heart rate.[28] In postoperative patients who have atrial pacing wires in place, atrial pacing at slightly higher rates than the rate of the JET will frequently establish AV synchrony. This may improve cardiac output. If these interventions are unsuccessful, cooling of the patient to 34 to 35°C has been effective in slowing the heart rate to allow sufficient cardiac output. To achieve hypothermia, neuromuscular blockade is often required to eliminate the shivering response. The postoperative form of JET is usually transient and resolves within a few days; however, it is associated with a high incidence of morbidity and mortality.

Ventricular Tachycardia

Ventricular tachycardia is defined as a tachycardia that originates below the bifurcation of the His bundle. It may be caused by reentry or increased automaticity. It is characterized by at least three beats with a wide QRS complex and distorted or nonvisible p waves (Fig. 8). If the ventricular tachycardia persists for more than 30 seconds, it is called sustained ventricular tachycardia. Single, early ventricular beats are called premature ventricular contractions (PVC). PVCs can increase in frequency and may eventually lead to ventricular tachycardia. Occasional PVCs may be a normal finding. Symptomatic and frequent PVCs (especially if polymorphic) may be treated with the same antiarrhythmic medications that are used for ventricular tachycardia. Ventricular tachycardia can be classified as monomorphic (all beats look alike), polymorphic (varying appearance of QRS complexes), or torsades de pointes (typical change in QRS amplitude between negative and positive over several beats). Differential diagnosis includes SVT in a patient with bundle branch block (typically a patient who has had open heart surgery in the past), SVT with aberrant conduction, and atrial flutter or fibrillation in a patient with Wolf-Parkinson-White syndrome. Nevertheless, *a wide complex tachycardia should always be treated as ventricular tachycardia*, unless another etiology can be proven. Depending on the heart rate during ventricular tachycardia, symptoms vary from mild unspecific discomfort to chest pain, palpitations, hypotension, signs of heart failure, or cardiovascular collapse.

Patients who have unstable vital signs in sustained ventricular tachycardia have to be treated emergently. If the pulse is still palpable, synchronized electric cardioversion with 0.5 to 2.0 J/kg is performed. If this is unsuccessful, repeat cardioversion with twice the energy is performed. Cardiopulmonary resuscitation (CPR) is started immediately in patients without pulse or without an adequate cardiac output. If the ventricular tachycardia has poorly identifiable QRS complexes (unable to deliver synchronized electric shock) or if no pulse is palpable, defibrillation with 2 to 4 J/kg is recommended. This may be repeated twice with increasing energies. One dose of epinephrine (10 μg/kg, 0.1 mL/kg of a 1:10,000 solution) is administered intravenously or via an endotracheal tube, if defibrillation is still unsuccessful.

If the patient is awake and has stable vital signs, or if the attempted electric interventions have been unsuccessful in an unstable patient, antiarrhythmic medications are started. In a stable patient, especially with previous history of open heart surgery or known bundle branch block on a baseline ECG, an attempt to restore normal sinus rhythm can be made with 100 to 200 μg/kg adenosine. Adenosine is unlikely to convert ventricular tachycardia, but will interrupt SVT, which may be present in this situation. Otherwise, intravenous lidocaine as a bolus of 1 mg/kg is recommended as the first-line agent.

In unstable patients, cardioversion/defibrillation should be repeated after the bolus of lidocaine. If there is return to normal sinus rhythm, a continuous lidocaine infusion at 20 to 50 μg/kg/min is started. Many pediatric cardiologists prefer procainamide over lidocaine, especially since it also has a positive effect on atrial arrhythmias (eg, SVT, atrial flutter). Procainamide is administered as a bolus of 5 to 15 mg/kg followed by a continuous infusion of 20 to 80 μg/kg/min. Procainamide is administered over 10 to 15 minutes, because hypotension may occur with rapid intravenous administration. The dosage of both medications (lidocaine and procainamide) should be monitored with blood levels several hours after starting the continuous infusion. If lidocaine and procainamide are not effective, bretylium (5 mg/kg) may be attempted. Another second-line medication is phenytoin, which is especially useful in digoxin toxicity. Phenytoin is administered as a bolus of 5 to 10 mg/kg over 20 to 30 minutes. For torsades de pointes, 50 mg/kg of magnesium sulfate has been effective. Intravenous amiodarone has recently been used, with good success, to treat resistant ventricular tachycardia. After an initial 5 mg/kg over 1 hour, a continuous infusion is started at 5 to 15 μg/kg/min. The loading dose may be substituted by several slow intravenous boluses of 1 mg/kg. Side effects of amiodarone include prolongation of the QT interval. If the corrected QT interval reaches 0.53 seconds (in normal sinus rhythm), the dose should be reduced. Monitoring of blood levels is recommended. Repeated attempts of electric defibrillation should be undertaken in unstable patients, until return of a more stable rhythm that results in an acceptable cardiac output.

After initial stabilization of the patient, serum electrolytes (K^+, Ca^{++}, Mg^{++}) should be measured, to exclude abnormal levels as a cause for the arrhythmia. Medications should be considered as causative agents (inotropic agents, digoxin, antiarrhythmics, tricyclic antidepressants). If previously healthy children present with ventricular tachycardia, serum and urine drug testing should always be performed. An echocardiogram is essential to exclude structural abnormalities and to evaluate cardiac function. Myocarditis should always be considered as a cause for the ventricular tachycardia. Ischemia and myocardial infarction are rare causes for ventricular tachycardia in the pediatric age range, but must be included in the differential diagnosis.

Ventricular Fibrillation

Ventricular fibrillation is characterized by uncoordinated contractions of different regions of the ventricular myocardium which result in no significant cardiac output and no palpable pulse. Affected patients are always apneic, unresponsive, and unconscious. On the cardiac rhythm strip or ECG, bizarre, rapid, and irregular ventricular activity is seen. Immediate electric defibrillation with 2 J/kg is required. The defibrillation should be repeated twice with increasing energies (up to 4 J/kg), if there is no success. The further emergent management is identical to the treatment of pulseless ventricular tachycardia as explained above. Underlying causes, such as hyperkalemia, severe hypoxia, myocarditis, digitalis toxicity, and other medications (antiarrhythmics), should be excluded.

Bradyarrhythmias

A heart rhythm originating from the sinus node that is slower than normal for the patient's age or slower than appropriate for the specific situation is called sinus bradycardia. Sinus bradycardia in an otherwise stable patient requires no treatment. It may be a normal variant, especially in well conditioned athletes (often during sleep). Centrally triggered bradycardia in patients with increased intracranial pressure is part of the Cushing's triad (altered respiratory pattern, bradycardia, hypertension). It resolves with correction of the underlying problem. Bradycardia due to hypoxia is treated by providing adequate ventilation and oxygenation. Many medications (digoxin, β-blockers, sedatives, etc.) cause bradycardia through direct cardiac or central nervous effects. Discontinuation of the medication, if possible, is the treatment of choice. If necessary, intravenous bolus doses of atropine (0.02 mg/kg/dose; minimum dose: 0.1 mg) or continuous intravenous administration of isoproterenol (0.05 to 2 μg/kg/min) are used to control the low heart rates until the underlying problems are corrected (Table 5). If medications are ineffective, temporary pacing may be required. This can be accomplished transvenously, although the quickest route is transcutaneously. All modern-day defibrillators have the capacity to perform transcutaneous pacing via surface-placed pads.

Patients who have a history of cardiac surgery (especially after Fontan or Mustard surgery) may have a condition called sick sinus syndrome, which results in inappropriate tachycardias, sinus bradycardia, or even sinus node arrest. Atropine, epinephrine, and isoproterenol may be helpful for initial management of symptomatic bradycardic episodes. These medications should be used cautiously, due to a risk of further paradoxic worsening of the bradycardia. Emergent placement of a temporary (and subsequently permanent) pacemaker may be required.

Patients who have Eisenmenger syndrome may experience acute onset of sinus

Table 5

Etiology of Sinus Bradycardia

Normal variant
Hypoxia
Medications (digoxin, β-adrenergic antagonist)
CNS disease (increased intracranial pressure, vagal tone)
Hypothermia
Hypothyroidism
Right atrial distention
Sick sinus syndrome

CNS = central nervous system.

bradycardia. This is caused by right atrial distention, due to volume overload, in the presence of the elevated pulmonary vascular resistance. Pulmonary artery thrombosis or embolization may be a triggering event. Besides management with atropine and isoproterenol, oxygen (via face mask) should be given to these patients, since it is a pulmonary vasodilator and may act to decrease right ventricular afterload and thereby decrease right atrial distention. Other more specific therapy is aimed toward improving right ventricular function with inotropic agents and possibly with the judicious use of diuretics. These bradycardia episodes in patients with Eisenmenger syndrome result in a high mortality rate.

Heart Block

First-degree AV block is the prolongation of the PR interval above the normal for age and heart rate (normal: <0.16 to 0.18). It may be a normal finding, which requires no treatment. New-onset first-degree AV block may be caused by myocarditis (including rheumatic fever) or by medications (digitalis). Besides routine evaluation of electrolytes and treatment of underlying causes, no treatment is necessary.

Second-degree AV block is characterized by frequent drops of the QRS complexes after preceding p waves. If the PR interval lengthens progressively until the drop of the QRS complex, it is classified as second-degree AV block, type Wenkebach (Mobitz I). If the QRS complexes are dropped regularly, without a change of the PR intervals, it is called second-degree AV block (Mobitz type II). Second-degree AV block (especially Mobitz type I) may be a rare finding in an otherwise healthy child. Etiologies of second-degree AV block are similar to those of first-degree AV block. Second-degree AV block, Mobitz type II, is more likely to progress to third-degree AV block. Emergency therapy is required when the ventricular rates are too low to maintain adequate cardiac output. In such a case, atropine or low-dose isoproterenol are the medications of choice. Treatment of an underlying cause may cure the arrhythmia.

Third-degree AV block (complete heart block) is complete dissociation of the atrial and ventricular contractions. This is apparent on the ECG by complete dissociation of p waves and QRS complexes, with the atrial rate faster than the ventricular rate (Fig. 8). Depending on the location of the block, the ventricular (escape) beats may have narrow or wide QRS complexes. The third-degree AV block may be congenital, in which case it is often due to structural heart disease (L-transposition, single ventricle, AV canal) or due to maternal lupus antibodies. Most patients with congenital heart block have an acceptable ventricular rate and can be followed conservatively for varying time periods. Acquired forms of complete heart block may be the result of previous cardiac surgery, medications, or myocarditis. Complete heart block in the immediate postoperative period is treated with an external pacemaker (leads placed at the time of surgery). If the ventricular heart rate is adequate, the pacemaker may be on standby mode. Many of the immediate postoperative heart blocks resolve within 7 to 10 days. If the heart block persists, implantation of a permanent pacemaker is required. Acutely symptomatic patients with acquired complete heart block are treated with intravenous atropine and/or isoproterenol until temporary pacing can be performed (transesophageal, transvenous, or transcutaneous). Underlying causes, such as myocarditis or medications, should be considered and treated appropriately. Maintenance of an appropriate heart rate in the presence of myocarditis is especially important, since cardiac output is even more rate-dependent in this situation.

Asystole

Asystole is defined as the absence of electrical activity and mechanical contraction of the heart. It is characterized by a "flat line" on ECG and rhythm strip. Patients with asystole are apneic, have no palpable pulse, and are unconscious. The most common cause for asystole in the pediatric age range is hypoxia. Besides CPR and assurance of adequate ventilation and oxygenation, administration of atropine and epinephrine (intravenous or via the endotracheal tube) is the first step in treatment. Electric defibrillation is not helpful, but emergent external pacing should be considered. If severe acidosis or hyperkalemia are possible causes for the asystole, sodium bicarbonate and calcium chloride should be administered. Repeat doses of epinephrine and atropine are given in regular intervals (about 3 to 5 minutes). Current recommendations for epinephrine dosing include an initial dose of 10 μg/kg and subsequent doses of 100 μg/kg. If there is any doubt about the heart rhythm, the ECG leads should be switched or replaced to assure appropriate treatment.

Pulseless Electrical Activity (Electromechanical Dissociation)

The electrical (and often mechanical) function of the heart is maintained during the pulseless electrical activity. The cardiac rhythm strip shows ventricular activity—often some form of bradycardia—but no pulse is palpable. Attempts to locate a weak pulse, by use of Doppler, should be undertaken. Hemodynamic insufficiency is often the result of mechanical obstruction to blood flow (pneumothorax, pericardial effusion, pulmonary embolism) or due to hypovolemia (Table 6). After start of CPR, epinephrine and atropine are administered as for asystole. Possible underlying causes are considered and treated appropriately. If hypovolemia is a consideration, multiple isotonic fluid boluses are administered.

Table 6

Etiology of Pulseless Electrical Activity

Hypovolemia
Hypoxia
Cardiac tamponade
Tension pneumothorax
Acidosis
Hypothermia
Pulmonary embolism
Drug overdose/intoxication
Hyperkalemia

Distant, muffled heart sounds may be due to a pericardial effusion/tamponade, which requires immediate drainage. Absent or decreased breath sounds suggest a pneumothorax. Repeat doses of epinephrine and atropine are given in 3- to 5-minute intervals. Sodium bicarbonate may be helpful for the treatment of acidosis and hyperkalemia.

Pacemaker Failure

There are multiple causes for pacemaker failure, most of which can be diagnosed by a routine 12-lead ECG. Single-lead rhythm strips alone are frequently misleading, because pacemaker spikes may be tiny and can be missed easily. A chest x-ray should be obtained to assess for possible fracture of pacemaker leads. Due to the complexity of modern pacemakers, diagnosis by a noncardiologist is often impossible, especially if the programmed pacemaker settings are unknown. Complete failure of the generator or battery is characterized by the absence of atrial or ventricular pacer spikes and a heart rate typically below the programmed low heart rate of the pacemaker. This should not be confused with a normally functioning pacemaker, where pacing spikes are often absent at higher heart rates. Here, the functioning pacemaker is sensing the spontaneous ventricular contractions but is programmed not to pace due to the appropriate heart rate. Failure to capture the ventricular myocardium is present when there is complete dissociation between the ventricular pacing spikes and the QRS complexes.

Many pediatric patients who have congenital heart disease or congenital third-degree AV block have a sufficient spontaneous heart rate. As long as the patients have good cardiac output and are in no acute distress, no emergent intervention is required. Symptomatic patients are treated with an atropine bolus or with continuous isoproterenol infusion, with the goal of achieving a heart rate high enough to maintain cardiac output. Very few select patients do not respond to chronotropic medications and require temporary external pacing.

Chapter 7 Appendix

Medications

Medication	Route	Dose	Side Effects
Adenosine	i.v. (rapid push)	50 to 250 µg/kg/dose. Maximum dose: 18 mg	bronchospasm,[26] complete AV block, chest pain
Amiodarone	i.v.	5 mg/kg load over 1 hour (or 1 mg/kg bolus, repeat up to 10 times), then 5 to 15 µg/kg/min	nausea, hypotension, arrhythmia, hypothyroidism, hepatotoxicity, wean dose if QTc >0.53 sec
Amrinone	i.v. infusion	Loading dose: 0.5 to 1.0 mg/kg Infusion: 5 to 20 µg/kg/min	tachycardia, hypotension, thrombocytopenia
Atenolol	PO	1 to 2 mg/kg/day: q day or BID	Fatigue, bradycardia, hypotension, bronchoconstriction
Atropine	i.v.	0.02 mg/kg/dose Minimum dose: 0.05 mg Maximum dose: 2 mg	tachycardia, paradoxical bradycardia, mydriasis
Bretylium	i.v. (slow bolus over 5 to 10 min)	5 mg/kg/dose Maximum: 15 mg/kg/dose	arrhythmia, hypotension
Captopril	PO	<6 mos: 0.3 mg/kg/day TID, ↑ slowly up to 2 mg/kg/day >6 mo: 0.5 to 4 mg/kg/day TID	hypotension, cough, renal impairment
Cardioversion (synchronized)		Initial 0.5 to 1 J/kg Repeat dose: 2 to 4 J/kg Maximum dose: 300 J	arrhythmia, burns
Carnitine	PO i.v.	500 to 100 mg/kg/day BID-TID 25 mg/kg/day BID-TID	none
Defibrillation		Initial dose: 2 J/kg Repeat dose: 4 J/kg Maximum dose: 300 J	arrhythmia, burns
Dobutamine	i.v. infusion	2 to 20 µg/kg/min	tachycardia, arrhythmia, hyper/hypotension
Dopamine	i.v. infusion	1 to 20 µg/kg/min Renal dose: 2 to 5 µg/kg/min	tachycardia, arrhythmia, hypertension, vasoconstriction
Enalapril	i.v. PO	0.02 to 0.1 mg/kg/day: BID 0.1 to 0.4 mg/kg/day: BID-QD	hypotension, renal impairment; start at low dose
Epinephrine	i.v./ETT (bolus) i.v. infusion	0.01 to 0.1 mg/kg/dose 0.01 to 1.0 µg/kg/min	tachycardia, hypertension, ischemia, vasoconstriction
Esmolol	i.v. infusion	Loading dose: 0.5 mg/kg Infusion: 50 to 500 µg/kg/min	hypotension, bradycardia

Chapter 7 Appendix (continued)

Medications

Medication	Route	Dose	Side Effects
Ibutilide	i.v. (in 50 cc NS over 10 min)	0.01 to 0.025 mg/kg over 10 min. Repeat ×1 in 10 min (stop infusion when in sinus rhythm). Maximum dose: 1 mg/dose	arrhythmia; long QTc (expected effect), do not use with class 1a or 3 antiarrhythmics[23-25]
Isoproterenol	i.v. infusion	0.01 to 1.0 µg/kg/min	hypotension, tachycardia
Lidocaine	i.v. (bolus ± infusion	Bolus: 1 mg/kg/dose Infusion: 20 to 50 µg/kg/min	seizures, hypotension, arrhythmia. Blood level: 2 to 5 µg/mL
Magnesium Sulfate	i.v. (slow bolus over 5 to 10 min)	50 mg/kg/dose Maximum dose: 2 grams	hypotension, apnea, neuromuscular blockade
Milrinone	i.v. infusion	Initial load: 50 to 100 µg/kg Infusion: 0.5 to 1.0 µg/kg/min	arrhythmia, hypotension
Nitroprusside	i.v. infusion	0.01 to 5 µg/kg/min	hypotension, nausea, cyanide and thiocyanate toxicity
Phenylephrine	i.v. (bolus) i.v. infusion	2 to 10 µg/kg/dose 0.1 to 1 µg/kg/min	hypertension, arrhythmia, decreased GFR, RBF
Phenytoin	i.v. bolus over 30 min	4 to 10 mg/kg/dose	nausea, hypotension, arrhythmias. Blood level: 5 to 20 µg/mL
Procainamide	i.v. infusion	Initial load: 5 to 10 mg/kg Infusion: 20 to 80 µg/kg/min	hypotension, arrhythmia. Blood levels: 4 to 10 µg/mL; procainamide + NAPA level: 10 to 30 µg/mL
Propranolol	i.v. PO	0.01 to 0.1 mg/kg/dose 1 to 4 mg/kg/day QID	hypotension, bradycardia, bronchoconstriction
Prostaglandin E$_1$	i.v. infusion	Start at 0.1 µg/kg/min then decrease to 0.05 µg/kg/min (lowest dose 0.01 µg/kg/min)	apnea, fever, hypotension, seizure, rash

References

1. Schamberger MS. Cardiac emergencies in children. *Pediatr Ann* 1996;25:339–344.
2. Rychik J, Gullquist SD, Jacobs ML, Norwood WI. Doppler echocardiographic analysis of flow in the ductus arteriosus of infants with hypoplastic left heart syndrome: Relationship of flow patterns to systemic oxygenation and size of interatrial communication. *J Am Soc Echocardiogr* 1996;9:166–173.
3. Barnea O, Austin EH, Richman B, Santamore WP. Balancing the circulation: Theoretic optimization of pulmonary/systemic flow ratio in hypoplastic left heart syndrome. *J Am Coll Cardiol* 1994;24:1376–1381.
4. Day RW, Tani LY, Minich LL, et al. Congenital heart disease with ductal-dependent systemic perfusion: Doppler ultrasonography flow velocities are altered by changes in the fraction of inspired oxygen. *J Heart Lung Transplant* 1995;14:718–725.
5. Jobes DR, Nicolson SC, Steven JM, et al.

Carbon dioxide prevents pulmonary overcirculation in hypoplastic left heart syndrome. *Ann Thorac Surg* 1992;54:150–151.
6. Broderick TW, Higgins CB, Guthaner DF, et al. Critical aortic stenosis in neonates. *Radiology* 1978;129:393–399.
7. Hascoet JM, Didier F, Monin P, Vert P. Efficiency of prostaglandin E_1 in a tiny baby with coarctation of the aorta and ligated ductus arteriosus. *Acta Paediatr* 1992;81:938–940.
8. Freed MD, Heymann MA, Lewis AB, et al. Prostaglandin E_1 in infants with ductus arteriosus dependent congenital heart disease. *Circulation* 1981;6:899–905.
9. Lewis AB, Freed MD, Heymann MA, et al. Side effects of therapy with prostaglandin E_1 in infants with critical congenital heart disease. *Circulation* 1981;64:893–898.
10. Barkin RM. Congestive heart failure in children. *J Emerg Med* 1986;4;379–382.
11. Martin AB, Webber S, Fricker FJ, et al. Acute myocarditis. Rapid diagnosis by PCR in children. *Circulation* 1994;90:330–339.
12. Smith SC, Ladenson JH, Mason JW, Jaffe AS. Elevations of cardiac troponin I associated with myocarditis. Experimental and clinical correlates. *Circulation* 1997;95:163–168.
13. Zales VR, Benson DW. Reversible cardiomyopathy due to carnitine deficiency from renal tubular wasting. *Pediatr Cardiol* 1995;16: 76–78.
14. Canter CE, Strauss AW. Cardiomyopathies: When to think of congenital causes. *Contemp Pediatr* 1995;12:25–40.
15. Kaplan S. New drug approaches to the treatment of heart failure in infants and children. *Drugs* 1990;39:388–393.
16. Parikh SR, Girod DA. Treatment of heart failure in the pediatric and young adult patient. *Contemp Treat Cardiovasc Dis* 1996;1:3–32.
17. McNamara DM, Rosenblum WD, Janosko KM, et al. Intravenous immune globulin in the therapy of myocarditis and acute cardiomyopathy. *Circulation* 1997;95:2476–2478.
18. Drucker NA, Colan SD, Lewis AB, et al. Gamma-globulin treatment of acute myocarditis in the pediatric population. *Circulation* 1994;89:252–257.
19. Camargo PR, Snitcowsky R, da Luz PL, et al. Favorable effects of immunosuppressive therapy in children with dilated cardiomyopathy and active myocarditis. *Pediatr Cardiol* 1995;16:61–68.
20. McKenna WJ, Davies MJ. Immunosuppression for myocarditis. *N Engl J Med* 1995;333: 312–313.
21. Del Nido PJ, Armitage JM, Fricker FJ, et al. Extracorporeal membrane oxygenation support as a bridge to pediatric heart transplantation. *Circulation* 1994;90:1166–1169.
22. Gagliardi MG, Bevilacqua M, Squitieri C, et al. Dilated cardiomyopathy caused by acute myocarditis in pediatric patients: Evolution of myocardial damage in a group of potential heart transplant candidates. *J Heart Lung Transpl* 1993;12:224–229.
23. Stambler BS, Beckman KJ, Kadish AH, et al. Acute hemodynamic effects of ibutilide in patients with or without reduced left ventricular function. *Am J Cardiol* 1997;80:458–463.
24. Foster RH, Wilde MI, Markham A. Ibutilide: A review of its pharmacological properties and clinical potential in the acute management of atrial flutter and fibrillation. *Drugs* 1997;54:312–330.
25. Stambler BS, Wood MA, Ellenbogen KA, et al. Efficacy and safety of repeated intravenous doses of ibutilide for rapid conversion of atrial flutter or fibrillation. *Circulation* 1996;94:1613–1621.
26. DeGroff CG, Silka MJ. Bronchospasm after intravenous administration of adenosine in a patient with asthma. *J Pediatr* 1994;125: 822–833.
27. Case CL, Gillette PC. Automatic atrial and junctional tachycardias in the pediatric patient: Strategies for diagnosis and management. *PACE* 1993;16:1323–1335.
28. Raja P, Hawker RE, Chaikitpinyo A, et al. Amiodarone management of junctional ectopic tachycardia after cardiac surgery in children. *Br Heart J* 1994;72:261–265.

Chapter 8

Postoperative Cardiac Care

Joseph D. Tobias, MD and William R. Wilson Jr., MD

Introduction

The postoperative care and support of the pediatric cardiac patient represents an integral step in the correction, treatment, and palliation of congenital heart defects. The initial step in the transition from the operative to the postoperative period begins with the safe transport of the patient from the operating room to the intensive care unit (ICU). Extreme vigilance is necessary during this critical time, and continued monitoring of vital signs including invasive hemodynamic parameters is required. Recent advances in transport monitor technology allow the cassette or module used to monitor the patient in the operating room to be removed and inserted into a transport module. This allows not only for continuous patient monitoring, but also for the storage of intraoperative data, such as blood pressures and filling pressures, in the event that later review of this information is necessary. If such equipment is not available, then a separate transport monitor capable of continuous electrocardiogram (ECG), oxygen saturation, and invasive hemodynamic monitoring should be used. Some means for the continuous auscultation of breath sounds, such as an esophageal or precordial stethoscope, is also recommended. Many newer models of transport monitors also allow for end-tidal carbon dioxide monitoring, which may be particularly valuable not only for demonstrating the intratracheal position of the endotracheal (ET) tube during transport, but also to allow for the appropriate level of carbon dioxide depending on the patient's underlying anatomy and the recent surgical procedure. Without such monitoring, it is virtually impossible to match the amount of ventilation that was previously provided by the mechanical ventilator, and significant alterations in arterial carbon dioxide may occur.[1] Resuscitation medications and equipment must be carried and readily available to those transporting the patient. This is especially relevant when transport involves a significant time and/or distance.

On arrival in the ICU, thorough communication and cooperation are required to ensure the safe transition from the intraoperative to the postoperative period. A multidisciplinary approach involving medical and surgical specialties as well as the nursing and respiratory therapy staff is required for the postoperative care of these patients. This chapter discusses the postoperative care of the pediatric cardiac patient by addressing each specific organ system and the issues that may arise during the postoperative period.

From: Tobias JD (ed): *Pediatric Critical Care: The Essentials.* ©Futura Publishing Co., Inc., Armonk, NY, 1999.

Surgical Techniques and Cardiopulmonary Bypass

Operations for congenital heart disease can be classified as closed or open heart procedures, palliative or total repair. Closed heart procedures are techniques that do not require entrance into the chambers of the heart and do not require cardiopulmonary bypass (CPB) to support the circulation during the surgery. Closed procedures were the first procedures developed to treat congenital heart disease, and usually employed vascular clamps placed on the great vessels to temporarily occlude a portion of the circulation. Ligation of a patent ductus arteriosus, creation of a systemic-to-pulmonary shunt (modified Blalock-Taussig), and application of a pulmonary artery band are examples of closed heart surgery.

Open heart surgery refers to procedures that require the use of the heart-lung machine or CPB in order to support the circulation for a period of time to allow reconstructive procedures within the cardiac chambers, upon the great vessels or cardiac valves. Current surgical techniques of CPB allow all of the major congenital heart defects to be repaired with favorable chances of long-term survival.

In most centers, the current approach is one of early total repair in order to avoid the long-term consequences of abnormal physiology associated with uncorrected congenital cardiac lesions. With early corrective surgery, hypoxia, pulmonary overcirculation, and volume or pressure overload of the heart and lungs can be avoided. Palliative procedures such as construction of a systemic-to-pulmonary-artery shunt or pulmonary artery banding continue to be performed in patients with lesions that are not suitable to early total repair. This may include patients with severe cardiorespiratory dysfunction or specific cardiac lesions such as a single ventricle.

Current systems of CPB are designed for temporary circulatory support during repair of congenital heart disease. The system consists of several basic components. Clear polyvinyl chloride tubing is connected to the systemic venous circulation and drains blood by gravity to a venous reservoir. Blood is then pumped by either a roller pump or centrifugal pump from the reservoir through a heat exchanger, which allows heating or cooling of the patient as dictated by the procedure. The flow of blood is regulated by the speed of the pump, to provide the patient with a cardiac output based on weight and body surface area. The speed with which the pump turns can be adjusted to regulate the flow or cardiac output. Blood is then passed through a membrane oxygenator where gas exchange takes place. Within the membrane oxygenator, blood flows on one side of the membrane and fresh gas along the other side. This allows the removal of carbon dioxide from and the addition of oxygen to the blood. Once oxygen has been added to and carbon dioxide removed from the blood, the blood is returned to the patient via a cannula placed in the aorta. Filters, pressure monitors, and various other safety and monitoring devices complete the circuit, which connects through the arterial line to return blood to the patients' circulation (Fig. 1).

Venous return is accomplished by siphon drainage. For intracardiac repairs, bicaval cannulation is typically used with one cannula directed into the superior vena cava and a second passed into the inferior vena cava. Caval tourniquets are tightened around the cannulae with the drainage tip positioned distally to exclude all blood return from entering the heart and to thereby provide a bloodless operative field. Arterial inflow is accomplished with direct cannulation of the distal ascending aorta. The arterial cannulae must be large enough to keep the pressure gradient from the aorta cannula to the aorta less than 100 mm Hg to avoid hemolysis of the blood. Prior to starting bypass, systemic anticoagulation is achieved with use of heparin. Ongoing anticoagulation is monitored by periodic measurement of activated coagulation times, with the administration of more heparin as needed to achieved the desired activated coagulation time range of greater than 400 seconds.

Hemodilution during CPB has improved overall patient outcomes. Organ perfusion during bypass is improved by better

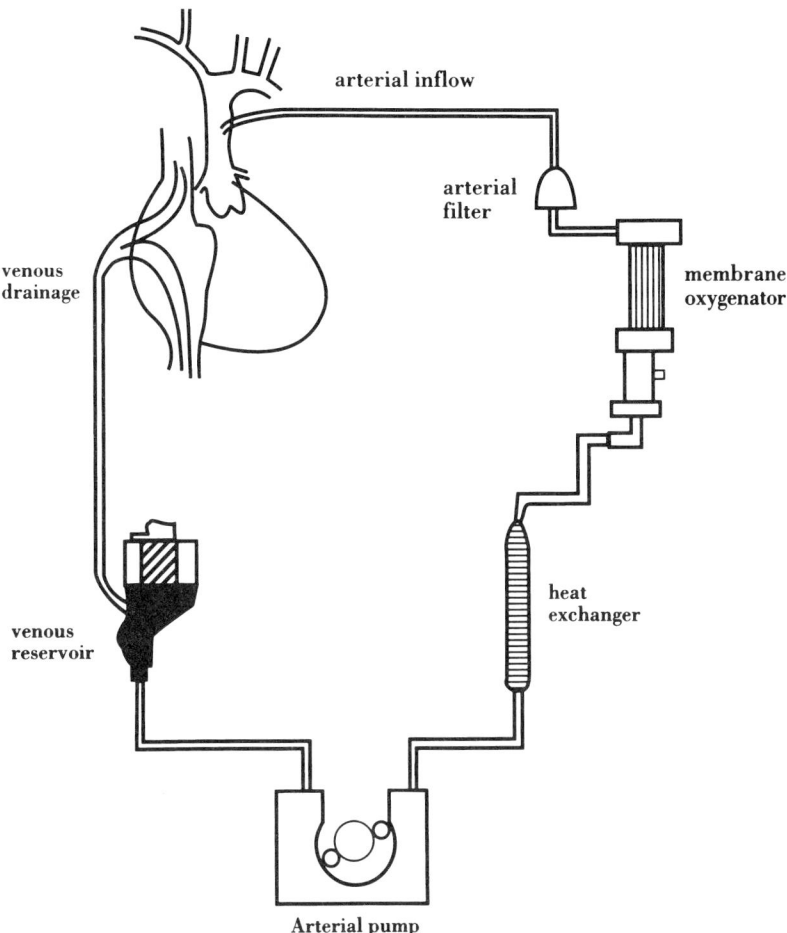

Figure 1. Diagram demonstrating the typical components of a cardiopulmonary bypass system used during correction of congenital heart defects; including a venous reservoir, roller pump, heat exchanger, membrane oxygenator, and arterial filter.

rheology of blood flow, lower shear stress, and lower viscosity when the hematocrit is lowered to 22% to 25%.[2] The use of hemodilution has lowered the incidence of renal insufficiency and neurologic problems following bypass. Current pediatric and neonatal bypass systems require a minimum priming volume of between 700 and 800 mL (roughly 2000 mL for adult circuits), dependent on the specific oxygenator, reservoir, and filters being used. The hematocrit on bypass can be predicted by using the patient's weight, prime volume required, preoperative hematocrit, and intravenous fluids given prior to bypass. Larger children and adults may receive a crystalloid prime with added colloid to maintain osmolarity to prevent excessive edema. Small infants and newborns receive a blood prime. Heparin, mannitol, and corticosteroids are also added to the CPB circuit.

Once the patient is placed on bypass, he or she is systemically cooled to a temperature determined by the requirements for the cardiac repair: typically to 26 to 32°C for moderate hypothermia. Induction of hypothermia reduces metabolism and oxygen consumption. This allows lower pump flows, better myocardial protection, improved organ perfusion, and improved overall results. Several repairs, such as the Norwood procedure, require the circulation be totally arrested. After cooling slowly to 16 to 18°C rectal temperature, corticosteroids and pentobarbital are given for cerebral protection, the head is packed in ice, and the bypass pump is stopped. Total circulatory arrest can be safely maintained for 30 to 60 minutes without adverse effects. Most other repairs are performed during CPB with moderate hypothermia.

Myocardial function depends on a continuous supply of oxygen to the myocyte. Ischemia results when there is an imbalance between oxygen supply and demand leading to accumulation of tissue metabolites of anaerobic metabolism including lactate, carbon dioxide, and H^+. A 45-minute period of unprotected global normothermic ischemia will result in reduction in postischemic myocardial function of 50% to 60%.[3] Many of the repairs required for complex congenital heart defects may require up to 120 minutes of ischemic arrest. Induction of a chemical hypothermic arrest of the heart, following the instillation of cardioplegia solution, allows a longer period of ischemic arrest and successful return of normal cardiac function. Typically a crossclamp is applied to the ascending aorta and a cold blood cardioplegia solution that is high in potassium (20 mEq KCl/L) and low in calcium is instilled in the proximal ascending aorta in an antegrade fashion. The hyperkalemia depolarizes the myocyte membrane and renders the myocardium unexcitable. The oxygen consumption of the heart is lowered by 80% to 90% in the arrested state.[3,4] Hypothermia further lowers the myocardial oxygen consumption. Repeat doses of antegrade cardioplegia (400 mL/m^2/dose) are given at 15- to 20-minute intervals during the period of crossclamping, to wash out accumulated metabolites and to maintain cardiac arrest. Retrograde cardioplegia through a coronary sinus catheter is also used. The heart is maintained in a decompressed state and topical ice slush is placed on the heart to lower myocardial temperature.

Once the cardiac repair has been accomplished, a warm dose of cardioplegia is administered and the crossclamp is removed. Gradually, the heart resumes a sinus rhythm and normal force of contraction. The patient is fully rewarmed to 37°C rectally, and an assessment of cardiac function and rhythm is made. The lungs are ventilated and the monitors calibrated. Pharmacologic support and epicardial pacing are added as needed. The venous line of the CPB circuit is gradually occluded to allow the heart to fill, and the flow from the CPB machine into the aortic cannula is reduced until the patient is off bypass.

Assessment of filling pressures, arterial pressure, force of cardiac contraction, requirements for pharmacologic support, and surgical bleeding is continually made during the early period following bypass. Once the patient is successfully off bypass, protamine is administered to reverse the residual effects of heparin, the cannulae are removed, and the sternum and skin are closed.

Care and Evaluation of the Postoperative Cardiac Patient

Initial Evaluation

The assessment of the pediatric cardiac patient begins with a systematic review of the preoperative history, the intraoperative course, and the surgical procedure. Particular attention should be paid to the length of CPB, the length of aortic crossclamping, and the difficulties encountered following discontinuation of CPB. The initial assessment should follow the ABCs of resuscitation (airway, breathing, circulation) with observation of adequate chest excursion with ventilation and auscultation for bilateral breath sounds. A chest x-ray is obtained to assess the placement of the ET tube, invasive hemodynamic lines, and chest tubes, as well as the quality of the lung fields.

This is followed by a preliminary assessment of perfusion and cardiac output. The initial assessment begins with a careful physical examination and evaluation of baseline vital signs. Aside from routine vital signs of heart rate, blood pressure, and respiratory rate, measurement of core temperature is an important part of the initial assessment of the child, following cardiac surgery. Although hypothermia is an integral part of cerebral protection during CPB and circulatory arrest, inadvertent hypothermia following the cessation of bypass or during closed heart procedures can have significant deleterious effects on cardiovascular function.

Several factors contribute to the high incidence of hypothermia in the pediatric patient. Heat loss occurs through four basic mechanisms: evaporation, conduction, convection, and radiation. Children and especially neonates have a larger surface-area-to-volume ratio, which increases heat loss to the environment. Regulation of body temperature and correction of hypothermia have significant implications in the postsurgical patient. Hypothermia has several deleterious physiologic effects including increase of myocardial irritability with cardiac arrhythmias, depression of myocardial contractility, altered drug metabolism, decreased glomerular filtration rate, and a leftward shift of the oxyhemoglobin dissociation curve. As such, hypothermia can severely compromise oxygen delivery to tissues through several different mechanisms. General anesthetic agents further aggravate hypothermia by inhibition of thermoregulation.[5] Measures to prevent hypothermia include humidification and warming of inspired gases, external heating by warming lights, a radiant warmer, forced air warming, and the warming of fluids and blood products. With such measures, rewarming of patients can usually be accomplished within the first few postoperative hours.

The Cardiovascular System

Evaluation of the cardiovascular system begins with an assessment of cardiac output. Although the placement of invasive hemodynamic monitors such as a pulmonary artery catheter allows the direct measurement of cardiac output, its use in the pediatric cardiac patient may be limited by size constraints and by the presence of residual cardiac shunts and malformations. With the use of standard pulmonary artery catheters that are placed percutaneously and advanced from the central circulation into the pulmonary artery, cardiac output is measured by thermodilution, which involves injection of a bolus of room-temperature saline into the right atrium (see chapter 2). Intracardiac shunting of blood (left to right or right to left) alters the accuracy of this technique and leads to difficulties with "floatation" of the catheter. Invasive hemodynamic monitors such as pulmonary artery catheters and left atrial lines may be used in certain situations (following the Fontan procedure or in patients at risk for pulmonary vasospasm), but the postoperative assessment of cardiac function primarily relies on physical assessment and laboratory values.

In high-risk patients, invasive hemodynamic lines may be placed prior to closure of the sternum. These may include pulmonary artery catheters and left atrial catheters. Catheters for monitoring central venous pressure (CVP) are generally placed percutaneously via either the jugular, subclavian, or femoral venous systems.[6,7] While subclavian or internal jugular venous lines are used most commonly in the adult population, an accurate measurement of CVP can be achieved with a catheter placed in the femoral venous system. With such placement, advancement to the junction of the right atrium and inferior vena cava is not necessary for an accurate assessment of CVP. CVP can be measured from the femoral system, provided that there are no pathologic conditions that are increasing intra-abdominal pressure. Pulmonary artery pressure monitoring may be used in patients who are at risk for pulmonary hypertension in the postoperative period. Normally pulmonary artery tone is controlled by the release of nitric oxide from the pulmonary endothelial cells. Patients with high pulmonary artery pressures preoperatively (total anomalous pulmonary venous return) and those with a large left-to-right shunt (large ventricular septal defect) are at risk for postoperative pulmonary hypertension. The incidence is particularly high in patients with trisomy 21. In such cases, a 3F or 4F catheter is placed directly into the main pulmonary artery for monitoring of pressure during the discontinuation of CPB and in the postoperative period. Special catheters can be used that contain an optical sensor that provides a continuous readout of mixed venous oxygen saturation. With this catheter in the pulmonary artery, an indirect estimation of cardiac output is possible by measurement of mixed venous oxygen saturation (see chapter 2 for a full discussion of mixed venous oxygen saturation). Although not as accurate as measurement in the pulmonary artery, mixed venous oxygen saturation can also be estimated by a sample drawn from a central venous catheter. In this setting the blood sample can be sent for blood gas analysis and the oxygen saturation can be used as an indirect means of assessing cardiac output. The latter may be affected by residual intracardiac shunting. A decline in the mixed venous oxygen saturation without a factor to suggest an increase in oxygen consumption or a decrease in the hemoglobin concentration or oxygen saturation implies a decrease in oxygen delivery. As oxygen delivery is determined by hemoglobin concentration, arterial oxygen saturation, and cardiac output, if the first two have not changed, a decline in cardiac output is the presumed etiology.

In many cases, the cardiac filling pressures are estimated by the using the CVP. While this is an indirect measurement of left-sided pressures, the correlation is generally sufficient to guide care in the postoperative patient. In specific circumstances, a more direct estimation of left-sided pressures may be needed. This is particularly relevant in the patient at risk for pulmonary hypertension or following the Fontan procedure. In such cases, a catheter may be placed directly into the left atrium. The left atrial pressure is used to estimate left ventricular preload or left ventricular end-diastolic volume (LVEDV). The left atrial pressure is analogous to the pulmonary capillary wedge pressure (PCWP), but is not influenced by factors that alter PCWP, such as changes in pulmonary vascular resistance (PVR) and alterations in alveolar pressure.

Cardiac output is also assessed on physical examination by noting peripheral perfusion, capillary refill, peripheral pulses, and blood pressure. Peripheral vasoconstriction may maintain blood pressure in the normal range despite a low cardiac output state, making arterial blood pressure a relatively poor reflection of cardiac output. Mental status may also be an indicator of cardiac output, but its use in the immediate postoperative period is limited by residual anesthetic agents. Additional tools used in the assessment of cardiac status include urine output and acid-base status. Although several factors may play a role in oliguria, especially following cardiac surgery, urine output is an end-organ measure of cardiac output. The acid-base status on arterial blood gas analysis and serum lactate levels may also reflect cardiac output. With inadequate tissue perfusion, anaerobic metabolism and the accumulation of lactate may occur.

In the immediate perioperative period, cardiorespiratory failure is the primary cause of mortality. Several factors may play a role in perioperative myocardial failure, including perioperative myocardial dysfunction, intraoperative events such as damage due to CPB, and residual cardiac lesions and shunts. Shortly after the introduction of CPB, it became apparent that low cardiac output was the primary cause of early postoperative death. Morales and associates[8] were the first to document scattered areas of myocardial necrosis in patients who died after CPB. Shortly thereafter, Najafi and colleagues[9] suggested that the diffuse myocardial necrosis was the result of damage related to CPB. Although various cardioplegia solutions have been investigated, none have been totally successful in preventing myocardial necrosis and the resultant postbypass myocardial dysfunction. Regardless of the type of cardioprotection that is used, there will be some areas of myocardial necrosis and additional areas that are still ischemic. The combination of these two result in postoperative depressions of myocardial contractility. Failure to reverse the problem, improve cardiac output, and decrease LVEDV can lead to further discrepancies in the myocardial oxygen delivery/demand ratio with the death of ischemic myocardium. Therefore, prompt recognition and treatment of the problem are necessary.

Concerns regarding myocardial preservation may be particularly relevant in the neonate; it has been suggested that the neonatal myocardium is particularly vulnerable to ischemic injury and that methods of protection used in adult patients may be ineffective in the pediatric population.[10,11] The increased sensitivity may be related to the limited glycogen stores and rapid intracellular lactate accumulation. In the perioperative period, part of the dysfunction may be reversible, and prevention of imbalances in myocardial oxygen demand and delivery may prevent further cardiac decompensation.

The balance of myocardial oxygen delivery and consumption may be precarious in the immediate postoperative period, and alterations in various parameters such as heart rate may not only increase oxygen demand but may also limit delivery. Myocardial oxygen consumption is determined primarily by heart rate, left ventricular end diastolic pressure (LVEDP), afterload, and contractility. Myocardial oxygen delivery occurs primarily during diastole and is determined by the coronary perfusion pressure (diastolic blood pressure minus LVEDP). An increase in heart rate not only increases oxygen consumption, but also decreases diastolic time and therefore coronary perfusion time. Excessive vasodilation may decrease diastolic blood pressure, impairing coronary perfusion pressure, while myocardial ischemia can lead to increases in LVEDP which further increase myocardial oxygen consumption and impair oxygen delivery. Such imbalances may be of particular relevance in patients with systemic-to-pulmonary shunts (either surgical or medical with prostaglandin E_1), since diastolic runoff may lead to significant decreases in diastolic pressure. Abnormalities of oxygen delivery and consumption may be further aggravated by anatomic abnormalities of the coronary vasculature. Although the use of inotropic agents is frequently necessary, agents that increase heart rate and systemic vascular resistance (SVR) excessively may increase myocardial oxygen consumption and lead to increased myocardial damage.[12] With such concerns, maintenance of adequate cardiac output and tissue oxygen delivery while limiting or decreasing factors that increase oxygen consumption should be the primary goal in the immediate postoperative period.

As in any other clinical situation, cardiac output is determined by the product of heart rate and stroke volume. Although alterations in heart rate may be of little clinical significance in older patients, bradycardia can lead to significant decrease in cardiac output in the neonate and infant. The impact of heart rate on cardiac output may be significant following CPB, because alterations in stroke volume may be limited by a relatively noncompliant myocardium. The latter can be a result of the underlying cardiac disorder and/or a result of CPB. In the noncompliant heart, ventricular relaxation (lusitropic function) is impaired. As such, a higher than normal filling pressure is needed to allow for ventricular filling, and cardiac output becomes heart-rate-dependent. Therefore, although excessive increases in heart rate should be avoided for the previously mentioned reasons, heart rates of 20% to 30% above the norm for the age are not uncommon in the postoperative period.

Alterations in cardiac rhythm with asynchrony of the atria and ventricles may also impair cardiac output. Although the atrial kick is responsible for only 10% to 15% of the cardiac output in the healthy state, alterations in ventricular compliance may leave the ventricle dependent on atrial contraction to ensure adequate ventricular preload. In such instances, loss of the synchrony between atrial and ventricular contraction may lead to significant decreases in cardiac output. Atrial arrhythmias may also be particularly detrimental following the Fontan procedure, in which the atrial contraction may be necessary to propel blood through the pulmonary artery to the left atrium.

In addition to alterations in rhythm that are related to CPB, dysrhythmias may be related to the surgical procedure and are commonly seen following closure of atrial septal defects (sinus venosus type) and following atrial shunt procedures (Mustard and Senning procedures). The treatment of dysrhythmias will be dependent on the type (atrial versus ventricular) as well as the underlying etiology. In patients who are at risk for atrioventricular (AV) block, pacing wires are sutured to the epicardium prior to sternal closure. The onset of AV block is treated by the initiation of sequential AV pacing or isolated ventricular pacing. The former is beneficial in patients who are dependent on atrial filling for optimal cardiac output. Postsurgical AV block may be the result of direct surgical damage during repair, but is more likely a transient phenomenon arising from swelling, or the residual effect of cardioplegia. Temporary AV sequential pacing via epicardial leads may be required. Permanent pacemaker placement is deferred for 7 to 14 days.

While the primary mechanisms of ventricular or atrial ectopy may be related to the surgical trauma, underlying causes including direct irritation from intravascular catheters, hypoxemia, hypercarbia, acidosis, myocardial ischemia, and electrolyte disturbances should be ruled out. Low levels of potassium and magnesium may be particularly common during the immediate postoperative period and may lead to ventricular irritability.[13] The immediate treatment of tachyarrhythmias is mandatory. Pharmacologic treatment is acceptable if the patient is hemodynamically stable, while synchronized cardioversion is indicated if cardiac decompensation occurs. In addition to dysrhythmias, sinus node dysfunction with bradycardia may be temporarily present following CPB. Low-dose isoproterenol (0.01 to 0.05 μg/kg/min) may be required to maintain an acceptable heart rate. After the establishment of a normal sinus rhythm and AV synchrony with a normal heart rate for age, manipulation of cardiac function depends on alterations in stroke volume.

Stroke volume is determined by LVEDV (preload), by afterload, and by contractility. In the immediate postoperative period, assessment of these three factors, of rhythm, and of heart rate allow for pharmacologic and fluid management to optimize the hemodynamic status of the patient. In the patient with acute decompensation, mechanical difficulties such as tension pneumothorax and cardiac tamponade should be ruled out. Once these factors are ruled out, fluid and inotropic agents are indicated to maintain and improve cardiac output. Fluid management should be guided by measurement of filling pressures via invasive monitoring when available. Although the CVP can be used to estimate right ventricular preload, its use to assess left ventricular preload is somewhat limited. This is especially true in the patient with alterations in ventricular function and elevated pulmonary vascular resistance.

An elevated ventricular preload may be required in the patient with compromised cardiac function or a noncompliant ventricle with diastolic dysfunction (impaired lusitropic function or ventricular relaxation). As such, left atrial pressures (PCWP) of 10 to 14 mm Hg, or CVP pressures of 15 to 18 mm Hg, may be required. Direct measurement of cardiac output and afterload is generally not available in the pediatric cardiac patient. Residual intracardiac shunts and the small size of many patients preclude the use of thermodilution measurements of cardiac output and calculation of afterload. Qualitative estimates can be obtained by monitoring mixed venous oxygen saturation and evaluating peripheral pulses and skin temperature.

Alterations in afterload may also affect cardiovascular function especially in the postoperative setting in the patient with compromised cardiac contractility. In addition to SVR, respiratory function may also affect afterload. In the healthy state, spontaneous ventilation leads to an increase in ventricular filling and increased cardiac output, with little or no increase in afterload. However, in the patient with respiratory distress, large negative increases in interpleural pressure may significantly increase afterload and decrease cardiac output. Therefore, an acute decompensation of cardiac output may respond most quickly to ET intubation, controlled ventilation, and the resultant decrease in afterload.

In patients who are not undergoing invasive hemodynamic monitoring, fluid and inotropic administration are titrated by clinical responses such as improvements in perfusion, capillary refill, urine output, and peripheral temperature. Once an adequate volume status is reached, the administration of inotropic agents is indicated to optimize cardiac contractility. Agents used to improve contractility act to increase intracellular calcium availability by increasing calcium release from the sarcoplasmic reticulum; this leads to increased muscle fibril crosslinking and contraction. Three basic choices are available:

1. exogenous administration of calcium
2. drugs that act through activation of adrenergic receptors
3. inhibitors of phosphodiesterase (PDE) III

Exogenous calcium administration improves contractility by increasing the transmembrane concentration and increasing intracellular accumulation when calcium channels are opened during action potential propagation. Although some evidence links increases in intracellular calcium with subsequent neuronal damage, several factors in the immediate postoperative period may lead to decreased serum ionized calcium, including the administration of citrate-preserved blood, administration of protamine to reverse the residual effects of heparin, low levels of serum magnesium, and alterations in parathyroid function. Exogenous calcium administration may be particularly relevant in the neonatal population, as their myocardial cells are relatively deficient in sarcoplasmic reticulum and therefore excitation-contraction coupling is more dependent on extracellular calcium. Exogenous calcium administration is indicated to achieve normal serum ionized calcium levels.

The choice of agent—calcium chloride versus calcium gluconate—is somewhat controversial. It is generally accepted that the administration of equimolar concentrations of either agent will normalize serum calcium. This may include either 0.1 mL/kg of 10% calcium chloride or 0.3 mL/kg of 10% calcium gluconate. Dosing of calcium replacement should be based on serial measurements of ionized calcium. Calcium replacement should be administered over 20 to 30 minutes to prevent alterations in heart rate and rhythm, such as bradycardia, which may occur with rapid administration.

The adrenergic agonists interact with specific cell receptors. Although several subclasses of the receptors exist, three are of predominant importance for inotropic administration. Alpha receptors are located primarily on vascular tissue, although recent evidence has also documented their presence on myocardial cells. Stimulation of these receptors leads to vasoconstriction. β_1 Receptors are located on myocardial cells. Stimulation leads to increased force of contraction (inotropy), increased heart rate (chronotropy), and increased speed of impulse conduction along the conduction pathways (dromotropy). Stimulation of β_1 receptors that increase force of contraction also impairs ventricular relaxation. As such, these agents may impair the diastolic function of the heart and make the ventricle less compliant. β_2 Receptor stimulation, present on vascular tissue, causes vasodilatation.

Controversy remains over the optimal inotropic agent to follow CPB.[14,15] Proponents of potent agents such as epinephrine believe that quick and prompt correction of the low cardiac output state is mandatory to prevent further cardiac decompensation and necrosis. Epinephrine, with equal effects at the alpha and beta receptors, will improve contractility with little or no change in SVR when used in doses of 0.01 to 0.1 μg/kg/min. However, venoconstriction may increase filling pressures, and a venodilator such as nitroglycerin may be needed to offset this effect. A second approach is the combination of norepinephrine with a vasodilator (phentolamine, nitroprusside). With these agents, the potent inotropic effects of norepinephrine may be achieved while its deleterious effects on SVR are minimized by the addition of the vasodilator. The PDE inhibitors can also be combined with norepinephrine. The potent vasodilatory effects of the PDE inhibitors are used to offset the vasoconstricting effects of norepinephrine or epinephrine.[16]

Although many centers use dopamine or dobutamine initially and then switch to epinephrine if these agents fail, studies in the adult population suggest that the dose-response curve to both dopamine and dobutamine are flat following CPB.[17] Additionally, the use of an indirect agent that relies on the release of endogenous catecholamines such as dopamine may be ineffective in a patient who has been chronically stressed in whom endogenous catecholamine stores are depleted. Regardless of the agent(s) chosen, serial measurements of cardiac output (when available) or repeated evaluation of cardiac output on clinical examination should be used to guide the administration of fluid as well as the inotropic agents. As in patients with shock of other etiologies, the choice of inotropic agent and treatment with fluid are based on the perceived or measured hemodynamic variables that control cardiac output including heart rate, preload, afterload, and contractility (see also chapter

2 for a full discussion of cardiovascular physiology and treatment of shock states).

The PDE inhibitors (amrinone, milrinone) are the newest class of inotropic agents in clinical practice.[18,19] These agents inhibit PDE III in cardiac cells, thereby increasing intracellular cyclic adenosine monophosphate (cAMP) concentrations, which results in an increase in the availability of intracellular calcium. The final common pathway of inotropic agents is an increase in intracellular cAMP levels. Since these agents bypass adrenergic receptors, they may be useful in patients who are receiving adrenergic agents for the long term, who have alterations in receptor number and function. The prototype of these agents, amrinone, is administered as a bolus (0.5 to 1.0 mg/kg) followed by a continuous infusion of 5 to 20 µg/kg/min. Cardiovascular effects include increased inotropy and vasodilatation. These effects combine to decrease filling pressures and afterload, thereby improving cardiac output and favorably affecting myocardial oxygen demand and delivery. One adverse effect, which has been related to the metabolite of amrinone, is thrombocytopenia. This may cause problems during the immediate postoperative period when other factors related to CPB may predispose the patient to thrombocytopenia. In this setting, similar cardiovascular effects can be achieved with milrinone. Dosing regimens include a loading dose of 50 to 100 µg/kg followed by an infusion of 0.5 to 1.0 µg/kg/min. Both agents can cause a significant drop in SVR and mean arterial pressure (MAP), especially in the immediate postbypass period. Treatment of the latter may require the addition of a drug that has α-adrenergic effects such as dopamine, norepinephrine, or epinephrine.

Regardless of the inotropic agents chosen, progressive myocardial dysfunction may lead to progressive cardiogenic shock. In such instances mechanical support of the circulation may be an option to maintain the circulation and prevent further myocardial damage while allowing time for myocardial recovery. Options include extracorporeal membrane oxygenation (ECMO), ventricular assist devices, and the intra-aortic balloon pump (IABP).[20-23] ECMO was originally introduced as salvage therapy for progressive respiratory failure. However, with arteriovenous ECMO, flow (cardiac output) is provided by the roller pump, and the circulation can be supported. The technique involves the placement of a venous cannula that drains blood into a reservoir. From there, blood is pumped through a membrane oxygenator and then returned to the patient via the arterial cannula placed into the aorta. This support may be instituted through the sternotomy incision, with cannulae placed directly in the right atrium and aorta or with percutaneous cannulae. The venous cannula may be placed percutaneously into either the internal jugular or the femoral vein, while the arterial cannula is generally placed into the ascending aorta through the carotid artery. The major disadvantage of this technique is carotid artery obstruction during the process and the resultant risk of neurologic complication. However, studies in neonatal ECMO have shown a very low risk of neurologic sequelae.

Ventricular assist devices have recently been used to support the failing heart in children.[21] These devices can be used to support either the right or the left ventricle. Blood is drained from either the right or the left atrium and then delivered via an extracorporeal pump into either the pulmonary artery or the aorta.

The third option for mechanical assist is the IABP. Although it is most commonly used in adults, a recent report documents its efficacy in children.[22,23] The IABP is placed through the femoral artery and positioned in the first part of the descending aorta, distal to the left subclavian artery. The balloon inflates during diastole and deflates prior to systole. This reduces afterload and improves flow during diastole. The improvement in diastolic flow augments myocardial perfusion while the decrease in afterload improves cardiac output. Although systolic pressure is slightly lowered, MAP and cardiac output increase. Despite the reported success in one pediatric series, mechanical problems with the device are particularly common in children.[23] The small size of many patients precludes its use, and the general elasticity of the aorta of an infant or child limits the IABP's ability to decrease afterload and augment diastolic flow. Additionally, the relatively rapid heart rate of children makes the timing of inflation and deflation more difficult. Complications inherent in the use of any of the mechanical devices include bleeding from heparinization, thromboembolic events, infection, hemolysis, and vascular compromise related to cannulae.

Respiratory System

Respiratory failure is second to cardiac failure as the most common cause of death in the immediate postoperative period. The initial assessment, following auscultation for breath sounds and documentation of bilateral, adequate excursion of the thoracic cavity, includes examination of the postoperative chest x-ray film for ET tube placement and ruling out of residual pneumothoraces. Following this, initial ventilator settings should be determined. The initial option includes either pressure- or volume-limited ventilation, depending on the patient's age and the compliance of the respiratory system. Patients with decreased compliance related to pulmonary edema of either a cardiac or noncardiac etiology may benefit from pressure-limited ventilation with a decreased incidence of barotrauma and improved oxygenation related to the decelerating flow pattern. The initial pressure limit, set as either the peak inflating pressure or pressure above positive end-expiratory pressure (PEEP) (the ΔP), is adjusted to achieve adequate chest excursion and returned or exhaled tidal volumes of 8 to 10 mL/kg. For patients with normal compliance and little or no alveolar space disease noted on the initial chest x-ray, volume-limited ventilation with delivered tidal volumes adjusted to produce an exhaled volume of 8 to 10 mL/kg is suggested. The delivered tidal volume may need to be greater than the exhaled volume of 8 to 10 mL/kg in patients with uncuffed ET tubes who have an airleak around the ET tube.

Other ventilator parameters include an initial FiO_2 of 1.0, an inspiratory time of 0.5 to 1.0 second, and PEEP of 3 to 5 cm H_2O. The initial FiO_2 of 1.0 is provided to all patients except those with a residual intracardiac shunt in whom the pulmonary vasodilation may lead to an increase in left-to-right shunt and a decrease in systemic cardiac output. One example is the patient following a stage I Norwood procedure. The Norwood procedure is performed in patients with a single ventricle, most commonly hypoplastic left heart syndrome, and involves a system whereby the single ventricle ejects blood to the lungs and also to the systemic circulation. As the ventricle can eject into either system, the blood flow is preferentially distributed based on the difference in vascular resistance of these two beds. If an FiO_2 of 1.0 is delivered, pulmonary vasodilation may occur, thereby increasing pulmonary blood flow. Although the oxygen saturation increases, there is excessive pulmonary blood flow and decreased flow to the systemic circulation that can result in tissue hypoxia and shock. In such patients, the oxygen is decreased to achieve a systemic saturation of 70% to 80%. In other patients, residual shunts may make the oxygen saturation relatively unresponsive to the increased FiO_2, and the FiO_2 should be weaned based on the acceptable arterial oxygen saturation determined by the patient's underlying anatomy. Patients who have had a complete repair are expected to have normal arterial oxygen saturations, while saturations of 75% to 80% may be acceptable in patients with residual shunts or single ventricles.

The inspiratory time and PEEP are adjusted as needed to maintain the mean airway pressure. With a relatively normal postoperative chest x-ray, physiologic levels of PEEP of 3 to 5 cm H_2O are provided. Higher levels of PEEP may be required in patients with pulmonary edema and alveolar space diseases that result in decreased pulmonary compliance. Regardless of the underlying lung disease, adjustments of PEEP and mean airway pressure may significantly impact on venous return, afterload, and cardiovascular status, especially in patients with diminished function. Increases in PEEP or mean airway pressure may lead to decreases in right ventricular preload and, hence, decreases in right-sided cardiac output. The increase in PVR also further decreases right ventricular output, leading to decreased blood flow to the left ventricle and thereby further decreasing LVEDV. The third effect of the increased mean airway pressure and

PEEP (which results in an increased PVR) that can further compromise LVEDV is known as ventricular interdependence. The right and left ventricles are constrained by the pericardium. The right ventricle is normally crescent shaped. As the PVR and the right ventricular end-diastolic pressure (RVEDP) increase, the septum bows into the left ventricular cavity. The bowing of the septum further impedes LVEDV and left ventricular cardiac output.

PEEP by itself does not increase PVR. Rather the relationship between PEEP and PVR is determined by the lung volume. PVR is lowest at a normal functional residual capacity (FRC). As overinflation occurs, the pulmonary vessels are distended and PVR increases. If atelectasis occurs, the pulmonary vessels become collapsed and distorted, thus increasing PVR. As such, increases in PEEP to 10 to 12 cm H_2O will increase PVR if there is no pulmonary parenchymal disease, with an end result of overdistention of the lung; however, the same amount of PEEP may increase lung volume closer to a normal FRC in a patient with noncardiogenic pulmonary edema, and thereby decrease PVR. The exact effects of mean airway pressure and PEEP on cardiac function vary according to: 1) the extent of the underlying lung disease, which determines how much of the alveolar pressure is transmitted to the pulmonary capillary bed; 2) the patient's intravascular volume status; and 3) the underlying function of the myocardium. No prediction can be made as to the patient's response to alterations in mechanical ventilation. As such, observation of invasive monitors, peripheral perfusion, MAP, and urine output are used to judge the response of the cardiovascular system to changes in ventilatory support.

Initial respiratory rate should be appropriate for age (30 to 40 breaths per minute for a neonate and 10 to 14 for an adolescent), with subsequent increases or decreases based on analysis of arterial blood gases and noninvasive monitors of ventilation. Higher rates may be required for patients in whom hypocapnia is required to control PVR.

The optimal duration of mechanical ventilation for the postoperative pediatric cardiac patient remains controversial. Twenty to 30 years ago, mechanical ventilation was arbitrarily continued for 24 to 48 hours in all patients. However, recent reports have suggested the safety of early (<12 hours) extubation following cardiac surgery in the adult population.[24,25] With this approach, earlier ICU discharge may be possible and morbidity related to ET intubation, such as mucus plugging, atelectasis, pulmonary infections, and tracheal trauma, may be decreased. Additionally, the deleterious hemodynamic effects of positive pressure ventilation may be avoided. Although the initial studies were performed in adults following coronary artery bypass grafting, the feasibility of early extubation for selected pediatric patients has also been demonstrated. Heard and coworkers[26] demonstrated a correlation of the duration of CPB with the probability of early extubation (within 6 hours). This correlation is not surprising, since histologic studies show interstitial and intra-alveolar edema, perivascular and intra-alveolar hemorrhage, and miliary atelectasis after prolonged CPB.[27,28] Early extubation appears appropriate for older patients (older than 6 to 12 months of age) who are undergoing relatively simple procedures such as repair of atrial or ventricular septal defects and coarctation of the aorta.

Early tracheal extubation may also be beneficial in patients with specific repairs and resultant anatomy. The purpose of repairs such as a Glenn shunt or Fontan procedure (see glossary of surgical procedures) is to treat conditions involving the absence of a ventricle on the pulmonary side of the circulation, and are dependent on the CVP to drive blood through the pulmonary circuit. The absence of the ventricle makes alterations in pulmonary blood flow very dependent on changes in interpleural and intrathoracic pressure. With positive pressure ventilation, these pressures increase, impede passive venous return, and thus decrease blood flow through the lungs and its return to the left side. With spontaneous ventilation, venous return and pulmonary blood flow are increased. Early return of spontaneous ventilation and tracheal extubation may be beneficial in these patients.

Neonates and those with more complex

lesions may require a more prolonged course of mechanical ventilation. As many as 40% of neonates undergoing cardiac surgery require prolonged ventilation. The etiologies for this postoperative respiratory dysfunction are both controversial and most likely multifactorial. Furthermore, physical examination and laboratory findings do not differentiate infants who will tolerate early extubation from those who will require prolonged ventilation. When an infant requires prolonged ventilation, a systematic approach to the possible mechanism(s) of the respiratory failure is helpful. These can be categorized into five groups: central nervous system (CNS) dysfunction, airway problems, neuromuscular weakness, residual cardiovascular dysfunction, and pulmonary parenchymal disease. CNS dysfunction may be related to residual anesthetic effects, ongoing administration of sedative drugs, metabolic derangements, or damage related to CPB and episodes of hypoperfusion. The evaluation of the infant who fails to wake up following surgery is discussed later in this chapter. Following a careful physical examination, metabolic work-up including serum electrolytes, calcium, phosphorous, magnesium, glucose, and ammonia will rule out many of the metabolic causes of altered mental status. Computed-tomography (CT) scanning of the head and electroencephalogram may also be indicated. Airway problems include postextubation stridor and airway edema. The latter is particularly common in infants and patients with trisomy 21.[29] Measures to minimize airway edema include use of an appropriately sized ET tube (uncuffed in patients <6 to 8 years of age), measurement of cuff pressures during the postoperative course when cuffed ET tubes are used, and adequate sedation during mechanical ventilation to prevent excessive movement. For patients with prolonged courses of ventilation without an audible leak around the ET tube, the administration of corticosteroids (dexamethasone 1 mg/kg/day divided every 6 hours) may decrease the incidence of postextubation stridor. Following tracheal extubation, an oxygen/helium mixture may decrease the work of breathing in infants with a compromised airway, allowing time for resolution of subglottic edema. If such measures fail and prolonged ventilation is required due to airway problems, direct laryngoscopy may be indicated to rule out vocal cord paralysis. This is especially true following surgical procedures that involve the aortic arch and great vessels, since inadvertent damage to the recurrent laryngeal nerve may occur.

Neuromuscular weakness may compromise postoperative respiratory function. Aside from the residual effects of neuromuscular blocking agents, several metabolic derangements including hypokalemia, hypomagnesemia, and hypophosphatemia may lead to generalized muscle weakness. Such derangements may occur in infants maintained on parenteral alimentation. The prolonged use of diuretics can cause significant depletion of body stores of potassium, magnesium, and phosphorous. Diuretics, aminoglycoside antibiotics, and several other medications may have neuromuscular blocking properties as a side effect, and their role in potentiating muscle weakness should be considered.

Inadequate cardiovascular function may also affect respiratory function. Poor cardiac output may lead to easy fatiguability of the diaphragm and to respiratory failure. In such instances inotropic support and improvement of cardiovascular function may permit weaning from mechanical ventilation. Additionally, diaphragmatic dysfunction may be related to phrenic nerve damage during surgical manipulation. Fluoroscopic examination of both diaphragms during spontaneous ventilation is required to ensure that diaphragmatic movement is normal. Ultrasound evaluation may be possible in the smaller infant and neonate. The advantage of the latter technique is that it may be done in the pediatric intensive care unit (PICU).

In the immediate postoperative period it is also necessary to consider the deleterious effects of pain, including decreased tidal volume, FRC, and forced expiratory volume. These changes, combined with decreased cough effort and the residual effects of anesthetic agents, can lead to ventilation-perfusion mismatch, postoperative hypoxemia, and respiratory failure.

Increased lung water, alveolar-capillary leak, inspissated secretions, alterations in airway reactivity, and recurrent pulmonary infections may affect postoperative respiratory function. Periodic examination of chest x-ray films and tracheal aspirates may be helpful in guiding diuretic therapy and the need for antibiotics to clear pulmonary infections. Edema of the chest wall or of the pulmonary interstitium may also lead to respiratory failure. Cardiac dysfunction with engorgement of pulmonary and bronchial veins may impinge on the airway space while residual cardiac shunts and increased pulmonary flow may lead to postoperative edema. Postoperative echocardiography or catheterization may be needed to define the presence of a residual shunt and its effect on cardiorespiratory function. In many cases, the etiology of the respiratory dysfunction is multifactorial and requires therapy to correct several different factors.

When an infant requires prolonged ventilation, an assessment of the five groups (see above) should be pursued, to evaluate the cause of the respiratory failure. In many cases optimization of cardiovascular function and the judicious use of diuretics to decrease lung water allow for a gradual wean from mechanical ventilation. The other component of respiratory failure that should be aggressively addressed is nutrition. Many of these infants and neonates have little or no nutritional reserve. This, compounded by a prolonged postoperative course, can have significant deleterious effects on the patient.

Aside from concerns regarding gas exchange, alterations in PVR and the development of pulmonary vasospasm can have significant implications during the postoperative period. Since the first report of pulmonary hypertension in 1897 by Eisenmenger, it has become increasingly clear that prevention and treatment of pulmonary hypertension can alter postoperative outcome. Although it is impossible to identify all patients who are at risk for postoperative pulmonary vasospasm, patients with high flows through the pulmonary vascular bed related to a high left-to-right shunt (preoperative Q_p/Q_s >2:1 to 3:1) or those with obstruction to venous return (anomalous pulmonary venous return with obstruction) are at risk. Patients with trisomy 21 appear to be at risk for developing pulmonary vascular changes despite low to moderate shunt ratios (Q_p/Q_s 1.5:1 to 2:1). Although additional information may be gained from the preoperative cardiac catheterization, PVR may be affected by the type and degree of sedation administered during the procedure.

Control of PVR may also be indicated in patients with a univentricular repair (Glenn shunt or Fontan procedure) who are dependent on the CVP to provide passive pulmonary blood flow. As there is no ventricle to augment pulmonary blood flow, small increases in PVR may significantly decrease pulmonary blood flow and, subsequently, left-sided cardiac filling. In these patients, monitoring of pulmonary artery pressure/left atrial pressure and early treatment of increases in PVR may be indicated.

Once the patients who are most at risk are identified, prevention of pulmonary vasospasm is particularly important in the immediate postoperative period. CPB may increase the chances of developing pulmonary hypertension. Several factors play a role in the propensity to develop pulmonary vasospasm following CPB; these include alterations in pulmonary endothelial function with decreased synthesis of endothelial-dependent relaxing factor (EDRF), now commonly known as nitric oxide, and alterations in platelet and leukocyte function with release of thromboxanes and leukotrienes. Prevention of pulmonary vasospasm is easiest with early detection. This requires invasive hemodynamic monitoring including intraoperative placement of pulmonary artery catheters and left atrial catheters. Treatment and prevention include both ventilator and pharmacologic management. Ventilator management includes modest hyperventilation with arterial carbon dioxide pressure of 30 to 35 mm Hg, maintenance of a normal to slightly alkalotic pH, and an arterial oxygen partial pressure of 90 to 100 mm Hg. Hyperventilation is continued for 2 to 3 days and slowly weaned as tolerated. The FiO_2 is decreased in increments of 3% to 5% every hour as long as the PaO_2 is greater than 90 to 100 mm Hg. In addition, metabolic acidosis and hypothermia should be aggressively treated, since either condition may lead to increases in PVR. Adequate sedation and analgesia are extremely important, as uncontrolled pain and the release of endogenous catecholamines can lead to irreversible episodes of pulmonary vasospasm and death. The synthetic opioids such as fentanyl appear to be particularly advantageous, since they provide analgesia with relative cardiovascular stability while having beneficial effects on the reactivity of the pulmonary vasculature. Initial doses of 5 to 10 μg/kg are followed by a continuous infusion of 5 to 10 μg/kg/h and increased as needed.

Vasodilator therapy may be helpful for patients who develop episodes of pulmonary vasospasm or increased PVR. Available pharmacologic agents include nitroglycerin, nitroprusside, tolazoline, prostacyclin, isoproterenol, and the PDE inhibitors. Although it has been suggested that some of these agents may be more specific for the pulmonary vascular bed, all of them will also cause some degree of peripheral vasodilatation. Of the available agents, the PDE inhibitors are helpful in that they augment cardiovascular function and improve cardiac output while decreasing PVR. In patients with invasive hemodynamic lines, the vasodilator may be infused directly into the pulmonary artery line to limit its effects on the systemic circulation. Most recently, the drug of choice to treat increased PVR following cardiovascular surgery has become nitric oxide.[30] Nitric oxide, is synthesized in pulmonary endothelial cells and leads to smooth muscle relaxation through interactions with the intracellular cyclic guanosine monophosphate system. The administration of inhaled nitric oxide (5 to 40 ppm) into the ventilator circuit leads to selective pulmonary vasodilatation. Since the agent is immediately inactivated by hemoglobin when it reaches the blood stream, no systemic effects occur. Early studies suggest that nitric oxide may have many therapeutic uses including the treatment of pulmonary hypertension following cardiac surgery. Based on its lack of systemic effects, limited adverse physiologic effects, and ease of administration, it currently represents the first choice for the treatment of pulmonary hypertension.

Reaction of nitric oxide with oxygen can lead to the generation of a toxic metabolite, nitrogen dioxide, which can damage the respiratory epithelium. The concentration of this gas is monitored from the ventilator circuit. Additionally, nitric oxide can cause methemoglobin formation in vivo, and methemoglobin levels are monitored every 6 to 8 hours during nitric oxide administration.

Central Nervous System

Although dysfunction of the cardiorespiratory system may have the greatest effect on mortality in the immediate perioperative period, CNS damage may have more prolonged consequences for the patient. CPB and surgery for congenital heart disease pose several embolic and hemodynamic threats to neurologic function. Despite several ongoing areas of research in the field, pharmacologic manipulation to prevent post-CPB neurologic dysfunction is still limited to the laboratory. Hypothermia and limitation of circulatory arrest time remain the mainstay of measures to provide CNS protection and prevent postoperative neurologic dysfunction.[31]

Although the incidence of CNS complications following CPB has decreased in the past 20 years, little or no change has occurred in the past 10 years. The difference from 20 years ago has been attributed to the use of filters in the extracorporeal part of the circuit to limit the risk of embolic events. Despite the accepted risks of CNS dysfunction following CPB, few if any preoperative or intraoperative events or risk factors have been shown to correlate with CNS damage in the pediatric population. CNS effects are more commonly seen following open heart procedures than closed heart procedures.

In the perioperative period, the first suggestion that a CNS event has occurred may be that the patient does not wake up following surgery. In such cases the residual effects of anesthetic agents should be ruled out. This may include either sedative/analgesic agents (opioids and benzodiazepines) or neuromuscular blocking agents. Peripheral nerve stimulation with a standard train-of-four, as used in the operating room, is helpful in the evaluation of residual neuromuscular blockade (see chapter 11 for a full discussion of sedative/analgesic and neuromuscular blocking agents). The effects of residual anesthetic agents are more difficult to evaluate. Although reversal agents exist for both opioids (naloxone) and benzodiazepines (flumazenil), their use in the perioperative period is not recommended because of the risks of precipitating acute withdrawal symptoms, cardiovascular effects such as hypertension and tachycardia, and seizures.

Following a thorough physical examination, laboratory evaluation of the patient should include a search for metabolic causes of altered mental status including serum electrolytes, blood urea nitrogen, glucose, calcium, magnesium, and ammonia. Further investigation may include CT scan or ultrasound (in neonates) of the head to rule out ischemic, hemorrhagic, or thrombotic damage. Changes on the CT scan may not be present for 3 to 5 days following thrombotic or embolic events. An electroencephalogram should be obtained to rule out subclinical seizures, which may present as altered mental status related to repeated periods of postictal states.

A second adverse neurologic event seen following CPB, especially circulatory arrest, is the onset of seizures. The incidence of seizures increases with the length of circulatory arrest and is greatest in patients with arrest times longer than 60 minutes. Although circulatory arrest with deep hypothermia is generally well tolerated in infants and neonates with little or no impairment of long-term outcome, perioperative seizures may occur in 5% to 10% of patients.[32,33] These seizures generally occur within the first 48 hours of the surgery and do not require long-term anticonvulsant therapy. Once metabolic causes of seizures are ruled out, therapy should be initiated with a single agent, either phenobarbital, phenytoin, or fosphenytoin. Anticonvulsants should be continued for 4 to 6 weeks, but can then be discontinued in patients with a normal electroencephalogram and no further evidence of seizure activity.

Gastrointestinal and Hepatic Systems

Several issues concerning both the gastrointestinal (GI) system and the liver affect perioperative care. The majority of patients, especially those requiring postoperative mechanical ventilation, should have a nasogastric (NG) tube passed to allow for continuous decompression of the stomach. The NG tube can be allowed to vent to gravity in most patients or can be connected to intermittent suction in patients with GI distention. The amount of NG drainage, its color, and the pH are noted.

GI ulceration in the critically ill patient is thought to occur not only from increased acid secretion but also from alterations in the normal protective barrier of the stomach. Few topics have gathered as much controversy as the role of various agents in the prevention of stress ulceration in the PICU patient. The reader is referred to chapter 21 for a discussion of these issues and of the various agents used for GI prophylaxis.

Nutritional concerns are not of paramount importance for the majority of patients with a brief postoperative course; however, these issues have significant impact on patients with prolonged postoperative courses, especially neonates and patients who were malnourished preoperatively. When oral feedings cannot be administered for more than 2 to 3 days, parenteral nutrition should be started. Although parenteral nutrition sustains the patient when enteral feeds are not possible, our approach is to use enteral feeds whenever possible. Even if full enteral feeds are not possible, the delivery of small amounts of food into the GI tract may prevent villous atrophy and decrease the risk of bacterial translocation and the development of multisystem organ failure. Once cardiovascular stability is achieved and the patient has evidence of GI activity, enteral feeds are started. A very cautious increase in enteral feeds is mandatory for patients who have had recent bouts of cardiovascular compromise that may have compromised GI perfusion. Such patients may develop necrotizing enterocolitis if feeds are advanced too quickly. Necrotizing enterocolitis is especially important following repair of coarctation of the aorta. These patients are at high risk for the development of mesenteric arteritis as the splanchnic circulation is now exposed to pulsatile flow. Slow advancement of feedings is suggested in this population, and immediate restriction of oral intake is necessary if abdominal pain, distention, or vomiting occur.

The need for fluid restriction may necessitate further restrictions of feedings. In such cases, calorie-dense formulas (30 calories/ounce) may provide adequate calories within the guidelines of the fluid restriction. The increase in caloric density should be achieved with the use of both carbohydrate and lipid. The overzealous administration of carbohydrate may lead to feeding intolerance and diarrhea due to carbohydrate malabsorption. Additionally, the increased carbon dioxide production from carbohydrate metabolism, regardless of whether parenteral or enteral nutrition is used, may lead to hypercarbia and respiratory failure.

Other factors, including pancreatic injury following CPB[34] and alterations in GI motility due to opioid administration, may affect the success of enteral feedings. The latter problem may respond to motility agents such as metoclopramide or cisapride. Our current practice for patients who are expected to spend 3 or more postoperative days in the ICU is to initiate a combination of parenteral nutrition on postoperative day 1 and to supplement it as tolerated with enteral feeds. The enteral feeds are administered via a soft feeding tube that is placed past the pylorus.

Several factors impact on hepatic function in the perioperative period. Preoperative drug therapy and abnormalities in cardiac output may result in preoperative compromise of hepatic function, which may be further complicated by the stress of CPB. Hepatic function may be further affected by infection (cytomegalovirus, Epstein-Barr virus, hepatitis B, C, and D) and by parenteral nutrition. Periodic monitoring of hepatic function and of the coagulation profile are suggested. Treatment of hepatic dysfunction is the same regardless of its etiology, and includes, whenever possible, reversal of the etiology (such as cardiovascular dysfunction) and supportive care including blood products to correct abnormalities of coagulation and treatment of hyperammonemia in severe hepatic failure. Histologic examination of patients with hepatic failure due to alterations in cardiac output reveals centrilobular necrosis. The patients at greatest risk include those with prolonged periods of hypoperfusion requiring inotropic support, especially in the setting of elevated right-sided filling pressures.[35]

Electrolyte and Fluid Considerations

Several factors impact on fluid and electrolyte balance in the perioperative period. Alterations in cardiovascular function, residual effects of CPB on pulmonary capillary integrity, and ongoing fluid shifts and losses make close monitoring of fluid status imperative. Although filling pressures (CVP and left atrial pressures) may be used to guide fluid administration, periodic physical examination and measurement of urinary output are also helpful. Fluid boluses of isotonic crystalloid or colloid (5% albumin) may be required during the first 24 to 36 postoperative hours. Third spacing and capillary leak, related to alterations induced by CPB, frequently occur during this time. Decreases in urine output require fluid administration with the understanding that third spacing and tissue edema may occur. Diuretics are rarely indicated during the first 12 to 24 postoperative hours.

Initial fluid management generally includes the administration of a hypotonic crystalloid with 5% glucose at half to full maintenance. Careful calculation of all fluid administered is imperative, especially in neonates and infants, since antibiotics and other fluids (inotropic agents, etc.) can account for a large percentage of the total daily requirements and must be taken into account into the total daily fluids. Periodic monitoring of serum electrolytes, ionized calcium, magnesium, and glucose are recommended. Avoidance of both hypoglycemia and hyperglycemia is important. Seizures, altered mental status, and permanent neurologic damage may result from prolonged hypoglycemia. On the other hand, hyperglycemia may also adversely affect neurologic outcome. Neurologic outcome may be worse following episodes of hypoxemia or hypoperfusion during hyperglycemia. This is thought to result from increased lactic acid production in neuronal cells during anaerobic metabolism in the presence of hyperglycemia.

Full maintenance fluids are generally required on postoperative day 2 or 3. Patients taking preoperative diuretics or those with residual intracardiac shunts or mixing lesions will generally require postoperative diuretic administration. For most patients, furosemide is an effective diuretic in a dose of 1 to 2 mg/kg every 8 to 12 hours. Furosemide should be administered slowly in the immediate postoperative period, as its chemical structure resembles the nitrates and it can result in vasodilation, decreases in ventricular filling, and a decrease in MAP. Some patients, in particular those requiring larger preoperative doses, may become resistant. Several options are available to the diuretic-resistant patient, including furosemide by continuous infusion, use of another loop diuretic (bumetidine or ethacrynic acid), or the addition of oral metolazone.[36,37] Our preference for resistant patients is the use of a furosemide/chlorothiazide infusion (1 mg furosemide per 5 mg chlorothiazide per 1 mL of normal saline administered at 0.1 mL/kg/h to provide 0.1 mg/kg/h of furosemide. The rate of the infusion is increased or decreased as needed to maintain the desired level of diuresis.

Diuretic administration can lead to electrolyte disturbances including hyponatremia, hypokalemia, hypochloremic alkalosis, and hypercalciuria. Significant hypokalemia may increase the risk of cardiac arrhythmias especially in patients receiving digoxin. Replacement may be required if serum potassium levels are less than 3.0 mEq/L. Intravenous replacement should be administered over 1 hour with no more than 0.25 mEq/kg/h, to a maximum of 10 mEq/h. Hypercalciuria is more a long-term problem; however, significant nephrocalcinosis and impairment of renal function may occur with the prolonged administration of loop diuretics. Periodic monitoring of the urinary calcium-to-creatinine ratio and the addition or substitution of thiazide diuretics for loop diuretics may be indicated. Thiazide diuretics such as chlorothiazide and hydrochlorothiazide limit the calcium loss in the urine and may prevent the development of nephrocalcinosis. Additionally, the addition of spironolactone (1 to 2 mg/kg/day) may be considered in order to eliminate the need for ongoing potassium supplementation.

Hyponatremia may be a problem when switching from parenteral to enteral nutrition. Most parenteral nutrition solutions contain anywhere from 30 to 60 mEq/L of sodium, while most formulas contain only 4 to 8 mEq/L. Periodic monitoring of serum sodium is recommended, especially when switching from enteral feeds. Patients receiving aggressive diuretic regimens may require sodium supplementation.

Hypochloremic metabolic alkalosis may develop following the prolonged use of diuretics, especially the loop diuretics, as these agents block the reabsorption of chloride. In response to this, the renal tubules reabsorb excessive amounts of bicarbonate to maintain electrical neutrality. Although this is generally of limited clinical significance, an excessive degree of metabolic alkalosis may depress the central respiratory drive in an attempt to develop hypercarbia to achieve a normal pH of 7.40. The mainstay of treatment for the metabolic alkalosis is to limit the use of diuretics and to provide adequate potassium chloride supplementation. When this does not succeed in correcting the metabolic alkalosis, options include the administration of a carbonic anhydrase inhibitor (acetazolamide), ammonium chloride, or a dilute solution of 0.1 N hydrochloric acid. Acetazolamide acts to inhibit carbonic anhydrase in the renal tubules, leading to bicarbonate loss in the urine. The dose is 5 to 10 mg/kg intravenously once a day. Our practice is to administer a one-time dose, follow serum electrolytes, and repeat the dose as needed to achieve a serum bicarbonate concentration of less than 30 mEq/L. Ammonium chloride, administered intravenously in doses of 1 to 2 mEq/kg over 1 to 2 hours, can also be used to correct the metabolic acidosis. It is metabolized to ammonia, free hydrogen ion, and chloride. Excessive accumulation of ammonia, especially in patients with hepatic dysfunction, may lead to hyperammonemia. Administration of a 0.1 N HCl solution can cause significant problems with thrombophlebitis and must be administered via a central line. While its use has been reported in the adult population, there are no reports in the pediatric age group.

Alterations in other serum anions and cations such as calcium, phosphorus, and magnesium may also follow cardiac surgery. Several factors may affect serum calcium, including dilution with CPB fluid, citrate in blood products, alterations in serum magnesium levels, and protamine administration. Impairment of parathyroid activity with an inability to mobilize calcium from bone may be seen in the neonate, in the stressed infant, and following asphyxia. Alterations in pH can affect the active fraction, ionized calcium. Increases in pH as can be seen in aggressive hyperventilation or base administration for the treatment of increased PVR can result in a decrease in the ionized fraction. Treatment consists of calcium supplementation with either calcium chloride or calcium gluconate. Either agent will increase serum calcium to the same extent provided equivalent doses of the calcium cation are administered (0.1 mL/kg of calcium chloride or 0.3 mL/kg of calcium gluconate). Addition of calcium to the maintenance intravenous fluids may be required to maintain calcium in the normal range.

Recent interest has focused on magnesium and its effects on cardiovascular function. Magnesium losses are increased by the administration of loop diuretics and aminoglycoside antibiotics. Although magnesium is required for parahormone synthesis and release, it also has effects on cardiovascular function separate from those of the calcium ion. Hypomagnesemia may occur following CPB in a significant percentage of patients, leading to decreased cardiac contractility and ventricular arrhythmias. Equipment is now available in many hospital laboratories to measure ionized magnesium levels. With magnesium, as with calcium, the ionized fraction represents the active moiety and, when available, ionized levels should be monitored. Replacement by bolus dosing and addition to maintenance intravenous fluids may be required. Bolus doses of 50 to 100 mg/kg intravenously (maximum dose of 2 g) are administered over 30 to 60 minutes. Rapid administration or excessive dosing with hypermagnesemia can result in hypotension due to vasodilation and potentiation of neuromuscular blockade with muscle weakness or paralysis.

Several physiologic effects have been ascribed to hypophosphatemia, including impaired cardiac contractility, muscle weakness, respiratory failure, and leftward shift of the oxyhemoglobin dissociation curve with impaired oxygen delivery at the tissue level. Diuretic therapy with increased urinary losses, NG drainage, dilution during CPB, and inadequate replacement in parenteral nutrition solutions are common causes of hypophosphatemia.

Hematologic Issues

Cardiac surgery and CPB can have significant effects on all three formed elements of the bone marrow: platelets, erythrocytes, and leukocytes. These effects include alterations not only in numbers, but also in function of the formed elements. Of primary concern in the immediate postoperative period are effects on platelet numbers and function as well as dilution of coagulation factors. Such effects may lead to severe postoperative hemorrhage and may further complicate the postoperative course.

There are many possible causes of thrombocytopenia in the immediate postoperative period. A decrease in the platelet count occurs during the initiation of CPB, due to dilution. Other effects include mechanical damage to platelets with activation and adherence to the surface of the oxygenator and the tubing. Such effects are less prevalent with the use of membrane oxygenators than with bubble oxygenators. Damage to platelets may also lead to alterations in platelet function without a decrease in number. These coagulation disturbances may be aggravated by other causes of postoperative coagulopathy including incomplete reversal of heparin or protamine overdose.

Excessive postoperative bleeding is noted by excessive output via chest and mediastinal tubes. Various formulas have been suggested to define the maximum amount of drainage allowed. Our preference is to define excessive bleeding as greater than 10% of the circulating blood volume per hour for 3 consecutive hours. Patients with excessive bleeding require an immediate evaluation, including a platelet count, prothrombin time/partial thromboplastin time, and fibrinogen concentration, to ascertain the possible etiologies of the bleeding. Although a thorough evaluation of coagulation status is indicated in patients with persistent bleeding, inadequate surgical hemostasis may also cause persistent hemorrhage. In such cases repeated surgical intervention is the only answer. Every attempt should be made to correct coagulation abnormalities as time permits. A normal PT with a prolonged PTT suggest inadequate reversal of heparin and may be corrected with incremental doses of protamine (0.1 to 0.2 mg/kg) given by slow intravenous infusion. Prolongation of both the PT and PTT suggests an abnormality in coagulation factors because of dilution, consumption, or inadequate hepatic synthesis. Correction with fresh frozen plasma (10 mL/kg) is indicated. Cryoprecipitate is indicated when fibrinogen levels are less than 100 to 150 mg/dL. Thrombocytopenia is treated with platelet infusions (0.2 U/kg of random donor platelets or 10 mL/kg of pheresed platelets).

An additional approach to the treatment of bleeding resulting from platelet dysfunction is the administration of desmopressin (0.3 µg/kg), a synthetic analogue of posterior pituitary hormone. This agent acts by increasing levels of factor VIII and factor VIII antigen and thereby improving platelet function. Prospective, controlled studies are still needed to define the exact role of this agent in the perioperative period. Adverse effects related to desmopressin include hypotension due to systemic vasodilation and hyponatremia due to its antidiuretic hormone actions. Other agents used to manage postoperative bleeding include antifibrinolytic agents such as ε-aminocaproic acid/tranexamic acid and the protease inhibitor, aprotinin. These agents act by inhibiting fibrinolysis. Reports of their efficacy have varied in the literature.

Anemia is also a common problem during the postoperative period. Dilution from CPB, ongoing losses through chest tubes, repeated phlebotomy for diagnostic laboratory investigation, and mechanical damage to erythrocytes from prosthetic valves and intracardiac materials contribute to the problem. Measurement of hematocrit every 4 to 6 hours is indicated during the immediate postoperative period. Although there is much controversy concerning the optimal hematocrit, our general practice is to keep it above 30% in patients with acyanotic lesions and above 40% in those with cyanotic lesions. Higher hematocrit levels may also be indicated in patients with compromised cardiovascular status, to optimize oxygen delivery to the tissues. In the immediate postoperative period, this may require daily transfusions, especially in infants and small children. Once enteral feeds are started, the addition of iron to the formula may limit the need for transfusions. An additional intervention that may play a role in the perioperative period is the administration of synthetic erythropoietin. This may be especially important for patients who have religious objections to the use of blood products.

Hemolysis may also contribute to the drop in hematocrit following CPB. Damage to erythrocyte membranes due to contact with the oxygenator leads to decreased erythrocyte life span. These effects are more common with bubble oxygenators than with the newer membrane oxygenators. Erythrocyte damage and hemolysis may also be seen with prosthetic devices such as heart valves, or with high-velocity flow through shunts or septal defects. Treatment includes repeated transfusions to maintain an acceptable hematocrit, and repair of the defect if the hemolysis persists.

Infectious Disease Issues

Alterations in both the number and the function of leukocytes in the postoperative period have been described. These factors, compounded by the need for intravascular devices, places affected patients at risk for nosocomial infections and sepsis. Outside of the immediate postoperative period, infectious complications remain one of the primary causes of delayed morbidity and mortality.[38] CPB leads to complement activation, leukopenia, and alterations in both humoral and cellular immune function. Hauser and associates[39] demonstrated similar alterations in immune function (both cellular and humoral) following open heart surgery in children. Alterations in complement and immunoglobulin levels persisted for 2 to 7 days following surgery, as did changes in T cell counts and lymphocyte transformation to antigenic stimulation. Such studies further document alterations not only in numbers, but also in the function of several components of the immune system, including leukocytes and lymphocytes. These effects may be especially deleterious in neonates, since their immune function is immature and significantly less efficient than in adults. Further studies are needed to investigate the various means of modulating the immune system, such as the perioperative administration of cytokines and/or immunoglobulins.

Regardless of the various factors that lead to immunodepression, an aggressive search for the cause of fever is required in the postoperative cardiac surgery patient. The appearance of more subtle signs, such as mild cardiovascular instability, glucose intolerance, thrombocytopenia, or alterations in the white blood cell count (neutropenia or leukocytosis), should be considered as sepsis until proven otherwise. Cultures from blood (from all intravascular catheters), urine, and tracheal aspirates should be obtained. Broad-spectrum antibiotic coverage should be instituted until cultures are negative. Initial coverage should include a combination of vancomycin for gram-positive species including *Staphylococcus epidermidis/aureus,* and a third-generation cephalosporin, semisynthetic penicillin (ticarcillin or piperacillin), or an aminoglycoside for *Pseudomonas spp.,* in addition to other gram-negative organisms. Antibiotic coverage may have to be tailored to the resistance pattern in the particular hospital. For patients receiving broad-spectrum antibiotics, the addition of imipenem/meropenem or tobramycin may be indicated to cover for resistant organisms. Antibiotic therapy is adjusted based on culture results. As important as early institution of antibiotic therapy is its prompt discontinuation if cultures remain negative at 72 hours. This discontinuation may be helpful for preventing the emergence of resistant organisms as well as for limiting the overgrowth of pathogenic organisms including fungal species. Persistent fever despite appropriate antibiotic coverage may indicate invasive fungal disease. Ophthalmologic examination as well as CT or ultrasonography of the liver, spleen, and kidneys may identify occult fungal disease. In patients with such disease, the empiric administration of amphotericin B may be indicated until cultures are negative.

Renal System

Alterations in renal function are common in the perioperative period. Drug therapy, alterations in hemodynamic status, and changes in renal blood flow during CPB affect renal function. The etiology of renal insufficiency in the perioperative period is generally multifactorial and control of several factors is needed to ensure proper renal function. Limitation of the use of nephrotoxic drugs and close monitoring of the renal function are of prime importance when such drugs are administered. Commonly used medications that may be nephrotoxic include antibiotics (especially aminoglycosides and amphotericin B), diuretics, and dyes used during cardiac catheterization.

If oliguria is present, a thorough investigation should be conducted to determine its cause. Prerenal, renal, and postrenal (obstructive) factors may contribute to postoperative oliguria. The judicious use of inotropic agents and fluid administration while following hemodynamic parameters is required to maintain adequate renal blood flow. When oliguria develops, the calculation of the fractional excretion of sodium may be useful when separating prerenal causes from renal causes. Recent use of diuretic agents will distort the normal values for fractional excretion of sodium and will invalidate its results. Ultrasonography of the kidneys may be indicated to rule out obstructive causes.

Although the early and aggressive restoration of cardiac output will restore renal function in most patients, this is more easily said than done in the postoperative cardiac patient. A persistently low cardiac output state may lead to acute tubular necrosis and renal insufficiency. Decreases in renal blood flow may be aggravated by diuretics, resulting in hypovolemia or the use of inotropic agents with vasoconstriction and decreases in renal blood flow. In such cases support of the patient with extracorporeal devices (see above) may be required.

The initial treatment of renal insufficiency is directed at the correction of metabolic abnormalities. Fluid restriction and withholding of exogenous potassium should be the first steps. Fluids should be limited to insensible losses plus urinary output. Insensible losses are generally 15% to 30% of normal maintenance fluids, but may be higher for patients with fever and increased respiratory losses due to tachypnea. Additional fluids may also be required to replace ongoing third space losses or drainage from NG or chest tubes. When treatment fails to reverse the etiology of the renal insufficiency, progressive renal failure with oliguria or anuria may result. Indications for dialysis include fluid overload, hyperkalemia, hyperphosphatemia, severe hyponatremia (serum sodium <120 mEq/L), and profound metabolic acidosis.

Although hemodialysis was previously the most commonly used means of supporting the oliguric or anuric patient, other options include peritoneal dialysis and hemofiltration. Continuous arteriovenous hemofiltration (CAVH) allows the removal of an ultrafiltrate composed of plasma, water, and nonprotein-bound small and middle weight molecules. The system uses the patient's own blood pressure (CAVH) or a roller pump (continuous venous-venous hemofiltration or [CVVH]) to drive the blood through an exogenous system with a semipermeable membrane. This allows the removal of excessive fluid without hemodialysis. CVVH, which uses a pump to move the blood through the system, obviates the need for arterial access and allows better control of flow through the system without dependence on the patient's intrinsic blood pressure to drive blood flow through the system. The infusion of dialysis fluid in a countercurrent direction across the membrane permits the more rapid removal of fluid and solutes including blood urea nitrogen and potassium. This method is known as continuous arteriovenous or venovenous hemodiafiltration. These techniques may totally replace hemodialysis or, more likely, decrease its use. Unlike hemodialysis, the removal of fluid is accomplished over a 24-hour period, thus limiting the cardiovascular effects. Adverse effects include the need for indwelling venous catheters and partial anticoagulation, as there is an extracorporeal component to the system.

Peritoneal dialysis or hemodialysis will also be required for some patients. Hemodialysis may be unsuitable in the perioperative period because of its deleterious effects on cardiovascular function. Peritoneal dialysis may be more efficacious in children because of the relatively large surface area of the peritoneum, but may require 2 to 3 days until full volumes of the peritoneal fluid can be used; therefore its efficacy is limited in the emergent or urgent situation. Cardiorespiratory compromise may occur with the intermittent filling of the peritoneal space. Recovery of renal function generally occurs in 3 to 10 days following acute tubular necrosis. The onset may be heralded by a polyuric phase, during which close attention to fluid and electrolyte replacement is required. The reader is referred to chapter 16 for a full discussion of the treatment of renal failure and renal replacement therapies.

Postoperative Analgesia/Sedation

There are several options for the provision of postoperative analgesia following thoracic surgery; these include systemic opioids (administered intermittently on an "as needed" (or prn) basis, by continuous infusion or by a patient-controlled analgesia device), intercostal nerve blocks, epidural local anesthetics or opioids, and intrathecal opioids. Of these options, systemic opioids remain the most frequently used because of the ease of administration and the limited requirement for experienced personnel. For a full discussion of the use of sedative and analgesic agents, the reader is referred to chapter 11.

The administration of parenteral opioids necessitates three choices: the route of administration, the opioid to be used, and the method of administration (continuous versus intermittent). Intravenous administration remains the primary route in the immediate postoperative period because of the variability in absorption and uptake associated with the other routes.

For most patients a continuous infusion supplemented with intermittent intravenous bolus doses provides the best level of analgesia. Although studies with children are limited, adult studies suggest that a continuous opioid infusion provides superior analgesia and fewer adverse effects than either as needed or fixed-interval dosing. Lynn and associates[40] evaluated the respiratory effects of continuous morphine infusion in children following cardiac surgery. They found that morphine infusions of 10 to 30 µg/kg/h provided adequate analgesia and did not impair weaning from mechanical ventilation.

For most patients, the choice of opioid is inconsequential provided that equipotent doses are used. However, in the patient with hemodynamic compromise or at risk for pulmonary vasospasm, the synthetic opioids (fentanyl, sufentanil) provide effective analgesia without compromising cardiovascular function. These agents also effectively block pulmonary vasospasm and may decrease morbidity and mortality in this high-risk population.[41,42]

Summary

Despite advances in techniques of surgery and CPB, significant physiologic compromise occurs following repair of congenital heart disease in children. Appropriate care of these patients begins with a smooth transition and transport from the operating room to the PICU setting with open communication and cooperation between the many services caring for them. The initial evaluation begins with the basic ABCs and then follows a logical organ-system-based evaluation. The multiorgan involvement that can be seen with such patients necessitates familiarity with the care and correction of problems in several different organ systems. This approach requires a thorough understanding of the concepts outlined not only in this chapter, but in the remainder of this volume.

Glossary of Surgical Procedures

arterial switch procedure: Also known as a Jateen procedure for transposition of the great arteries, it involves transection of the aorta and pulmonary artery with re-anastomosis of these vessels to the appropriate ventricles. The coronary arteries are also removed from the aorta arising from the right ventricle and reanastomosed to the aorta or posterior great vessel that has been attached to the left ventricle.

Fontan procedure: Procedure performed in patients with univentricular anatomy such as tricuspid atresia. It involves the separation of the two circulations by anastomosing the right atrium directly to the pulmonary artery and using the single ventricle to pump blood to the systemic circulation. The driving pressure for blood to the lungs is central venous pressure with some assist from right atrial contraction.

Glenn shunt: Shunt also used for palliation of patients with univentricular anatomy. It involves anastomosis of the superior vena cava to the pulmonary artery. It is currently used as a "bidirectional shunt" which provides blood flow to both pulmonary vascular beds. This procedures is usually followed in 1 to 2 years by a formal Fontan procedure.

Norwood Procedure: Procedure used for patients with univentricular anatomy, most commonly hypoplastic left heart syndrome. The procedure includes stage I, which is performed during the neonatal period, during which the right ventricle is connected to a neo-aorta that is constructed out of the main segment of the pulmonary artery and synthetic material. The right ventricle is used as the systemic pumping ventricle as the neo-aorta is connected to the aortic arch. Pulmonary blood flow is provided by a central neo-aorta to right/left pulmonary artery shunt. An atrial septectomy is also performed to allow for mixing of blood at the atrial level. The first stage is followed 1 to 2 years later by stage II, which is a classic Fontan procedure. The latter may be staged into a Glenn procedure (stage II) and completion of the Fontan procedure (stage III).

Potts Shunt: Anastomosis of the descending aorta to the left or main pulmonary artery. The procedure was formally used to provide pulmonary blood flow in patients with cyanotic lesions who were too small for the Blalock-Taussig shunt. Problems included excessive pulmonary blood flow and the risk of early development of pulmonary vascular changes.

Ross procedure: As a result of problems related to the life expectancy of prosthetic valves, the Ross procedure involves using the patient's own pulmonary valve in the systemic-to-pulmonary-artery place of the aortic valve and then placing a homograft in the pulmonary circulation. Due to the lower pressures, the homograft valve lasts longer in the pulmonary circuit.

systemic-pulmonary-artery or Blalock-Taussig shunt: Also known as a BT shunt, the procedure involves an end-to-side anastomosis of the subclavian artery to the pulmonary artery. The procedure is used palliatively to provide pulmonary blood flow to patients with cyanotic lesions with diminished pulmonary blood flow.

modified Blalock-Taussig Shunt: Modification of the above described technique. The modified version uses a gortex graft to provide a side-to-side connection of the subclavian artery and the pulmonary artery. As the diameter of the graft is known, problems with excessive or diminished pulmonary blood flow which can be seen with the original BT shunt procedure are limited.

Waterston Shunt: Anastomosis of the ascending aorta to the right or main pulmonary artery. The procedure was formally used to provide pulmonary blood flow in patients with cyanotic lesions who were too small for the Blalock-Taussig shunt. Problems included excessive pulmonary blood flow and the risk of early development of pulmonary vascular changes.

References

1. Tobias JD, Lynch A, Garrett J. Alterations of carbon dioxide during the intrahospital transport of children. *Pediatr Emerg Care* 1996;12:249–251.
2. Messmer K. Hemodilution. *Surg Clin North Am* 1975;55:658–678.
3. Robertson JM, Vinten-Johansen J, Buckberg GD, et al. Safety of prolonged aortic clamping with blood cardioplegia. I: Glutamate enrichment of normal hearts. *J Thorac Cardiovasc Surg* 1984;88:395–401.
4. Vinten-Johansen J, Hammon JW. Myocardial protection during cardiac surgery. In Gravlee GP, Davis RF, Utley JR (eds): *Cardiopulmonary Bypass: Principles and Practice*. Baltimore: Williams and Wilkins; 1998:171–172.
5. Sessler DI, Rubinstein EH, Maoyeri A. Physiologic responses to mild perianesthetic hypothermia in humans. *Anesthesiology* 1991;75:594–610.
6. Berg RA, Lloyd TR, Donnerstein RL. Accuracy of central venous pressure monitoring in the intra-abdominal inferior vena cava: A canine study. *J Pediatr* 1992;120:67–71.
7. Reda Z, Houri S, Davis AL, et al. Effect of airway pressure on inferior vena cava pressure as a measure of central venous pressure in children. *J Pediatr* 1995;126:961–965.
8. Morales AR, Fine G, Taber RE. Cardiac surgery and myocardial necrosis. *Arch Pathol* 1967;83:71–79.
9. Najafi H, Henson D, Dye WS, et al. Left ventricular hemorrhagic necrosis. *Ann Thorac Surg* 1969;7:550–561.
10. Coles JG, Watanabe T, Wilson GJ, et al. Age-related differences in the response to myocardial ischemic stress. *J Thorac Cardiovasc Surg* 1987;94:526–534.
11. Wittnich C, Peniston C, Ianuzzo, D et al. Relative vulnerability of neonatal and adult hearts to ischemic injury. *Circulation* 1987;76:156–160.
12. Mueller HS, Evans R, Ayres SM. Effect of dopamine on hemodynamics and myocardial metabolism in shock following acute myocardial infarction in man. *Circulation* 1978;57:361–365.
13. Yurvati AH, Sanders SP, Dullye LJ, et al. Anti-arrhythmic response to intravenously administered magnesium after cardiac surgery. *South Med J* 1992;85:714–717.
14. Kapur PA. Con: Epinephrine and norepinephrine are the inotropes of choice: An opposing viewpoint. *J Cardiothorac Anesth* 1987;3:259–262.
15. Tinker J. Pro: Strong inotropes (i.e. epinephrine) should be drugs of first choice during emergence from cardiopulmonary bypass. *J Cardiothorac Anesth* 1987;3:256–258.
16. Royster RL, Butterworth JF 4th, Prielipp RC, et al. Combined inotropic effects of amrinone and epinephrine after cardiopulmonary bypass in humans. *Anesth Analg* 1993;77:662–672.
17. Steen PA, Tinker JH, Pluth JR, et al. Efficacy of dopamine, dobutamine, and epinephrine during emergence from cardiopulmonary bypass in man. *Circulation* 1978;57:378–384.

18. Berner M, Jaccard C, Oberhansli I, et al. Hemodynamic effects of amrinone in children after cardiac surgery. *Intensive Care Med* 1990;16:85–88.
19. Lawless S, Burckart G, Diven W, et al. Amrinone in neonates and infants after cardiac surgery. *Crit Care Med* 1989;17:751–754.
20. Rogers AJ, Trento A, Siewers RD, et al. Extracorporeal membrane oxygenation for post-cardiotomy cardiogenic shock in children. *Ann Thorac Surg* 1989;47:903–906.
21. Louis PT, Bricker JT, Frazier OH, et al. Nonpulsatile left ventricular support in pediatric patients. *Crit Care Med* 1992;20:704–707.
22. Veasy LG, Webster HF, McGough EC. Intra-aortic balloon pumping: Adaptation for pediatric use. *Crit Care Clin* 1986;2:237–249.
23. Christensen DW, Veasy G, McGough J, et al. Intra-aortic balloon counterpulsation in children: A review of 29 patients. *Crit Care Med* 1991;19:S75.
24. Prakash O, Jonson B, Meij S, et al. Criteria for early extubation after intracardiac surgery in adults. *Anesth Analg* 1977;59:703–708.
25. Quasha AL, Leober N, Feeley TW, et al. Postoperative respiratory care: A controlled trial of early and late extubation following coronary-artery bypass grafting. *Anesthesiology* 1980;52:135–141.
26. Heard GG, Lamberti JJ Jr., Park SM, et al. Early extubation following surgical repair of congenital heart disease. *Crit Care Med* 1985;13:830–832.
27. Connell RS, Page US, Bartley TD, et al. The effect on pulmonary ultrastructure of dacron-wool filtration during cardiopulmonary bypass. *Ann Thorac Surg* 1973;15:217–229.
28. DiCarlo JV, Raphaely RC, Steven JM, et al. Pulmonary mechanics in infants after cardiac surgery. *Crit Care Med* 1992;20:22–27.
29. Sherry KM. Postextubation stridor in Down's syndrome. *Br J Anaesth* 1983;55:53–55.
30. Moncada S, Higgs A. The L-arginine nitric oxide pathway. *N Engl J Med* 1993;329:2002–2012.
31. Crittenden MD, Roberts CS, Rosa L, et al. Brain protection during circulatory arrest. *Ann Thorac Surg* 1991;51:942–947.
32. Brunberg JA, Reilley EL, Doty DB. Central nervous system consequences in infants of cardiac surgery using deep hypothermia and circulatory arrest. *Circulation* 1974;50 (suppl 2):1160–1168.
33. Ehyai A, Fenichel GM, Bender HW Jr. Incidence and prognosis of seizures in infants after cardiac surgery with profound hypothermia and circulatory arrest. *JAMA* 1984;252:3165–3167.
34. Fernandez-del Castillo C, Harringer W, Warshaw AL, et al. Risk factors for pancreatic cellular injury after cardiopulmonary bypass. *N Engl J Med* 1991;325:382–387.
35. Jenkins JG, Lynn AM, Wood AE, et al. Acute hepatic failure following cardiac operation in children. *J Thorac Cardiovasc Surg* 1982;84:865–871.
36. Segar JL, Robillard JE, Johnson KJ, et al. Addition of metolazone to overcome tolerance to furosemide in infants with bronchopulmonary dysplasia. *J Pediatr* 1992;120:966–973.
37. Singh NC, Kissoon N, al Mofada S, at al. Comparison of continuous versus intermittent furosemide administration in postoperative pediatric cardiac patients. *Crit Care Med* 1992;20:17–21.
38. Pollock EM, Ford-Jones EL, Rebeyka I, et al. Early nosocomial infections in pediatric cardiovascular surgery patients. *Crit Care Med* 1990;18:378–384.
39. Hauser GJ, Chan MM, Casey WF, et al. Immune dysfunction in children after corrective surgery for congenital heart disease. *Crit Care Med* 1991;19:874–881.
40. Lynn AM, Opheim KE, Tyler DC. Morphine infusion after pediatric cardiac surgery. *Crit Care Med* 1984;12:863–866.
41. Hickey PR, Hansen DD, Wessel DL, et al. Pulmonary and systemic hemodynamic responses to fentanyl in infants. *Anesth Analg* 1985;64:483–486.
42. Hickey PR, Hansen DD, Wessel DL, et al. Blunting of stress responses in the pulmonary circulation of infants by fentanyl. *Anesth Analg* 1985;64:1137–1142.

Chapter 9

Status Epilepticus

Joseph E. Segeleon, MD and Steven E. Haun, MD

Introduction

Status epilepticus (SE) is a common pediatric emergency. In a recent prospective population-based study in Richmond, Virginia, the incidence of SE was found to be 41 patients per year per 100,000 population.[1] The same study went on to project 126,000 to 195,000 SE events with 22,200 to 42,000 deaths annually in the United States. It is imperative that health care workers who care for children be able to recognize and treat SE. An established therapeutic plan for seizure termination, as well as meticulous supportive care, will greatly benefit the patient and will limit the detrimental effects of prolonged seizure activity. This chapter reviews the definition, classification, epidemiology, morbidity, mortality, and treatment of SE in children.

SE is a clinical diagnosis. It is defined as continuous seizure activity for at least 30 minutes or recurrent seizures without a return to baseline level of consciousness between seizures. Although the definition of SE is time-based, the exact duration of seizure activity is often impossible to ascertain, and therefore efforts to terminate seizure activity should not be withheld until the "time definition" is fulfilled. It is generally recommended that antiepileptic drugs be administered whenever seizure activity extends beyond 10 minutes.[2]

Any seizure may evolve into SE. Generalized convulsive SE is the most common type in the pediatric population and is the primary focus of this chapter. The classification of epilepsy, epileptic syndromes, and SE is complex. An accepted system, based on the work of Gastaut,[3] is presented in Table 1. For a more in-depth discussion of the classification and distinction between individual types of epilepsy and epileptic syndromes, the reader is referred to Reference 4.

SE is likely to be encountered by all pediatric health care providers. According to Hauser,[5] 70% of children with epilepsy diagnosed prior to 1 year of age will have an episode of SE either on presentation or soon after diagnosis. Additionally, 20% of individuals with epilepsy will experience SE within 5 years of the initial diagnosis. In a recent study to determine risk factors for SE in children with symptomatic epilepsy, it was found that those children with focal background electroencephalogram (EEG) abnormalities, partial seizures with secondary generalization, generalized abnormalities on neuroimaging, and patients whose first seizure was SE, were at higher risk of SE when compared to the control group.[6] In individuals with and without underlying epilepsy, fever remains a common cause of SE. Of the estimated 2% to 5% of the US population who will have a febrile seizure, 5% will have an episode of SE.[5]

The etiology of SE is diverse and differs

From: Tobias JD (ed): *Pediatric Critical Care: The Essentials.* ©Futura Publishing Co., Inc., Armonk, NY, 1999.

between children and adults. There is a long list of potential etiologies including fever, acute central nervous system (CNS) infections, trauma, toxin exposure, hypoxic-ischemic encephalopathy, and metabolic abnormalities (Table 2). The etiologies of SE can be organized into four broad categories: 1) atypical febrile seizures; 2) acute CNS disorders such as trauma, meningitis, encephalitis, or tumors; 3) idiopathic or remote symptomatic epilepsy; and 4) chronic or progressive neurologic disorders that may be either congenital or acquired.[7]

A recent population-based study that included children and adults noted that 50% of pediatric cases of SE were caused by systemic infections, with congenital malformations, anoxia, metabolic disorders, subtherapeutic antiepileptic drug levels, CNS infections, and trauma contributing as additional major causes of SE.[8] The same study found cerebrovascular accidents, subtherapeutic antiepileptic drug levels, alcohol withdrawal, anoxia, and idiopathic and metabolic diseases as major causes in adults.

In two large series of pediatric patients,[9,10] idiopathic epilepsy and febrile SE each accounted for approximately one quarter of the cases. An acute and potentially treatable cause was identified in 23% to 41% of the study patients. Consequently, it is imperative that an underlying precipitant be sought in the infant or child with SE (see below). In a review of 193 children, 75% of episodes of SE in children younger than 1 year were associated with an acute cause. The majority of these cases were caused by either meningitis or metabolic abnormalities and, hence, were treatable.[10]

Infants with SE often have an acute CNS process, underlying metabolic abnormality, or a congenital malformation. Older infants and toddlers commonly present with episodes related to fever, trauma, and toxin ingestion. Nonaccidental trauma, or child abuse, must be considered, particularly in the infant with seizures, retinal hemorrhages, and without evidence of external trauma. During adolescence, SE may be associated with drug ingestion, trauma, or noncompliance with antiepileptic drugs. Malignancy, infections, subtherapeutic drug levels, and idiopathic may occur at any age.

Seizures in the neonatal period are unique in that the diagnosis, evaluation, treatment, and prognosis remain controversial. A comprehensive discussion on neonatal SE is beyond the scope of this chapter. A few issues are discussed, as neonates with

Table 1

Classification of Status Epilepticus

Generalized
  Convulsive
    tonic-clonic
    tonic
    clonic
    myoclonic
  Nonconvulsive
    absence
Partial
  Elementary
    somatomotor
    dysphasic
    other
  Complex
Unilateral
Erratic
Neonatal

From Reference 3.

Table 2

Etiology of Status Epilepticus

Idiopathic
Febrile seizures
Trauma
Malignancy
Toxin exposure
Infection
  meningitis
  encephalitis
  brain abscess
Hypoxic-ischemic
  encephalopathy
Cerebrovascular
  disease
    stroke
    subarachnoid
      hemorrhage
    vasculitis
Hypertension
Neurocutaneous
  syndromes
Nutritional deficiencies
Degenerative brain
  disorders
Metabolic disturbances
  hypoglycemia
  hyperglycemia
  hyponatremia
  hypernatremia
  hypomagnesemia
  hypocalcemia
  uremia
Thyroid disorders
Cerebral malformations
Noncompliance with
  antiepileptic drugs
Drug withdrawal

seizures are cared for in the pediatric intensive care unit. The classification of neonatal seizures is complex and the reader is referred to Mizrahi's paper[11] for further discussion. Possible etiologies include hypoxic-ischemic encephalopathy, intracranial hemorrhage, trauma, metabolic and electrolyte abnormalities, infection, drug withdrawal, and developmental malformation. Clearly, one of the controversial issues is the underestimation and overestimation of seizures based on clinical observation. Seizure activity often goes unrecognized in infants who are pharmacologically paralyzed and in those with evidence of electroencephalographic seizures without clinical correlation. Conversely, there are a variety of perceived abnormal motor movements that are incorrectly thought to be seizure activity, and thus the infant is exposed to unnecessary diagnostic tests and treatments.[12] In a retrospective analysis of neonates with EEG-confirmed seizures in a large obstetric hospital, only 45% of preterm infants and 53% of full-term infants with electroencephalographic seizures had identifiable clinical correlation.[13] Consequently, the recognition of neonatal seizures can be challenging, and the literature supports the use of early diagnostic intervention with EEG while treatment, prognostication, and follow-up should be done in conjunction with a pediatric neurologist.

Morbidity and Mortality of Status Epilepticus

The morbidity and mortality associated with SE have decreased over the past two decades.[5] The likely explanation for this improvement is early and aggressive intervention together with specialized supportive care. Morbidity and mortality are affected by several factors; the two most important are the underlying disorder and the duration of seizure activity. Logically, morbidity is more likely in individuals with severe CNS pathology (trauma and meningitis) than in patients with idiopathic or atypical febrile seizures. Maytal et al[9] noted morbidity to be more likely in those younger than 1 year and in patients with an acute CNS process or progressive encephalopathy. Furthermore, they noted that only 2 of 137 children with idiopathic, remote symptomatic, or atypical febrile status suffered neurologic sequelae. In the same study, 29% of infants younger than age 1, 11% of children aged 1 to 3 years, and 6% of children older than 3 years had residual neurologic deficits. All of the mortality and 88% of neurologic sequelae were noted in patients with acute or progressive CNS insults.

Seizures of prolonged duration may be associated with increased morbidity. In a retrospective review of 57 children with febrile SE, 24% were observed to have mild to severe neurologic deficits.[14] Data analysis revealed two risk factors for neurologic sequelae including a longer seizure duration and the need for two different drugs for seizure termination. Similarly, in a prospective study of 114 convulsive SE episodes in 97 children, it was found that the duration of status was twice as long in those who died or were left with a new deficit.[15] In addition to the underlying etiology and the duration of status, other factors may contribute to morbidity. Systemic stresses such as hypoxia, hyperpyrexia, cardiopulmonary dysfunction, and a host of other deleterious side effects may significantly contribute to the morbidity of SE.

Mortality resulting from SE is lower in children than in adults. A recent population-based study revealed mortality rates for pediatric, adult, and elderly populations to be 2.5%, 14%, and 38%, respectively.[16] The same study noted the highest mortality in the pediatric population to be associated with tumors. As previously noted, mortality is often related to the underlying etiology, and therefore is more frequent in the very young, who are more likely to have acute or progressive CNS disorders than older children. Additionally, when evaluating children and adults, DeLorenzo et al[8] found individuals with prolonged seizures (seizure duration >1 hour) had a mortality rate of 34.8% within 1 month of the SE episode, whereas those with nonprolonged seizures had a rate of 3.7%.

Despite these recent findings, the mortality and perhaps the morbidity of SE continues to decline. Progress in pharmacotherapeutics, diagnostic techniques, supportive care, and use of monitoring technology, as well as advances in the treatment of underlying disease, have contributed to the decrement of mortality rates over the years.

Pathophysiology of Status Epilepticus

The pathophysiology of SE has been well studied in a variety of animal models. The pathophysiologic characteristics of SE can be divided into three parts. First, there are unique events at the cellular level that enable seizure activity to begin, self-propagate, and lead to cell injury and death when seizure activity is not terminated. Second, the dynamics of the entire brain are important, as there are adaptive mechanisms which attempt to limit injury and, with continued status, may contribute to its pathology. Finally, SE has profound systemic effects that may affect morbidity and mortality. Termination of seizure activity and meticulous supportive care may circumvent much of the potential deleterious pathophysiology and limit morbidity and mortality.

Excessive excitation at the cellular level is likely to be the fundamental pathophysiologic event that serves to initiate, propagate, and deter inhibition of seizure activity. Glutamate, a prominent excitatory amino acid, along with other neurotransmitters, is important to the pathophysiology of SE because it has the ability to excite neurons and, in certain circumstances, destroy them. The inhibitory neurotransmitter γ-aminobutyric acid (GABA) is also important, as impairment of GABA transmission may augment seizure activity. Indeed, animal studies have shown a reduced rate of GABA synthesis in the substantia nigra in rats with pilocarpine-induced SE.[17]

Glutamate receptors are classified according to their ability to bind to certain substances. Glutamate binding to the N-methyl-D-aspartate (NMDA) channel results in an influx of calcium. Additionally, non-NMDA-gated channels, such as those activated by kainic acid and α-amino-3-hydroxy-5-methyl-4-isoxazole-propionic acid (AMPA), when stimulated, also allow the influx of calcium, leading to further depolarization of the cell. A third class of glutamate receptors are known as metabotropic receptors. These receptors, when activated, perpetuate their actions via a second-messenger system culminating in an increase in intracellular calcium.

Glutamate agonism has been shown in animal models to produce experimental SE.[18] Similarly, seizure activity may be inhibited by glutamate antagonists.[19,20] Excitatory amino-acid-induced increases in intracellular calcium may lead to stimulation of a number of deleterious pathways including activation of protein kinase C, protein phosphatases, proteases, phospholipases (leading to arachidonic acid formation), and nitric oxide synthase, and may result in neuronal cell death.[21] The reader is referred to the recent review by Fountain and Lothman[22] for information on this subject. In summary, excitatory amino acid stimulation may perpetuate seizure activity and, in doing so, may allow dangerous and potentially toxic levels of intracellular calcium to accumulate, thus contributing to cell injury and necrosis.

Brain injury in SE may be secondary to direct neurotoxic cellular effects and/or the systemic consequences of ongoing seizure activity such as hypoxemia and cardiovascular compromise. As with many disorders in the critically ill, initial homeostatic adaptive mechanisms may eventually contribute to injury, morbidity, and cell death. Human and animal studies have identified specific areas in the brain that appear to be vulnerable.[23] The hippocampus, neocortex, and cerebellum are often included, although Meldrum and Brierley[24] have shown that cerebellar injury may be inhibited when hyperpyrexia and shock are controlled in a bicuculline-induced baboon model of SE. Convulsive and nonconvulsive generalized SE may result in permanent neuronal injury; thus it is imperative to terminate both clinical and electroencephalographic seizure activity.

Figure 1 illustrates various electroencephalographic, cerebral, and systemic pathophysiologic factors that contribute to the overall pathology of SE.[25] Electroencephalographically, early SE is characterized by isolated seizure activity that becomes more frequent and eventually merges into continuous EEG seizure activity. EEG find-

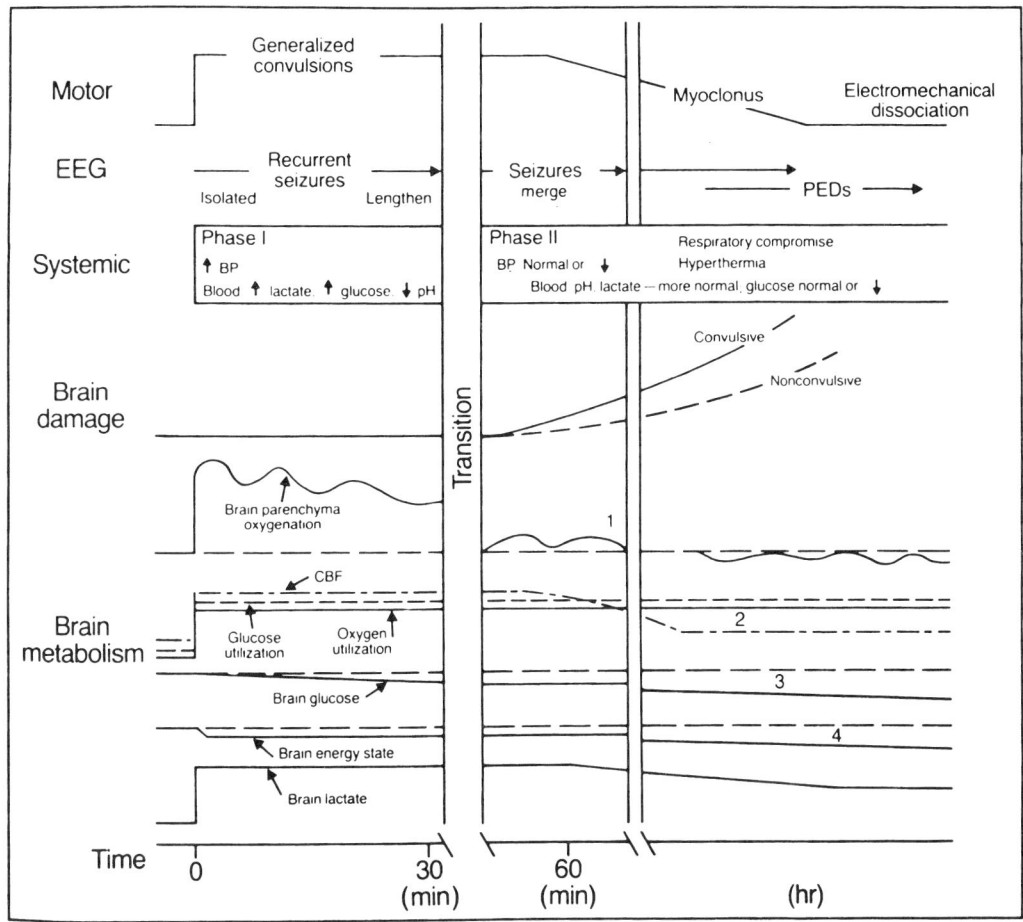

Figure 1. Summary of cerebral metabolism and systemic events associated with status epilepticus. Reproduced from Reference 25, with permission.

ings are paralleled clinically by discreet motor seizures progressing to nonstop generalized convulsive activity. During the first 30 minutes, adaptive mechanisms prevail, resulting in elevated catecholamines leading to a rise in systemic blood pressure and hyperglycemia. Additionally, prolonged muscle activity results in hyperpyrexia and increased lactate production. Excessive muscle activity and anaerobic metabolism, often coupled with inadequate ventilation, may lead to significant acidosis.

At the cerebral level one sees adaptive mechanisms attempting to keep up with the tremendous metabolic demands of SE. Early on, cerebral blood flow is elevated to accommodate increased use of glucose and oxygen. Systemic hypertension aids in the meeting of this demand even if cerebral vascular autoregulation is in jeopardy.[22] Ultimately, substrate utilization and energy states decline, resulting in lactic acid accumulation and acidosis.

Lothman's comprehensive work[25] identifies a "transition phase" occurring after 30 minutes of convulsive activity that may be seen as a failure of adaptive mechanisms. Often this heralds the onset of cerebral and systemic decompensation. Typically, blood pressure normalizes or decreases, serum glucose may be normal or low, and hyperthermia is observed. Respiratory compromise or failure frequently complicate this phase. In spite of a persistently high cerebral metabolic demand, cerebral blood flow may fall, resulting in a mismatch of substrate supply and demand which may contribute to overall pathology. Irreversible brain damage in convulsive and nonconvulsive SE may occur at this time. At the cellular level, amino acid excitotoxicity may lead to ongoing neuronal injury via the aforementioned cascades, which culminate in alterations of calcium homeostasis.

Finally, there are numerous systemic effects that result from SE that may lead to further neuronal injury and morbidity.[26] Elevated circulating catecholamines result in tachycardia, hyperglycemia, and hypertension. Cardiac arrhythmias, pulmonary edema, aspiration, hyperkalemia, peripheral leukocytosis, and cerebrospinal fluid pleocytosis have been observed in patients with SE.[23] Additionally, prolonged convulsive activity can result in rhabdomyolysis, myoglobinuria, and acute renal failure. Obviously, hypoxia and cerebral ischemia may contribute to brain injury. A multitude of cellular, cerebral, and systemic processes contribute to the pathophysiology of SE. The management is directed toward termination of all seizure activity while providing meticulous supportive care to limit the cerebral and systemic effects of SE (see below).

Management of Status Epilepticus

The management of SE necessitates a well organized therapeutic plan that attempts to terminate seizure activity and simultaneously provide constant assessment and supportive care. There are four primary goals of therapy:

1. Ensure adequate systemic and cerebral oxygen delivery.
2. Terminate seizure activity.
3. Prevent seizure recurrence.
4. Establish a diagnosis and initiate therapy for treatable underlying disorders.

Although emergency stabilization, pharmacotherapeutics, and diagnostic evaluation are discussed separately below, it is necessary that all three take place concurrently when providing care to children with SE.

Initial Stabilization

The child who presents to the emergency department or intensive care unit may already be in a state of decompensation. As previously discussed, the effects of prolonged seizure activity may be significant and the initial presentation may reflect the neuronal and systemic pathology discussed in the prior section. Additionally, many children exhibit the effects of sedating medications administered by parents or emergency personnel. Consequently, it is important that the health care team be ready to provide full support to the child on initial presentation. As with all critically ill children, initial efforts should be directed toward the ABCs (airway, breathing, and circulation). The actively convulsing child is visually captivating, and it is essential that attempts to obtain vascular access and to stop seizure activity not preclude assessment and support of the ABCs. Table 3 provides a guide for this phase of management.

While initial vital signs are obtained, electrocardiogram (ECG) and pulse oximetry monitoring should be established. Adequate oxygenation and ventilation should be the first priority when confronted with a patient in SE. The airway should be evaluated for patency, and airway reflexes should be assessed. Often airway patency may be

Table 3

Emergency Stabilization

Assessment	Intervention
Adequate airway	Positioning Triple airway maneuver Suction oropharynx 100% oxygen
Adequate breathing	Bag/mask ventilation 100% oxygen Establish i.v. access Endotracheal intubation Mechanical ventilation
Adequate circulation	Isotonic fluid boluses Antipyretics Vasoactive agents
Ongoing reassessment of ABCs	Physical exam ECG Pulse oximetry

achieved by suctioning material from the oropharynx and by performing a triple airway maneuver (jaw thrust, chin lift, head tilt). It is essential that the team be ready to assist ventilation and intubate the trachea in the event of respiratory compromise. Furthermore, many of the drugs used in the treatment of SE cause respiratory depression, hence ongoing seizure activity and the medications used to terminate SE may lead to respiratory failure in a patient who initially had satisfactory spontaneous efforts. Therefore, assessment of the respiratory system must be continuous in the patient with SE. Cervical spine protection should be used if indicated by history or physical examination; otherwise the patient may be positioned on his or her side to prevent aspiration of gastric contents.

Oxygen via high-flow nonrebreathing mask to provide as close to an FiO_2 of 1.0 as possible should be administered to all patients, and oxygenation should be monitored by continuous pulse oximetry. Hypoxemia is a preventable cause of CNS morbidity. Physical examination findings suggestive of inadequate oxygenation and/or ventilation include nasal flaring, poor chest rise, apnea, intercostal retractions, abdominal muscle recruitment, diminished breath sounds, and cyanosis. Objective data may be obtained by pulse oximetry and arterial blood gas analysis. The patient breathing 100% oxygen via a nonrebreather face mask, who has oxygen saturation of 90% or less, ineffective respiratory effort, or frank cyanosis, requires endotracheal intubation. Airway intervention should not be delayed, as hypoxemia and poor ventilation may have grave consequences.

Once the decision has been made to intubate the trachea, a quick review of assembled personnel and equipment should be taken. See also chapter 1 for a full review of airway management. Intravenous access should be established as soon as possible. Central venous or intraosseous access may be used if attempts at peripheral access are not successful. Available equipment should include a large suction catheter, suction, oxygen, laryngoscope and blades, appropriately sized masks, endotracheal tubes, and a self-inflating resuscitation bag or standard Ambu bag. A Broselow Tape® (Armstrong Medical Industries Inc., Lincolnshire, IL) may be useful for guiding the health care team with regard to the appropriate tube sizes, drug dosages, and weight estimation. Clearly, the effectiveness of equipment is predicated on the individuals directing its use, and it is vital that the health care team comprise personnel skilled in pediatric airway management.

Often, the patient has already received sedatives that were administered for their antiepileptic properties, and further sedatives may or may not be necessary. If additional sedatives are necessary, one may administer a benzodiazepine (lorazepam 0.1 mg/kg or midazolam 0.1 mg/kg intravenously) or the short-acting barbiturate sodium thiopental (3 to 5 mg/kg). All sedatives, particularly barbiturates, may reduce the blood pressure, and therefore drug choice and dosage must be tailored to the patient's hemodynamic status. With the administration of sedatives and the transition to positive pressure ventilation, many patients will require blood pressure augmentation in the form of volume and possibly vasoactive medications. Assisted ventilation is often required as one readies to intubate the trachea. Use of bag/mask ventilation with cricoid pressure (Sellick maneuver) can effectively ventilate most patients and prevent regurgitation and aspiration of gastric contents. A short-acting neuromuscular blocking agent is usually required to facilitate tracheal intubation. Available drugs include rocuronium (0.6 to 1.2 mg/kg intravenously), vecuronium (0.1 to 0.2 mg/kg), and succinylcholine (1.0 to 2.0 mg/kg). The clinician using neuromuscular blocking agents must be familiar with the side effects and contraindications of each drug, and must be skilled at pediatric airway management. Finally, one must be cognizant that neuromuscular blocking agents will mask ongoing seizure activity and prevent clinical assessment. The reader is referred to chapter 11 for a full discussion of the use of neuromuscular blocking agents.

Finally, emergency stabilization must include assessment of the patient's circulatory status. Tachycardia, cool extremities, diminished pulses, decreased urine output, and prolonged capillary refill are signs of inadequate perfusion to vital organs. Patients may be hypovolemic secondary to the underlying illness and may have increased losses due to hyperpyrexia, vomiting, diarrhea, or other sources. Isotonic fluid boluses (normal saline 10 to 20 mL/kg) may augment perfusion and replenish volume status. After each bolus, the patient should be assessed for a decrease in heart rate, an improvement in peripheral circulation, and an increase in urine output. These patients are often hyperpyrexic, and aggressive treatment of fever may reduce tachycardia, improve the physical examination, and may potentially inhibit neuronal injury and lessen the chances of recurrence of SE.

In summary, the management of SE is challenging because emergency stabilization, seizure termination, and diagnostic evaluation must take place concurrently. The importance of initial and ongoing assessment cannot be overemphasized. As seizures persist and sedating drugs are administered, the clinician should recognize that cardiorespiratory embarrassment is a common occurrence. A well organized aggressive therapeutic strategy will aid in seizure termination and prevent secondary injury due to cardiorespiratory compromise.

Pharmacotherapeutics

A number of drugs exist for the treatment of SE, although no single drug is sufficient. The goals of therapy are to terminate seizure activity and to prevent recurrence. Common errors in the management of SE include delay in drug administration, inappropriate dosing (usually low) of antiepileptic drugs, and failure to recognize and treat systemic complications. Table 4 lists commonly used drug preparations.

Benzodiazepines remain the first-line drugs in the treatment of SE. Benzodiazepines exert their anticonvulsant effect by binding to the GABA receptor. Lorazepam, midazolam, and diazepam are commonly used in the treatment of SE. Although diazepam has been used for years, lorazepam and midazolam are now more frequently used as first-line drugs. Lorazepam is less lipophilic than diazepam and therefore has a slower onset and longer duration. Duration for diazepam is often less than 1 hour, whereas lorazepam's anticonvulsant effect may last longer than 3 hours. Both drugs have a rapid onset and have been proven efficacious in the treatment of SE.[27–29] Both drugs may be given via the intravenous or intraosseous route, and diazepam may also be given rectally. The dose of lorazepam is 0.1 mg/kg/dose and may be repeated every 10 minutes. The intravenous and intraosseous dose of diazepam is 0.1 to 0.3 mg/kg/dose and may be given every 10 minutes. The rectal dose of diazepam is 0.2 to 0.5 mg/kg (the intravenous preparation is used for rectal administration) delivered via a lubricated tuberculin syringe placed 4 to 5 centimeters into the rectum,[30] a Foley catheter with the end bulb inflated,[31] or a lubricated 14F suction catheter. All of the benzodiazepines may produce respiratory depression, although there have been reports that suggest that the need for endotracheal intubation is greater with diazepam.[32]

Midazolam is a short-acting benzodiazepine with a rapid onset that has been gaining widespread use in the treatment of SE. It may be given via the intravenous, intramuscular, intraosseous, or rectal route. It has been used in intermittent dosages as well as by continuous infusion in the treatment of refractory SE.[33,34] An advantage of midazolam is its short duration, which allows for a quicker return to baseline neurologic status. Like other benzodiazepines, midazolam may contribute to respiratory depression and sedation and may lower systemic blood pressure.

Phenytoin is our preferred long-acting anticonvulsant. It exerts its effect by stabilizing the neuronal membrane. It is less lipid-soluble than the benzodiazepines and it achieves therapeutic CNS levels in approximately 20 minutes.[35] A loading dose of 20 mg/kg may be infused via a secure peripheral or central venous catheter at a rate no faster than 1 mg/kg/min (adults: 50 mg/min). ECG and blood pressure must be monitored, as arrhythmias and hypotension are the most common adverse side effects. Dextrose-containing solutions should be avoided because they may cause precipitation. The high alkalinity of phenytoin merits caution in its use via a peripheral i.v., and warrants constant assessment during the infusion, as infiltration and/or extravasation may cause tissue necrosis.

Table 4

Anticonvulsants

Drug	Dosage	Onset	Duration
Lorazepam	i.v./IO: 0.1 mg/kg/dose every 10 minutes. maximum: 4 mg/dose	2–3 min	≥3 hours
Midazolam	i.v./IO/IM: 0.05–0.2 mg/kg/dose every 10 minutes maximum: 5 mg/dose infusion 1 μg/kg/min (increase as necessary) PR: 0.5–1.0 mg/kg/dose	2–5 min	30–60 min
Diazepam	i.v./IO: 0.1–0.3 mg/kg/dose every 10 minutes maximum: 10 mg/dose PR: 0.3–0.5 mg/kg/dose	3–5 min	60–90 min
Phenytoin	i.v.: loading dose 20 mg/kg 1 mg/kg/min up to 50 mg/min monitor ECG, blood pressure, i.v. site	15–30 min	≥10 hours
Fosphenytoin	i.v./IM: loading dose 20 mg/kg 3 mg/kg/min up to 150 mg/min monitor ECG, blood pressure	10–30 min (IM ≥ 30 min)	≥10 hours
Phenobarbital	i.v./IM: loading dose 20 mg/kg 1 mg/kg/min up to 100 mg/min monitor blood pressure and respiratory status	20–30 min	≥50 hours
Pentobarbital	i.v.: loading dose 5 mg/kg 1 mg/kg/min up to 50 mg/min infusion: 1 mg/kg/h monitor ECG, EEG, blood pressure	1 min	≥50 hours

i.v. = intravenous; IM = intramuscular; IO = intraosseous; PR = per rectum.

Fosphenytoin, a relatively new anticonvulsant, is a water-soluble disodium phosphate ester of phenytoin that is converted in plasma to phenytoin.[36,37] It is compatible with most intravenous solutions, can be administered intramuscularly, and is devoid of propylene glycol, a significant contributor to the cardiovascular effects of phenytoin. Its development is a major advance in the treatment of epilepsy and SE. Studies in children aged 5 to 18 years have found fosphenytoin to be effective and safe when administered intravenously at a rate of up to 3 mg/kg/min to a maximum of 150 mg/min.[38] Moreover, it offers great advantage over phenytoin in that it can be given intramuscularly and can be administered safely intravenously without concerns of local irritation and tissue necrosis.[38,39] Developed to replace intravenous phenytoin, its only current deterrent to widespread usage is its much higher cost when compared to phenytoin. Fosphenytoin is administered in a dose similar to phenytoin (20 mg/kg), but should be prescribed in PEs (phenytoin equivalents), since 750 mg of fosphenytoin is equivalent to 500 mg of phenytoin. Discussion with the pharmacy service and an agreement on how to write the desired amount will help in preventing problems. Phenytoin and fosphenytoin, unlike the benzodiazepines and phenobarbital, do not cause sedation or respiratory depression.

Phenobarbital has a long track record as an effective antiepileptic drug. It may be given via the intravenous route, the intramuscular route, or intraosseous route. The intravenous loading dose is 20 to 25 mg/kg and should be infused no faster than 1 mg/kg/min (maximum of 100 mg/min) unless the patient's ventilation is already controlled. Cumulative dosages as high as 120 mg/kg have been used in cases of refractory SE.[40] Potential side effects of phenobarbital include respiratory depression, prolonged sedation, hypotension, and bradycardia. The combined therapy of benzodiazepines and phenobarbital commonly leads to respiratory compromise. In the patient in whom the

SE has been controlled with benzodiazepine, but in whom it is decided to administer a loading dose of phenobarbital, an alternative that will limit the incidence of respiratory depression is to divide the loading dose into two 10 mg/kg doses and administer each over 1 hour separated by 1 hour. The latter is only recommended once SE has been controlled.

In summary, as detailed in the following section, the first-line drug for the patient in SE should be a benzodiazepine followed quickly by a longer-acting antiepileptic. We use lorazepam or midazolam as the benzodiazepine. Phenytoin is our preferred long-acting anticonvulsant because it does not cause sedation or respiratory depression. Furthermore, fosphenytoin reduces potential adverse effects of phenytoin and enhances safety characteristics when compared to phenobarbital. Phenobarbital may heavily sedate the patient and lead to prolonged mechanical ventilation, increased length of stay in the intensive care unit, and unnecessary diagnostic testing. Consequently, we reserve the use of phenobarbital for those who are allergic to phenytoin or who continue to have seizure activity in spite of appropriate benzodiazepine and phenytoin administration.

Treatment Strategy

There are a number of approaches that may be used in the treatment of SE.[2,41–46] The following strategy, outlined in Tables 3 and 5, is intended to provide a practical approach to the treatment of SE. We suggest that a strategy be developed ahead of time so that the clinician has an organized plan that can be implemented effectively and in a timely fashion.

First, the patient's cardiorespiratory system must be assessed, and supportive care provided as illustrated in Table 3. It is important to remember that the patient with SE may have been convulsing for a prolonged length of time (beyond the 30-minute transition phase), and he or she may possibly have received medications prior to hospital arrival that may sedate and impede effective oxygenation and ventilation. Early interventions may include jaw thrust, head positioning, oral/nasal airways, and the application of high-flow oxygen. Throughout the management, the clinician must constantly reassess the ABCs to assure adequate oxygen delivery and diminish secondary systemic complications.

Next, vascular access is obtained, ideally with two peripheral intravenous catheters. Intraosseous access may be used in children under 8 years. Alternatively, central venous access may be used if personnel skilled in pediatric vascular access are available and peripheral access cannot be obtained. Next, a bedside Chemstrip should be performed and 25% dextrose solution (2 to 4 mL/kg) should be administered if the patient is hypoglycemic. Routine administration of high dextrose solutions is not recommended and should only be used in patients with documented hypoglycemia. Laboratory tests that may be helpful are listed in Table 6, although tests should be tailored to the patient's history and physical examination. Anticonvulsant levels should be measured in patients on chronic antiepileptic therapy. Most patients will require a complete blood count, electrolytes, blood urea nitrogen, creatinine, calcium, magnesium, and phosphorous levels. Blood culture should be obtained for those with a possible infectious etiology. Similarly, if the history and physical examination suggest toxin exposure, a toxicology screen may prove useful. Although laboratory data may provide the diagnosis, it is essential that the clinician not delay treatment while waiting for test results.

The approach to drug therapy is outlined in Table 5. After venous access is obtained, lorazepam or midazolam is given at a dose of 0.1 mg/kg i.v.. Midazolam, given intramuscularly at 0.2 mg/kg has been found to be effective and is a suitable alternative if intravenous access is delayed or if it cannot be obtained.[47] The benzodiazepine may be repeated every 10 minutes. We recommend administration of a loading dose of phenytoin immediately after the initial benzodiazepine dose. The loading dose of phenytoin is 20 mg/kg and should be given through a secure i.v. at a rate no faster than 1 mg/kg/min. ECG, blood pressure, and i.v. site must be monitored during the infusion. Alternatively, intravenous fosphenytoin can be used (20 mg/kg at a rate of 3 mg/kg/min to a maxi-

Table 5

Strategy for the Treatment of Status Epilepticus

A. Assess ABCs. Apply oxygen, establish airway and ventilation.
   Continuous reassessment of ABCs.
B. Establish i.v. access. Labs for initial studies.
   Administer dextrose if hypoglycemic. Isotonic fluid boluses as necessary for perfusion and/or hypotension.
C. Pharmacotherapy for SE:
   1. Administer lorazepam 0.1 mg/kg i.v. or midazolam 0.1 mg/kg i.v.
      May repeat benzodiazepines every 10 min up to 4 doses.
      Alternatives: midazolam 0.2 mg/kg IM or diazepam 0.5 mg/kg PR.
   2. Administer phenytoin 20 mg/kg i.v. no faster than 1 mg/kg/min with a maximum rate of 50 mg/min immediately after initial dose of benzodiazepine.
      Monitor ECG, blood pressure, and i.v. site.
      Note: An additional 5 mg/kg of phenytoin may be give prior to initiation of phenobarbital therapy if seizures persist.
      Alternative: fosphenytoin 20 mg/kg i.v. no faster than 150 mg/min.
   3. If seizures persist after initial benzodiazepine and phenytoin, administer phenobarbital 20 mg/kg i.v. no faster than 1 mg/kg/min up to a maximum rate of 100 mg/min. Monitor blood pressure.
   4. If seizures persist, initiate refractory SE treatment.
      Midazolam bolus of 0.15 mg/kg and begin infusion of 1 µg/kg/min and increase until seizures are terminated. Monitor ECG, blood pressure, and EEG.
   5. If seizures persist, administer pentobarbital 5 mg/kg i.v. up to a maximum rate 50 mg/min. Begin infusion at 1 mg/kg/h. May give additional 5 mg/kg boluses to achieve either burst-suppression or suppression pattern on EEG. Monitor ECG, blood pressure, and EEG. Consider PA or CVP monitoring.
   6. Clinical seizure activity may cease but nonconvulsive SE may persist. EEG evaluation is strongly recommended in patients who do not return to baseline neurological status.
D. Continue diagnostic evaluation.
   Treat underlying causes and systemic complications.

CVP = central venous pressure; ECG = electrocardiogram; EEG = electroencephalogram; IM = intramuscular; i.v. = intravenous; PA = pulmonary artery; PR = per rectum; SE = status epilepticus

mum of 150 mg/min).[38] Although fosphenytoin may be given intramuscularly, intravenous administration is preferred because it achieves therapeutic levels significantly sooner. Additional dosages of benzodiazepines may be given while the phenytoin is infused; however, multiple benzodiazepine doses should not be substituted for phenytoin. The early administration of phenytoin may reduce the need for multiple doses of benzodiazepines and may prevent respiratory compromise and prolonged sedation.

Patients who continue to have seizures after receiving benzodiazepines and phenytoin should receive a loading dose of 20 mg/kg of phenobarbital. Recall that the combination of benzodiazepines and phenobarbital often leads to respiratory compromise and patients who are not already mechanically ventilated will likely require endotracheal intubation at this point. Some centers will give an additional 5 mg/kg of phenytoin prior to phenobarbital. Once the airway is secured and mechanical ventilation established, additional dosages of phenobarbital in 5 to 10 mg/kg increments may be administered. Prolonged obtundation and cardiovascular compromise commonly occur with large doses of phenobarbital. Obviously, treatment for metabolic and electrolyte abnormalities should be initiated as test results become available. Furthermore,

Table 6

Laboratory Evaluation and Imaging

Complete blood count	Cerebrospinal fluid
Electrolytes	glucose, protein, cell
Glucose	count
Magnesium	gram stain
Calcium	bacterial, viral, fungal
Phosphate	culture
Blood urea nitrogen	PCR for herpes
Creatinine	simplex virus
Urinalysis	Anticonvulsant
Blood culture	levels
Cervical spine films	Computed tomography
Toxicology screen	of head
Ammonia	Magnetic resonance
Metabolic screen	imaging of brain
(infants)	

PCR = polymerase chain reaction.

antimicrobial therapy should be given if an infectious etiology is suspected. Finally, if seizure activity continues in spite of benzodiazepine, phenytoin, and phenobarbital administration, treatment for refractory SE should be initiated as discussed below.

Refractory Status Epilepticus

Refractory SE is defined as ongoing seizure activity that fails to respond to initial doses of benzodiazepines and loading doses of phenytoin and phenobarbital. There is no general consensus on management, and a number of approaches are used. A recent survey of intensivists in the United Kingdom found that phenobarbital, general anesthetics, paraldehyde, benzodiazepines, and thiopental were among therapies used in responding pediatric intensive care units.[48] It is imperative that clinicians have a predetermined plan for refractory SE just as they do for the initial treatment. The patient with refractory SE should have continuous EEG monitoring. Treatment should be directed through a collaborative effort between the intensive care team and a pediatric neurologist. The goal of therapy is complete eradication of all clinical and electroencephalographic (nonconvulsive) seizures. We use midazolam (continuous infusion) as our first-line agent, and progress to pentobarbital if midazolam does not succeed in terminating seizure activity.

A number of studies have used midazolam for the treatment of children with refractory SE, and have encountered minimal adverse effects.[33,34,39,49] Midazolam is administered as a 0.15 mg/kg bolus and is followed with an infusion of 1 µg/kg/min. The dose is increased by 1 µg/kg/min every 15 minutes until seizures are controlled. The patient should have continuous EEG monitoring during this therapy. In one series of patients cared for in a pediatric intensive care unit setting,[33] seizures were controlled in a mean time of 0.78 hours with a mean infusion rate of 2.3 µg/kg/min (range 1 to 18). Astonishingly, no patients in the above study experienced cardiovascular or respiratory compromise during the midazolam infusion. We recommend maintaining the infusion for 12 hours after the last seizure before beginning to taper the drug. Obviously, prior anticonvulsants should be continued and maintained at therapeutic levels during the therapy of refractory SE.

If seizure termination is not accomplished with midazolam, one should proceed to pentobarbital-induced coma. Barbiturates are well established in the treatment of refractory SE and phenobarbital,[40] thiopental,[50] and pentobarbital[51] have been used in this clinical setting. It has been our practice to use pentobarbital in patients whose seizure activity has failed to respond to benzodiazepines, phenytoin, and phenobarbital. Most patients will have already have received endotracheal intubation and those who are not should undergo endotracheal intubation prior to the initiation of pentobarbital. The goal of therapy is to produce a burst suppression or complete suppression (flat) pattern on EEG. Hence, constant EEG monitoring is required. Titration to burst suppression may not be necessary, and pentobarbital may be titrated to seizure termination in units that have personnel skilled in EEG interpretation present 24 hours per day. Pentobarbital is administered as a 5 mg/kg bolus and followed with an infusion of 1 mg/kg/h. Further boluses of 5 mg/kg are administered every 10 to 15 minutes until a burst suppression or complete suppression pattern is noted. Myocardial depression and hypotension are common occurrences, and central venous pressure monitoring or pulmonary artery catheterization may be required to guide the administration of intravenous volume expanders and vasoactive medications. After 12 hours of burst suppression or a flat EEG, pentobarbital is tapered and the patient is closely monitored for recurrent clinical or electroencephalographic seizures. If seizures recur, pentobarbital is resumed at the previous infusion rate that achieved burst suppression pattern, and another 12 hours is allowed to transpire before attempts are made to discontinue the pentobarbital. Meticulous supportive care and avoidance of complications are key factors for successful outcomes.

Diagnostic Evaluation

A diagnostic evaluation must occur simultaneously with the stabilization and management of the patient in SE. A brief history should be obtained when possible, as it often gives clues to the underlying etiology. Table 6 lists frequent laboratory tests and imaging studies that may prove useful in the evaluation. Laboratory and radiologic studies should be tailored to the patient and based on history and physical examination findings. Anticonvulsant levels should be drawn on all patients with known epilepsy. Likewise, cervical spine evaluation and precautions should be utilized on any patient where trauma is a possibility.

Computed tomography (CT) of the head should be obtained on all patients presenting with history or physical findings consistent with head trauma, focal neurologic deficit, focal seizure, evidence of increased intracranial pressure, and first-time seizure. Many clinicians will obtain a head CT in any patient who presents with decreased sensorium and/or diminished ability to perform an adequate neurologic exam. Shaken baby syndrome, a clinical entity consisting of brain injury, retinal hemorrhages, and the absence of signs of external trauma, may present as SE and the clinician should image the brain of infants in whom this diagnosis is considered.

A lumbar puncture is indicated on all febrile patients, since the presence or absence of meningeal signs is often hard to interpret in light of decreased sensorium. Additionally, a lumbar puncture should be done in those presenting with meningeal signs, immunodeficiency, or first-time seizure. Contraindications include thrombocytopenia, marked coagulopathy, hydrocephalus, and increased intracranial pressure. An imaging study of the brain should be done prior to lumbar puncture in those with focal seizures or residual focal deficits. The lumbar puncture may be delayed because of cardiopulmonary instability or due to the above contraindications. In these cases, empiric antimicrobial coverage should be started and continued until meningitis is no longer an etiologic possibility. Acyclovir should be considered if there are any concerns about the possibility of herpes encephalitis. These concerns may be no more than SE, focal findings, and fever. Acyclovir is relatively devoid of adverse effects, and failure to treat herpes encephalitis is disastrous. The history and physical examination, in conjunction with basic laboratory and imaging studies, will often provide the etiology. Finally, the clinician must not delay treatment while awaiting lab results, and specific anticonvulsant therapy and cardiopulmonary supportive care should continue while the diagnostic evaluation takes place.

Summary

SE is a common pediatric emergency. Common errors in management include failure to recognize and treat cardiopulmonary decompensation, inappropriate drug dos-ages, and delays in drug administration. A predetermined, well organized therapeutic plan will aid the clinician in treatment of the patient, and will serve to diminish potential complications and reduce inherent morbidity and mortality. Focusing solely on seizure termination will cause one to ignore vital supportive care interventions that are necessary for limiting morbidity and preventing ongoing neuronal injury. Airway control and resuscitative measures are often necessary, and the health care team must be able to manage these effectively and expeditiously. The treatment strategy should include four goals: 1) maintenance of adequate cardiorespiratory function; 2) termination of seizure activity; 3) prevention of seizure recurrence; and 4) identification and treatment of any underlying etiologies. Aggressive treatment of the child with SE may limit the time-dependent cerebral injury and deter its associated systemic complications.

Acknowledgment: The authors would like to thank Kaitlyn Furst for her ongoing inspiration.

References

1. DeLorenzo RJ, Hauser WA, Towne AR, et al. A prospective, population-based epidemiologic study of status epilepticus in Richmond, Virginia. *Neurology* 1996;46:1029–1035.
2. Working Group on Status Epilepticus. Treatment of convulsive status epilepticus. Recommendations of the Epilepsy Foundation of America's Working Group on Status Epilepticus. *JAMA* 1993;270:854–859.
3. Gastaut H. Classification of status epilepticus. *Adv Neurol* 1994;34:15–35.
4. Commission on Classification and Terminology of the International League Against Epilepsy. Proposal for revised classification of epilepsies and epileptic syndromes. *Epilepsia* 1989;30:389–399.
5. Hauser WA. Status epilepticus: Epidemiologic considerations. *Neurology* 1990;40 (suppl 2):9–13.
6. Novak G, Maytal J, Alshansky A, Ascher C. Risk factors for status epilepticus in children with symptomatic epilepsy. *Neurology* 1997;49:533–537.
7. Mitchell WG. Status epilepticus and acute repetitive seizures in children, adolescents, and young adults: Etiology, outcome, and treatment. *Epilepsia* 1996;37:S74–S80.
8. DeLorenzo RJ, Towne AR, Pellock JM, Ko D. Status epilepticus in children, adults, and the elderly. *Epilepsia* 1992;33:S15–S25.
9. Maytal J, Shinnar S, Moshe SL, Alvarez LA. Low morbidity and mortality of status epilepticus in children. *Pediatrics* 1989;83:323–331.
10. Phillips SA, Shannahan RJ. Etiology and mortality of status epilepticus in children. A recent update. *Arch Neurol* 1989;46:74–76.
11. Mizrahi EM. Clinical diagnosis and management of neonatal seizures. *Int Pediatr* 1994;9:94–101.
12. Scher MS, Painter MJ. Controversies concerning neonatal seizures. *Pediatr Clin North Am* 1989;36:281–310.
13. Scher MS, Aso K, Beggarly ME, et al. Electrographic seizures in preterm and full-term neonates: Clinical correlates, associated brain lesions, and risk for neurologic sequelae. *Pediatrics* 1993;91:128–134.
14. van Esch A, Ramlal IR, van Steensel-Moll HA, et al. Outcome after febrile status epilepticus. *Dev Med Child Neurol* 1996;38:19–24.
15. Dunn DW. Status epilepticus in children: Etiology, clinical features, and outcome. *J Child Neurol* 1988;3:167–173.
16. DeLorenzo RJ, Pellock JM, Towne AR, Boggs JG. Epidemiology of status epilepticus. *J Clin Neurophysiol* 1995;12:316–325.
17. Wasterlain CG, Baxter CF, Baldwin RA. GABA metabolism in the substantia nigra, cortex, and hippocampus during status epilepticus. *Neurochem Res* 1993;18:527–532.
18. Mayat E, Lerner-Natoli M, Rondouin G, et al. Kainate-induced status epilepticus leads to a delayed increase in various specific glutamate metabotropic receptor responses in the hippocampus. *Brain Res* 1994;645:186–200.
19. Fujikawa DG, Daniels AH, Kim JS. The competitive NMDA receptor antagonist CGP 40116 protects against status epilepticus-induced neuronal damage. *Epilepsy Res* 1994;17:207–219.
20. Young D, Dragunow M. MK-801 and NBQX prevent electrically induced status epilepticus. *Neuroreport* 1994;5:1481–1484.
21. Lipton SA, Rosenberg PA. Excitatory amino acids as a final common pathway for neurologic disorders. *N Engl J Med* 1994;330:613–622.
22. Fountain NB, Lothman EW. Pathophysiology of status epilepticus. *J Clin Neurophysiol* 1995;12:326–342.
23. Wasterlain CG, Fujikawa DG, Penix L, Sankar R. Pathophysiological mechanisms of brain damage from status epilepticus. *Epilepsia* 1993;34(suppl 1):S37–S53.
24. Meldrum BS, Brierley JB. Prolonged epileptic seizures in primates: Ischemic cell change and its relation to ictal physiological events. *Arch Neurol* 1973;28:10–17.
25. Lothman E. The biochemical basis and pathophysiology of status epilepticus. *Neurology* 1990;40(suppl 2):13–23.
26. Walton NY. Systemic effects of generalized convulsive status epilepticus. *Epilepsia* 1993;34:S54–S58.
27. Lacey DJ, Singer WD, Horwitz SJ, Gilmore H. Lorazepam therapy of status epilepticus in children and adolescents. *J Pediatr* 1986;108:771–774.
28. Giang DW, McBride MC. Lorazepam ver-

sus diazepam for the treatment of status epilepticus. *Pediatr Neurol* 1988;4:358–361.
29. Crawford TO, Mitchell WG, Snodgrass SR. Lorazepam in childhood status epilepticus and serial seizures: Effectiveness and tachyphylaxis. *Neurology* 1987;37:190–195.
30. Dieckmann RA. Rectal diazepam for prehospital pediatric status epilepticus. *Ann Emerg Med* 1994;23:216–224.
31. Ramsay RE. Treatment of status epilepticus. *Epilepsia* 1993;34:S71–S81.
32. Chiulli DA, Terndrup TE, Kanter RK. The influence of diazepam or lorazepam on the frequency of endotracheal intubation in childhood status epilepticus. *J Emerg Med* 1991;9:13–17.
33. Rivera R, Segnini M, Baltodano A, Perez V. Midazolam in the treatment of status epilepticus in children. *Crit Care Med* 1993;21:991–994.
34. Koul RL, Aithala GR, Chacko A, et al. Continuous midazolam infusion as treatment of status epilepticus. *Arch Dis Child* 1997;76:445–448.
35. Browne TR. The pharmacokinetics of agents used to treat status epilepticus. *Neurology* 1990;40(suppl 2):28–32.
36. Ramsay RE, DeToledo J. Intravenous administration of fosphenytoin: Options for the management of seizures. *Neurology* 1996;46:S17–S19.
37. Browne TR, Kugler AR, Eldon MA. Pharmacology and pharmacokinetics of fosphenytoin. *Neurology* 1996;46:S3–S7.
38. Pellock JM. Fosphenytoin use in children. *Neurology* 1996;46:S14–S16.
39. Uthman BM, Wilder BJ, Ramsay RE. Intramuscular use of fosphenytoin: An overview. *Neurology* 1996;46:S24–S28.
40. Crawford TO, Mitchell WG, Fishman LS, Snodgrass SR. Very high-dose phenobarbital for refractory status epilepticus in children. *Neurology* 1988;38:1035–1040.
41. Segeleon JE, Haun SE. Status epilepticus in children. *Pediatr Ann* 1996;25:380–386.
42. Weise KL, Bleck TP. Status epilepticus in children and adults. *Crit Care Clin* 1997;13:629–646.
43. Walsh GO, Delgado-Escueta AV. Status epilepticus. *Neurol Clin* 1993;11:835–856.
44. Shepherd SM. Management of status epilepticus. *Emerg Med Clin North Am* 1994;12:941–961.
45. Roberts MR, Eng-Bourquin J. Status epilepticus in children. *Emerg Med Clin North Am* 1995;13:489–507.
46. Tunik MG, Young GM. Status epilepticus in children. *Pediatr Clin North Am* 1992;39:1007–1030.
47. Chamberlain JM, Altieri MA, Futterman C, et al. A prospective, randomized study of comparing intramuscular midazolam with intravenous diazepam for the treatment of seizures in children. *Pediatr Emerg Care* 1997;13:92–94.
48. Walker MC, Smith JM, Shorvon SD. The intensive care treatment of convulsive status epilepticus in the U.K. *Anaesthesia* 1995;50:130–135.
49. Parent JM, Lowenstein DH. Treatment of refractory generalized status epilepticus with continuous infusion of midazolam. *Neurology* 1994;44:1837–1840.
50. Tasker RC, Boyd SG, Harden A, Matthew DJ. EEG monitoring of prolonged thiopentone administration for intractable seizures and status epilepticus in infants and young children. *Neuropediatrics* 1989;20:147–153.
51. Kinoshita H, Nakagawa E, Iwasaki Y, et al. Pentobarbital therapy for status epilepticus in children: Timing and tapering. *Pediatr Neurol* 1995;13:164–168.

Chapter 10

Increased Intracranial Pressure/Intracranial Pressure Monitoring

Steven E. Haun, MD and Joseph E. Segeleon, MD

Introduction

The foundation of neurointensive care is excellent supportive care. Several therapies that were commonly used to treat intracranial hypertension in the recent past are now believed to be of limited value or even deleterious. Meticulous attention to the maintenance of adequate oxygenation, ventilation, and blood pressure comprises the majority of what modern intensive care has to offer patients with acute brain injury. This chapter reviews the basic principles of intracranial pressure (ICP) monitoring, the pathophysiology of the intracranial vault, the regulation of cerebral blood flow (CBF), and the management of increased ICP.

Intracranial Pressure Monitoring

The goal of ICP monitoring is to provide real-time measurement of cerebral perfusion pressure (CPP). CPP is defined as the mean arterial blood pressure (MAP) minus the ICP.

$$CPP = MAP - ICP$$

CBF, and therefore cerebral oxygen delivery, is dependent on an adequate CPP (see below). The primary goal of therapy in the acutely brain-injured child is to ensure adequate cerebral oxygen delivery. Maintaining an adequate CPP is absolutely essential to achieving this goal. This section reviews the indications, techniques, and complications of ICP monitoring.

Indications for Intracranial Pressure Monitoring

The indications for ICP monitoring remain controversial. ICP monitoring has achieved widespread use in the management of traumatic brain injury in spite of the lack of a randomized, controlled trial documenting that ICP monitoring improves outcome. One approach to ICP monitoring in traumatic brain injury is to monitor patients who have a Glasgow Coma Scale (GCS) of 8 or less and an abnormal computed-tomography (CT) scan of the head.[1] An abnormal CT scan is defined as one that demonstrates hematomas, contusions, edema, or compression of basal cisterns. Patients who have a GCS of 8 or less and a normal CT scan should also be considered for ICP monitoring if they have had episodes of hypotension prior to admission to the intensive care unit or if they exhibit unilateral or bilateral motor posturing.

Other types of brain injuries in which ICP monitoring has been applied include hydrocephalus, subarachnoid hemorrhage, intracerebral hemorrhage, hepatic encephalopathy, Reye's syndrome, central nervous system infections (meningitis and encephalitis), and hypoxic-ischemic encephalopathy. Again, there is no randomized, controlled trial documenting the efficacy of ICP monitoring in any of these conditions and, ultimately, the decision to monitor ICP will be made by the intensivist and neurosurgeon managing the patient, based on the patient's status and GCS, and the physician's personal experience and preference. In general, ICP monitoring is not performed unless the patient is sufficiently comatose (ie, GCS ≤8). With this level of neurologic function, there is little left of the neurologic exam to determine if the patient's level of consciousness is improving. In hypoxic-ischemic encephalopathy, ICP monitoring and treatment of increased ICP have not been demonstrated to result in an improved outcome.[2,3] Increased ICP in this setting appears to be an epiphenomenon of cell death. Thus, most centers no longer monitor ICP in patients with hypoxic-ischemic brain injury.

Techniques of Intracranial Pressure Monitoring

ICP monitoring devices are classified by their location and the method of pressure transduction.[4] ICP monitors can be placed in the following locations: lateral ventricles, the brain parenchyma, or the subarachnoid, subdural, and epidural spaces. There are three different methods of pressure transduction: fluid-coupled to an external strain gauge, catheter tip strain gauge, and catheter tip fiber optic. Fluid-coupled devices have a continuous column of fluid extending from the intracranial location being monitored to an external strain gauge. The external strain gauges are extremely accurate and can be recalibrated. The major drawback to this method is that any obstruction to the fluid couple can lead to inaccurate measurements. Catheter tip devices are calibrated prior to insertion and cannot be recalibrated after insertion. Measurement drift has been a problem for both types of catheter tip technologies.[4]

Intraventricular catheters fluid-coupled to an external strain gauge are the gold standard against which all other ICP monitors are compared. An added advantage of ventricular catheters is that they are therapeutic devices, which allow drainage of cerebrospinal fluid (CSF) to lower ICP (see below). Intraparenchymal catheter tip transducers (fiber optic and strain gauge) have gained popularity over the last decade. The parenchymal location offers the advantage of ease of placement, especially when the lateral ventricles are compressed, making placement of a ventricular catheter difficult. Disadvantages of intraparenchymal catheter tip monitors include the inability to drain CSF, the inability to recalibrate the monitor, measurement drift, and the cost. Monitoring in the other locations (subarachnoid, subdural, and epidural spaces) has been fraught with problems of inaccuracy and has largely been abandoned.

Complications of Intracranial Pressure Monitoring

Complications from ICP monitoring include malposition, malfunction, obstruction, infection, and hemorrhage. Obstruction can occur in ventricular catheters, but is not an issue with intraparenchymal monitors. Clinically significant intracranial infections associated with ICP monitoring devices are unusual,[5,6] although bacterial colonization of devices is common. Bacterial colonization of ventricular catheters occurs at a rate of 5%, whereas intraparenchymal monitors are colonized at a rate of 14%.[4] The use of prophylactic antibiotics to prevent colonization of ICP monitors is controversial, but most centers use an antistaphylococcal antibiotic such as oxacillin, nafcillin, or a third-generation cephalosporin. ICP monitor-associated hematomas occur with an incidence of 1.1% for ventricular devices and 2.8% for intraparenchymal devices.[4] While complications resulting from ICP monitoring are not uncommon, serious long-term morbidity is rare.

Pathophysiology of the Intracranial Vault

The foundation of our understanding of the intracranial vault was developed approximately 200 years ago by Monro[7] and Kellie.[8] The Monro-Kellie doctrine states that the volume of the intracranial vault is relatively constant (ie, the skull is a rigid structure). Under normal conditions, the intracranial vault contains three major components: brain, blood, and CSF. Under pathologic conditions, the intracranial vault may contain additional components resulting from the disease process, such as foreign bodies, air, pus, tumors, and extravascular blood. If the ICP is to remain constant, an increase in volume of one component must be accompanied by a corresponding decrease in volume of another. For example, when a patient suffers an epidural hematoma, there is a compensatory decrease in CSF volume and cerebral blood volume (CBV). If the volume of the epidural hematoma exceeds the compensatory decrease in CSF volume and CBV, the ICP will rise. The volume-pressure relationship of the intracranial vault is illustrated in Figure 1. As the volume of the intracranial contents increases, a critical point is reached where a small increase in volume causes a dramatic rise in ICP. The steep portion of this curve represents failure of compensatory mechanisms (decreases in CSF volume and CBV).

Treatment of increased ICP in this example consists of evacuation of the epidural hematoma. The following section reviews each of the components of the intracranial vault (brain, CSF, CBV) and their role in the pathophysiology of increased ICP (Table 1).

Brain volume can increase as the result of brain edema. Many different disease states result in cerebral edema (traumatic brain injury, meningitis, encephalitis, brain abscesses, brain tumors, hypoxic-ischemic brain injury, Reye's syndrome, hepatic encephalopathy, diabetic ketoacidosis, and hydrocephalus). There are three different types of brain edema: vasogenic, cytotoxic, and interstitial.[9] Vasogenic edema results from increased capillary permeability which leads to fluid accumulation in the extracellular space. It commonly occurs in inflammatory states such as traumatic brain injury, encephalitis, and meningitis. It also occurs in areas surrounding tumors and abscesses. Vasogenic edema typically responds to osmotic agents such as mannitol. There may also be a role for corticosteroids in specific types of vasogenic edema. Cytotoxic edema results from failure of brain cells (neurons and glia) to maintain their transmembrane ionic gra-

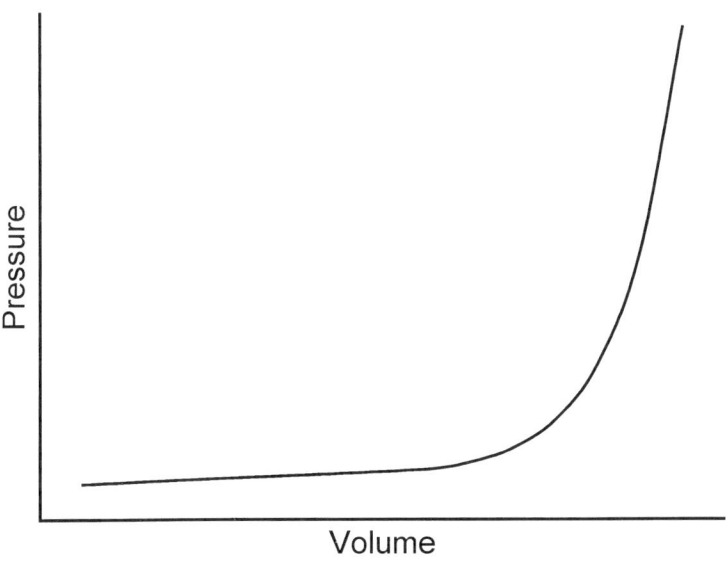

Figure 1. Volume-pressure curve of the intracranial vault. Volume of the intracranial contents is on the x axis and intracranial pressure is on the y axis. As the volume of intracranial contents increases, a critical point is reached where intracranial pressure rises dramatically with small increases in volume.

Table 1

Pathophysiology of Increased Intracranial Pressure

Increased brain volume
  vasogenic edema
  cytotoxic edema
  interstitial edema

Increased cerebral blood volume
  hypercapnia
  hypoxia
  hypotension
  hyperthermia
  seizures

Increased CSF volume
  communicating hydrocephalus
  obstructive hydrocephalus

Pathological space-occupying lesions
  tumor
  hematoma
  abscess
  foreign body
  air

CSF = cerebrospinal fluid.

---

dients. Sodium accumulates in the intracellular space and the cells swell. This type of cerebral edema is the result of severe cellular dysfunction and/or cell death and is resistant to therapy. Cytotoxic edema is most commonly encountered in the setting of hypoxic-ischemic brain injury, but can result from brain injury of any etiology providing the insult is severe enough. Interstitial edema results from increased CSF hydrostatic pressure in the setting of hydrocephalus. Interstitial edema typically occurs in periventricular regions of the brain and responds well to CSF drainage.

The volume of CSF present in the central nervous system is the result of the equilibrium between production and absorption. CSF is produced by the choroid plexus and absorbed by the arachnoid villi. Increased ICP can result from CSF overproduction or decreased absorption. CSF overproduction is extremely rare, but can result from tumors of the choroid plexus. Decreased CSF absorption is relatively common and can result from impaired CSF circulation (obstructive hydrocephalus) or impaired absorption (communicating hydrocephalus). Treatment of increased ICP resulting from hydrocephalus can be achieved by draining CSF via a temporary external ventricular drain or a permanent internal ventricular drain such as a ventriculoperitoneal shunt.

CBV is defined as the volume of intravascular blood contained within the intracranial vault at any given time. Vasodilation of the cerebral vasculature increases CBV whereas vasoconstriction decreases CBV. It is important to understand that CBF and CBV do not necessarily change in the same direction. In patients with traumatic brain injury, there appears to be no correlation between CBF and CBV.[10] In patients with intact pressure-flow autoregulation (see below), a low CPP causes cerebral vasodilation[11] leading to increased CBV and increased ICP.[12] Increased ICP can, in turn, lead to decreased CBF. CBV can be minimized by maintaining an adequate CPP (see below). Hyperventilation can also be used to reduce CBV,[13] as hypocapnia causes cerebral vasoconstriction. However, hypocapnia also decreases CBF, which may lead to ischemic injury (see below). Hypoxia and hypercapnia also lead to cerebral vasodilation and should be meticulously avoided in the patient with increased ICP (see below).

Regulation of Cerebral Blood Flow

As stated above, the primary goal of therapy in the acutely brain-injured child is to ensure adequate cerebral oxygen delivery. Ensuring adequate cerebral oxygen delivery provides an optimal environment for healing and prevents secondary brain injury (ischemia). Cerebral oxygen delivery is the product of CBF and arterial oxygen content (CaO_2).

Cerebral oxygen delivery = CBF × CaO_2

As described in chapter 2, CaO_2 is primarily a function of hemoglobin concentration and arterial oxygen saturation (SaO_2). Thus, cerebral oxygen delivery is dependent on CBF, hemoglobin concentration, and SaO_2. This section reviews the four major determinants of CBF: CPP, cerebral metabolic rate for oxygen ($CMRO_2$), partial pressure of arterial carbon dioxide ($PaCO_2$), and partial pressure of arterial oxygen (PaO_2). Also briefly discussed is monitoring of the oxygen saturation of blood obtained from the jugular bulb (SjO_2) as a measure of the adequacy of cerebral oxygen delivery.

Pressure-Flow Autoregulation

Pressure-flow autoregulation refers to the ability of a vascular bed to maintain constant blood flow over a wide range of perfusion pressures. The relationship between CBF and CPP is demonstrated in Figure 2. Under normal conditions the brain can maintain a constant CBF over CPP ranging from 50 to 150 mm Hg.[14] This is accomplished by varying cerebrovascular resistance (vasoconstriction or vasodilation) at the level of medium to small arteries and arterioles.[15] At the lower end of autoregulation (50 mm Hg), vessels are maximally vasodilated and further reductions in CPP will result in pressure-passive decreases in flow and subsequent ischemic injury. At the upper level of autoregulation (150 mm Hg), further increases in CPP will result in pressure-passive increases in flow.

Pressure-flow autoregulation can be impaired following traumatic brain injury.[10]

In the setting of increased ICP, it is important to maintain an adequate CPP regardless of whether autoregulation is intact or defective.[16] If pressure-flow autoregulation is intact, an inadequate CPP will result in cerebral vasodilation leading to increases in CBV and ICP. If pressure-flow autoregulation is defective, a low CPP will result in an inadequate CBF because CBF is pressure-passive. Current recommendations for adults with severe head injury suggest maintaining a minimum CPP of 70 mm Hg (see below).[17]

Metabolism

CBF and $CMRO_2$ are normally tightly coupled. For example, an increase in $CMRO_2$ is normally accompanied by an increase in CBF. The coupling between flow and metabolism is achieved by vasoconstriction and vasodilation of arterioles. Coupling of CBF and $CMRO_2$ has important clinical implications. Fever and seizures result in increased $CMRO_2$ and thus increased CBF. Resultant vasodilation may lead to increases in CBV and ICP. Thus, prompt and effective treatment of fever and seizures is imperative in the patient with acute brain injury. Hypothermia and barbiturates are therapeutic

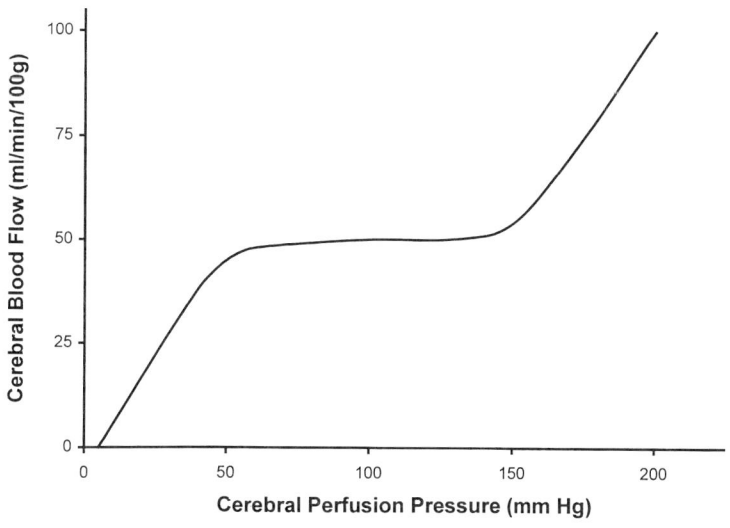

Figure 2. Pressure-flow autoregulation in the cerebral circulation. Cerebral blood flow is held constant over a wide range of cerebral perfusion pressures by varying cerebrovascular resistance. Cerebral blood flow is pressure-passive at cerebral perfusion pressures above 150 mm Hg and below 50 mm Hg, the limits of pressure-flow autoregulation.

maneuvers that lower the $CMRO_2$. These maneuvers may be helpful when cerebral oxygen delivery is inadequate despite standard therapies.

Traumatic brain injury can result in uncoupling of metabolism and flow,[18] and patients who exhibit uncoupling appear to have worse outcomes.[19] Inadequate cerebral oxygen delivery (ischemia) is a common finding during the first 24 hours following traumatic brain injury[20,21] and may contribute to secondary injury. Adequacy of cerebral oxygen delivery can be assessed using SjO_2 monitoring (see below).

Carbon Dioxide

Carbon dioxide is a potent modulator of the cerebral circulation. Carbon dioxide readily crosses the blood-brain barrier and induces changes in the perivascular pH which, in turn, alters vasomotor tone.[22] High $PaCO_2$ levels cause vasodilation leading to increased CBF, whereas low $PaCO_2$ levels cause vasoconstriction leading to decreased CBF.[23] The relationship between CBF and $PaCO_2$ is shown in Figure 3. Hypocapnia also rapidly lowers ICP by causing cerebral vasoconstriction, which decreases CBV.[23] It is important to note that these changes in vasomotor tone occur relatively independent of $CMRO_2$ or CPP. In brain-injured patients, it is possible to induce cerebral ischemia by vigorous hyperventilation.[18,24] Hypoventilation can result in cerebral vasodilation which, in turn, can lead to increases in CBV and ICP. Thus, both hypocapnia and hypercapnia can result in inadequate cerebral oxygen delivery which underscores the importance of maintaining normocapnia in patients with increased ICP.

Oxygen

Hypoxia causes cerebral vasodilation and increased CBF. This is a protective mechanism that attempts to preserve cerebral oxygen delivery. The relationship between CBF and PaO_2 is illustrated in Figure 4. As the PaO_2 falls below 50 mm Hg, the CBF begins to rise dramatically. This threshold effect occurs because the SaO_2 (and thus CaO_2) falls precipitously with a PaO_2 ≤50 mm Hg. Recall that the steep portion of the oxyhemoglobin dissociation curve is between 10 and 40 mm Hg. It is extremely important to maintain an adequate PaO_2 in brain-injured patients to prevent cerebral

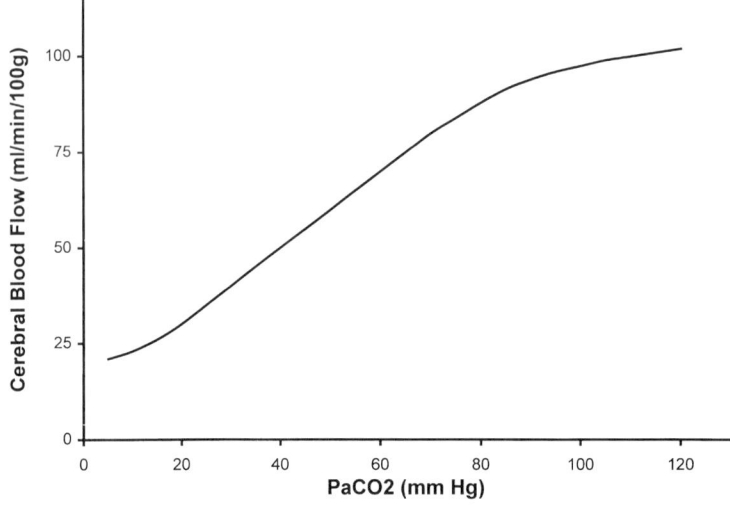

Figure 3. Relationship between partial pressure of arterial carbon dioxide ($PaCO_2$) and cerebral blood flow. There is a linear relationship between $PaCO_2$ and cerebral blood flow over the range of clinically relevant $PaCO_2$ values. Hypocapnia causes cerebral vasoconstriction and decreases cerebral blood flow whereas hypercapnia causes vasodilation and increases cerebral blood flow.

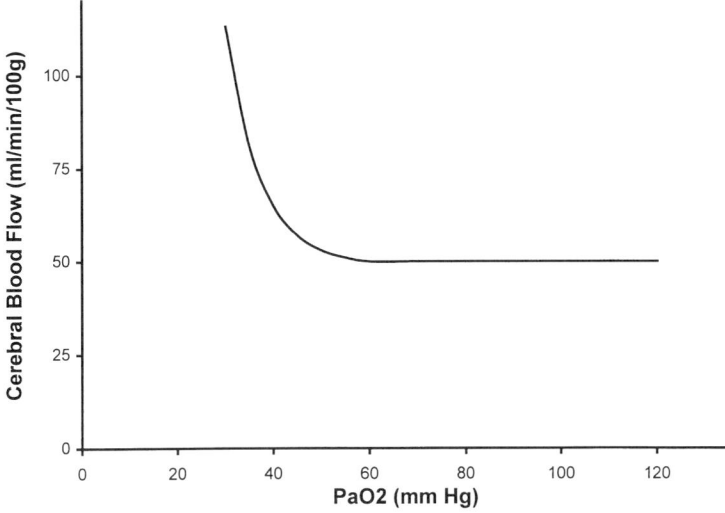

Figure 4. Relationship between arterial oxygen pressure (PaO$_2$) and cerebral blood flow. Hypoxia (PaO$_2$ <50 mm Hg) causes cerebral vasodilation and increases cerebral blood flow.

vasodilation and resultant increases in CBV and ICP.

SjO$_2$ Monitoring

Unfortunately, cerebral oxygen delivery is rarely measured in the clinical setting because bedside measurement of CBF is fraught with technical limitations.[16] Recently, xenon-enhanced CT scanning has been used to measure CBF in the clinical setting.[21,24] This technique provides accurate CBF measurements including regional blood flows. Xenon-enhanced CT scanning combined with SjO$_2$ monitoring allows calculation of cerebral oxygen delivery and CMRO$_2$. However, the major limitation of this method is the need to transport the patient to the CT scanner to measure CBF. Obviously, the logistics involved in repetitive transports limits the availability of serial measurements. How, then, can the clinician determine whether cerebral oxygen delivery is adequate to meet the metabolic demands of the brain? A more easily applied method is to measure the SjO$_2$, which allows an estimation of cerebral oxygen extraction ratio (cerebral oxygen use divided by cerebral oxygen delivery). This is analogous to measuring the oxygen saturation of mixed venous blood obtained from the pulmonary artery (see chapter 2). A simplified method for calculating the cerebral oxygen extraction ratio is shown below:

$$\text{Cerebral oxygen extraction ratio} = \frac{(SaO_2 - SjO_2)}{SaO_2}$$

The brain normally uses about 40% of the oxygen delivered to it (cerebral oxygen extraction ratio=0.4). Accordingly, normal SjO$_2$ is approximately 62%, with a range of 55% to 71%.[25] Thus, SjO$_2$ less than 55% implies inadequate cerebral oxygen delivery. Indeed, jugular venous desaturation (SjO$_2$ <50% for more than 10 minutes) in head-injured patients is strongly associated with poor neurologic outcomes and increased mortality.[26]

It is our practice to place a jugular bulb catheter in children who have traumatic brain injury and GCS of 8 or less. The jugular bulb is catheterized by inserting a catheter retrogradely through the internal jugular vein.[27] It is common practice to cannulate the internal jugular vein with dominant venous drainage which, in most patients, is the right internal jugular vein.[25] Intracranial position of the catheter tip must be confirmed radiographically. We use a 3F central venous catheter, which allows intermittent sampling, although some centers use a fiber optic catheter to obtain continuous measurement of SjO_2. We strive to maintain the SjO_2 at 60% or greater. Anything that reduces cerebral oxygen delivery will decrease the SjO_2. Recall that cerebral oxygen delivery is dependent on CBF, hemoglobin concentration, and SaO_2. Common causes of jugular venous desaturation include hypocapnia, hypotension, hypoxemia, and increased ICP.[26]

There are two limitations to this methodology. First, if the tip of the catheter is not located within the intracranial vault or if the blood sample is withdrawn too rapidly, contamination with extracranial venous blood may lead to erroneously high SjO_2 values. Second, as cerebral oxygen extraction ratio as measured by SjO_2 is a global measure, it is possible for focal areas of ischemia to be missed by this monitoring method. Thus, a normal SjO_2 does not exclude regional ischemia. However, inadequate cerebral oxygen delivery is definitely present when the SjO_2 is low. Despite its limitations, SjO_2 monitoring can provide valuable information regarding the adequacy of cerebral oxygen delivery. It may be particularly helpful in cases of refractory increases in ICP when therapeutic interventions are limited and lowering of $PaCO_2$ is considered.

Management of Increased Intracranial Pressure

As stated in the introduction to this chapter, excellent supportive care is the foundation of neurointensive care. In our discussion regarding regulation of CBF, we have emphasized the importance of maintaining normal CPP, PaO_2, and $PaCO_2$ in an effort to ensure adequate cerebral oxygen delivery. Novel therapies will come and go, but the basic priorities of critical care (airway, breathing, circulation) remain constant. The importance of excellent supportive care cannot be overemphasized. For example, it has been clearly demonstrated in both children[28] and adults[29] with traumatic brain injury, that hypotension during initial resuscitation is associated with sig-

Table 2

Management of Increased Intracranial Pressure

Decrease brain volume
  mannitol
  steroids
  resect injured brain

Decrease cerebral blood volume
  elevate head of bed 15–30°
  head in midline position
  avoid hypoxia
  avoid hypercapnia
  avoid hypotension
  avoid hyperthermia
  treat seizures
  mannitol
  pentobarbital
  hypothermia
  hyperventilation

Decrease CSF volume
  CSF drainage via intraventricular catheter
  ventriculoperitoneal shunt

Decrease volume of pathological components
  resect tumor
  evacuate hematoma
  drain abscess
  remove foreign body

Increase Intracranial Volume
  decompressive craniectomy

CSF = cerebrospinal fluid.

nificantly increased mortality. This section reviews principles of supportive care for patients at risk for increased ICP, and therapeutic maneuvers purported to reduce ICP (Table 2). Also presented is an integrated approach to the patient with increased ICP. The reader is cautioned that most of these therapies have been studied primarily in the setting of traumatic brain injury and their extrapolation to other clinical settings, (meningitis) may not be based on sound clinical evidence.

Airway Management

The reader is referred to chapter 1 for a detailed discussion of airway management of patients with increased ICP. In general, patients with a GCS of 8 or less require endotracheal intubation to protect the airway and control the ventilatory pattern. In trauma patients, the cervical spine should be immobilized with in-line stabilization during endotracheal intubation. Oral intubation is the preferred route in trauma patients because of the risk of intracranial intubation associated with nasotracheal intubation. It is vital that patients be adequately anesthetized for intubation because laryngoscopy can dramatically increase ICP. In hemodynamically stable patients, thiopental and propofol are acceptable choices for induction, as both decrease the $CMRO_2$ and the ICP. In hemodynamically unstable patients, etomidate is the drug of choice because it lowers $CMRO_2$ and ICP but is less likely to cause hypotension. Intravenous lidocaine administered prior to intubation will further blunt increases in ICP associated with laryngoscopy. Muscle relaxants that are appropriate for this setting include succinylcholine, rocuronium, and vecuronium. Hypotension during or following intubation can be largely prevented by appropriate selection of pharmacologic adjuncts to intubation. If hypotension develops, it must be corrected aggressively.

Ventilator Management

Principles of mechanical ventilation are covered in detail in chapter 4. The goal of mechanical ventilation in the patient with increased ICP is to provide normoxia (PaO_2 of 80 to 120 mm Hg) and normocapnia ($PaCO_2$ of 35 to 40 mm Hg). Hypoxia and hypercapnia are to be meticulously avoided because both cause cerebral vasodilation and resultant increases in CBV and ICP. Hypocapnia causes cerebral vasoconstriction, which can result in cerebral ischemia in brain-injured patients.[18,24] Hyperventilation as a modality to decrease ICP is discussed below.

High mean airway pressures can cause elevated ICP by impeding jugular venous drainage. This does not imply that positive end-expiratory pressure should not be used in patients at risk for increased ICP. Positive end-expiratory pressure should be titrated to achieve oxygenation goals and minimize the toxic effects of inspired oxygen. Positive end-expiratory pressure to levels of 10 cm H_2O appears to have minimal effect on ICP.[30] Endotracheal suctioning can result in acute increases in ICP. Suctioning-associated increases in ICP can be minimized or prevented by lidocaine (1 mg/kg) administered intravenously several minutes prior to suctioning. Coughing and biting the endotracheal tube can also cause elevations in ICP and can be minimized by adequate sedation and, if necessary, neuromuscular blockade.

Hemodynamic Management

Hemodynamic management is an area of management that has undergone dramatic change over the past decade. Until recently, brain-injured patients were fluid-restricted and diuresed to the point of hypovolemia, and the target CPP was a minimum of 50 mm Hg. Recent guidelines for adults with traumatic brain injury suggest that the CPP should be maintained at a minimum of 70 mm Hg[17] and the endpoint for intravascular volume be euvolemia or mild hypervolemia.[31] The target CPP that should be used in infants and young children is unclear, as blood pressure and hence the normal CPP rises with age.[32] It is our approach to maintain CPP of 50 mm Hg or greater in infants up to 1 year of age, 60 mm Hg or greater in children from 1 to 10 years of age, and 70 mm Hg or greater in patients older than 10 years of age. As CPP is a function of both MAP and ICP, it is also important to have a clear threshold for treatment of increased ICP. Again, recent guidelines for adults with traumatic brain injury suggest that treatment for increased ICP be initiated at an upper threshold of 20 to 25 mm Hg.[33]

To achieve this higher target CPP, many patients will require vasopressors to raise the MAP.[31] It is our practice to use dopamine as a first-line agent, followed by norepinephrine if greater support is needed. Monitoring of central venous filling pressures in these patients is extremely useful. Central venous pressure monitoring is adequate for most patients, although a pulmonary artery catheter can be very helpful. The importance of maintaining adequate filling pressures cannot be overemphasized. Mannitol can rapidly decrease intravascular volume, and urine output may need to be replaced to avoid hypovolemia. It is our practice to maintain the central venous pressure or pulmonary artery wedge pressure between 8 and 12 mm Hg, while other authors advocate even higher filling pressures.[31]

Initial intravenous fluids should be isotonic to prevent decreases in plasma osmolality.[34] Hypo-osmolality can worsen existing brain edema and increase ICP. Dextrose-containing fluids should be administered with great caution because hyperglycemia is associated with more severe brain injury in animal models of global cerebral ischemia[35] and poor neurologic outcomes in adults with head trauma.[36] The initial intravenous fluid of choice for patients at risk for increased ICP is 0.9% NaCl. Dextrose can be added to the maintenance fluids after hyperglycemia has resolved or has been corrected with insulin. Hyponatremia must be avoided; serum sodium should be maintained between 140 and 150 mEq/L. As the serum sodium rises, hypotonic fluids can be administered, usually in the form of enteral feedings or parenteral nutrition.

Head Positioning

Our practice is to elevate the head of the bed to 15 to 30° to augment jugular venous drainage and optimize CPP.[37] More recently, the practice of elevating the head of the bed has been questioned. With the head of the bed elevated, the distance from the heart to the head increases, thereby decreasing CPP. If the head of the bed is elevated, the ICP and MAP should be measured at the level of the external auditory meatus and the CPP maintained, as mentioned previously, according to the patient's age. The head should be kept midline to prevent jugular compression. Inadvertent jugular vein compression from cervical collars and endotracheal tube ties should be meticulously avoided to optimize jugular venous outflow.

Temperature Control

Hyperthermia causes increased $CMRO_2$ and cerebral vasodilation. Cerebral vasodilation in turn increases CBF, CBV, and ICP. Increases in ICP may prevent compensatory increases in CBF, leading to inadequate cerebral oxygen delivery. Thus, in patients at risk for increased ICP, body temperature should be monitored continuously and hyperthermia should be treated aggressively. Body temperature can be lowered with acetaminophen and cooling blankets. Shivering can be prevented by neuromuscular blockade.

Seizure Management

Seizures increase $CMRO_2$, causing cerebral vasodilation, which leads to increases in CBF, CBV, and ICP. Increases in ICP may prevent compensatory increases in CBF, leading to ischemia. Thus, seizure activity should be treated aggressively in patients at risk for increased ICP. Lorazepam 0.1 mg/kg can be administered intravenously every 10 minutes until seizures are terminated. An intravenous loading dose of phenytoin (20 mg/kg) should be initiated as soon as possible and administered over 20 minutes (1 mg/kg/min). Maintenance dosing of phenytoin should be based on serum drug levels. Prophylactic anticonvulsant therapy after traumatic brain injury is controversial.[38] Continuous electroencephalographic (EEG) monitoring should be considered for patients with seizure activity, especially if neuromuscular blockade is required for ICP control.

Analgesia, Sedation, and Neuromuscular Blockade

Head-injured patients commonly have other injuries that can result in significant pain (eg, femur fracture). Adequate analgesia and sedation are essential to control increased ICP. The reader is referred to chapter 11 for an in-depth discussion of analgesia and sedation in the pediatric intensive care unit. Analgesia is usually achieved with an intravenous infusion of an opioid such as fentanyl or morphine. Benzodiazepines such as midazolam or lorazepam are commonly used for sedation in this setting and can be administered either as a bolus or by continuous infusion. Caution should be exercised with the administration of opioids and sedatives, as both classes of drug can cause hypotension, especially when administered as a bolus.

If ICP is not lowered with adequate analgesia and sedation, neuromuscular blockade can be added. Pancuronium and vecuronium are used most commonly for this purpose and may be administered as intermittent boluses or as an infusion. Neuromuscular blockade should be used only when other means to control ICP are unsuccessful. The use of prophylactic neuromuscular blockade in head-injured patients has been shown to increase the incidence of pneumonia and sepsis and lengthen stay in the intensive care unit.[39] Neuromuscular blockade should be stopped daily in order to examine the patient and assess ongoing need for neuromuscular blockade.

Specific Therapies to Lower Intracranial Pressure

Surgical Evacuation

Evacuation of mass lesions (epidural hematoma) can lower ICP and definitively address the etiology of the intracranial hypertension. However, not all mass lesions require emergent evacuation. Emergent neurosurgical consultation should be obtained in all patients with acute alterations in mental status and mass lesion identified on CT scan.

Cerebrospinal Fluid Drainage

Emergent drainage of CSF can be lifesaving in patients with hydrocephalus. However, intraventricular drains can also be used to lower ICP in patients without hydrocephalus. In patients with a "tight" vault (ie, on the steep portion of the volume-pressure curve [Fig. 1]), draining a small amount of CSF can result in dramatic lowering of ICP. This is most commonly used in the treatment of traumatic brain injury, but can be helpful in other settings (eg, meningitis). CSF drainage is achieved by opening the intraventricular catheter to drain into a closed collection system. It is important to note that ICP measurement is not accurate while the intraventricular catheter is open for drainage. ICP measurements should be obtained when the drainage system is closed.

Mannitol

Mannitol is an osmotic diuretic that effectively lowers increased ICP.[40] The use of mannitol is supported by recent clinical guidelines for the treatment of traumatic brain injury in adults.[41] There is still controversy regarding the mechanisms by which mannitol lowers ICP. Mannitol appears to work by two different mechanisms: rheologic and osmotic. Mannitol has a plasma-expanding effect, which occurs within minutes of administration. This, in turn, reduces hematocrit, reduces blood viscosity, increases CBF, and increases cerebral oxygen delivery. Mannitol may lower ICP by increasing CPP and decreasing blood viscosity, both of which cause cerebral vasoconstriction and reductions in CBV. The osmotic effect of mannitol results from the osmotic gradient that develops between the intravascular space and the extracellular space of the brain. Theoretically, this causes a small reduction in brain water content, leading to reductions in brain volume and ICP.[42]

Mannitol (0.25 to 1.0 g/kg) is administered as an intravenous bolus over 10 to 30 minutes. Some centers administer mannitol on a scheduled basis (every 2 to 6 hours), whereas others administer mannitol on an "as needed" basis (in response to elevations in ICP). Adverse effects of mannitol include intravascular volume depletion and acute renal failure. Careful attention to filling pressures and adequate fluid replacement is essential when mannitol is administered. The risk of renal failure is greater in patients with a serum osmolality greater than 320 mOsm. Serum osmolality should be measured prior to each dose of mannitol, and the dose held when osmolality exceeds 320 mOsm.[40]

Barbiturates

As described above, CBF is normally tightly coupled with $CMRO_2$. Barbiturates are thought to lower ICP by decreasing the $CMRO_2$ which, in turn, results in cerebral vasoconstriction and decreases in CBV and CBF.[43] Prophylactic barbiturate coma appears to be of no value in the treatment of traumatic brain injury.[44,45] However, barbiturates do appear to reduce mortality in head-injured patients with increased ICP refractory to conventional therapy.[46] Recent guidelines for adult patients with traumatic brain injury call for the use of barbiturates in "patients with intracranial hypertension refractory to maximal medical and surgical ICP-lowering therapy."[47] The value of barbiturates for lowering increased ICP in other clinical settings (meningitis) remains unclear.

There are many different regimens of barbiturate administration for ICP control. Pentobarbital is the barbiturate most commonly used to lower ICP. Ideally, patients receiving high-dose barbiturates should have continuous EEG monitoring. Our approach to pentobarbital therapy is to administer a loading dose of 5 mg/kg intravenously over 15 minutes. The loading dose can be repeated until the ICP is lowered or an EEG pattern of burst suppression is achieved. Burst suppression correlates well with maximal metabolic suppression and, thus, further increases in pentobarbital levels are unlikely to lower ICP but may increase systemic toxicity.[43] Burst suppression refers to a flat line on the EEG with periodic episodes (bursts) of activity. The pentobarbital is administered to maintain 4 to 6 bursts per minute. After the ICP is lowered, a maintenance infusion of pentobarbital can be administered at a dose of 1 to 2 mg/kg/h. Subsequent episodes of increased ICP can be treated by repeating the loading dose as described above. Again, the endpoint of therapy is ICP control or an EEG pattern of burst suppression.

Barbiturates have two detrimental effects: hypotension and impaired leukocyte function.[43] It is important to note that hypotension and resultant cerebral vasodilation may negate any beneficial effect of barbiturates. Hypotension can largely be avoided by maintaining an adequate intravascular volume, although vasopressors are usually required to maintain an adequate CPP. Our practice is to, at a minimum, monitor central venous pressure. A pulmonary artery catheter can be very helpful in this setting.

Hypothermia

Hypothermia is thought to lower ICP in a fashion analogous to barbiturates: by decreasing the $CMRO_2$, which results in cerebral vasoconstriction and decreases CBV and CBF. Hypothermia appears to have neuroprotective effects in addition to its effect on ICP. Hypothermia has been shown to improve outcome in animal models of global cerebral ischemia and traumatic brain injury.[48] Preliminary clinical studies that subjected head-injured patients to moderate hypothermia (32 to 33°C) for 24 to 48 hours have yielded promising results,[49-51] and a prospective randomized controlled trial of moderate hypothermia for traumatic brain injury is under way. Although moderate hypothermia was well tolerated in the preliminary clinical studies cited above, there are potential adverse effects of hypothermia, including arrhythmias, coagulopathy, and sepsis. The risk of adverse effects appears to be dependent on the depth and the duration of hypothermia.

Hyperventilation

Hyperventilation has been recommended as a first-line therapy for increased ICP for more than 20 years. Hyperventilation lowers ICP by causing cerebral vasoconstriction, which decreases CBV.[13] Patients were commonly subjected to hyperventilation ($PaCO_2$ <30 mm Hg) for days despite evidence that hyperventilation-induced cerebral vasoconstriction is short-lived, lasting only 4 to 6 hours.[52] The biggest risk of hyperventilation as a modality to lower ICP is that hyperventilation lowers CBF independent of the metabolic needs of the brain. Thus, it is possible to induce ischemia with hyperventilation.[18,24] CBF is reduced by nearly 50% during the first 24 hours following traumatic brain injury, and then increases over the next several days.[19-21,53,54] Hence, the risk of causing cerebral ischemia with hyperventilation appears to be greatest during the first 24 hours post injury. Long-term prophylactic hyperventilation in the setting of traumatic brain injury has been studied in a prospective, randomized, clinical trial and has been shown to result in worse outcome at 3 and 6 months post injury.[55] Recent guidelines for adult patients with traumatic brain injury suggest that prophylactic hyperventilation be avoided, especially during the first 24 hours following injury.[56]

Short-term hyperventilation, however, can be life-saving in the management of acute neurologic deterioration while awaiting emergent CT scanning and/or evacuation of mass lesions (eg, epidural hema-toma).[57] Hyperventilation should be initiated in the presence of clinical signs of impending herniation including Cushing reflex (bradycardia and hypertension), asymmetric pupillary reactivity, ipsilateral or bilateral pupillary dilation, and ipsilateral or bilateral motor posturing. Some clinicians continue to advocate the use of prolonged hyperventilation in the management of increased ICP that is unresponsive to conventional measures such as sedation, paralysis, CSF drainage, and mannitol.[56] If hyperventilation is deemed necessary, the patient's CBF and/or SjO_2 should be monitored to identify the presence of ischemia. Prolonged hyperventilation should be abandoned if SjO_2 falls below 55% or if ischemia is noted on xenon-enhanced CT scanning. We prefer to use prolonged hyperventilation as a last resort (see below), recognizing that prophylactic hyperventilation reduces CBF independent of the brain's metabolic needs. It uncouples cerebral oxygen delivery and $CMRO_2$.

Corticosteroids

Corticosteroids do not appear to have any effect on outcome following traumatic brain injury and are not recommended in this setting.[58] When used in patients with traumatic brain injury, corticosteroids lead to an increased incidence of nosocomial infections and gastrointestinal bleeding. However, corticosteroids can be used to lower ICP in patients with mass lesions such as tumors and abscesses.[59] Corticosteroids appear to lower ICP in this setting by reducing vasogenic edema surrounding the mass lesion.

Decompressive Craniectomy

Decompressive craniectomy lowers ICP by increasing intracranial volume. Clearly, this is an extraordinary therapeutic measure. A preliminary report of decompressive craniectomy in patients with post-traumatic intracranial hypertension refractory to conventional treatment yielded encouraging results.[60] However, efficacy of this modality must be demonstrated in a prospective, randomized, controlled trial before widespread application can be recommended.

Integration of Therapy

In this section, we present a pragmatic approach to therapy for increased ICP. Our therapeutic approach is a modification of the clinical pathways developed by the American Association of Neurological Surgeons and the Brain Trauma Foundation for the treatment of traumatic brain injury.[61] We have attempted to provide a general approach that is applicable to all settings in which it is reasonable to attempt to lower ICP. Again, as discussed above, measures to lower ICP after global hypoxic-ischemic brain injury do not appear to alter outcome, and it is our opinion that measures other than supportive care are not indicated in this setting.

The algorithm for treatment of increased ICP is presented in Figure 5. This algorithm assumes that CT scanning has been performed, mass lesions have been evacuated, and an ICP monitor has been placed. The first step in management of increased ICP is to ensure an adequate CPP. Vasopressors are often required to maintain an adequate CPP. The use of vasopressors is guided by invasive hemodynamic monitoring, which may include central venous pressure and pulmonary artery catheters. Mechanical ventilation should be titrated to achieve normoxia and normocapnia. The head of the bed should be elevated 15 to 30°. Seizures and hyperthermia should be aggressively treated. Adequate sedation and analgesia should be provided, and if the ICP remains elevated, neuromuscular blockade should be established. If ICP is not lowered with the above measures, CSF drainage should be performed and mannitol should be administered. Mannitol may be repeated as long as serum osmolality is 320 mOsm or less. The importance of maintaining ade-

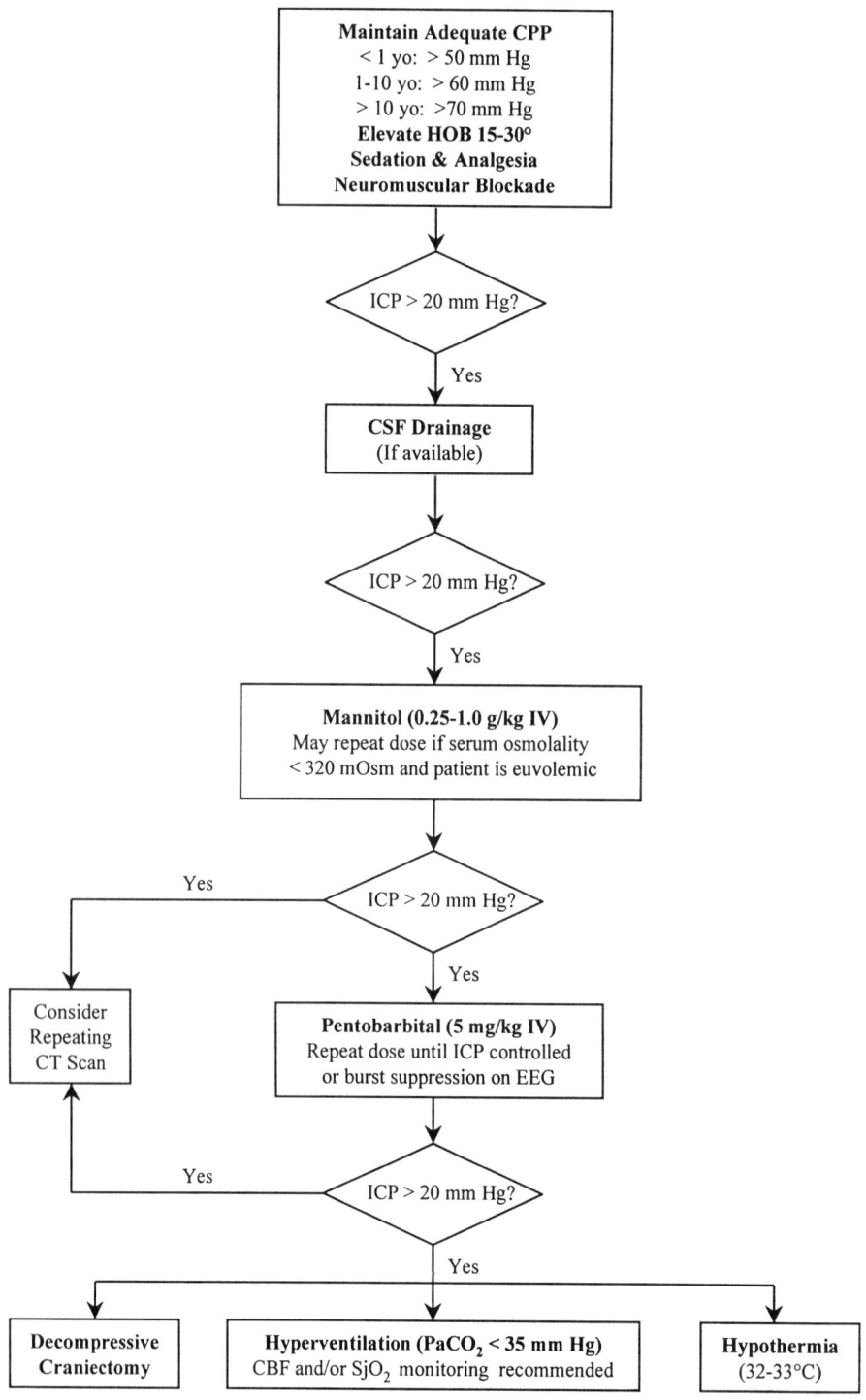

Figure 5. Treatment of increased intracranial pressure. CBF=cerebral blood flow; CPP=cerebral perfusion pressure; CSF=cerebrospinal fluid; CT=computed tomography; EEG=electroencephalogram; HOB=head of bed; ICP=intracranial pressure; yo=years old. Modified from Reference 61.

quate intravascular volume during mannitol therapy cannot be overemphasized. Steroids should be considered in patients with tumors and abscesses.

"Second-tier" therapies[31] should be considered if ICP is not controlled with sedation, paralysis, CSF drainage, and mannitol. Repeat CT scanning should always be considered when ICP is difficult to control or if abrupt ICP spikes occur in a patient in whom ICP had been previously well controlled. We would proceed next to high-dose barbiturate therapy, recognizing that other centers might use prolonged hyperventilation prior to barbiturates. It is our opinion that the danger of cerebral ischemia from hyperventilation outweighs the risks of barbiturates. Again, if prolonged hyperventilation is used, CBF and/or SjO_2 should be monitored. Hypothermia and decompressive craniectomy are second-tier therapies that are still under investigation. Some centers may advocate the use of hypothermia prior to barbiturates and certainly prior to decompressive craniectomy.

Summary

This chapter has reviewed the basic principles of ICP monitoring, the pathophysiology of the intracranial vault, the regulation of CBF, and management of increased ICP. Most of the advances in our understanding of the pathophysiology and treatment of increased ICP are based on research in traumatic brain injury. Recent advances have contradicted several of the previously held dogmas of neurointensive care, including hypovolemic dehydration and prolonged hyperventilation, and have reemphasized the importance of excellent supportive care in the management of increased ICP. Hopefully, our enhanced understanding of the pathophysiology and treatment of increased ICP will translate into improved outcomes for children with acute central nervous system pathology.

References

1. Indications for intracranial pressure monitoring. Brain Trauma Foundation. *J Neurotrauma* 1996;13:667–679.
2. Bohn DJ, Biggar WD, Smith CR, et al. Influence of hypothermia, barbiturate therapy, and intracranial pressure monitoring on morbidity and mortality after near-drowning. *Crit Care Med* 1986;14:529–534.
3. Sarniak AP, Preston G, Lieh-Lai M, Eisenbrey AB. Intracranial pressure and cerebral perfusion pressure in near-drowning. *Crit Care Med* 1985;13:224–227.
4. Ghajar J. Intracranial pressure monitoring techniques. *New Horizons* 1995;3:395–399.
5. Mayall CG, Archer NH, Lamb VA, et al. Ventriculostomy-related infections. A prospective epidemiologic study. *N Engl J Med* 1984;310:553–559.
6. Narayan RK, Kishore PR, Becker DP, et al. Intracranial pressure: To monitor or not to monitor. *J Neurosurg* 1982;56:650–659.
7. Monro A. *Observations on the Structure and Function of the Nervous System*. Edinburgh: Creech and Johnson; 1783.
8. Kellie G. An account of the appearances observed in the dissection of two of three individuals presumed to have perished in the storm of 3rd, and whose bodies were discovered in the vicinity of Leith on the morning of the 4th November 1821 with some reflections on the pathology of the brain. *Trans Med Chir Sci Edinb* 1824;1:84–169.
9. Fishman RA. Brain edema. *N Engl J Med* 1975;293:706–711.
10. Bouma GJ, Muizelaar JP. Cerebral blood flow, cerebral blood volume, and cerebrovascular reactivity after severe head injury. *J Neurotrauma* 1992;9(suppl 1):333–348.
11. Kontos HA, Wei EP, Navari RM, et al. Responses of cerebral arteries and arterioles to acute hypotension and hypertension. *Am J Physiol* 1978;234:H371-H383.
12. Bouma GJ, Muizelaar JP, Bandoh K, Marmarou A. Blood pressure and intracranial pressure-volume dynamics in severe head injury: Relationship with cerebral blood flow. *J Neurosurg* 1992;77:15–19.
13. Greenberg JH, Alavi A, Reivich M, et al. Local cerebral blood volume response to carbon dioxide in man. *Circ Res* 1978;43:324–331.
14. Paulson OB, Strandgaard S, Edvinsson L. Cerebral autoregulation. *Cerebrovasc Brain Metab Rev* 1990;2:161–192.
15. Kontos HA. Regulation of the cerebral circulation. *Ann Rev Physiol* 1981;43:397–407.
16. Bouma GJ, Muizelaar JP. Cerebral blood flow in severe clinical head injury. *New Horizons* 1995;3:384–394.
17. Guidelines for cerebral perfusion pressure. Brain Trauma Foundation. *J Neurotrauma* 1996;13:693–697.
18. Obrist WD, Langfitt TW, Jaggi JL, et al.

Cerebral blood flow and metabolism in comatose patients with acute head injury: Relationship to intracranial hypertension. *J Neurosurg* 1984;61:241–253.
19. Jaggi JL, Obrist WD, Gennarelli TA, Langfitt TW. Relationship of early cerebral blood flow and metabolism to outcome in acute head injury. *J Neurosurg* 1990;72:176–182.
20. Bouma GJ, Muizelaar JP, Choi SC, et al. Cerebral circulation and metabolism after severe traumatic brain injury: The elusive role of ischemia. *J Neurosurg* 1991;75:685–693.
21. Bouma GJ, Muizelaar JP, Stringer WA, et al. Ultra-early evaluation of regional cerebral blood flow in severely head-injured patients using xenon-enhanced computerized tomography. *J Neurosurg* 1992;77:360–368.
22. Kontos HA, Raper AH, Patterson JLJ. Analysis of vasoactivity of local pH, PCO_2, and bicarbonate on pial vessels. *Stroke* 1977;8:358–360.
23. Reivich M. Arterial PCO_2 and cerebral hemodynamics. *Am J Physiol* 1964;206:25–35.
24. Skippen P, Seear M, Poskitt K, et al. Effect of hyperventilation on regional cerebral blood flow in head-injured children. *Crit Care Med* 1997;25:1402–1409.
25. Feldman Z, Robertson CS. Monitoring of cerebral hemodynamics with jugular bulb catheters. *Crit Care Clin* 1997;13:51–77.
26. Gopinath SP, Robertson CS, Contant CF, et al. Jugular venous desaturation and outcome after head injury. *J Neurol Neurosurg Psychiatry* 1994;57:717–723.
27. Gayle MO, Frewen TC, Armstrong RF, et al. Jugular venous bulb catheterization in infants and children. *Crit Care Med* 1989;17:385–388.
28. Pigula FA, Wald SL, Shackford SR, Vane DW. The effect of hypotension and hypoxia on children with severe head injuries. *J Pediatr Surg* 1993;28:310–316.
29. Chesnut RM, Marshall LF, Klauber MR, et al. The role of secondary brain injury in determining outcome from severe head injury. *J Trauma* 1993;34:216–222.
30. Cooper KR, Boswell PA, Choi SC. Safe use of PEEP in patients with severe head injury. *J Neurosurg* 1985;63:552–555.
31. Chesnut RM. Medical management of severe head injury: Present and future. *New Horizons* 1995;3:581–593.
32. Report of the second task force on blood pressure control in children-1987. *Pediatrics* 1987;79:1–25.
33. Intracranial pressure treatment threshold. Brain Trauma Foundation. *J Neurotrauma* 1996;13:681–683.
34. Zornow MH, Prough DS. Fluid management in patients with traumatic brain injury. *New Horizons* 1995;3:488–498.
35. Pulsinelli WA, Waldman S, Rawlinson D, Plum F. Moderate hyperglycemia augments ischemic brain damage: A neuropathologic study in the rat. *Neurology* 1982;32:1239–1246.
36. Lam AM, Winn HR, Cullen BF, Sundling N. Hyperglycemia and neurological outcome in patients with head injury. *J Neurosurg* 1991;75:545–551.
37. Feldman Z, Kanter MJ, Robertson CS, et al. Effect of head elevation on intracranial pressure, cerebral perfusion pressure, and cerebral blood flow in head-injured patients. *J Neurosurg* 1992;76:207–211.
38. The role of antiseizure prophylaxis following head injury. Brain Trauma Foundation. *J Neurotrauma* 1996;13:731–734.
39. Hsiang JK, Chesnut RM, Crisp CB, et al. Early, routine paralysis for intracranial pressure control in severe head injury: Is it necessary? *Crit Care Med* 1994;22:1471–1476.
40. Bullock R. Mannitol and other diuretics in severe neurotrauma. *J Neurotrauma* 1995;3:448–452.
41. The use of mannitol in severe head injury. Brain Trauma Foundation. *J Neurotrauma* 1996;13:705–709.
42. Paczynski RP. Osmotherapy: Basic concepts and controversies. *Crit Care Clin* 1997;13:105–129.
43. Wilberger JE, Cantella D. High-dose barbiturates for intracranial pressure control. *New Horizons* 1995;3:469–473.
44. Ward JD, Becker DP, Miller JD, et al. Failure of prophylactic barbiturate coma in the treatment of severe head injury. *J Neurosurg* 1985;62:383–388.
45. Schwartz ML, Tator CH, Rowed DW, et al. The University of Toronto head injury treatment study: A prospective, randomized comparison of pentobarbital and mannitol. *Can J Neurol Sci* 1984;11:434–440.
46. Eisenberg HM, Frankowski RF, Constant CF, et al. High-dose barbiturate control of elevated intracranial pressure in patients with severe head injury. *J Neurosurg* 1988;69:15–23.
47. The use of barbiturates in the control of intracranial hypertension. Brain Trauma Foundation. *J Neurotrauma* 1996;13:711–714.
48. Clifton GL. Hypothermia and hyperbaric oxygen as treatment modalities for severe head injury. *New Horizons* 1995;3:474–478.
49. Clifton GL, Allen S, Barrodale P, et al. A phase II study of moderate hypothermia in

severe brain injury. *J Neurotrauma* 1993;10: 263–271.
50. Marion DW, Obrist WD, Carlier PM, et al. The use of moderate therapeutic hypothermia for patients with severe head injuries: A preliminary report. *J Neurosurg* 1993;79:354–362.
51. Marion DW, Penrod LE, Kelsey SF, et al. Treatment of traumatic brain injury with moderate hypothermia. *N Engl J Med* 1997; 336:540–546.
52. Raichle ME, Posner JB, Plum F. Cerebral blood flow during and after hyperventilation. *Arch Neurol* 1970;23:394–403.
53. Muizelaar JP, Marmarou A, DeSalles AA, et al. Cerebral blood flow and metabolism in severely head-injured children. Part 1: Relationship with GCS score, outcome, ICP and PVI. *J Neurosurg* 1989;71:63–71.
54. Marion DW, Darby J, Yonas H. Acute regional cerebral blood flow changes caused by severe head injury. *J Neurosurg* 1991;74: 407–414.
55. Muizelaar JP, Marmarou A, Ward JD, et al. Adverse effect of prolonged hyperventilation in patients with severe head injury: A randomized clinical trial. *J Neurosurg* 1991; 75:731–739.
56. The use of hyperventilation in the acute management of severe traumatic brain injury. Brain Trauma Foundation. *J Neurotrauma* 1996;13:699–703.
57. Marion DW, Firlik A, McLaughlin MR. Hyperventilation therapy of severe traumatic brain injury. *New Horizons* 1995;3:439–447.
58. The role of glucocorticoids in the treatment of severe head injury. Brain Trauma Foundation. *J Neurotrauma* 1996;13:715–718.
59. Miller JD, Sakalas R, Ward JD, et al. Methylprednisolone treatment in patients with brain tumours. *Neurosurgery* 1977;1:114–117.
60. Polins RS, Shaffrey ME, Bogaev CA, et al. Decompressive bifrontal craniectomy in the treatment of severe refractory posttraumatic cerebral edema. *Neurosurgery* 1997; 41:84–89.
61. Critical pathway for the treatment of established intracranial hypertension. Brain Trauma Foundation. *J Neurotrauma* 1996;13: 719–720.

Chapter 11

The Use of Sedative/Analgesic and Neuromuscular Blocking Agents in Children in the Pediatric Intensive Care Unit

Joseph D. Tobias, MD

Introduction

Several factors may cause anxiety, fear, and pain in children during their stay in the pediatric intensive care unit (PICU). Precipitating factors include separation from parents, invasive procedures, disruption of the usual day-night cycle, and the presence of unfamiliar people and machines. Although reassurance and parental presence may alleviate some of the distress associated with the PICU,[1] pharmacologic intervention is frequently required.

Despite the use and trial of several different sedative agents (Table 1), no single agent can be expected to be effective in all patients and to meet all of the criteria of the ideal agent (Table 2). Therefore, physicians caring for children in the PICU should attempt to become familiar with several different agents, which will allow them to switch from one agent to another when the first-line drug is either ineffective or leads to adverse effects.

The importance of aggressive sedation and analgesia cannot be overemphasized. The importance of adequate relief of pain and anxiety is highlighted by recent investigations that have demonstrated the impact of postoperative analgesia on patient outcome. While many of these reports may be considered preliminary, they are part of what may be considered a revolution in the recognition and treatment of pain and anxiety in children.[2] The issues of pain management extend beyond the obvious humanitarian issues, with recent clinical studies demonstrating that the level of analgesia (both intraoperatively and postoperatively) may impact on postoperative outcome. These studies focus on the adverse effects of the postsurgical stress response, which has been characterized as a metabolic, hormonal, and hemodynamic response to major injury or surgery.[3] The neuroendocrine cascade with the release of catecholamines, cortisol, glucagon, and other catabolic hormones results in increased oxygen consumption, increased carbon dioxide production, hyperglycemia, and a generalized catabolic state with a negative nitrogen balance.[4] Additional effects, including tachycardia, systemic hypertension, and increases in pulmonary artery pressure, may result from the liberation of endogenous catecholamines. Anand et al[5] have demonstrated that the postsurgical stress response occurs even in preterm infants, and that its magnitude is greatest in groups of patients

Table 1

Agents for Sedation in the PICU

Inhalational anesthetic agents
Nitrous oxide
Benzodiazepines
Opioids
Phenothiazines
Antihistamines
Chloral hydrate
Etomidate
Ketamine
Barbiturates
Propofol

PICU = pediatric intensive care unit.

Table 2

Suggested Properties of the Ideal Agent for PICU Sedation

1. Rapid onset
2. Predictable duration of activity
3. No active metabolites
4. Effects dissipate rapidly when agent discontinued
5. Multiple options for route of delivery
6. Easy to titrate by continuous infusion
7. Limited effects on cardiorespiratory function
8. Effects and duration not altered by renal or hepatic disease
9. No interference with effect or metabolism by other drugs
10. Wide therapeutic index

PICU = pediatric intensive care unit.

with the highest mortality.[6] These investigators were also the first to demonstrate that alterations in intraoperative and postoperative analgesic techniques may influence patient outcome.[5,7] A prospective comparison of high-dose sufentanil versus halothane-morphine anesthesia was performed in infants undergoing cardiac surgery.[7] Neonates were randomized to receive anesthesia with either high-dose sufentanil followed by continuous sufentanil infusion for 24 hours following surgery, or halothane-morphine intraoperatively followed by intermittent morphine and diazepam for postoperative sedation and analgesia. There was a significant decrease in the parameters of the postsurgical stress response in infants who received sufentanil, as well as a significant reduction in the incidence of metabolic acidosis, sepsis, disseminated intravascular coagulation, and postoperative mortality (0 of 30 in the sufentanil group versus 4 of 15 in the halothane-morphine group).

In addition to effects mediated by the postsurgical stress response, pain following thoracic and abdominal surgery can have significant deleterious effects on respiratory function including decreased tidal volume, functional residual capacity, and forced expiratory volume.[8,9] These changes, combined with decreased cough effort and the residual effects of anesthetic agents, may result in ventilation-perfusion mismatch with postoperative hypoxemia and respiratory failure. Inadequate analgesia may also delay postoperative ambulation and, thus, further compromise postoperative pulmonary function and further increase the risk of postoperative pulmonary complications.[10,11] An additional benefit of adequate postoperative analgesia is that it partially prevents the deleterious effects of pain on pulmonary function and encourages earlier postoperative ambulation.[12,13] With such effects in mind, the need for providing postoperative analgesia becomes readily apparent.

The recent clinical investigations emphasize the need for the aggressive treatment of anxiety and pain, even in our youngest patients. Although the majority of studies have focused on a single group of patients (ie, postoperative cardiac patients), the PICU physician is faced with a much more diverse group of patients with various medical and postsurgical problems. Several unanswered questions exist concerning the stress response and its relationship to the PICU patient, including: does it even exist in this group of patients or is it merely a postoperative phenomenon? Which agents blunt it most effectively? Should we use synthetic opioids as Anand and colleagues have done, or are other agents equally effective in blunting the consequences of the stress response? Further studies are certainly needed to address many of these issues.

Prior to the use of sedative or analgesic agents, physiologic causes of agitation such as hypoxemia, hypercarbia, and cerebral hypoperfusion from a low cardiac output state should be excluded. Although the PICU setting provides the optimal environment for monitoring patients, any of the agents used for sedation and analgesia can have deleterious effects on cardiorespiratory function, and therefore close monitoring of patients in accordance with the guidelines of the American Academy of Pediatrics is recommended.[14]

Due to the diversity in patient population and the varied indications for these agents, it is not possible to provide a "cookbook" with definite guidelines for sedation and analgesia. Sedative and analgesic agents should not be dosed strictly on a per-kilogram basis like other medications such as antibiotics. Dosing recommendations are meant as guidelines for starting doses. The actual amount administered should be titrated up or down to achieve the desired effect. The need to titrate the dose up and/or down is illustrated by a recent study evaluating fentanyl infusion rates required to achieve sedation in the PICU patient.[15] The authors noted a wide variability in infusion requirements (0.47 to 10.3 μg/kg/h) needed to achieve the desired level of sedation.[15] Wide interpatient variability was also noted in regard to the volume of distribution and terminal elimination half-life.

Aside from the interpatient variability in dosing requirements, there is a wide range of indications for analgesic and sedative agents in the PICU. While analgesia is certainly required for postoperative patients, sedation and analgesia may also be required during the performance of various invasive or diagnostic procedures, to improve the efficacy of mechanical ventilation and to alleviate the distress associated with acute medical illnesses. Sedation during mechanical ventilation is becoming increasingly important with newer modalities of mechanical ventilation for patients with severe lung disease including permissive hypercapnia, reverse inspiratory-to-expiratory (I:E) ratio ventilation, and high-frequency techniques. Sedation may also be used as a therapeutic tool in the treatment of raised intracranial pressure (ICP) or to prevent pulmonary vasospasm following cardiac surgical procedures.

Significant variability is also present when considering the length of time during which sedation is needed. The duration of sedation may be brief (<15 minutes) for an invasive procedure or more commonly, it may be required for days or weeks during mechanical ventilation or following acute traumatic injuries. While the intravenous route is usually chosen in the PICU patient, in certain situations alternative, nonintravenous routes may be necessary. In addition to the choice of drug and the route of administration, the mode (continuous or intermittent) must be determined. This chapter reviews the various agents available for sedation and analgesia in the PICU patient and the options for route of administration and mode of delivery. This is followed by a review of indications and applications of neuromuscular blocking agents (NMBAs) in the PICU patient.

Agents for Sedation

While opioids and benzodiazepines remain the most frequently used agents for sedation,[16] several alternatives are available including the inhalational anesthetic agents, nitrous oxide, ketamine, propofol, and the barbiturates. Lessons learned from previously used agents such as etomidate emphasize the need for the careful evaluation of new agents. While etomidate was chosen due to its lack of adverse effects on cardiovascular function, its use by continuous infusion for prolonged sedation has been abandoned following the discovery of increased mortality related to its depressant effects on adrenocortical function. Despite this effect, etomidate remains a useful agent, because of its lack of effects on cardiovascular function and its beneficial effects on the cerebral metabolic rate for oxygen, for providing sedation during endotracheal intubation in the patient with increased ICP and altered cardiovascular function (see chapter 1).

Inhalational Anesthetic Agents

The inhalational anesthetic agents in common clinical use include halothane, enflurane, isoflurane, sevoflurane, and desflurane. Although their use is limited in this country, certain centers in Europe have significant experience with these agents (most commonly isoflurane).[17,18] While halothane, enflurane, and isoflurane have all been used for sedation in ICU patients, only the latter is now commonly used. Problems with halothane include its direct negative inotropic effects, arrhythmogenic properties especially in the setting of increased catecholamines or when used in conjunction with other medications (aminophylline), and most importantly, hepatitis, related to an immunologic reaction directed against an oxidative metabolite, trifluoroacetic acid. Although the latter problem has been reported with the other inhalational agents including isoflurane, its incidence is much less common with isoflurane due to its limited metabolism.

Concerns about enflurane relate to its similar negative inotropic effect and the release of significant amounts of fluoride during its metabolism. Fluoride, at increased concentrations (>50 μmol/L), can be nephrotoxic, resulting in decreases in glomerular filtration rate and nephrogenic diabetes insipidus. As less than 1% of isoflurane is metabolized, the issues of fluoride toxicity are minimal.

The major cardiovascular action of isoflurane is peripheral vasodilatation; it therefore maintains cardiac output better than either halothane or enflurane. Reflex tachycardia can lead to increases in myocardial oxygen demand and an imbalance in the myocardial oxygen delivery/demand ratio in susceptible patients. Coronary steal has also been suggested to occur in susceptible patients. It should therefore be used cautiously in patients who are at risk for myocardial ischemia or in whom tachycardia and a decrease in systemic vascular resistance may be detrimental.

Advocates of the use of inhalational anesthetic agents emphasize their benefits, including a rapid onset, rapid awakening upon discontinuation, and ease of control of the depth of sedation. Despite their apparent efficacy and benefits, several logistical problems may limit the usefulness of these agents outside of the operating room. Rules and regulations abound as to who should regulate the inspired concentration of the agent and, in most centers, the nursing staff is not permitted to alter the vaporizer setting. Effective scavenging devices are needed to prevent environmental pollution. Aside from this concern, delivery of these agents requires specialized equipment. Since moving an anesthesia machine into the ICU is not always practical, most ICUs use an ICU ventilator with a vaporizer attached to it. These ventilators can be equipped to permit effective scavenging of the exhaled agent by attaching to conventional wall suction.

The inhalational anesthetic agents are triggering agents for malignant hyperthermia. Cerebral vasodilatation may be seen, leading to increases in ICP. This effect is least common with isoflurane and may be partially prevented by hyperventilation ($PaCO_2$ 25 to 30 mm Hg).[19,20] However, with the availability of other agents (see below), the inhalational anesthetic agents cannot be recommended for continuous sedation in patients with altered intracranial compliance. One beneficial effect of isoflurane on the central nervous system (CNS) is a reported cerebral protective effect during periods of hypoxemia related to alterations in cerebral blood flow or arterial oxygenation.[21] Due to these effects, isoflurane remains the inhalational agent of choice for neuroanesthesia. Aside from these physiologic actions, the inhalational agents alter the metabolism of lidocaine, β-adrenergic blocking agents, benzodiazepines, local anesthetics, and other agents administered in the PICU setting.[22]

Additionally, there is limited clinical experience with these agents in the pediatric population. Arnold et al[23] administered isoflurane for sedation during mechanical ventilation in 10 patients, ranging in age from 3 weeks to 19 years. Effective sedation was achieved in all patients without notable adverse effects on end-organ function. The highest fluoride concentration was 26.1 μmol/L and no evidence of renal toxicity was noted. Despite their anecdotal success in children, the above mentioned concerns of delivery and scavenging with these agents will limit their routine use for sedation in the PICU. Cost issues must also be considered. Aside from the cost of the specialized equipment, isoflurane is quite expensive, with an average daily cost ranging from $50 to $150 per day depending on the inspired concentration and the size of the patient. Due to their beneficial effects on airway reactivity, these agents may be used as therapeutic agents in the treatment of refractory status asthmaticus.[24] Additional reports suggest their therapeutic potential for refractory status epilepticus.[25]

Nitrous Oxide

Nitrous oxide meets many of the criteria for desirable characteristics of the ultimate agent for sedation (Table 2). It has a rapid onset of action, is easy and inexpensive to use, and most importantly, its effects dissipate rapidly once it is discontinued. Due to its relative insolubility in blood with a low blood-gas partition coefficient, nitrous oxide reaches a steady-state alveolar concentration in 5 to 10 minutes, thereby accounting for its rapid onset of action. In the operating room it is delivered via an anesthesia machine in varying concentrations mixed with oxygen. For use outside of the operating room, it may delivered as a preset concentration from a tank that contains a mixture of nitrous oxide and oxygen, or it can be blended with oxygen from separate tanks. The premixed tanks are commercially available as a 50% nitrous oxide/50% oxygen mixture. If such tanks are not available, nitrous oxide and oxygen may be blended together to achieve the desired concentration. When this is done, the machines must have the same safety measures as used in the operating room. These include a failsafe mechanism so that the nitrous oxide flow is shut off when the oxygen pressure falls. Without such a safety feature it is possible to deliver 100% nitrous oxide! A second safety feature is an interlocking connection between the oxygen and nitrous oxide flow meters so that a hypoxic mixture of the two gases cannot be delivered. This permits, at most, the delivery of 70% nitrous oxide, thereby ensuring the delivery of an FiO_2 of at least 0.3.

Issues of environmental pollution are a definite concern with nitrous oxide, and scavenging devices are required. Reported problems associated with prolonged exposure to nitrous oxide include reduced fertility with a increased risk of spontaneous abortion,[26] chronic myeloneuropathy, and megaloblastic anemia. The latter two problems are related to the effects of nitrous oxide on vitamin B_{12} metabolism. Due to its potential for abuse, certain precautions are required for storing nitrous oxide that may add logistical problems due to the size of the tanks.

Aside from its effects on health care workers, repeated or prolonged exposure impacts on the patient. Short-term exposure of nitrous oxide may cause alterations in cardiorespiratory function, and its use is contraindicated in patients with altered mental status or respiratory failure. Effects on the CNS include alterations in cerebral blood flow and increases in ICP. Although the reports are somewhat conflicting, nitrous oxide generally has little effect on cardiac function in patients with normal myocardial function, while decreases in both cardiac output and blood pressure may occur in patients with myocardial dysfunction.[27] More importantly, significant increases in pulmonary artery pressure have been reported with nitrous oxide administration.[28] Since concentrations of 40% to 70% are needed to provide analgesia, nitrous oxide cannot be used in patients who require a high concentration of inspired oxygen.

An additional concern is the effect of prolonged exposure of nitrous oxide on the hematopoietic system, including bone marrow suppression, megaloblastic anemia, and alterations in white cell function/motility.[29-32] These effects and the chronic myelopathy are related to nitrous oxide's inhibitory effects on vitamin B_{12} metabolism that lead to defective function of the enzyme methionine synthetase.

Due to its low solubility in blood, nitrous oxide will rapidly diffuse into air-containing spaces. It is therefore contraindicated in the presence of a loculated collection of air such as a pneumothorax or pneumocephalus. Nitrous oxide will also diffuse into the middle ear and will increase pressure in patients with eustachian tube dysfunction, and it will also diffuse into the cuff of the endotracheal tube. Due to these limitations, the prolonged use of nitrous oxide is not recommended and therefore has little role for prolonged sedation in the PICU patient. It may have some application for sedation during brief invasive or painful procedures in older children and adolescents. It should only be used by persons trained in its administration and with the proper monitoring, including a measure of the inspired oxygen concentration and of the patient's oxygen saturation, as the delivery of a hypoxic gas mixture is possible with improper use or with malfunction of the equipment.

Benzodiazepines

In many institutions, benzodiazapines remain the most commonly used drugs for sedation in the PICU. Their mechanism of action is through the facilitation, in the CNS, of the activity of the inhibitory neurotransmitter, γ-aminobutyric acid (GABA). Binding of the benzodiazepine molecule to the α-subunit of the GABA receptor facilitates binding of GABA to the β-subunit, leading to increased chloride conduction across the neuronal membrane and subsequent hyperpolarization.[33] Benzodiazepines have no intrinsic analgesic properties[34]; therefore the concomitant administration of an opioid is necessary in situations requiring analgesia.

Three benzodiazepines are commonly used in this country for sedation: diazepam, midazolam, and lorazepam. For many years, diazepam was the agent of choice for sedation in the ICU. Its high lipid solubility results in a rapid onset of action and it is effective by both the oral and intravenous route. However, due to its low solubility in water, it is administered in a solution of propylene glycol, which can cause pain on injection and thrombophlebitis when administered through a peripheral infusion. This has recently become less of a problem, with the introduction of a newer preparation that eliminates the propylene glycol diluent and delivers diazepam in a lipid base. More importantly, prolonged sedation may follow repeated administration due to its long elimination half-life and hypnotically active metabolites (oxazepam and n-desmethyldiazepam). Both of these agents have elimination half-lives that far exceed that of the parent compound and thereby limit their use for repeated administration in the PICU population.

Midazolam is an imidazobenzodiazepine with a rapid onset of action and a short elimination half-life. Due to its short half-life, the use of midazolam generally requires its administration by continuous infusion, except in brief invasive procedures. Several investigations have documented the efficacy of midazolam infusions for sedation in the ICU in starting doses ranging from 0.05 to 0.2 mg/kg/h.[35-37]

Certain medications or underlying conditions may potentiate the effects of midazolam through either alterations in metabolism or decreases in protein binding. Midazolam is metabolized by the P450 system of the liver, and is subject to possible drug interactions with other agents such as cimetidine that may inhibit its metabolism and thereby increase its serum concentration. Alterations in protein binding may also alter the effect of midazolam. Heparin increases the free fraction of midazolam by displacing it from protein binding sites. The free fraction is also increased by a factor of 2 to 3 in patients with hepatic and/or renal dysfunction,[38,39] necessitating adjustments of the loading dose and infusion regimens. The major disadvantage of midazolam is the cost, ranging from $50 to $100 per day, in a 20-kg patient requiring an infusion of 0.1 to 0.2 mg/kg/h.

While intravenous administration is generally the route chosen in the PICU, several investigators have described novel routes of delivery for midazolam including oral, transmucosal (nasal, rectal), sublingual, and subcutaneous.[40-43] Due to limited absorption, increased doses are required for these alternative routes of delivery (Table 3). These alternative routes are rarely used for ongoing sedation in the PICU, but may have some role for one-time sedation for brief diagnostic/invasive procedures. One drawback of the nonintravenous administration is the need to use the intravenous preparation, which contains the preservative benzyl alcohol. This has a bitter taste, necessitating mixture of the drug in a solution in an attempt to mask its flavor. Benzyl alcohol can also cause significant discomfort when applied to mucous membranes, causing burning and discomfort with intranasal administration.

Lorazepam is the other water-soluble

Table 3

Suggested Dosing Guidelines for Midazolam Administration

Route	Dose (mg/kg)	Maximum Dose (mg)	Reference Number
Oral	0.5–0.7	20	41
Rectal	1.0	20	40
Nasal	0.2–0.4	10	42,43
Sublingual	0.2	10	42
Intravenous	0.03–0.05	2*	35–37

*With intravenous administration, the dose can be repeated every 3 minutes and titrated to effect.

benzodiazepine that may find some role in PICU sedation. While midazolam's short half-life necessitates its administration by continuous infusion, lorazepam's duration of action is 2 to 4 hours, allowing for a longer duration of action following intermittent, on-demand (prn) dosing. A second advantage of lorazepam over other benzodiazepines including midazolam is that it is metabolized by glucoronyl transferase and not by the P450 system. Medications known to alter the P450 system (anticonvulsants, rifampin, cimetidine) have no effect on the pharmacokinetics of lorazepam. In patients with advanced liver disease, phase II reactions (glucoronyl transferase) are better preserved than phase I reactions (P450 system). Additionally, lorazepam has no active metabolites. Therefore, its serum concentrations (and hence its sedative effects) should be less variable than those of midazolam, especially in patients with altered hepatic and renal function.

While there is little information concerning lorazepam use in children, both intermittent and continuous infusion techniques may be used for sedation. For intermittent administration, 0.025 to 0.05 mg/kg (maximum starting dose of 2 mg) can be administered every 2 to 4 hours. For continuous infusions, the starting dose is 0.025 mg/kg/h (maximum of 2 mg/h). As with other sedative agents, the infusion rate should be supplemented with prn bolus doses, and adjusted accordingly.

While the benzodiazepines are generally well tolerated with limited effects on cardiorespiratory function,[44] certain situations may arise that necessitate the administration of a reversal agent. Flumazenil is a GABA antagonist and has been marketed as a reversal agent for the benzodiazepines. In a recent clinical trial, reversal of sedation was observed following the administration of flumazenil in 14 of 15 patients sedated with midazolam.[45] However, since the half-life of flumazenil is less than that of midazolam, resedation occurred in seven of the patients. Therefore, continued observation of patients is necessary when flumazenil is used to reverse life-threatening adverse effects. Additionally, seizures may occur due to flumazenil's antagonistic effects at the GABA receptor. Seizures may be more common in patients receiving long-term benzodiazepines or other medications that are known to lower the seizure threshold.[46] In such situations the use of flumazenil is contraindicated.

As with opioids (see below), the prolonged administration of benzodiazepines may result in physical dependency with the development of an abstinence syndrome if these agents are abruptly discontinued.[47,48] This can be prevented by slowly tapering the intravenous administration of the drug or switching from intravenous midazolam to an orally active agent with a longer half-life, such as lorazepam, which eliminates the need for intravenous access.[49] Another option is to slowly taper the infusion of midazolam, but to switch to subcutaneous administration at an equivalent dose and thereby eliminate the need to maintain intravenous access,[50] which may become problematic following prolonged admissions to the PICU.

Ketamine

Ketamine, an intravenous anesthetic agent that is chemically related to phencyclidine, was first described for clinical use by Domino et al[51] in 1965. One of the unique properties of ketamine that makes it particularly attractive is the provision of both amnesia and analgesia. It was initially used as an induction agent for general anesthesia and then later applied as an intraoperative anesthetic[52,53] and postoperative analgesic.[54,55]

Ketamine is a racemic mixture of the

two optical (+,-) isomers. Metabolism occurs primarily by hepatic N-methylation to norketamine with further metabolism by hydroxylation pathways and subsequent urinary excretion. The hepatic metabolic product, norketamine, retains roughly one third of the analgesic and sedative properties of the parent compound. As ketamine is primarily dependent on hepatic metabolism, doses should be reduced in patients with hepatic dysfunction.

Additional advantages of ketamine include preservation of cardiovascular function and limited effects on respiratory mechanics in the majority of patients.[56,57] Ketamine produces a dose-related increase in heart rate and blood pressure, which are thought to be mediated through the sympathetic nervous system and the release of endogenous catecholamines.[58] Although the indirect sympathomimetic effects generally overshadow ketamine's direct negative inotropic properties, hypotension may be seen in patients with diminished myocardial contractility.[59,60] In these patients, it is postulated that ketamine's direct negative inotropic properties predominate because endogenous catecholamine stores have been depleted.

An issue of utmost importance for children with congenital heart disease is the effect of ketamine on pulmonary vascular resistance (PVR). This issue is somewhat controversial, as mixed reports have appeared in the literature. Increased PVR has been reported in adults, and avoidance of ketamine has been recommended for patients with pulmonary hypertension.[61] These initial studies, however, were performed with spontaneous ventilation, and the alterations in PVR may have been related to increases in $PaCO_2$ and not the direct result of ketamine on the pulmonary vasculature. Morray et al[62] found statistically significant increases in pulmonary artery pressure (20.6 to 22.8 mm Hg) and PVR after ketamine administration in spontaneously breathing patients. In contrast, Hickey et al[63] found no change in PVR in intubated infants with minimal ventilatory support (4 breaths per minute and FiO_2 of 0.4). The latter study included 14 patients: 7 with normal and 7 with elevated baseline PVR. Pending further investigations, ketamine should be used cautiously in patients with pulmonary hypertension, especially during spontaneous ventilation.

Respiratory function is generally well maintained during ketamine administration. Functional residual capacity, minute ventilation, and tidal volume have been reported to be unchanged following ketamine administration,[64] while other studies have demonstrated improved pulmonary compliance and decreased bronchospasm.[65] These effects have also been attributed to the release of endogenous catecholamines.[65] Although minute ventilation is generally well maintained, elevations of $PaCO_2$ and a shift to the right of the carbon dioxide response curve may occur.[66] Furthermore, in higher doses, ketamine can cause apnea. Controversy remains, concerning ketamine's effects on protective airway reflexes. Although clinical use and experimental studies suggest that these reflexes are maintained,[67] aspiration and laryngospasm have been reported following ketamine in spontaneously breathing patients without a protected airway.[68] An additional effect that may impact on airway patency is increased oral secretions. The concomitant administration of an antisialogogue such as atropine or glycopyrrolate is recommended because ketamine increases salivary and bronchial gland secretion through stimulation of central cholinergic receptors.

Ketamine may also increase ICP and therefore should be avoided in patients who are at risk for intracranial hypertension.[69] Increases in ICP result from direct cerebral vasodilatation, mediated through central cholinergic receptors and not secondary to alterations in cerebral metabolic rate or changes in $PaCO_2$.[70-72] The adverse effect related to ketamine that receives the most attention is the occurrence of emergence phenomena or hallucinations. Emergence phenomena, which are dose-related, are more common in older patients, and their incidence can be decreased by the preadministration of a benzodiazepine.[73] Emergence phenomena are thought to be the result of an alteration of auditory and visual relays in the inferior colliculus and the medical geniculate nucleus that lead to the misinterpretation of visual and auditory stimuli.[73] The administration of a benzodiazepine (lorazepam or midazolam) 5 minutes prior to the administration of ketamine is generally effective for preventing emergence phenomena and allows the use of ketamine even in older patients.

Due to its favorable effects on cardiorespiratory function, ketamine may be quite useful for patients who require sedation during mechanical ventilation and develop myocardial depression with opioids or benzodiazepines. For this purpose, a bolus dose of 1 to 2 mg/kg is followed by a continuous infusion of 1.0 mg/kg/h and increased or decreased as needed.[74] An additional option is to combine ketamine and midazolam in a single solution (ketamine 10 mg/mL and midazolam 1 mg/mL). The infusion is then started at 0.1 mL/kg/h, which provides ketamine 1 mg/kg/h and midazolam 0.1 mg/kg/h. Ketamine also proves to be a useful agent to provide sedation and analgesia during the performance of painful invasive procedures, especially in spontaneously breathing patients. For this purpose, an anticholinergic agent (glycopyrrolate 5 µg/kg) and midazolam (0.03 to 0.5 mg/kg) are administered intravenously followed by incremental boluses of ketamine (0.5 mg/kg) every 2 to 3 minutes as needed.

Propofol

Propofol is an intravenous anesthetic agent of the alkyl phenol family that is chemically unrelated to barbiturates and other commonly used anesthetic induction agents.[75] Like the barbiturates, it is a sedative/amnestic agent and possesses no analgesic properties. As such, it should be combined with an opioid infusion in patients who require analgesia. Due to its rapid onset, rapid recovery time, and lack of active metabolites, it remains a popular agent for sedation in adult ICUs.[76,77] When compared with midazolam for sedation in adult patients, propofol was found to have shorter recovery times, more rapid titration efficiency, and reduced posthypnotic obtundation with faster weaning from mechanical ventilation.[76] Favorable effects on CNS dynamics include a decreased cerebral metabolic rate for oxygen and ICP. The latter effect is much the same as that seen with the barbiturates and etomidate.

With its increased use for sedation and anesthetic induction in the ICU, certain adverse effects have been reported (Table 4). Its cardiovascular effects are similar to those of the barbiturates and include peripheral vasodilation and negative inotropic properties.[78] These effects are particularly prominent following bolus administration. Although well tolerated in patients with adequate cardiovascular function, propofol should be used cautiously in hemodynamically unstable patients. In addition to its negative inotropic properties, it may increase central vagal tone leading to bradycardia and even asystole when combined with other medications that are known to alter cardiac chronotropic function (fentanyl, succinylcholine).[79] Although the relative bradycardia is generally considered a beneficial effect in patients at risk for myocardial ischemia, it may be a significant deterrent to the use of propofol in patients with fixed stroke volumes whose cardiac output is heart rate-dependent.

Additional concerns regarding use of propofol include the reports of unusual neurologic manifestations including opisthotonic posturing, myoclonic movements (especially in children), and convulsions.[80-83] More recently, unexplained metabolic acidosis and fatal cardiac failure have been reported in children with respiratory infections

Table 4

Adverse Effects Described with Propofol

Hypotension:
   negative inotropic effects
   vasodilation
   bradycardia
Neurologic sequelae:
   opisthotonic posturing
   seizures
   myoclonus
Anaphylactoid reactions
Metabolic acidosis and caridac failure
Pain on injection
Bacterial contamination of solution
Hyperlipidemia

who received propofol.[84,85] Although the patients in the initial report were receiving higher than recommended doses (up to 13.6 mg/kg/h), pending further evaluation, use of propofol can no longer be recommended for continuous infusion in the PICU patient younger than 10 to 12 years of age. Due to the above mentioned beneficial properties, it may have some role in providing short-term sedation (24 to 48 hours) in older patients.

Additional problems relate to the delivery of propofol in a lipid emulsion. Significant pain on injection is commonly seen with administration through a peripheral infusion. Variable success in decreasing the incidence of pain has been reported with various maneuvers including the preadministration of lidocaine, mixing the lidocaine and propofol in a single solution, diluting the concentration of the propofol, or cooling it prior to bolus administration. More importantly, anaphylactoid reactions have occasionally been reported.[86] These may be more likely in patients with a history of egg allergy. Unlike other medications used for continuous sedation, the initial production of propofol did not contain preservatives. Laboratory investigation has demonstrated that the lipid emulsion serves as a suitable culture media for bacteria[87] while systemic bacteremia and wound infections have been linked to extrinsically contaminated propofol.[88] A recent change in the preparation has included the addition of edetic acid (EDTA) as a preservative, which may limit the risk of bacterial contamination and growth. Despite the recent changes, meticulous aseptic technique is required when using propofol, and opened but unused vials should be disposed of promptly and not saved for later use. The infusion vial and tubing should be changed every 12 hours during continuous infusion for ICU sedation. Due to its short half-life and brief duration of action, except for the during briefest of procedures, propofol is used as a continuous infusion.

Other problems related to the high lipid content of the solution have included hypertriglyceridemia[89] and, more recently, its anecdotal association with increasing $PaCO_2$ during mechanical ventilation.[90] The latter report describes a patient who required up to 200 μg/kg/min of propofol to maintain an adequate level of sedation. This resulted in a total caloric intake of 4500 calories per day (53% from the lipid in the propofol diluent). The $PaCO_2$ increased from 67 mm Hg to a maximum value of 78 mm Hg despite increasing the minute ventilation from 11 to 13 L/min. The lipid content of propofol should be taken into consideration when calculating the patient's daily caloric intake. Propofol infusions at 2 mg/kg/h provide roughly 0.5 g/kg/day of fat.

Barbiturates

The barbiturates are one of the oldest classes of agents used for sedation in the PICU. As with many of the agents described, their effects on cardiorespiratory function are dose-dependent. In healthy patients, sedative doses have minimal effects on respiratory drive and airway protective reflexes while excessive doses can produce apnea and hypotension. The cardiorespiratory depressant effects are additive when the barbiturates are used with other agents (ie, opioids). Cardiovascular depression is related to both peripheral vasodilation and a direct negative inotropic effect.

Several different barbiturate agents are available and are most easily classified according to the duration of activity. Short-acting agents include methohexital, thiopental, and thiamylal. These agents have a duration of action of 5 to 10 minutes and are usually used by intravenous bolus administration for brief procedures such as endotracheal intubation. When a more prolonged effect is needed, a continuous infusion may be used to maintain constant plasma levels. Longer acting agents with half-lives of 6 to 12 hours include pentobarbital and phenobarbital.

Beneficial physiologic effects include decrease of the cerebral metabolic rate for oxygen with a reduction in cerebral blood flow and ICP. The barbiturates are potent anticonvulsants and may be used to treat status epilepticus that is unresponsive to other agents. While still controversial, it has also been suggested that they may provide some degree of cerebral protection during periods of hypoxia or hypoperfusion.

Although the barbiturates are most commonly used for their therapeutic effects (as anticonvulsants or to decrease ICP), these agents may provide an effective alternative for providing sedation in the PICU when the usual combination of benzodiazepines and opioids, either alone or in combination, fails to provide adequate sedation.[91] One particularly difficult situation is the provision of sedation during extracorporeal membrane oxygenation (ECMO). While fentanyl is the most commonly used agent, rapid tolerance and the need for dose escalation has been noted so that doses of 30 to 50 µg/kg/min are not uncommon. Pentobarbital may be an effective alternative to more conventional agents for sedating pediatric patients during ECMO. For PICU sedation, a loading dose of pentobarbital (1 to 2 mg/kg) is followed by a continuous infusion of 1 to 2 mg/kg/h.

As these agents do have negative inotropic effects, they should be used cautiously in patients with cardiovascular dysfunction. The risks of adverse cardiovascular effects can be limited by slow administration (over 5 minutes) of the bolus doses. Another problem that may limit the use of barbiturates is that the solution is alkaline (pH 9 to 11), and is thus incompatible with other medications and parenteral alimentation solutions. Therefore, the barbiturates should be administered separately from other medications. Significant local erythema can occur with subcutaneous infiltration. Despite such problems, pentobarbital may be effective if the usual benzodiazepine/opioid combination becomes ineffective.

Opioids

Although generally used for analgesia, opioids also possess sedative properties and are often chosen as first-line drugs for sedation in the PICU patient, even when true analgesia is not required. This may be especially relevant depending on the age of the patient. Clinical experience suggests that the opioids may be more efficacious in neonates and infants. This may relate to the well developed endogenous opioid receptor system of the neonate. Opioids provide analgesia and not amnesia, even with high-dose fentanyl (50 to 75 µg/kg) techniques commonly used during repair of congenital heart defects. Additional agents are needed when amnesia is desired (ie, for the toddler or older child who is receiving NMBAs; see below).

With the administration of opioids, three choices must be made, including: 1) the opioid to be used; 2) the mode of administration; and 3) the route of administration. While the mode of administration is usually given little emphasis, it may be the most important of the three choices. Sedative and/or analgesic agents are most effective when administered in such a manner as to maintain a steady-state serum concentration. Without a serum concentration of the drug, an effect cannot occur, and sedation or analgesia will be inadequate. Choices for mode of administration include intermittent, on-demand (commonly known as prn dosing), fixed interval dosing whereby a fixed amount of the medication is administered at predetermined intervals not in response to the patient's need, a continuous infusion, or the use of a patient-controlled analgesia (PCA) device. The prn mode is generally considered antiquated and is the least likely to provide adequate sedation and analgesia for the patient. More efficacious modes include a PCA device or a continuous infusion supplemented by bolus doses.

While the intravenous route is generally chosen for the PICU patient, certain situations may arise that preclude or interfere with intravenous administration. One novel nonintravenous route to opioid delivery is the development of transdermal fentanyl. Although its efficacy has been demonstrated in adults,[92,93] its use in children is still relatively anecdotal.[94] The transdermal delivery system allows the continuous administration of fentanyl at four different doses including 25, 50, 75, and 100 µg/h. Following application, a steady-state serum concentration is achieved in 8 hours and lasts for 72 hours with a single patch. Although the dosing options may limit its use in smaller patients, this technique of delivery is useful in patients with limited intravenous access who require several different medications that are incompatible with the opioid infusion.[94] An example of such a patient cared for in our PICU is presented to illustrate this point. The patient was a neonate with complex congenital heart disease who required prolonged postoperative mechanical ventilation. The only venous access that could be maintained was through a Broviac catheter. Sedation was provided by a continuous infusion of fentanyl at 45 µg/h. Fungal sepsis necessitated the use of amphotericin which required administration over a 4-hour period. As amphotericin and fentanyl are not compatible in the same solution, it became necessary to discontinue the fentanyl during the amphotericin infusion, which resulted in inadequate sedation and agitation. A fentanyl patch was applied and 12 hours later the fentanyl infusion was discontinued. After the course of antifungal therapy, the fentanyl infusion was restarted.

A recent episode of respiratory depression (outlined in a letter from Jansen Pharmaceuticals) with the use of the fentanyl patch for routine postoperative analgesia in a child stresses its potential complications. These problems have led the Jansen Pharmaceutical group to advise against its use in children less than 12 years of age. We have used it in younger children, but only in special circumstances when the options for route of opioid administration are limited.[94]

Subcutaneous administration is another possibility when drug incompatibilities preclude the intravenous route. While this route has generally been reserved for the terminal cancer patient,[95] Bruera et al[96] have recently described their experience with subcutaneous infusions of opioids in the adult ICU population. Opioids were administered by either intermittent subcutaneous dosing or by continuous infusion to 13 patients for a total of 60 patient days. The infusions were delivered through a 25-gauge butterfly needle inserted subcutaneously in subclavicular area or the anterior abdominal wall. The site was changed if erythema, swelling, or leakage was observed or at 7-day intervals. No infectious complications were noted and the insertion site was changed only three times due to local problems such as erythema. The authors expressed a theoretical concern over possible delays in onset of activity or decreased absorption in patients with decreased peripheral perfusion, although they noted no such problems in their patients.

The subcutaneous route is also a possible alternative for the PICU patient, similar to that described above in which drug incompatibilities limit the intravenous route[97] or during the recovery period when a slow taper of the opioid infusion is necessary to prevent withdrawal (see below).[50] In either circumstance, the technique is the same. Concentrated solutions of opioids are used so that the total volume is limited to 3 mL/h or less. The subcutaneous infusion is started at the same time that the intravenous infusion is discontinued. Either a standard 22-gauge angiocath or a butterfly needle can be used. Prior to placement, the tubing and needle are flushed with the opioid solution and after sterile preparation of the area, the needle is inserted subcutaneously and covered with a bio-occlusive dressing. The same infusion pumps that are used for intravenous drug administration can be used for subcutaneous administration. The pressure limit may need to be adjusted to allow for subcutaneous administration. Several different opioids are suitable for subcutaneous administration including morphine, hydromorphone, and fentanyl. Methadone, on the other hand, causes significant tissue reaction with erythema and is not recommended for subcutaneous administration.

Despite the success of the above mentioned techniques, the intravenous route is usually the most feasible and most readily accessible method for opioid administration, especially in the PICU. For the majority of patients, a continuous infusion supplemented with intermittent, prn bolus doses provides the best level of analgesia and sedation. Although studies are limited in children, adult studies suggest that a continuous narcotic infusion provides superior postoperative analgesia with fewer adverse effects than either prn or fixed interval dosing.[98,99]

For sedation or analgesia in the younger patient, continuous infusions are often combined with as-needed doses of either an opioid or a benzodiazepine. In older, cooperative patients, an alternative to continuous infusion or intermittent intravenous administration is PCA. This technique for opioid delivery allows the patient to administer a preset amount of opioid as needed at preselected intervals. With appropriate instruction and patient selection, PCA may be used in children as young as 5 to 6 years of age. Prior to starting PCA, opioid is administered incrementally to the patient until the desired level of comfort is achieved. Advantages of PCA include improved analgesia and patient satisfaction with decreased total narcotic use.[100-102] PCA can be used with any opioid (see below); however, in most institutions, morphine is the most commonly used opioid for postoperative analgesia. Starting doses for morphine include 0.02 mg/kg every 8 to 10 minutes as needed.

A second option with PCA is to include a low basal infusion rate. This represents one of the most controversial areas of PCA. It should be remembered that the use of a basal infusion rate is contradictory to the "safety factor" of PCA: "if a patient is too sleepy to push the button, no opioid is infused." With the basal infusion rate, opioid is infused regardless of patient demands. Studies in adults suggest no improvement in analgesia with the basal infusion and an increased incidence of adverse effects such as sedation and respiratory depression.[103,104] Somewhat different results have been reported in pediatric patients depending on the dosing regimen of the basal infusion rate. Doyle et al[105] compared PCA (0.02 mg/kg every 5 minutes as needed) with and without a basal infusion rate of 0.02 mg/kg/h. There was no difference in the pain scores between the two groups, while there were more adverse effects including nausea, sedation, and hypoxemia in the patients who received the basal infusion rate. In a follow-up study the same investigators compared three different regimens of PCA, one of which included a significant decrease in the dose used for basal infusion.[106] The PCA included 0.02 mg/kg every 5 minutes as needed with: 1) no basal infusion rate; 2) basal infusion rate of 0.01 mg/kg/h; or 3) basal infusion rate of 0.004 mg/kg/h. Pain scores were equivalent in the three groups. The investigators noted an increased time spent asleep the first 2 postoperative nights in both of the basal infusion groups while there was no difference in time asleep during the day. There was an increased incidence of nausea and vomiting in the group that received the basal infusion rate of 0.01 mg/kg/h. The authors concluded that a low basal infusion of 0.004 mg/kg/h improved the sleep pattern when compared with no basal infusion rate, without increasing the occurrence of adverse effects.

Since PCA requires an awake, cooperative patient who is able to comprehend its purpose and push the button when additional analgesia is required, its use may be limited in many of the patients admitted to the PICU, due to either age or underlying illness. In these patients, the PCA device may be activated by the bedside nurse, thereby eliminating the delay in opioid administration that occurs as the nurse signs out the medication and draws it up. The PCA device also allows the delivery of the medication through a closed system, thereby decreasing the number of times the intravenous line is entered (which may be an issue in patients with central venous access or alterations in immune function). However, when used in this fashion, the inherent safety factor of PCA is again lost (see above).

Although routes of administration have been systematically evaluated by several different investigators, there appears to be little information concerning the optimal opioid for PICU sedation or postoperative analgesia. In the patient who has compromised cardiovascular status or who is at risk for pulmonary hypertension, such as an infant with a large preoperative systemic-to-pulmonary shunt, the synthetic opioids (fentanyl, sufentanil) provide cardiovascular stability, beneficial effects on PVR, and blunting of the sympathetic stress. Due to their prompt redistribution and resultant short plasma half-lives following a bolus administration, synthetic opioids must be administered by a continuous infusion to maintain plasma concentrations adequate to provide analgesia. When comparing the different synthetic opioids (fentanyl, sufentanil, alfentanil, remifentanil), there does not seem to be an inherent advantage with regard to any agent of these agents. Fentanyl, however, is the least expensive. While fentanyl, sufentanil, and alfentanil, like other opioids, are dependent on hepatic metabolism, remifentanil is metabolized by nonspecific esterases in the plasma with a resultant clinical half-life of 5 to 10 minutes. Its rapid onset and offset of activity offers some advantage for providing intraoperative analgesia; however, it will have limited role in the postoperative care of the PICU patient.

Two caveats of any of the synthetic opioids are their effects on ICP and the idiosyncratic occurrence of chest wall rigidity. While still controversial, recent evidence suggests that the synthetic opioids may increase ICP in patients with altered intracranial compliance.[107] Sperry et al[107] and Milde et al[108] also noted a moderate decrease in mean arterial pressure which, when combined with the increase in ICP, further decreased cerebral perfusion pressure. The mechanism underlying the effect on ICP is thought to be a reflex vasodilation in response to the decrease in mean arterial pressure. Further studies have demonstrated that if the drop in mean arterial pressure is treated with a direct-acting vasoconstrictor, no change in ICP is noted.

Another possibly deleterious effect that has been described with the synthetic opioids is chest wall rigidity.[109] Although Pokela et al[109] noted significant decreases in compliance and oxygen saturation in four infants receiving alfentanil and concluded that these agents should not be used without concomitant neuromuscular blockade, chest wall rigidity does not routinely occur in all patients receiving synthetic opioids. This is especially true in the doses used for sedation in the ICU. In fact, Irazuzta et al[110] demonstrated improved compliance in the majority of patients receiving fentanyl. Chest wall rigidity can be reversed with naloxone or it can be interrupted with NMBAs.

Other opioids, such as morphine, are acceptable and cheaper alternatives for patients with normal cardiovascular function. Morphine causes some venodilation and may thereby decrease blood pressure in hypovolemic patients. However, for the majority of patients, morphine is generally chosen as the first choice opioid for PICU sedation and analgesia.

Alternatives to morphine include hydromorphone, meperidine, and methadone. Hydromorphone may be advantageous when adverse effects related to histamine release, such as pruritus, occur with morphine.[111] The equipotent dose of hydromorphone can be determined by considering the potency ratio of the two opioids with hydromorphone, 5 to 7 times as potent as morphine (Table 5).

Meperidine appears to be a relatively poor choice for analgesia due to relatively high incidence of adverse CNS effects including dysphoria, agitation, and seizures.[112] In older children and adults, the dysphoric response may manifest itself as complaints of "not feeling well" and restlessness while agitation and uncontrollable crying may be the only manifestation in the younger child or infant. CNS toxicity (including seizures) results from the accumulation of normeperidine following hepatic N-methylation of the parent compound. Normeperidine has a long half-life (15 to 20 hours) and is dependent on renal excretion. High or toxic levels occur more commonly in the setting of renal insufficiency, with the coadministration of drugs such as phenobarbital that stimulate hepatic microsomal enzymes, and with large doses (>2 g/day in an adult). The latter issue becomes problematic in the patient who is receiving opioids for the long term, in whom dose escalations are needed to provide effective analgesia. Due to these considerations and since meperidine offers no particular advantage over other opioids, morphine or fentanyl are commonly used as the first-line agents.

Another opioid that may have some role in the treatment of acute pain is methadone. Methadone's potency is roughly equivalent to that of morphine; however, its half-life is 12 to 24 hours. Therefore, a single dose of methadone results in a prolonged serum con-

Table 5

Potency and Half-Lives of Opioids

Agent	Potency	Half-Life (hours)*
Morphine	1	2–3
Merperidine	0.1	2–3
Hydromorphone	5	2–4
Methadone	1	12–24
Fentanyl	100	0.3–0.5
Sufentanil	1000	0.2–0.4
Alfentanil	20	0.2–0.3
Remifentanil	100	0.1

*The reported half-life refers to the initial redistribution phase following a single bolus administration.

centration, resulting in a prolonged duration of action without the need for a continuous infusion. Berde et al[113] evaluated the efficacy of methadone for postoperative analgesia in children aged 3 to 7 years. Children who received methadone (0.2 mg/kg following the induction of anesthesia) had lower pain scores and required fewer doses of supplemental opioid analgesics over the ensuing 36 hours. Although limited experience exists with the use of methadone in children, its longer duration of action offers certain advantages over the intermittent administration of agents with shorter half-lives. Oral methadone may also be used to slowly taper opioid therapy in patients who have developed tolerance following prolonged opioid administration (see below).

Despite recent clinical studies and advances in the understanding of pediatric pain, inadequate analgesia still occurs, especially in younger children and infants, due to unfounded fears of adverse effects and addiction. Fear of respiratory depression or a possible inability to wean from mechanical ventilation are often cited as reasons to avoid opioids especially in the postoperative patient. Lynn et al[114] evaluated the respiratory effects of continuous morphine infusion in children following cardiac surgery. Morphine infusions of 10 to 30 µg/kg/h resulted in serum concentrations of 10 to 22 ng/mL, provided adequate analgesia, and did not impair weaning from mechanical ventilation.

The incidence of addiction in patients receiving opioid analgesic agents for postoperative pain control has been shown to be exceedingly rare.[115] What can be seen following the prolonged administration of opioids and sedative agents is tolerance and physical dependency.[116,117] Tolerance is the need to increase the dose of a drug over time to achieve the same effect. It can occur with any sedative/analgesic agent and occurs due to changes at or distal to the receptor. It is not related to increased metabolism or clearance of the drug. Physical dependency is a physiologic state whereby signs and symptoms of withdrawal occur if the drug is abruptly discontinued. Withdrawal refers to the constellation of signs and symptoms that may occur in a dependent patient when the sedative/analgesic agent is abruptly discontinued. Addiction implies a psychologic dependency on a drug with drug-seeking and antisocial behavior.

Arnold et al[116] described and investigated what they termed "the neonatal abstinence syndrome (NAS)" in infants sedated with fentanyl during ECMO. They undertook a retrospective chart review of 37 neonates who required ECMO for respiratory failure and found that the infants at risk for opioid tolerance and withdrawal included those who required ECMO for greater than 5 days or who received a total dose of fentanyl greater than 1.6 mg/kg. They also reported that plasma concentrations of fentanyl increased as the infusion rate was increased, demonstrating that the increased infusion requirements were the result of tolerance and were not related to increased metabolism or clearance.

Katz et al[117] prospectively evaluated the incidence of opioid withdrawal in 23 infants and young children (age 1 week to 22 months) following the use of fentanyl for sedation during mechanical ventilation. The symptoms of opioid withdrawal were quantified using a scale described by Finnegan et al.[118] Both the total dose of fentanyl and the duration of infusion correlated with the incidence of withdrawal, while the maximum fentanyl infusion rate did not. Infants who received fentanyl for 5 days or a total dose of greater than 1.5 mg/kg had a 50% incidence of withdrawal while patients who received fentanyl for 9 days or a total dose of greater than 2.5 mg/kg had an incidence of withdrawal of 100%. The major strengths of this most recent report are the use of a standardized scoring system to identify opioid withdrawal symptoms and the identification of the "at-risk" group. It should be noted that Katz et al tapered the fentanyl infusion quickly so that all infants were theoretically at risk for withdrawal. The infusion was decreased by half every 24 hours times two and then stopped. The author does not recommend this practice in the at-risk group. A slow taper of the infusion or the use of orally equivalent agents may prevent withdrawal symptoms.

The importance of the NAS is not to limit the use of opioids in infants, but rather to emphasize the need to slowly wean the infusion once the acute illness has subsided. For patients who are at risk of withdrawal, several options are available, including slowly weaning or switching to subcutaneous administration. Oral administration is suggested for patients who are receiving high-dose opioid infusions in whom the weaning process may require weeks.[49,119] Advantages of methadone are an oral bioavailability of 75% to 80%, which allows for oral administration, and a prolonged half-life of 12 to 24 hours, allowing twice-a-day dosing. With the switch from intravenous to oral methadone, the patients can be discharged to home on a tapering schedule that is easily followed by their parents.[119] The conversion from intravenous fentanyl to oral methadone is based on the differences of potency and serum half-life of the two drugs. Although, fentanyl is 100 times more potent than methadone, its half-life is 50 to 100 times shorter. This allows for relatively easy conversion from the total fentanyl dose (mg/day) to an equivalent amount of methadone. A 10-kg patient who is receiving an infusion of 10 μg/kg/h of fentanyl receives 2.4 mg/day of fentanyl. This patient would be started on methadone 1.2 mg, orally, twice a day. Following the second dose the infusion is decreased by 50%, by 50% again following the third dose, and then discontinued after the fourth dose. Symptoms of opioid withdrawal are treated with intravenous rescue doses of morphine and the daily dose of methadone is increased accordingly. Oral administration is also possible for patients sedated with benzodiazepines or barbiturates.[49]

Another option that allows for the slow tapering of opioid/sedative administration is a switch to subcutaneous administration. The technique for subcutaneous administration has been previously described in this chapter. Subcutaneous administration is possible for opioids and benzodiazepines and is generally chosen for patients receiving moderate doses of either agent and in whom the weaning process will not prolong hospitalization.[50] Subcutaneous administration eliminates the need for maintaining intravenous access and allows the removal of central lines when they are no longer needed for other medications.

Miscellaneous Agents

Several other agents or combinations of agents have been used with varying degrees of success for sedation in the PICU patient (Table 6). Phenothiazines and butyrophenones are considered the "major tranquilizers" and are generally used in the treatment of psychiatric disturbances or for their antiemetic properties. Neither of these types of agents has found great popularity as a sedative in the PICU; however, they continue to be used with regularity in adult ICUs. Of the many agents available, haloperidol appears to the most frequently chosen of the butyrophenones. While not approved by the FDA for intravenous administration, there is an abundance of clinical experience with its use by this route. Riker et al[120] reported their experience with haloperidol by continuous intravenous infusion (range: 3 to 25 mg/h) for sedation in eight adult ICU patients. The authors cited many benefits of haloperidol including a rapid onset, minimal respiratory depression, and no active metabolites. Adverse effects associated with the butyrophenones and phenothiazines include hypotension related to α-blockade and peripheral vasodilatation, dystonic and extrapyramidal effects, lowering of the seizure threshold, and, in rare cases, the neuroleptic malignant syndrome. Of even greater concern are possible cardiac events such as cardiac arrest and torsades de pointes, which have been reported with haloperidol. In the study of Riker et al, cardiac events included atrial dysrhythmias, prolongation of the QT interval, and ventricular tachycardia in one patient. Alterations in repolarization may be particularly dangerous in patients with altered sympathetic function related to fever, pain, or the stresses of an acute illness.

Table 6

Miscellaneous Agents for ICU Sedation

Phenothiazines
Butyrophenones
Chloral hydrate
Clonidine
Antihistamines

ICU = intensive care unit.

More commonly, health care providers have, in the past, used the phenothiazines in combination with other agents (ie, DPT: demerol, phenergan, and thorazine) for invasive procedures. This practice is no longer recommended, since the combination may result in prolonged sedation and the risk of respiratory depression and apnea.[121] If such combinations are used, careful and prolonged postprocedure monitoring is suggested.

Chloral hydrate, a sedative-hypnotic agent, is metabolized in the liver to its active form, trichloroethanol, which has a half-life of 8 to 12 hours. As there is no parenteral formulation, oral or rectal administration is needed, which may result in a slow onset of action of up to 20 minutes, limiting its utility in controlling the acutely agitated patient in the PICU. More importantly, repeated administration can lead to the accumulation of active metabolites and prolonged sedation that may persist following its discontinuation. However, chloral hydrate is a valuable agent for brief, nonpainful procedures such as computed-tomography imaging. For this indication, 75 to 80 mg/kg is administered per rectum. Its use is not recommended for infants younger than 3 months of age or for patients with hepatic dysfunction. Additionally, the active metabolite, trichloroethanol, is related to the halogenated hydrocarbons and has been associated with the occurrence of ventricular arrhythmias especially in patients at risk for such problems (tricyclic antidepressant ingestions).

Although diphenhydramine is most commonly used for its antihistamine effects, the associated sedative properties may be beneficial in the PICU patient. This agent may be useful in the spontaneously breathing patient in whom a sedative agent is required (eg, the toddler with bronchiolitis or status asthmaticus). In such situations, use of chloral hydrate (30 to 40 mg/kg per rectum) or diphenhydramine (0.5 mg/kg i.v., repeated every 4 to 6 hours) has proven to be effective, with limited effects on respiratory function.

Clonidine, a centrally acting α_2-agonist that decreases central sympathetic outflow, was initially introduced for the treatment of hypertension.[122] Recent work has demonstrated its efficacy as a premedicant for the operating room.[123] Beneficial effects include sedation, anxiolysis, decreased anesthetic requirements, cardiovascular stability, and the potentiation of opiate-induced analgesia.[124] To date, its use for sedation in the ICU has appeared only as anecdotal case reports.[125] In addition to sedative properties, clonidine and other α_2-adrenergic agonists possess intrinsic analgesic effects that are thought to be mediated at the spinal level (dorsal horn) through the interaction with specific adrenergic receptors. Activation of presynaptic receptors (first-order neurons) results in decreased release of the nociceptive transmitter substance P, while postsynaptic activation decreases the rate of depolarization of second-order neurons. Although the clinical use of these agents is currently limited, their beneficial physiologic properties suggest their potential for future use both as sedatives and analgesics in the PICU patient.

Neuromuscular Blocking Agents

Several situations may arise that necessitate the use of NMBAs in children (Table 7).[126] NMBAs should be used only when absolutely indicated and should only be prescribed by those who have received

Table 7

Indications for Neuromuscular Blockade in Children

Facilitate procedures/diagnostic studies:
  endotracheal intubation
  central line placement
  radiologic imaging (MRI, CT scanning)
Immobilization during transport:
  interhospital
  intrahospital
Intensive care indications:
  facilitate mechanical ventilation
  control increased intracranial pressure
  eliminate shivering/decrease peripheral oxygen utilization
  control severe agitation unresponsive to adequate sedation
  maintain immobilization status post specific surgical procedure

MRI = magnetic resonance imaging; CT = computed tomography.

appropriate training in their pharmacology and possess the knowledge and capability to treat adverse effects related to them. The term muscle relaxant should not be used to describe these agents. Rather, they should be thought of as agents of neuromuscular blockade. These agents have absolutely no amnestic, analgesic, or sedative properties, and should not be used without the coadministration of an amnestic agent (ie, benzodiazepine or barbiturate). In the absence of underlying systemic illnesses that alter the sensorium, patients receiving NMBAs will be unable to move but will be totally aware. An additional caveat is that these agents should be used only by physicians trained in airway management. As these agents inhibit neuromuscular transmission, resulting in muscle paralysis, respiratory paralysis also occurs, mandating the institution of mechanical ventilation. The inability to manage the airway and provide controlled ventilation will result in hypoxia and death. NMBAs should not be used if there is any question as to the the normalcy of the airway and the ability to successfully accomplish endotracheal intubation.

Normal neuromuscular transmission results from the release of acetylcholine from the nerve terminal, movement across the synaptic cleft, and binding to the postsynaptic nicotinic receptor on the sarcolemma of the skeletal muscle. The acetylcholine receptor (nicotinic receptor on the sarcolemma) is a pentameric protein composed of five subunits and is responsible for the conversion of the chemical stimulus (acetylcholine) into an electrical impulse (depolarization of the sarcolemma). Stimulation of the acetylcholine receptors opens ion channels allowing the movement of small, positively charged cations such as sodium, potassium, and calcium. The sodium influx depolarizes the muscle membrane leading to excitation-contraction coupling with the release of calcium from the sarcoplasmic reticulum and muscle contraction. Cessation of muscle contraction and repolarization occurs when acetylcholine is metabolized by a specific enzyme, acetylcholinesterase, which is present in the synaptic cleft.

Depolarizing Agents

The major difference between the two general classes of NMBAs (depolarizing agents and nondepolarizing agents) is their basic mechanism of action. Depolarizing agents such as succinylcholine mimic acetylcholine and bind to the acetylcholine receptor at the neuromuscular junction. As these agents are resistant to degradation by acetylcholinesterase, there is sustained occupation of the receptor and sustained depolarization resulting in muscle paralysis. The action of succinylcholine accounts for the clinical effects seen, including muscle fasciculations followed by flaccid paralysis. The onset of action of succinylcholine is more rapid than any nondepolarizing agent, with total muscle paralysis occurring in 30 to 45 seconds thereby allowing for rapid control of the airway with endotracheal intubation. Succinylcholine undergoes rapid redistribution and metabolism by the plasma enzyme, pseudocholinesterase (plasma cholinesterase). This limits its clinical duration to 5 to 10 minutes. In rare individuals, congenital or acquired deficiency of the enzyme can lead to a prolonged duration. Disease states that lead to a quantitative decrease in pseudocholinesterase levels include severe liver disease, myxedema, pregnancy, protein-calorie malnutrition, and certain malignancies. Drugs, including chemotherapeutic agents (cyclophosphamide) and echothiopate ophthalmic drops, can also affect pseudocholinesterase levels.

The hereditary form of pseudocholinesterase deficiency is related to an abnormal variant of the enzyme. This disorder is an autosomal recessive trait (1:2500 to 3500) so that only homozygotes have a clinically significant prolongation of the effect of succinylcholine. Homozygotes may have paralysis for up to 4 hours following a single dose of succinylcholine. Although the enzyme is contained in fresh frozen plasma, its use is not recommended because of the risk of infectious disease. Treatment is aimed at early recognition with continuation of ventilatory support until the patient's muscle strength returns. Additionally, provision of amnesia with a benzodiazepine is required, because although the patient cannot move, he or she is aware and awake.

Despite its rapid onset, the adverse effects of succinylcholine can be devastating and even fatal (Table 8). Alterations in cardiac rhythm have been described following the administration of succinylcholine; these include bradycardia, tachycardia, and atrial or ventricular ectopy. Succinylcholine has a chemical structure similar to that of two molecules of acetylcholine, and most commonly causes bradycardia from activation of cardiac muscarinic receptors. This effect is especially common in infants and children. Therefore, in this population, succinylcholine should always be preceded by an anticholinergic agent such as atropine. The bradycardic effects of succinylcholine may be accentuated following repeated doses, in the presence of hypoxemia, hypothermia, and increased ICP.

The effects of succinylcholine on ICP are somewhat more controversial. Succinylcholine increases ICP through a direct cholinergic mechanism that is unrelated to the fasciculations.[127] However, since its onset is rapid (30 to 45 seconds), succinylcholine allows for rapid endotracheal intubation and control of arterial oxygenation and ventilation, which are the primary determinants of ICP.

As succinylcholine activates the acetylcholine receptor prior to producing muscle paralysis, depolarization of the muscle endplate occurs, leading to contraction of the muscle fascicles or fasciculations. These fasciculations are responsible for the myalgias that can occur following succinylcholine. The severity of the fasciculations can be prevented by the administration of a small dose of a nondepolarizing agent (eg, curare 0.03 mg/kg) prior to the succinylcholine. This is referred to as a "defasciculating dose." The technique is used in the operating room when succinylcholine is administered to adults. However, it is not commonly used in the pediatric population for several reasons: 1) children younger than 6 years of age do not fasciculate; 2) the use of the defasciculating dose delays the onset of paralysis and increases the dose of succinylcholine needed; and 3) in patients with severe cardiorespiratory compromise, the defasciculating dose can cause a significant degree of muscle paralysis and lead to respiratory insufficiency or laryngeal incompetency with the risk of aspiration.

The primary concern with succinylcholine is the occurrence of lethal hyperkalemia in patients who have certain underlying disorders (Table 9). While many of these disorders are readily apparent, the oc-

Table 8

Adverse Effects of Succinylcholine

Arrhythmias:
  bradycardia
  tachycardia
  asystole
  atrial and ventricular ectopy
Hypertension
Increased intraocular pressure
Increased intragastric pressure
Increased intracranial pressure
Diffuse myalgias, myoglobinuria
Malignant hyperthermia
Prolonged paralysis with pseudocholinesterase deficiency
Hyperkalemia

Table 9

Conditions Associated with Hyperkalemia After Succinylcholine

Hyperkalemia
Muscular dystrophy
Burns
Metabolic acidosis
Paraplegia/quadriplegia
Denervation injury
Metastatic rhabdomyosarcoma
Parkinson's disease
Disuse atrophy/prolonged bedrest
Polyneuropathy
Degenerative CNS disorders
Purpura fulminans
Tetanus
Guillain-Barré
Myotonia dystrophy
Prolonged administration of nondepolarizing NMBA

CNS = central nervous system; NMBA = neuromuscular blocking agents.

currence of cardiac arrest following succinylcholine administration to apparently healthy children has led to a restructuring of the recommendations for its use. The problem is that some children with muscular dystrophy may not manifest symptoms until later in life (>10 years of age). If succinylcholine is administered to these children during anesthetic induction, potentially lethal degrees of hyperkalemia can occur. Because of such problems, succinylcholine should only be used for emergency airway management when rapid endotracheal intubation is necessary.

In emergency situations when intravenous access cannot be readily obtained, succinylcholine can be administered intramuscularly (4 to 5 mg/kg). Intramuscular administration will result in paralysis sufficient to allow for endotracheal intubation in 2 to 3 minutes. This route is not recommended in patients who have conditions that decrease cardiac output or blood flow to the muscles. In such a situation, the onset of action will be significantly delayed and intraosseous administration (1.5 to 2.0 mg/kg) should be considered.[128] Outside of the emergent situation, the routine use of succinylcholine is not recommended. More importantly, if problems occur following the administration of succinylcholine, hyperkalemia should be suspected and the resuscitation tailored to include the possibility of hyperkalemia.

Nondepolarizing Agents

The nondepolarizing NMBAs act as competitive antagonists at the neuromuscular junction, and block the actions of acetylcholine at the receptor. As the name implies, these agents do not activate the acetylcholine receptor. Nondepolarizing NMBAs are used intraoperatively to facilitate endotracheal intubation and also to provide ongoing muscle relaxation for specific surgical procedures (eg, exploratory laparotomy). When used to provide ongoing neuromuscular blockade in the operating room or the ICU, these agents can be administered by intermittent bolus dosing or continuous infusions (see below).

The first nondepolarizing NMBAs (curare, gallamine, metocurine) were introduced in the 1940s. The past 10 years, however, have seen a rapid growth in the number of nondepolarizing agents that are available. There are two basic chemical structures of the nondepolarizing NMBAs: aminosteroid compounds and benzylisoquinolinium compounds (Table 10). The differences in their chemical structure have limited clinical significance. Of more importance are differences in: 1) onset; 2) duration of action; 3) cardiovascular effects; 4) metabolism; 5) metabolic products; and 6) cost.

With the heightened awareness of the problems caused by succinylcholine, the search continues for an NMBA whose onset of action parallels that of succinylcholine. Of the currently available nondepolarizing NMBAs, only rocuronium has an onset of action that approaches that of succinylcholine. The remainder of the NMBAs require 90 to 120 seconds to provide conditions acceptable for endotracheal intubation. Doses of rocuronium of 1 mg/kg provide acceptable intubating conditions within 60 seconds in the majority of patients.[129] However, with the more rapid onset of the higher dose, there is also a prolonged duration of action (60 to 80 minutes), unlike that of succinylcholine (5 to 10 minutes). Therefore, although rocuronium provides an onset time close to that of succinylcholine, its duration of action is markedly longer.

Pancuronium is an aminosteroid compound. Doses of 0.1 to 0.15 mg/kg provide adequate intubating conditions in 120 seconds with a duration of action of 60 to 75

Table 10

Classification of nondepolarizing NMBAs

Aminosteroid compounds:
  pancuronium
  rocuronium
  vecuronium
  pipecuronium

Benzylisoquinolinium compounds:
  mivacurium
  atracurium
  cis-atracurium
  doxacurium

NMBA = neuromuscular blocking agent.

minutes, making it a long-acting agent (Table 11). Pancuronium causes an increase in heart rate and blood pressure via its vagolytic activity. This effect can be used to balance the negative chronotropic effects of certain anesthetic agents such as fentanyl and halothane. Metabolism is primarily renal (80%), resulting in a significantly prolonged effect in patients with renal insufficiency. Hepatic metabolism is primarily hydroxylation with production of an active 3-OH metabolite which has roughly half of the neuromuscular blocking effects of the parent compound. The 3-OH metabolite is also dependent on renal excretion.

Like pancuronium, vecuronium is an aminosteroid compound. It was released for clinical use in the 1980s. In doses of 0.1 to 0.15 mg/kg, acceptable intubating conditions are provided in 90 seconds, with a duration of action of 20 to 40 minutes, making it an intermediately acting agent. Increasing the dose to 0.3 mg/kg speeds the onset time to 60 to 75 seconds, but also prolongs the duration of neuromuscular blockade to 60 to 90 minutes. Even with higher doses, vecuronium is devoid of cardiovascular effects. Metabolism is primarily hepatic (70%); however, hepatic metabolism results in the production of active desacetyl metabolites, which are dependent on renal excretion. These metabolites possess roughly half of the neuromuscular blocking effects of the parent compound. This combined with the 30% renal excretion of the parent compound results in a prolonged clinical duration in patients with renal and/or hepatic insufficiency.

Rocuronium is the newest of the aminosteroid NMBAs. As mentioned previously, it has the most rapid onset of the NMBAs, providing acceptable intubating conditions in 60 seconds following a dose of 0.6 to 1.0 mg/kg. Because of its rapid onset, it may be the drug of choice for rapid-sequence intubation and should be used in place of succinylcholine if there is any concern that succinylcholine may be contraindicated (see above). Following the usual intubating dose of 0.6 mg/kg, the duration of action is 20 to 40 minutes, making it an intermediately acting agent. As with other agents, the duration of action increases when larger doses are administered so that 50 to 60 minutes of paralysis may be seen following the use of 1.0 mg/kg for rapid-sequence intubation. Rocuronium undergoes primarily hepatic metabolism without the production of active metabolites. Although initially reported to have no cardiovascular effects, later studies revealed a mild vagolytic effect with increases in heart rate of 10 to 20 beats per minute following bolus dosing.[130]

Pipecuronium is structurally related to the other aminosteroids including pancuronium and vecuronium. Like vecuronium, it is devoid of cardiovascular effects. Following an intubating dose of 0.07 mg/kg, onset times vary from 2 to 3 minutes, and the duration of action (70 to 80 minutes) is longer than that of pancuronium. Pipecuronium is eliminated primarily by the kidneys (80%), with the remainder of the elimination dependent on hepatic metabolism. Unlike the other previously mentioned aminosteroid NMBAs, there is little enthusiasm for or clinical information concerning the use of pipecuronium in the pediatric population.

Atracurium and cis-atracurium are related compounds that belong to the other group of nondepolarizing NMBAs, the benzylisoquinolinium derivatives. Atracurium was released for use in the 1980s. A dose of 0.6 mg/kg achieves acceptable intubating conditions in 2 to 3 minutes, with a duration of action of 20 to 30 minutes, making it an intermediately acting agent. As with other benzylisoquinoliniums, atracurium can lead to histamine release and hypotension. Atra-

Table 11

Duration of Action of NMBAs

Short-acting (10 minutes):
   succinylcholine
   mivacurium

Intermediate-acting (20–40 minutes):
   atracurium
   vecuronium
   cis-atracurium
   rocuronium

Long-acting (60–90 minutes):
   pancuronium
   pipecuronium
   doxacurium

NMBA = neuromuscular blocking agent.

curium undergoes spontaneous degradation via a process known as Hofmann elimination, as well as through ester hydrolysis. Therefore, its duration of action is unchanged by either renal or hepatic insufficiency. Because of these properties, it has become one of the favorite agents of neuromuscular blockade for ICU patients. For this purpose, it is most commonly administered by continuous infusion (see below). The metabolites of atracurium do not possess significant neuromuscular blocking properties. However, one of the metabolic byproducts of Hofmann degradation, laudanosine, has been shown to be epileptogenic. The actual concentrations required to cause seizures in humans is unknown and no formal study has ever documented problems from high laudanosine levels. Laudanosine is renally excreted and its accumulation in patients with renal insufficiency is at least a theoretical concern.

Because of the concerns about histamine release with atracurium, Glaxo-Wellcome has recently introduced cis-atracurium for clinical use. Cis-atracurium is an isomer of atracurium that is 6 to 8 times as potent but devoid of clinically significant histamine release. Like atracurium, cis-atracurium is an intermediately acting NMBA with a duration of action of 20 to 30 minutes following an initial dose of 0.2 mg/kg. Onset of action for acceptable intubating conditions is 2 to 3 minutes.

Mivacurium, another benzylisoquinolinium, is the shortest acting of the nondepolarizing NMBAs. Following a dose of 0.2 mg/kg, onset times vary from 2 to 3 minutes, with a duration of action of 10 minutes. Like the other benzylisoquinoliniums, mivacurium can produce histamine release. In children, however, this is generally of limited clinical significance. Mivacurium is metabolized by pseudocholinesterase, the same enzyme that degrades succinylcholine. Therefore, prolonged blockade can occur in the same clinical situations as described for succinylcholine (see above). The metabolites of mivacurium, which are renally excreted, have limited neuromuscular blocking properties. Mivacurium is used for brief procedures (<10 minutes) either in the operating room or in the PICU. Mivacurium can be a useful agent to provide a brief duration of neuromuscular blockade for direct laryngoscopy in the PICU patient, to follow the progress of epiglottitis or some other airway problem. Mivacurium may also be advantageous in patients with underlying neuromuscular disorders (ie, muscular dystrophy). In this group of patients, even the intermediately acting agents can have prolonged effects (4 to 6 hours). Therefore, the use of an agent with the shortest clinical duration may be beneficial.[131]

Doxacurium is a benzylisoquinolinium derivative that has the longest duration of clinical activity. Like pipecuronium, it has a duration of action of 80 to 90 minutes following an initial dose of 0.05 mg/kg. Elimination is primarily renal with a small percentage dependent on hepatic excretion. The duration of action is prolonged in patients who have either hepatic or renal insufficiency. Despite that fact that it is a benzylisoquinolinium derivative, it is primarily devoid of histamine-releasing properties and cardiovascular effects.

Monitoring Neuromuscular Blockade

In the operating room, NMBAs may be used in a single dose at the start of the case to facilitate endotracheal intubation, or in repeated doses or a continuous infusion to provide ongoing neuromuscular blockade. Some means of monitoring neuromuscular blockade is necessary, as administration of excessive doses may mandate the use of postoperative mechanical ventilation until neuromuscular blockade has worn off or can be reversed.

The technique that is most commonly used by anesthesiologists in the operating room to monitor the degree of neuromuscular blockade is peripheral nerve stimulation, or train-of-four (TOF) monitoring. As this is painful, it should only be performed in patients who are anesthetized or sedated. The technique involves placement of standard electrocardiographic electrodes over a peripheral nerve. The nerves most commonly used are the facial, ulnar, or common peroneal nerves. The electrodes are then connected to a hand-held peripheral nerve stimulator, which delivers two stimuli per second for 2 seconds; a total of four stimuli, hence the term train-of-four. Depending on the number of acetylcholine receptors that are occupied by the nondepolarizing NMBA, there will be anywhere from zero to four responses or twitches. While other, more sophisticated techniques and neuromuscular stimulating devices are available, none are in common clinical use in the operating room or the PICU. In clinical practice, the TOF monitoring is combined with clinical assessment at the end of the case to ensure that the patient is strong enough for extubation. When there is some degree of neuromuscular function present (one twitch or more), reversal of residual neuromuscular blockade is possible (see below). Following reversal of neuromuscular blockade, clinical assessment of strength is combined with neuromuscular monitoring. Clinical assessment may include measurement of negative inspiratory force (NIF), which should be greater than -30 cm H_2O, strong hand grip, ability to maintain head-lift for 5 seconds, or contraction of the hip flexors and maintaining hip flexion. The latter is a valuable sign in neonates and infants, who are unable to follow commands.

Reversal of Neuromuscular Blockade

Although neuromuscular blockade is necessary for many surgical procedures, even a small amount of residual blockade may compromise ventilation or upper airway patency in the immediate postoperative period. With the dosing of NMBAs according to TOF monitoring, an adequate amount of surgical relaxation can be provided to allow for the successful completion of the surgical procedure while maintaining the ability to reverse residual neuromuscular blockade at the completion of the procedure.

Reversal of neuromuscular blockade is possible only with nondepolarizing agents. The drugs used to reverse neuromuscular blockade inhibit the activity of the enzyme, acetylcholinesterase. This, in turn, provides more acetylcholine to compete with the NMBA at the nicotinic receptor of the neuromuscular junction. The commonly used acetylcholinesterase inhibitors or "reversal agents" include neostigmine and edrophonium. These agents should always be preceded by an anticholinergic agent such as atropine or glycopyrrolate since the inhibition of acetylcholinesterase occurs not only at nicotinic receptors (neuromuscular junction), but also at muscarinic receptors. Therefore, unless preceded by an anticholinergic (antimuscarinic) agent, bradycardia and asystole can occur.

Neuromuscular Blocking Agents in the Pediatric Intensive Care Unit

In addition to their use in the operating room, specific situations may arise which mandate the use of NMBAs in the PICU (Table 7). NMBAs should be used only when aggressive attempts at sedation have failed to provide the desired level of patient immobilization. Several adverse effects may be noted with the use of NMBAs including decreased/absent cough, decreased functional residual capacity, and increased ventilation-perfusion mismatch. All of these may increase ventilatory demands, oxygen requirement, and the incidence of respiratory tract infections. However, NMBAs may be necessary especially when caring for critically ill patients with severe respiratory failure in whom newer modes of ventilation are being used to limit iatrogenic lung injury, such as permissive hypercapnia and reverse I:E ratio ventilation.

In the operating room, these agents are generally administered as intermittent bolus doses. However, in the PICU, a more stable baseline level of neuromuscular blockade may be desired. In this setting, a continuous infusion may be used. The major issues to consider when choosing an agent for use in the ICU population include cardiovascular effects, metabolism, and cost. Since many of the patients in the ICU have some degree of hemodynamic instability, agents that cause excessive histamine release should be avoided. Additionally, the presence of hepatic or renal insufficiency may affect dosing requirements of certain agents.

In the absence of end-organ dysfunction, pancuronium offers an inexpensive means of achieving neuromuscular block-

Table 12
Estimated Daily Cost of NMBAs in a 20-kg Patient*

Agent	Infusion Rate (mg/kg/h)	Cost	Unit Price
Pancuronium	0.08 mg/kg/h	$5.11	10 mg: $1.33
Vecuronium	0.1 mg/kg/h	$52.08	10 mg: $11.00
Rocuronium	0.8 mg/kg/h	$102.34	100 mg: $26.65
Atracurium	1 mg/kg/h	$197.95	100 mg: $41.24
Cis-atracurium	0.2 mg/kg/h	$67.20	200 mg: $140.00

*Cost estimates are based on the retail price to the pharmacy as of June 1996 at the University of Missouri. The costs will vary according to current pricing and regional pricing. NMBA = neuromuscular blocking agent.

ade (Table 12). Although pancuronium increases heart rate through a mild vagolytic effect, this is generally not a concern in the pediatric population. In a prospective evaluation in the PICU patient, pancuronium was administered by continuous infusion to 25 children who required neuromuscular blockade.[132] The patients ranged in age from 3 months to 17 years and in weight from 3.2 to 68 kg. The pancuronium infusion was adjusted to maintain a single twitch on a TOF monitor over a peripheral nerve. Infusion requirements varied in all patients from 0.03 to 0.22 mg/kg/h. However, 85% of the time, the infusion requirements varied from 0.03 to 0.09 mg/kg/h with a mean of 0.07 mg/kg/h.

While pancuronium is inexpensive and effective in patients without end-organ dysfunction, significant alterations in infusion requirements occur in patients with renal failure. Atracurium or cis-atracurium may be a more appropriate choice for patients with hepatic or renal failure, since such problems do not alter dosing requirements of either agent.[133,134] A prospective study evaluated cis-atracurium dosing requirements in 15 PICU patients ranging in age from 10 months to 11 years and in weight from 4 to 28 kg.[134] Cis-atracurium was dosed using TOF monitoring. Infusion requirements varied from 2.1 to 3.8 µg/kg/min on day 1, from 2.9 to 8.1 µg/kg/min on day 3, and from 1.4 to 22.7 µg/kg/min during all patient days. The highest infusion requirements were noted following administration of the drug for prolonged periods.

Regardless of the agent chosen, in the PICU setting like in the operating room, adjustment of the dose based on monitoring with a peripheral nerve stimulator is highly recommended. Regardless of the agent used, significant interpatient variability with up to tenfold variations in infusion requirements may be noted.[131-135] The variability results not only from interpatient variability but also from various associated conditions which may increase or decrease the sensitivity to NMBAs (Tables 13 and 14). Based on this knowledge, the recommended

Table 13
Factors that Increase Sensitivity to NMBAs

Drugs:
  inhalation anesthetic agents
  local anesthetics
  antibiotics (aminoglycosides)
  antiarrhythmic agents (quinidine, procainamide)
  calcium channel blockers
  β-adrenergic antagonists
  chemotherapeutic agents (cyclophosphamide)
  diuretics (furosemide)
  dantrolene
  lithium, magnesium
  cyclosporin

Underlying disorders:
  eletrolyte disturbances (hypokalemia, hypermagnesemia, hypocalcemia)
  hypothermia
  respiratory acidosis
  metabolic alkalosis
  myasthenia gravis
  Eaton-Lambert syndrome
  muscular dystrophy
  multiple sclerosis
  amyotrophic lateral sclerosis
  poliomyelitis

NMBA = neuromuscular blocking agents.

Table 14

Factors that Decrease the Sensitivity to NMBAs

Drugs:
  phenytoin
  aminophylline
  carbamazepine
  corticosteroids

Underlying conditions:
  hypercalcemia
  burns
  prolonged administration of NMBAs

NMBA = neuromuscular blocking agent.

doses (Table 15) for the various NMBAs are starting guidelines and the infusion should be increased or decreased as needed to maintain one twitch of the TOF. In patients with excessive movement or two or more twitches on the TOF, a bolus dose equivalent to the currently hourly infusion rate is administered and the infusion is increased by 10% to 15%. If no response is noted on the TOF, it should be ascertained that there are no technical problems with the monitor or with lead placement. Faulty batteries and monitors can result in false results, as can inappropriate lead placement or excessive tissue edema or obesity, which precludes access to the peripheral nerve.

An additional problem that occurs in the ICU patient who receives NMBAs for a prolonged period of time is the development of tachyphylaxis or an increased dose requirement over time. The primary cause is an upregulation of acetylcholine receptors in patients who are exposed to NMBAs for a long period of time. Dodson et al[135] demonstrated an increased density of acetylcholine receptors in muscle of patients who had received prolonged infusions of NMBAs. Prolonged neuromuscular blockade, like partial or complete deafferentation, leads to proliferation of acetylcholine receptors at the neuromuscular junction. This problem requires

Table 15

Suggested Guidelines for Dosing of Sedative, Analgesic, and Neuromuscular Blocking Agents

Agent	Dose	Comments
Fentanyl	2–3 μg/kg/h	modulates stress response and pulmonary vascular resistance
Morphine	10–30 μg/kg/h	inexpensive, venodilation
Midazolam	0.05–0.15 mg/kg/h	abundant clinical experience, expensive, P450 metabolism
Lorazepam	0.025–0.05 mg/kg/h	limited clincial experience, inexpensive, metabolism: glucoronyl transferase
Ketamine	1–2 mg/kg/h	endogenous catecholamine release, bronchodilation, cardiovascular stability, can be mixed 10:1 with midazolam
Pentobarbital	1–2 mg/kg/h	alternative to benzodiazepine/opioid, incompatible with other medications, vasodilation/negative inotropic effects
Propofol	1–3 mg/kg/h	not recommended for patients less than 10 years of age, rapid awakening, high lipid content of solution
Pancuronium	0.06–0.08 mg/kg/h	vagolytic effect, renal excretion
Vecuronium	0.1–0.15 mg/kg/h	no cardiovascular effects, hepatic metabolism to active metabolites that are renally excreted
Rocuronium	0.6–0.8 mg/kg/h	mild vagolytic effect, hepatic metabolism
Atracurium	1–1.5 mg/kg/h	mild histamine release, non-organ-dependent elimination
Cis-atracurium	0.2 mg/kg/h	no cardiovascular effects, non-organ-dependent elimination

that the dose of the NMBA be increased over time to maintain the same amount of neuromuscular blockade.

An additional problem that has recently been reported is persistent paralysis following the prolonged administration of NMBAs to critically ill patients.[136,137] Although many of the initial reports were related to excessive dosing, absence of appropriate monitoring to guide drug dosing, and failure to adjust doses in patients with renal or hepatic insufficiency, even with appropriate monitoring and dosing some patients will develop a persistent weakness following the discontinuation of NMBAs. The weakness may be profound enough to mandate prolonged mechanical ventilation or intensive physical therapy. As a full discussion of this problem is beyond the scope of this chapter, readers are referred to References 136 through 138 for a full discussion of this problem.

Summary

Due to the diversity of patients and clinical scenarios in the PICU, a cookbook approach to sedation remains impossible. Physicians caring for PICU patients must be facile with several different medications and routes of administration to ensure adequate sedation and analgesia in this diverse patient population. Initial choices for the provision of amnesia may include the continuous infusion of a benzodiazepine. While several options exist, lorazepam offers a cost-effective alternative to midazolam and eliminates the concerns regarding active metabolites. In situations that require analgesia, an opioid by either continuous infusion or a PCA device can be used. Although fentanyl is frequently chosen as the first-line opioid, morphine is an acceptable and cost-effective alternative for patients with stable cardiovascular function. The synthetic opioids are recommended for neonates, especially following cardiac surgical procedures and those at risk for pulmonary vasoconstriction. In this setting the use of the synthetic opioids may decrease postoperative morbidity and mortality and modulate the deleterious effects of pain and the stress response on the pulmonary vasculature. Opioids may also be used for the treatment of agitation in those situations that do not necessarily require analgesia. Clinical experience suggests that opioids may be more effective for sedation than benzodiazepines in children younger than 1 year of age. Regardless of the agent used, the infusion should be supplemented with as-needed doses. Patients requiring frequent bolus doses should have the baseline infusion rate increased. As the infusion rate is increased, the bolus doses should be increased to equal the hourly rate.

When the above agents fail to be effective or are associated with adverse effects, alternatives include ketamine or pentobarbital. Ketamine may be useful for the unstable patient or those with a bronchospastic component to their disease process. Pentobarbital may be effective when the combination of benzodiazepines and opioids fails to provide the desired level of sedation. Suggested starting guidelines for dosing of sedative and analgesic agents are listed in Table 15.

Various situations may arise which necessitate the use of NMBAs. These agents are used most frequently intraoperatively to facilitate endotracheal intubation and/or to provide ongoing muscle paralysis for specific surgical procedures. Several different agents are available whose differences include onset time, duration of clinical activity, metabolism, and cardiovascular effects. With the recent concerns over the use of succinylcholine in children, increased interest remains for the development of a nondepolarizing agents with an onset time that parallels that of succinylcholine. To date, rocuronium offers the most rapid onset of the nondepolarizing NMBAs, providing acceptable conditions for intubation in 60 seconds. For maintenance of NMBA in the operating room or the ICU, there are many appropriate agents. Regardless of the agent used, the ability to secure and maintain the airway must be assured prior to the administration of an NMBA. Additionally, although these agents provide a motionless patient, they possess no amnestic or analgesic properties.

References

1. Shovelton DS. Reflection on an intensive therapy unit. *Br Med J* 1979;1:737–742.
2. Mather L, Mackie J. The incidence of postoperative pain in children. *Pain* 1983;15:271–282.

3. Weissman C. The metabolic response to stress: An overview and update. *Anesthesiology* 1990;73:308–327.
4. Buckingham JC. Hypothalamic-pituitary responses to trauma. *Br Med Bull* 1985;41:203–211.
5. Anand KJS, Sippell WG, Aynsley-Green A. Randomised trial of fentanyl anaesthesia in preterm babies undergoing surgery: Effects on the stress response. *Lancet* 1987;2:243–247.
6. Anand KJS, Hansen DD, Hickey PR. Hormonal-metabolic stress responses in neonates undergoing cardiac surgery. *Anesthesiology* 1990;73:661–670.
7. Anand KJS, Hickey PR. Halothane-morphine compared with high-dose sufentanil for anesthesia and postoperative analgesia in neonatal cardiac surgery. *N Engl J Med* 1992;326:1–9.
8. Marshall BE, Wyche MQ. Hypoxia during and after anesthesia. *Anesthesiology* 1972;37:178–209.
9. Craig DB. Postoperative recovery of pulmonary function. *Anesth Analg* 1981;60:46–52.
10. Lanz E, Theiss D, Reiss W, Sommer U. Epidural morphine for postoperative analgesia: A double-blind study. *Anesth Analg* 1982;61:236–240.
11. Rawal N, Sjostrand U, Dahlstrom B. Postoperative pain relief by epidural morphine. *Anesth Analg* 1981;60:726–731.
12. Tyler DC. Respiratory effects of pain in a child after thoracotomy. *Anesthesiology* 1989;70:873–874.
13. Rawal N, Sjostrand U, Christoffersson E, et al. Comparison of intramuscular and epidural morphine for postoperative analgesia in the grossly obese: Influence on postoperative ambulation and pulmonary function. *Anesth Analg* 1984;63:583–592.
14. The Committee on Drugs of the American Academy of Pediatrics. Guidelines for monitoring and management of pediatric patients during and after sedation for diagnostic and therapeutic procedures. *Pediatrics* 1992;89:1110–1115.
15. Katz R, Kelly HW. Pharmacokinetics of continuous infusions of fentanyl in critically ill children. *Crit Care Med* 1993;21:995–1000.
16. Hansen-Flaschen JH, Brazinsky S, Basile C, Lanken PN. Use of sedating drugs and neuromuscular blocking agents in patients requiring mechanical ventilation for respiratory failure. *JAMA* 1991;266:2870–2875.
17. Kong KL, Willatts SM, Prys-Roberts C. Isoflurane compared with midazolam for sedation in the intensive care unit. *Br Med J* 1989;298:1277–1280.
18. Breheny FX, Kendall PA. Use of isoflurane for sedation in intensive care. *Crit Care Med* 1992;20:1062–1064.
19. Adams RW, Cucchiara RF, Gronert GA, et al. Isoflurane and cerebrospinal fluid pressure in neurosurgical patients. *Anesthesiology* 1981;54:97–99.
20. Drummond JC, Todd MM, Scheller MS, Shapiro HM. A comparison of the direct cerebral vasodilating potencies of halothane and isoflurane in the New Zealand White Rabbit. *Anesthesiology* 1986;65:462–467.
21. Newberg LA, Michenfelder JD. Cerebral protection by isoflurane during hypoxemia or ischemia. *Anesthesiology* 1983;59:29–35.
22. Reilly CS, Wood AJJ, Koshakji RP, Wood M. The effect of halothane on drug disposition: Contribution of changes in intrinsic drug metabolizing capacity and hepatic blood flow. *Anesthesiology* 1985;63:70–76.
23. Arnold JH, Truog RD, Rice SA. Prolonged administration of isoflurane to pediatric patients during mechanical ventilation. *Anesth Analg* 1993;76:520–526.
24. Revell S, Greenhalgh D, Absalom SR, Soni N. Isoflurane in the treatment of asthma. *Anaesthesia* 1988;43:477–479.
25. Kofke WA, Snider MT, Young RSK, Ramer JC. Prolonged low flow isoflurane anesthesia for status epilepticus. *Anesthesiology* 1985;62:653–656.
26. Rowland AS, Baird DD, Weinberg CR, et al. Reduced fertility among women employed as dental assistants exposed to high levels of nitrous oxide. *N Engl J Med* 1992;327:993–997.
27. Eisele JH, Smith NT. Cardiovascular effects of 40% nitrous oxide in man. *Anesth Analg* 1972;51:956–962.
28. Schulte-Sasse U, Hess W, Tarnow J. Pulmonary vascular responses to nitrous oxide in patients with normal and high pulmonary vascular resistance. *Anesthesiology* 1982;57:9–13.
29. Suzuki KS, Konno M, Kirikae T, et al. Effects of prolonged nitrous oxide exposure on hemopoietic stem cells in splenectomized mice. *Anesth Analg* 1990;71:389–393.
30. Schilling RF. Is nitrous oxide a dangerous anesthetic for vitamin B_{12}-deficient subjects? *JAMA* 1986;255:1605–1606.
31. Koblin DD, Tomerson BW, Waldman FM, et al. Effect of nitrous oxide on folate and vitamin B_{12} metabolism in patients. *Anesth Analg* 1990;71:610–617.
32. Nunn JF, O'Morain C. Nitrous oxide decreases motility of human neutrophils in vitro. *Anesthesiology* 1982;56:45–48.
33. Reves JG, Fragan RJ, Vinik R, et al. Midazo-

lam: Pharmacology and uses. *Anesthesiology* 1985;62:310–317.
34. Rosland JH, Hole K. 1,4-Benzodiazepines antagonize opiate-induced antinociception in mice. *Anesth Analg* 1990;71:242–248.
35. Lloyd-Thomas AR, Booker PD. Infusion of midazolam in paediatric patients after cardiac surgery. *Br J Anaesth* 1986;58:1109–1115.
36. Booker PD, Beechey A, Lloyd-Thomas AR. Sedation of children requiring artificial ventilation using an infusion of midazolam. *Br J Anaesth* 1986;58:1104–1108.
37. Silvasi DL, Rosen DA, Rosen KR. Continuous intravenous midazolam infusion for sedation in the pediatric intensive care unit. *Anesth Analg* 1988;67:286–288.
38. Trouvin JH, Farinotti R, Haberer JP, et al. Pharmacokinetics of midazolam in anesthetized cirrhotic patients. *Br J Anaesth* 1988; 60:762–767.
39. Vinik HR, Reves JG, Greenblatt DJ, et al. The pharmacokinetics of midazolam in chronic renal failure patients. *Anesthesiology* 1983;59: 390–394.
40. Beebe DS, Belani KG, Chang P, et al. Effectiveness of preoperative sedation with rectal midazolam, ketamine, or their combination in young children. *Anesth Analg* 1992;75:880–884.
41. McMillan CO, Spahr-Schopfer IA, Sikich N, et al. Premedication of children with oral midazolam. *Can J Anaesth* 1992;39:545–550.
42. Karl HW, Rosenberger JL, Larach MG, Ruffle JM. Transmucosal administration of midazolam for premedication of pediatric patients: Comparison of the nasal and sublingual routes. *Anesthesiology* 1993;78: 885–891.
43. Theroux MC, West DW, Corddry DH, et al. Efficacy of midazolam in facilitating suturing of lacerations in preschool children in the emergency department. *Pediatrics* 1993;91: 624–627.
44. Fragen RJ, Meyers SN, Barresi V, Caldwell NJ. Hemodynamic effects of midazolam in cardiac patients. *Anesthesiology* 1979;51:172–176.
45. Breheny FX. Reversal of midazolam sedation with flumazenil. *Crit Care Med* 1992;20: 736–739.
46. McDuffee A, Tobias JD. Seizure following flumazenil administration in a child. *Pediatr Emerg Care* 1995;11:186–187.
47. Hughes J, Gill A, Leach HJ, et al. A prospective study of the adverse effects of midazolam on withdrawal in critically ill children. *Acta Paediatr* 1994;83:1194–1199.
48. Sury MJR, Billingham I, Russell GN, et al. Acute benzodiazepine withdrawal. *Crit Care Med* 1989;17:301–302.
49. Tobias JD, Deshpande JK, Gregory DF. Outpatient therapy of iatrogenic drug dependency following prolonged sedation in the pediatric intensive care unit. *Intensive Care Med* 1994;20:504–507.
50. Tobias JD. Subcutaneous administration of fentanyl and midazolam to prevent withdrawal following prolonged sedation in children. *Crit Care Med* 1999. In press.
51. Domino EF, Chodoff P, Corssen G. Pharmacologic effects of CI-581, a new dissociative anesthetic in man. *Clin Pharmacol Ther* 1965;6:279–291.
52. Jastak JT, Goretta C. Ketamine as a continuous drip anesthesia for outpatients. *Anesth Analg* 1973;52:341–344.
53. Rees DI, Howell ML. Ketamine-atracurium by continuous infusion as the sole anesthetic for pulmonary surgery. *Anesth Analg* 1986; 65:860–864.
54. Clausen L, Sinclair DM, Van Hasselt CH. Intravenous ketamine for postoperative analgesia. *S Afr Med J* 1975;49:1437–1440.
55. Ito Y, Ichivanagi I. Postoperative pain relief with ketamine infusion. *Anaesthesia* 1974;29: 222–229.
56. Sheref SE. Ketamine and bronchospasm. *Anaesthesia* 1985;40:701–702.
57. Saegusa K, Furukawa Y, Ogiwara Y. Pharmacologic analysis of ketamine-induced cardiac actions in isolated, blood-perfused canine atria. *J Cardiovasc Pharmacol* 1986;8:414–419.
58. Chernow B, Laker R, Creuss D, et al. Plasma, urine, and cerebrospinal fluid catecholamine concentrations during and after ketamine sedation. *Crit Care Med* 1982;10:600–603.
59. Wayman K, Shoemaker WC, Lippmann M. Cardiovascular effects of anesthetic induction with ketamine. *Anesth Analg* 1980;59: 355–358.
60. Spotoft H, Korshin JD, Sorensen MB, et al. The cardiovascular effects of ketamine used for induction of anesthesia in patients with valvular heart disease. *Can Anaesth Soc J* 1979;26:463–467.
61. Gooding JM, Dimick AR, Travakoli M, et al. A physiologic analysis of cardiopulmonary responses to ketamine anesthesia in non-cardiac patients. *Anesth Analg* 1977;56:813–816.
62. Morray JP, Lynn AM, Stamm SJ, et al. Hemodynamic effects of ketamine in children with congenital heart disease. *Anesth Analg* 1984;63:895–899.
63. Hickey PR, Hansen DD, Cramolini GM, et al. Pulmonary and systemic hemodynamic responses to ketamine in infants with normal and elevated pulmonary vascular resistance. *Anesthesiology* 1985;62:287–293.

64. Mankikian B, Cantineau JP, Sartene R, et al. Ventilatory and chest wall mechanics during ketamine anesthesia in humans. *Anesthesiology* 1986;65:492–499.
65. Hirshman CA, Downes H, Farbood A, Bergman NA. Ketamine block of bronchospasm in experimental canine asthma. *Br J Anaesth* 1979;51:713–718.
66. Bourke DL, Malit LA, Smith TC. Respiratory interactions of ketamine and morphine. *Anesthesiology* 1987;66:153–156.
67. Lanning CF, Harmel MH. Ketamine anesthesia. *Annu Rev Med* 1975;26:137–141.
68. Taylor PA, Towey RM. Depression of laryngeal reflexes during ketamine administration. *Br Med J* 1971;2:688–689.
69. Shapiro HM, Wyte SR, Harris AB. Ketamine anesthesia in patients with intracranial pathology. *Br J Anaesth* 1972;44:1200–1204.
70. Gardner AE, Dannemiller FJ, Dean D. Intracranial cerebrospinal fluid pressure in man during ketamine anesthesia. *Anesth Analg* 1972;51:741–745.
71. Reicher D, Bhalla P, Rubinstein EH. Cholinergic cerebral vasodilator effects of ketamine in rabbits. *Stroke* 1987;18:445–449.
72. Oren RE, Rasool NA, Rubinstein EH. Effect of ketamine on cerebral cortical blood flow and metabolism in rabbits. *Stroke* 1987;18:441–444.
73. White PR, Way WL, Trevor AJ. Ketamine-its pharmacology and therapeutic uses. *Anesthesiology* 1982;56:119–136.
74. Tobias JD, Martin LD, Wetzel RC. Ketamine by continuous infusion for sedation in the pediatric intensive care unit. *Crit Care Med* 1990;18:819–821.
75. Sebel PS, Lowdon JD. Propofol: A new intravenous anesthetic. *Anesthesiology* 1989;71:260–277.
76. Harris CE, Grounds RM, Murray AM, et al. Propofol for long-term sedation in the intensive care unit. A comparison with papaveretum and midazolam. *Anaesthesia* 1990;45:366–372.
77. Beller JP, Pottecher T, Lugnier A, et al. Prolonged sedation with propofol in ICU patients: Recovery and blood concentration changes during periodic interuption in infusion. *Br J Anaesth* 1988;61:583–588.
78. Brussel T, Theissen JL, Vigfusson G, et al. Hemodynamic and cardiodynamic effects of propofol and etomidate: Negative inotropic properties of propofol. *Anesth Analg* 1989;69:35–40.
79. Egan TD, Brock-Utne JG. Asystole and anesthesia induction with a fentanyl, propofol, and succinylcholine sequence. *Anesth Analg* 1991;73:818–820.
80. Trotter C, Serpell MG. Neurological sequelae in children after prolonged propofol infusions. *Anaesthesia* 1992;47:340–342.
81. Saunders PRI, Harris MNE. Opisthotonic posturing and other unusual neurological sequelae after outpatient anesthesia. *Anaesthesia* 1992;47:552–557.
82. Collier C, Kelly K. Propofol and convulsions-The evidence mounts. *Anaesth Intensive Care* 1991;19:573–575.
83. Finley GA, MacManus B, Sampson SE, et al. Delayed seizures following sedation with propofol. *Can J Anaesth* 1993;40:863–865.
84. Parke TJ, Stevens JE, Rice ASC, et al. Metabolic acidosis and fatal myocardial failure after propofol infusion in children: Five case reports. *Br Med J* 1992;305:613–616.
85. Strickland RA, Murray MJ. Fatal metabolic acidosis in a pediatric patient receiving an infusion of propofol in the intensive care unit: Is there a relationship? *Crit Care Med* 1995;23:405–409.
86. Laxenaire MC, Mata-Bermejo E, Moneret-Vautrin DA, Gueant JL. Life-threatening anaphylactoid reactions to propofol. *Anesthesiology* 1992;77:275–280.
87. Sosis MB, Braverman B. Growth of Staphylococcus aureus in four intravenous anesthetics. *Anesth Analg* 1993;77:766–768.
88. Postsurgical infections associated with extrinsically contaminated intravenous anesthetic agent-California, Illinois, Maine, and Michigan, 1990. *MMWR Morb Mortal Wkly Rep* 1990;39:426–427, 433.
89. Gottardis M, Khunl-Brady KS, Koller W, et al. Effect of prolonged sedation with propofol on serum triglyceride and cholesterol concentrations. *Br J Anaesth* 1989;62:393–396.
90. Valente JF, Anderson GL, Branson RD, et al. Disadvantages of prolonged propofol sedation in the critical care unit. *Crit Care Med* 1994;22:710–712.
91. Tobias JD, Deshpande JK, Pietsch JB, et al. Pentobarbital sedation in the pediatric intensive care unit patient. *South Med J* 1995;88:290–294.
92. Miser AW, Narang PK, Dothage JA, et al. Transdermal fentanyl for pain control in patients with cancer. *Pain* 1989;37:15–21.
93. Holley FR, van Steenis C. Postoperative analgesia with fentanyl: Pharmacokinetics and pharmacodynamics at constant intravenous and transdermal delivery. *Br J Anaesth* 1989;63:56–69.
94. Tobias JD. Transdermal fentanyl: Applications and indications in the pediatric patient. *Pain Management* 1992;2:30–33.
95. Bruera E, Brenneis C, Michaud M, et al. Use of the subcutaneous route for the adminis-

tration of narcotics in patients with cancer pain. *Cancer* 1988;62:407–411.
96. Bruera E, Gibney N, Stollery D, Marcushamer S. Use of the subcutaneous route of administration of morphine in the intensive care unit. *J Pain Symptom Manage* 1991; 6:263–265.
97. Tobias JD, O'Connor TA. Subcutaneous administration of fentanyl for sedation during mechanical ventilation in an infant. *Am J Pain Manage* 1996;6:115–117.
98. Rutter PC, Murphy D, Dudley HAF. Morphine: Controlled trial of different methods of administration for postoperative pain relief. *Br Med J* 1980;280:12–16.
99. Nayman J. Measurement and control of postoperative pain. *Ann R Coll Surg Engl* 1979;61:419–422.
100. Berde CB, Lehn BM, Yee JD, et al. Patient-controlled analgesia in children and adolescents: A randomized, prospective comparison with intramuscular administration of morphine for postoperative analgesia. *J Pediatr* 1991;118:460–466.
101. Lawrie SC, Forbes DW, Akhtar TM, Morton NS. Patient controlled analgesia in children. *Anaesthesia* 1990;46:1074–1076.
102. Gaukroger PB, Omkins DP, Van Der Walt JH. Patient-controlled analgesia in children. *Anaesth Intensive Care* 1989;17:264–268.
103. Parker RK, Holtmann B, White PF. Patient-controlled analgesia: Does a concurrent opioid infusion improve pain management after surgery? *JAMA* 1991;266:1947–1952.
104. Parker RK, Holtmann B, White PF. Effects of a nighttime opioid infusion with PCA therapy on patient comfort and analgesic requirements after abdominal hysterectomy. *Anesthesiology* 1992;76:362–367.
105. Doyle E, Robinson D, Morton NS. Comparison of patient controlled analgesia with and without a background infusion after lower abdominal surgery in children. *Br J Anaesth* 1993;71:670–673.
106. Doyle E, Harper I, Morton NS. Patient-controlled analgesia with low dose background infusions after lower abdominal surgery in children. *Br J Anaesth* 1993;71: 818–822.
107. Sperry RJ, Bailey PL, Reuchman MV, et al. Fentanyl and sufentanil increase intracranial pressure in head trauma patients. *Anesthesiology* 1992;77:416–420.
108. Milde LN, Milde JH, Gallagher WJ. Effects of sufentanil on cerebral circulation and metabolism in dogs. *Anesth Analg* 1990;70:138–146.
109. Pokela ML, Ryhanen PT, Koivisto ME, et al. Alfentanil-induced rigidity in newborn infants. *Anesth Analg* 1992;75:252–257.
110. Irazuzta J, Pascucci R, Perlman N, Wessel D. Effects of fentanyl administration on respiratory system compliance in infants. *Crit Care Med* 1993;21:1001–1004.
111. Rosow CE, Moss J, Philbin DM, Savarese JJ. Histamine release during morphine and fentanyl anesthesia. *Anesthesiology* 1982;56:93–96.
112. Shochet RB, Murray GB. Neuropsychiatric toxicity of meperidine. *J Intensive Care Med* 1988;3:246–252.
113. Berde CB, Beyer JE, Bournaki MC, et al. Comparison of morphine and methadone for prevention of postoperative pain in children. *J Pediatr* 1991;119:136–141.
114. Lynn AM, Opheim KE, Tyler DC. Morphine infusion after pediatric cardiac surgery. *Crit Care Med* 1984;12:863–866.
115. Porter J, Jick J. Addiction rare in patients treated with narcotics (letter). *N Engl J Med* 1980;302:123.
116. Arnold JH, Truog RD, Orav EJ, et al. Tolerance and dependence in neonates sedated with fentanyl during extracorporeal membrane oxygenation. *Anesthesiology* 1990;73: 1136–1140.
117. Katz R, Kelly HW, Hsi A. Prospective study on the occurrence of withdrawal in critically ill children who receive fentanyl by continuous infusion. *Crit Care Med* 1994;22:763–767.
118. Finnegan LP, Kron RE, Connaughton JF Jr, et al. A scoring system for evaluation and treatment of the neonatal abstinence syndrome: A new clinical and research tool. In Morselli PL, Garattini S, Sereni F (eds): *Basic and Therapeutic Aspects of Perinatal Pharmacology*. New York: Raven Press; 1975:139–152.
119. Tobias JD. Outpatient therapy of iatrogenic opioid dependency following prolonged sedation in the pediatric intensive care unit. *J Intensive Care Med* 1996;11:284–287.
120. Riker RR, Fraser GL, Cox PM. Continuous infusions of haloperidol controls agitation in critically ill patients. *Crit Care Med* 1994;22:433–440.
121. Nahata MC, Clotz MA, Krogg EA. Adverse effects of meperidine, promethazine, and chlorpromazine for sedation in pediatric patients. *Clin Pediatr* 1985;24:558–560.
122. Maze MM, Tranquilli W. Alpha-2 agonists: Defining the role in clinical anesthesia. *Anesthesiology* 1991;74:581–591.
123. Mikawa K, Maekawa N, Nishina K, et al. Efficacy of oral clonidine premedication in children. *Anesthesiology* 1993;79:926–931.
124. De Kock MF, Pichon G, Scholtes JL. Intraoperative clonidine enhances postoperative morphine patient-controlled analgesia. *Can J Anaesth* 1992;39:537–544.

125. Bohrer H, Bach A, Layer M, Werning P. Clonidine as a sedative adjunct in intensive care. *Intensive Care Med* 1990;16:265–266.
126. Sharpe MD. The use of muscle relaxants in the intensive care unit. *Can J Anaesth* 1992;39:949–962.
127. Minton MD, Grosslight K, Stirt JA, Bedford RF. Increases in intracranial pressure from succinylcholine: Prevention by prior non-depolarizing block. *Anesthesiology* 1986;65:165–169.
128. Tobias JD, Nichols DG. Intraosseous succinylcholine for endotracheal intubation. *Pediatr Emerg Care* 1990;6:108–109.
129. Cooper R, Mirakhur RK, Clarke RSJ, Boulex Z. Comparison of intubating conditions after administration of rocuronium and suxamethonium. *Br J Anaesth* 1992;69:269–273.
130. Tobias JD. Continuous infusion of rocuronium in a paediatric intensive care unit. *Can J Anaesth* 1996;43:353–357.
131. Tobias JD, Atwood R. Mivacurium in children with Duchenne muscular dystrophy. *Paediatr Anaesthes* 1994;4:57–60.
132. Tobias JD, Lynch A, McDuffee A, Garrett JS. Pancuronium infusion for neuromuscular blockade in children in the pediatric intensive care unit. *Anesth Analg* 1995;81:13–16.
133. Tobias JD. Neuromuscular blockade in the pediatric intensive care unit: Pancuronium, vecuronium, rocuronium, or atracurium. *J Intensive Care Med* 1997;12:213–217.
134. Tobias JD. A prospective evaluation of the continuous infusion of cis-atracurium for neuromuscular blockade in the pediatric ICU patient: Efficacy and dosing requirements. *Am J Therapeutics* 1997;4:287–290.
135. Dodson BA, Kelly BJ, Braswell LM, Cohen NH. Changes in acetylcholine receptor number in muscle from critically ill patients receiving muscle relaxants: An investigation of the molecular mechanisms of prolonged paralysis. *Crit Care Med* 1995;23:815–821.
136. Segredo V, Caldwell JE, Matthay MA, et al. Persistent paralysis in critically ill patients after long term administration of vecuronium. *N Engl J Med* 1992;327:524–528.
137. Watling SM, Dasta JF. Prolonged paralysis in intensive care unit patients after the use of neuromuscular blocking agents: A review of the literature. *Crit Care Med* 1994;22:884–893.
138. Sladen RN. Neuromuscular blocking agents in the intensive care unit: A two edged sword. *Crit Care Med* 1995;23:423–428.

Chapter 12

Traumatic Injury and Burns

Joseph D. Tobias, MD

The Pediatric Trauma Patient

In the United States, traumatic injuries are the number one cause of death in children aged 1 to 10 years. Trauma accounts for 50% of deaths in this age range, with more than 20,000 deaths per year. The financial, psychologic, and social impact of trauma is even greater, because for each childhood trauma-related death, there are four survivors who are left with severe central nervous system (CNS) sequelae. Immediate stabilization and the expeditious transport of these patients to regional facilities can impact on both survival and the risks of debilitating sequelae. The successful management of the pediatric trauma patient depends on the expertise of physicians, nurses, and emergency medical personnel who are familiar with a systematic approach to the stabilization and treatment of patients with traumatic injuries.

The evaluation of the pediatric trauma patient is divided into the primary survey and secondary survey. The primary survey usually occupies the first 15 to 20 minutes and includes an assessment of the patient's airway, respiratory function, and cardiovascular function followed by the initial process of resuscitation and stabilization. During the primary survey, life-threatening injuries are identified and treatments are initiated to prevent further deterioration of the patient.

The most immediate concern in the management of any resuscitation, including trauma, is airway assessment with assisted or controlled ventilation as needed. Other attempts at resuscitation will fail if airway control and restoration of ventilation/oxygenation is delayed or ineffective. During the first 45 to 60 seconds, the airway is evaluated and the need for support of the respiratory system is identified. The reader is referred to chapter 1 for a full discussion of airway management. During the primary survey, other members of the team will help the physician in charge by gaining intravenous access and drawing the initial laboratory evaluation for the trauma patient, including a complete blood count, coagulation profile, basic laboratories (electrolytes, blood urea nitrogen, creatinine, glucose, calcium), and a type and cross.

Following major trauma, gas exchange may be compromised as a result of CNS injury, increased abdominal pressure, an unstable chest wall, pulmonary parenchymal injury (pulmonary contusion, aspiration, barotrauma), or cardiovascular instability (direct myocardial injury, tamponade, hemorrhagic shock). Patients who do not resume or maintain effective ventilation following relief of anatomic causes of airway obstruction and those with an altered level of consciousness (Glasgow coma score [GCS] of 8 or less) require endotracheal intubation. All patients should receive a fraction of inspired oxygen (FiO_2) of 1.0 by a high-flow mask system until the primary survey is completed and cardiorespiratory function is evaluated.

Airway intervention in the trauma setting may be fraught with difficulties.[1] Nakayama et al[1] reviewed airway management and its associated problems in 63 pediatric trauma patients. Complications were noted in 16 patients (25.4%), 13 of which were life-threatening, including right mainstem intubation, barotrauma, failure of adequate preoxygenation, esophageal intubation, and attempts at nasotracheal intubation in a patient with an open facial fracture. Airway management in the trauma setting is somewhat different from, and at times exceedingly more difficult than, the non-trauma setting due to the emergent nature of the need for airway control, the risk of acid aspiration and resultant pulmonary damage, associated maxillofacial injuries, associated CNS injury with increased intracranial pressure (ICP), associated cardiovascular instability, and the ever present risk of cervical spine instability. In addition to airway control and assisted ventilation, protection of the cervical spine is mandatory. This starts with the assumption that all pediatric trauma patients have a cervical spine injury until proven otherwise. While a thorough physical examination and radiologic investigation are helpful in excluding an injury, in the emergent setting there may be inadequate time to embark on such investigations. Therefore, as mentioned above, the airway is managed with the assumption that there is a cervical spine injury and techniques are used to control the airway and intubate the trachea (see below) that will not be harmful if a cervical spine injury is found during the subsequent evaluation.

Cervical spine injuries occur in 2% to 3% of adult trauma patients.[2] More importantly, it has been estimated that inappropriate treatment and ineffective cervical spine stabilization results in extension of the injury in 3% to 25% of patients.[3,4] Davis et al[2] prospectively evaluated the investigations used to rule out cervical spine injury and the etiology of missed injuries in adult trauma patients. The diagnosis was missed or delayed in 34 of 740 patients (4.6%). Ten of the 34 patients suffered permanent sequelae as a result of the missed diagnosis. The most common reason for missed diagnosis was failure to obtain an adequate radiographic evaluation. The authors concluded that the delay in diagnosis would have been avoided in 31 of 34 injuries if a standard three-view (anteroposterior, lateral, and odontoid views) cervical spine series had been obtained. Misinterpretation of the obtained films ranked as the second cause of missed injuries.

Controversy remains concerning the appropriate series of films that should be obtained to evaluate the cervical spine.[5,6] A single lateral cervical spine film will miss up to 15% of injuries,[7] while the five-view trauma series has a sensitivity of 92%[8] and is currently the standard in most institutions. The five-view trauma series includes a lateral film to include C_7 and the top of T_1, an anterior-posterior (AP) film, an open-mouth view of the odontoid, coned-down view of C_{1-2}, and a swimmer's view. Since the latter three may be difficult in the intubated patient, it may be more appropriate and technically easier to obtain a lateral and AP view plus computed tomography (CT) through C_{1-2}. The latter can most conveniently be performed during CT imaging of the head as long as the patient's cardiorespiratory status is stable.

"Clearing the cervical spine" should never take priority over resuscitation and the basic ABCs of trauma care. In many trauma patients, it may not be possible to absolutely clear the cervical spine. In such patients, immobilization must be maintained. One dilemma is encountered in the patient with an altered sensorium who has a normal five-view trauma series. It is recommended that the cervical collar not be removed until the physical examination documents no neck pain and no neurologic deficit. Oblique films may be obtained in these patients and if normal, the incidence of an occult injury, in the adult population, is small (no patient in the series of 1331 of Gerrelts et al[4]). Flexion-extension films are indicated when the patient complains of persistent neck pain despite a normal five-view trauma series and oblique views.

When there is a doubt concerning the presence of a cervical spine injury, CT scanning (of the entire cervical spine) has been reported to have a sensitivity of 99% to 100%[5] and is still considered the gold standard. Although the CT scan may add to the accuracy of identifying cervical spine injuries, obtaining a CT scan on all trauma patients is neither time effective nor cost effective. Therefore, the CT scan should be reserved for patients in whom there is a questionable injury based on the routine radiographic evaluation or in whom the physical examination is limited by an altered mental status or associated ("distracting injury") painful injury. The latter is included because the pain of a severe associated injury may limit the patient's ability to perceive neck pain related to a cervical spine injury.

Additional factors may cloud the issue of clearing the cervical spine in children. The first is age and its resultant effects on the ability to effectively communicate and/or complain of pain. The level of injury in children less than 8 years of age differs from that of the adult population.[9] The usual level of bony injury is C_{2-4} in infants and toddlers while a lower level of injury (C_{6-7}) is more common in adults. Another confounding factor is the increased ligamentous laxity in infants and children, which can lead to spinal cord injury without radiographic abnormality.[10] Therefore, a complete neurologic examination is mandatory in children, to rule out focal deficits prior to removing the cervical collar/restraint. Patients with neurologic deficits, persistent neck pain, or torticollis should be assumed to have a spinal cord injury and should be treated as such.

Based on the above mentioned problems of adequately clearing the cervical spine, especially in the younger pediatric population, compounded by the urgency for airway management in many patients, the usual routine is to proceed with airway management with the assumption that there is a cervical spine injury. Protection of the cervical spine is provided by the application of manual in-line axial stabilization. An assistant stands at the head of the patient with his or her hands on the patient's mastoid processes. The head and neck are stabilized, keeping the mastoid process in line with the axis of the head, preventing movement of the cervical spine. Traction force should be avoided as this may also result in trauma to the spinal cord in patients with bony injuries. The maneuver is designed to prevent extension or flexion of the cervical spine during laryngoscopy and tracheal intubation. Once in-line axial traction is applied and anesthesia induced, the front half of the rigid collar can be removed. This permits adequate mouth opening and facilitates oral endotracheal intubation.

Decisions regarding airway management include both the route of tracheal intubation (oral versus nasal) and the medications used for sedation/analgesia and neuromuscular blockade. An assessment is also made concerning the normalcy of the airway and the ability to successfully perform endotracheal intubation. The preferred route for endotracheal intubation in the pediatric trauma patient is oral. Attempts at nasal intubation can result in bleeding, which can obstruct visualization and make further attempts at endotracheal intubation difficult or impossible. Awake nasal intubation can lead to significant increases in ICP and is absolutely contraindicated in patients with closed-head injuries. Nasal intubation is also contraindicated in patients with evidence of facial trauma, cerebrospinal fluid leaks, or suggestion of basilar skull fracture (Battle's sign, raccoon eyes, hemotympanum). Any of the above are suggestive of disruption of the cribriform plate and the usual barrier between the nasopharynx and the intracranial vault. Additional implications related to blind nasotracheal intubation may include passing dislodged adenoidal tissue into the trachea, a high rate of a failure especially in infants and toddlers, and an inability to safely manipulate the head due to concerns of a possible cervical spine injury. The reader is referred to chapter 1 for complete details of the medications used and techniques for airway management.

Following successful endotracheal intubation, confirmation of correct endotracheal tube placement is mandatory and should begin with the auscultation of bilateral breath sounds. No method of confirming the intratracheal location of an endotracheal tube is 100% sensitive except for the direct observation of tracheal rings when a bronchoscope is passed through the endotracheal tube. The availability of end-tidal carbon dioxide is suggested whenever airway management is performed, as an additional means of confirming correct endotracheal tube placement.

Once endotracheal intubation is performed and confirmed, the focus of attention should shift to the provision of oxygenation and ventilation. Initial tidal volumes of 8 to 12 mL/kg are provided with respiratory rates adjusted according to the patient's age and the desired arterial carbon dioxide. The peak inflating pressure (PIP) should be noted with the initial setting of a tidal volume of 8 to 12 mL/kg. Monitoring of the PIP provides an ongoing assessment of the patient's respiratory compliance and of the need for investigation and intervention when altered compliance is noted. Patients who have an initially high PIP or progressively increasing PIPs require investigation into the etiology of the high PIP and into the appropriate treatment of the cause. The first step should be auscultation of breath sounds to rule out mainstem intubation. Auscultation will also reveal other treatable causes such as bronchospasm. A suction catheter should be passed through the endotracheal tube to ensure that the endotracheal tube is not kinked or that secretions/blood have not blocked the tube. A chest x-ray is indicated to rule out a pneumothorax or progressive alveolar space disease related to acid aspiration or progressive acute respiratory distress syndrome. If a pneumothorax is suspected, either because of lack of movement of the chest wall or absence of breath sounds, needle aspiration should be carried out followed by thoracostomy tube placement. There may not be time to obtain a chest film if the child's ventilatory or cardiovascular function is deteriorating. Once the cause of the increasing PIP is identified and easily treatable problems are corrected, if high pressures are still required to deliver an acceptable tidal volume, alternative means of ventilation may be necessary. Initial maneuvers to deliver an acceptable tidal volume and provide adequate ventilation while limiting the PIP include pressure-limited ventilation, a decelerating flow pattern, and lengthening out the inspiratory time. The reader is referred to chapters 4 and 5 for a full discussion of mechanical ventilation of patients with altered respiratory compliance.

All patients should receive an FiO_2 of 1.0 during the initial phases of evaluation, stabilization, and transport to either the pediatric intensive care unit (PICU) or the operating room. There is no risk of using an FiO_2 of 1.0 in the emergency setting. An adequate oxygen supply must be ensured prior to starting transport. An extra tank should be brought along if there is any question that the transport time will be prolonged.

Following airway management and stabilization of respiratory function, the primary survey continues with attention directed toward resuscitation and stabilization of the cardiovascular system. For a full discussion of cardiovascular physiology, use of inotropic agents, and invasive hemodynamic monitoring, the reader is referred to chapter 2. Cardiovascular instability in the pediatric trauma patient may result from hypovolemia from fluid and blood loss, disruption of the integrity of the vascular system (aortic transection, ventricular perforation), external factors affecting the contractile function of the myocardium (tension pneumothorax, excessive airway pressures during mechanical ventilation, pericardial tamponade), inadequate systemic vascular resistance (neurogenic shock), or myocardial pump failure (cardiac contusion, sedative/anesthetic agents) (Table 1). The prompt recognition of treatable causes and the immediate control of ongoing losses is the first priority. Although blood loss is easily recognized with external hemorrhage, fractures of long bones or of the pelvis can produce hidden losses that may total up to 2 L in adults. Control of obvious hemorrhage in most situations can be accomplished by direct pressure over the site. Although controversial, control of massive abdominal hemorrhage or hemorrhage from pelvic and long bone fractures can be controlled by application of military antishock trousers. In extreme situations, abdominal or thoracic bleeding may require thoracotomy and aortic crossclamping.

Spinal shock due to disruption of the descending sympathetic fibers in association with cervical spine trauma should be

Table 1

Etiology of Cardiovascular Dysfunction in Pediatric Trauma

Hypovolemia
Obstructive lesions:
   pericardial tamponade
   hemo/pneumothorax
   aortic disruption
   increased mean airway pressure

Cardiogenic:
   myocardial contusion
   valvular disruption
   ventricular septal defect
   coronary artery injury
   arrhythmias
   sedative/anesthetic agents

Metabolic:
   hypothermia
   hypocalcemia
   hypoglycemia
   acidosis

Distributive:
   neurogenic
   anaphylaxis

suspected in the patient with neurologic deficits (areflexia, paralysis), hypotension, and bradycardia. While most patients will demonstrate tachycardia from other forms of shock including hypovolemia, disruption of the sympathetic innervation to the cardioaccelatory fibers (T_{1-4}) results in bradycardia. Treatment of spinal shock requires first recognition of the problem, and second the use of inotropic agents such as phenylephrine to restore vascular tone.

Inotropic/vasopressor agents should never be used in place of adequate volume resuscitation. However, the recognition of dysfunction of the cardiovascular system (cardiac contractility, vascular integrity) or spinal shock is mandatory during the immediate phase of resuscitation and during subsequent hospital care. At times inotropic agents are necessary to maintain an acceptable mean arterial pressure while rapid repletion of the intravascular status is achieved.

Although most of the cardiovascular instability seen in the immediate phase of trauma is related to ongoing losses and hypovolemia, other causes of cardiovascular instability exist and must be identified, since many of them require surgical intervention. Although volume resuscitation may be needed in a patient with pericardial tamponade, fluid administration, no matter how aggressive, does not solve the problem. Likewise, fluid administration may be detrimental in patients with cardiogenic failure from myocardial contusion, infarction, or valvular disruption.

The most sensitive monitor of cardiac output and volume status in children is the heart rate. The adequacy of cardiac output is assessed by noting the quality, regularity, and rate of the pulse, and, secondarily, by obtaining a blood pressure. Children are able to vasoconstrict to a significant degree to maintain blood pressure in the setting of significant hypovolemia (up to 25% of total blood volume). The classification of shock according to blood volume loss is outlined in Table 2.

Before appropriate fluid resuscitation can be accomplished, vascular access must be established. The simplest, safest, and often the most rapid means of obtaining ve-

Table 2

Classification of Blood Loss and Associated Signs/Symptoms

Class I (loss of 10%–15% of total blood volume):
   increased heart rate
   normal blood pressure
   normal peripheral pulses

Class II (loss of 20%–25% of total blood volume):
   increased respiratory rate
   peripheral vasoconstriction/cool extremities
   decreased peripheral pulses
   pallor
   cyanosis
   decreased capillary refill

Class III (loss of 30%–35% of total blood volume):
   poor peripheral pulses
   altered sensorium
   decreased end-organ perfusion
   oliguria

Class IV (loss ≥40% of total blood volume):
   nonpalpable pulses/blood pressure
   obtundation, coma

nous access is by percutaneous peripheral vein cannulation. Because of the smaller size of veins in children and the fact that veins usually collapse when a child is in shock, percutaneous peripheral cannulation may be difficult and time-consuming. If peripheral venous cannulation cannot be accomplished within 60 to 90 seconds, initial access to the circulation can be rapidly obtained by placement of an intraosseous cannula. The preferred site is the medial aspect of the tibia, 2 to 4 cm below the anterior tibial tuberosity. While there are several commercially available intraosseous needles, a 16- or 18-gauge spinal needle can also be used. Fluid and medications can be administered through the intraosseous needle. When necessary, sedative and neuromuscular blocking agents can be administered via the intraosseous route for airway management and endotracheal intubation. Once appropriate fluid resuscitation has been carried out via the intraosseous route, cannulation of a peripheral vein is often possible.

One area of active debate in shock resuscitation is the type of fluid that should be used: crystalloid or colloid.[11,12] Only 25% of the volume of crystalloid that is administered will remain in the intravascular compartment. The remainder will fill the interstitial and extracellular fluid compartments. The tendency for crystalloids to leave the vascular compartment along with the dilution of plasma proteins may theoretically predispose patients to the development of pathologic extravascular fluid such as pulmonary edema. While this principle makes sense based on the Starling forces that control fluid movements across the vascular compartment, clinical studies do not provide evidence for the superiority of colloid over crystalloid for volume expansion in shock resuscitation.

The commercially available colloid solutions include 5% albumin, 6% hydroxyethyl starch, and low molecular weight dextran (Dextran 40). Adverse effects including platelet dysfunction, interference with crossmatching of blood, and renal failure limit the use of dextran preparations. Albumin is a naturally occurring plasma protein that provides approximately 80% of the intravascular colloid oncotic pressure in normal subjects. The albumin molecule has a molecular weight of 69,000 and is relatively impermeable to the vascular membrane under normal conditions. The intravascular half-life of albumin is 24 hours, with hemodynamic improvement persisting for up to 36 hours after administration.[13,14] As albumin is heat treated, there are limited infectious disease risks with its use. Another protein product derived from blood, plasma protein fraction or Plasminate, is not recommended for resuscitation in shock as it can occasionally cause hypotension due to the presence of activated mediators of the kininogen pathway that are present in the solution.

Hydroxyethyl starch is a synthetic colloid that consists of a hydroxyethyl-substituted, branched-chain amylopectin with a molecular weight similar to that of albumin. Although its elimination half-time is 17 days, its clinical effects persist for only 24 to 36 hours.[15] Adverse effects include inhibition of platelet aggregation following the administration of more than 15 to 20 mL/kg.

There also remains controversy as to which particular crystalloid is most appropriate for volume expansion. Without a doubt, an isotonic fluid should be used: normal saline, Ringer's lactate, or Plasmalyte. Ringer's lactate has a chloride concentration (109 mEq/L) that is roughly equivalent to the plasma chloride, while the lactate provides a source of buffer. One problem with Ringer's lactate is that the sodium concentration of 130 mEq/L is somewhat hypotonic compared to normal plasma, making it a relatively inappropriate fluid for patients with CNS trauma who are at risk for increased ICP.

Aside from the isotonic crystalloids, recent attention has shifted to the possible beneficial effects of hypertonic crystalloids with or without the addition of colloid. These agents were used in clinical practice as early as World War I. The principle behind their use is to restore effective circulating blood volume with a lower volume of fluid (4 to 5 mL/kg). This can be accomplished because hypertonic saline increases serum osmolarity and promotes the movement of endogenous fluid from the extravascular space into the intravascular space. Additional effects demonstrated in laboratory animals include an increase in inotropic function of the heart, constriction of capacitance vessels, decrease in resistance vessels, and dilatation of precapillary sphincters.[16–18] The initial clinical studies in humans have shown similar beneficial effects. Holcroft et al[19] and Vassar et al[20] have demonstrated successful resuscitation of trauma patients with hypertonic saline (250 mL of 7.5% sodium chloride) without adverse effects except for transient hypokalemia. These agents may have particular benefit for patients with associated closed-head injuries who are at risk for cerebral edema. The initial clinical studies in adult trauma victims have demonstrated improved survival following resuscitation with hypertonic saline as compared with Ringer's lactate.[21,22]

Although the ideal resuscitation fluid for the pediatric trauma victim has not yet been clearly identified, the initial studies in adults support the superiority of hypertonic saline solutions (ie, 7.5% NaCl). These solutions restore intravascular volume with a rapid mobilization of endogenous fluid, reduce vascular resistance, and improve myocardial contractility. Hypertonic saline may be particularly beneficial to the patient with associated closed-head injury. As with other crystalloid solutions, the hypertonic solutions are inexpensive and have a long shelf life.

Regardless of the fluid chosen, an initial 20 to 30 mL/kg of an isotonic crystalloid solution is given as quickly as possible. Additional crystalloid is infused and titrated against urine output, skin perfusion, heart rate, and blood pressure. For Class III or Class IV patients, the administration of blood will be necessary to restore adequate cardiac output and tissue oxygen delivery. Isotonic crystalloid and inotropic agents should not be used as substitutes for blood in Class III or IV patients. The ideal colloid in such patients would be fresh whole blood, which has clotting factors, normal to 2,3-DPG (diphosphoglycerate) levels, and normal pH, and therefore duplicates what is being lost. However, since fresh whole blood is rarely available, component therapy is used.

During the emergent resuscitative phase of Class III and IV patients, time may not allow for a full type and crossmatch to be completed. In these patients, if time allows for a type and screen to be completed, then type-specific blood should be administered. If time does not permit even a type and screen to be accomplished, then type O Rh-negative, noncrossmatched blood is administered. Type O blood lacks both the A and B antigens on the red cells and therefore is not hemolyzed by anti-A or anti-B antibodies that may be present in the recipient's plasma. Once resuscitation with ≥20 mL/kg of type O Rh-negative blood has started, it should be continued even when the type and crossmatch is available, since the antibodies which may be present in the type O (anti-A, anti-B antibodies) blood may cause hemolysis if type A or B blood is subsequently infused.

Whenever blood or large volumes of fluid are being administered to the pediatric trauma patient, blood warmers should be used to prevent hypothermia. Hypothermia can have significant deleterious physiologic effects, especially in the pediatric trauma patient. The reader is referred to chapter 15 for a full discussion of the use of blood and blood component therapy.

With the exception of factors V and VIII, plasma coagulation factors are relatively stable in banked blood. With the transfusion of large volumes of blood (>2 blood volumes in a child), hemostatic defects may occur. The hemostatic defects are related to a dilution of both platelets and circulating protein coagulation factors. The level of platelets necessary for adequate hemostasis has been widely debated. Although hemostatic function may be adequate in patients who have a slow decrease in their platelet count to 10,000/mm^3, the abrupt decrease in the platelet level to less than 50,000/mm^3 is generally considered an indication for the transfusion of platelet concentrates, especially when associated with clinical evidence of bleeding. In addition to thrombocytopenia, a dilution of coagulation factors may occur with the administration of packed red blood cells. Following the replacement of 1.5 to 2 blood volumes, coagulation parameters should be evaluated. The latter should include a prothrombin time (PT), partial thromboplastin time (PTT), and fibrinogen level. Abnormalities in the PT and PTT can be corrected with the administration of fresh frozen plasma, while low levels of fibrinogen should be treated with the administration of cryoprecipitate.

In addition to fluid therapy, correction of the metabolic abnormalities may improve cardiac output and may correct shock. With tissue hypoperfusion, metabolic acidosis frequently develops. This can be partially compensated for by endotracheal intubation and controlled ventilation. While fluid administration and cardiovascular resuscitation is mandatory for the elimination of the ongoing anaerobic processes that lead to lactate production, buffer administration is frequently required to rapidly correct the problem. Persistent acidosis (pH <7.20) not only profoundly depresses myocardial contractility, it also impairs the effectiveness of exogenous catecholamines. Bicarbonate administration, when necessary, should be administered slowly in a dose that is dependent on the base deficit (mEq sodium bicarbonate = 0.3 × weight (kg) × base deficit).

Sodium bicarbonate is administered slowly over 3 to 5 minutes, because its rapid administration may abruptly increase pH and lower ionized calcium levels due to alterations in protein binding. Low ionized calcium levels may be further aggravated by the citrate used as an anticoagulant in blood. Since many patients in shock may have low ionized calcium levels, measurement and correction of this cation may be indicated. Hypocalcemia impairs cardiac contractility and limits the vasopressor effect of catecholamines. Since the free or ionized fraction is the physiologic active moiety, measurement of ionized calcium is suggested. Hypocalcemia is treated by the administration of either calcium chloride or calcium gluconate.

During the initial evaluation, a quick check of serum glucose is suggested, with a rapid, bedside analyzer. The value can be confirmed by formal laboratory evaluation of serum glucose. Children, especially toddlers and infants, have limited glycogen stores and rapidly develop hypoglycemia during periods of stress. Severe hypoglycemia with subsequent CNS damage may occur if hypoglycemia is not identified and treated promptly. There is also some evidence to suggest that severe hypoglycemia may impair cardiovascular function. Serum glucose levels less than 60 mg/dL should be promptly treated with the administration of 1 mL/kg of 25% glucose or 2 mL/kg of 10% glucose. In the patient with associated closed-head injury, hyperglycemia related to the sympathetic stress response from the tissue trauma may be seen. Normal serum glucose levels should be maintained, as hyperglycemia has been shown to result in a worse neurologic outcome in patients with regional or global cerebral hypoperfusion. The suggested etiology of this phenomenon is the production of increased levels of lactate from the high glucose supply during periods of ischemia and anaerobic metabolism.

Once the cardiovascular system has been stabilized, the last step in the primary survey includes a rapid neurologic evaluation. A key component of the neurologic evaluation is the assignment of a GCS. The neurologic examination concentrates on the patient's level of consciousness, the GCS, and a search for signs of increased ICP that might necessitate endotracheal intubation and controlled ventilation. A more thorough neurologic exam is performed later as part of the secondary survey.

The basic principles of resuscitation and the primary survey are to begin treating life-threatening organ injuries and to not wait for a complete evaluation of the child. The primary survey focuses on those derangements, such as respiratory and cardiovascular insufficiency, that require immediate treatment to prevent morbidity and even mortality. During the primary survey, careful attention must be paid to prevent hypothermia. Since the patient is frequently undressed and placed in a cold environment, a rapid loss of body heat can occur. Measures to conserve body heat in children include use of external heating lamps, warming of intravenous fluids and blood products, and wrapping exposed body parts in materials such as plastic bags to prevent heat loss.

While the physician team leader is addressing the ABCs and completing the primary survey, the nursing staff involved should record the baseline findings, the fluids and drugs administered, and the ongoing responses of the patient to the therapy. Following the initial stabilization of the cardiorespiratory system, the identification and treatment of life-threatening injuries, and the reversal of shock, a complete physical examination should be accomplished. This is referred to as the secondary survey and generally takes 15 to 20 minutes. The secondary survey is accomplished in a head-to-toe fashion with preference to the evaluation of injuries in descending order of urgency.

The pediatric trauma victim should be assessed using a protocol in which all body areas are evaluated systematically. For those not involved in trauma care every day, this can be accomplished by having standardized in-hospital protocols and data sheets that can be easily followed. The evaluation should always be undertaken with particular care to avoid manipulation of the spinal axis until injuries are ruled out. Even during performance of the secondary survey, an ongoing assessment and reevaluation of the patient's status and vital signs is mandatory, since acute changes that require immediate intervention may occur.

The secondary survey begins with an evaluation of the head. This starts with the eyes, including the conjunctivae, pupillary size and reaction to light, fundoscopic examination, and assessment of the vision if the child is conscious. The face and scalp are then carefully examined. Maxillofacial trauma, including fractures and scalp lesions, should be palpated. Localized hematomas, especially in the periorbital region and behind the ears, are indicative of a basilar skull fracture. The tympanic membrane and nose are examined for blood and signs of cerebrospinal fluid leakage. The scalp, including the back of the head, should be carefully examined for lacerations or underlying soft tissue injury.

The neck is examined for subcutaneous emphysema, hematomas, or localized pain. Following the lateral cervical spine film, the cervical spine is palpated for evidence of bony trauma or pain. The location of the trachea is assessed to make sure it is midline. The neck is examined for discoloration, and the neck veins are inspected for distention which may be indicative of cardiac tamponade or tension pneumothorax.

A chest examination follows the head and neck examination. In addition to adequacy and rate of ventilation, any asymmetry in chest wall excursion and any painful areas should be observed with particular attention to the presence of a flail segment. After observation, a more thorough pulmonary and cardiovascular examination is performed using auscultation, percussion, and palpation. An examination of the abdomen is next. The specific diagnosis of an intra-abdominal injury is not necessary at this point. What must be determined here is whether surgical intervention is urgent or emergent. The initial examination of the abdomen consists of inspection, careful palpation, and auscultation. If the child is conscious, gentle palpation may identify areas of tenderness. A rapidly expanding abdominal girth is indicative of ongoing hemorrhage and is an indication for further diagnostic studies. At this point, there remains controversy in the surgical literature as to the value of the various diagnostic tests and their utility in identifying the need for surgical intervention. Diagnostic tests for evaluating the presence of intra-abdominal pathology include peritoneal lavage, CT scanning, and ultrasound evaluation. Gastric decompression with a nasogastric or orogastric tube is indicated in patients with abdominal trauma. Nasogastric tubes are contraindicated in patients with associated closed-head injuries, due to the risks of increasing ICP, as well as the possibility of intracranial placement should there be a disruption of the cribriform plate with a basilar skull fracture.

Following the abdominal examination, the patient is turned for evaluation of the entire posterior aspect of the body. This is an integral part of the examination, as the back is a frequent source of missed injuries. Also included in the abdominal examination is the examination of the pelvis and rectum. The bony prominences of the pelvis are palpated for tenderness and instability. The perineum is examined for lacerations, hematomas, or active bleeding. If a pelvic fracture is suspected or seen on a radiograph, a rectal examination should be carried out to evaluate the possibility of bony fragment injury to the pelvic structures. Although genitourinary tract injury is common in the pediatric trauma patient, the majority of these injuries are not apparent on the initial examination. The child with a pelvic fracture, perineal swelling or discoloration, flank pain or tenderness, rib fracture, or abdominal tenderness should be considered to have a genitourinary injury until proven otherwise. If an injury to the genitourinary tract is suspected, a urinary catheter should be inserted. Bladder decompression via a catheter provides a means to measure urine output, provides urine for examination, prevents urinary obstruction from blood clots in the bladder, and provides a route for contrast radiographic studies.

Next, the extremities are examined for abrasions, contusions, or hematomas. Bony instability is noted, and a neurovascular examination is performed to assess the presence of compromised blood flow and the development of a compartment syndrome. Disruption of blood flow to an extremity results in the so-called four P's: pulselessness, pallor, paresthesia, and paralysis. Lack of recognition of an injury to the neurovascular bundle of an extremity can lead to unnecessary morbidity. The blood vessels in injured limbs are vulnerable to compression or laceration. These blood vessels can continue to bleed and exacerbate hypovolemic shock or they can bleed into an intact fascial space, resulting in a compartment syndrome. If there is a suspicion of a compartment syndrome, muscle compartment pressures can be evaluated during the secondary survey using an 18 gauge needle and a water manometer. Compartment pressures of ≥40 cm of water should cause concern, while pressures of ≥60 cm of water require an immediate fasciotomy.

Next, a neurologic examination is performed. A thorough neurologic exam is carried out in a stepwise fashion, including assessment of the cranial nerves as well as a peripheral motor and sensory evaluation. In all patients with an abnormal initial GCS, ongoing examination is extremely important in order to identify those with a deteriorating neurologic status who may require further investigation or treatment of increasing ICP.

The final step in the secondary survey is to obtain a history of the onset of the injury or illness. This is often best obtained from accompanying family members or the emergency medical technicians. Knowledge of the forces of injury that resulted in the child's trauma can be important for determining the extent of injury and can be useful in the management of the pediatric trauma patient. In addition to the pertinent information concerning the acute event, relative past medical history should be obtained. Following this, the patient's current status and vital signs are reassessed prior to transport. At this stage, the child's airway and respiratory system should be stable. If the hemodynamic status is stable, the child is prepared for transport to the PICU. Specialized radiographic studies including CT imaging should be performed prior to transport to the PICU. If there is progressive deterioration of the hemodynamic status despite ongoing resuscitation with blood and fluids or if there is evidence of life-threatening injuries, the child should be prepared for transport to the operating room for immediate surgical intervention. In either case, prior to transport, the airway and respiratory function should be stabilized. During transport there should be continuous monitoring, including pulse oximetry, noninvasive blood pressure monitoring, and continuous electrocardiography. Additionally, ongoing monitoring of invasive hemodynamic monitors is appropriate. In addition to monitoring, a full complement of resuscitative drugs and airway equipment should be brought during the transport.

Thermal Injury

The initial care of the burn victim is directed at assessment for airway compromise, stopping the burning the process, and beginning fluid resuscitation. All clothing should be removed to prevent ongoing burning of the patient, and sites of chemical burns should be flushed with large amounts of water for 20 to 30 minutes. Patients who demonstrate any sign of airway compromise, burns to the face or airway, or abnormalities with air movement such as stridor, should receive early elective tracheal intubation. Airway management follows the basic principles outlined in chapter 1. Patients with significant thermal injuries will have delayed gastrointestinal motility and are at risk for acid aspiration during airway management. In the immediate 48 hours following a burn injury, both depolarizing and nondepolarizing neuromuscular blocking agents can be used safely. However, 48 to 72 hours after a body surface area (BSA) burn of greater than 10% to 15%, there is a significant upregulation in acetylcholine receptors and the administration of succinylcholine will result in an exaggerated hyperkalemic response. In such patients, a nondepolarizing neuromuscular blocking agent should be used during airway management. The upregulation of the acetylcholine receptors results in a resistance to the effect of the nondepolarizing neuromuscular blocking agents, which in turn results in a longer time to peak effect and the need to use larger doses.

Following the basic ABCs of resuscitation, an estimate is made of the burn size and depth. First-degree burns include superficial injuries such as sunburns which are characterized by erythema, pain, and occasionally mild blistering. Tissue loss is restricted to the epithelial layer. No treatment is generally necessary except for mild oral analgesics. Second-degree burns include tissue damage and death through the epidermis and into a variable portion of the dermis. The extent of injury to the dermis layer will determine the length of time it takes for the wound to heal and the presence or absence of scar formation. With deep partial-thickness burns with tissue necrosis through most of the dermis, healing may take up to 6 weeks and may be accompanied by scarring. Regardless of the depth of the initial burn, if there is infection or inadequate nutrition, conversion to a third-degree burn may be seen. A third-degree burn is a full-thickness injury in which all layers of the skin are destroyed. Third-degree burns, except for small ones, require surgical closure.

Assessment of the degree of injury includes estimation of the size and depth of burns, as previously outlined. A brief history of the mechanism of injury provides clues to associated trauma, history of electrical injury and the risk of cardiac damage, or the presence of inhalation injury with airway or respiratory compromise. Using standardized charts, an estimate is made of the percent of BSA that has been burned.[23] The most commonly used formula for patients greater than 14 years of age is the rule of 9's whereby 9% is accounted for by each arm and the head, and 18% by each leg, the front of the torso, and the back. Because of differences in surface area in children of various ages, other formulas may be more accurate in younger aged patients.[24] A generalized estimate can be obtained by considering the surface area of the palm of the hand to account for 1% of the BSA. Hospital admission is generally required for patients with burns greater than 15% to 20% BSA, for those with full-thickness burns, burns to the hands, feet, face, or perineum, and for those with complicating factors such as suspected child abuse, electrical and chemical burns, or airway injuries. Patients with electrical injuries including those associated with lightening require continuous electrocardiography monitoring due to the risk of delayed cardiac arrhythmias as well as monitoring for rhabdomyolysis and hemoglobinuria.

Following placement of an intravenous cannula, blood samples are sent for a complete blood count, type and crossmatch, carboxyhemoglobin level, as well as standard blood chemistries. Patients who are treated with intravenous fluids should have a bladder catheter placed for accurate measurement of urine output as a guide to the adequacy of ongoing fluid replacement. Intravenous opioid analgesics are administered as needed to treat pain. Initial wound care is limited to application of a clean, dry dressing. Blisters are left intact. Tetanus prophylaxis should be administered as needed according to the patient's immunization status. If there are any questions concerning the patient's immunization status, tetanus immune globulin should be administered in addition to routine tetanus immunization.

Based on recommendations from the American Burn Association, the following cases should be referred to a regional burn center:

1. Partial-thickness and third-degree burns that involve more than 10% of the BSA in patients less than 10 years of age.
2. Partial-thickness and third-degree

burns that involve more than 20% of the BSA.
3. Partial-thickness or third-degree burns that involve the face, eyes, ears, hands, feet, genitalia, perineum, and/or major joints.
4. Third-degree burns greater than 5% of the BSA.
5. Electrical burns including lightening.
6. Chemical burns.
7. Associated inhalation injury or airway compromise.
8. Patients with significant underlying associated health problems.

Following stabilization of the airway and respiratory system, aggressive intravenous hydration is mandatory to prevent hypovolemia and inadequate tissue perfusion and its resultant sequelae. Once the patient's cardiovascular system has been resuscitated from the initial trauma of the thermal injury, a determination is made of ongoing rates for fluid administration. Several formulas have been devised to estimate the fluid volumes that are required to replace ongoing losses in the pediatric burn patient. Regardless of the formula used, modifications are necessary to allow for alterations in the rate of fluid administration to provide a urine output of 0.5 to 1 mL/kg/h. Diuretics are seldom, if ever, indicated to augment urine output in the burn patient, except when there has been significant rhabdomyolysis with hemoglobinuria. Placement of a central venous catheter may be beneficial when burns exceed 25% to 30% of the BSA. However, fluid resuscitation should still be guided by urine output, since arbitrary attempts to produce high normal central venous filling pressures may result in the administration of excessive volumes of fluid, which may lead to increased edema formation.

The most widely used formula to estimate fluid administration during the first 24 hours is the Parkland formula, which provides 4 mL/kg per percent BSA burned. Despite the widespread use of the Parkland formula, it frequently results in an underestimation of fluid needs in the pediatric burn patient unless maintenance intravenous fluids are added to the infusion rates. Using the Parkland formula plus maintenance intravenous fluids, one half of the volume is given in the initial 8 hours with the second half delivered over the ensuing 16 hours. An isotonic fluid, most commonly lactated Ringer's, is used, although some controversy exists regarding the optimal fluid to be used during the first 24 hours following a burn. Most agree that there is no proven benefit to adding colloids such as albumin to the resuscitation fluids during the first 24 hours. However, more recently, some investigators have advocated the use of hypertonic saline solutions in hopes of decreasing fluid administration and tissue edema.[25] While some of the early studies in adults suggest the efficacy of this approach, future prospective studies are needed to evaluate its efficacy in the pediatric population. During the second 24 postburn hours, maintenance fluids are started with a glucose-containing hypotonic fluid such as D5 ½NS + maintenance potassium. Albumin, 12.5 g/L, may be added to each liter of i.v. fluid to maintain a normal serum albumin level.

In addition to providing fluid to the burn patient, an aggressive approach for providing nutrition is necessary. Following a thermal injury, there is a significant increase in the basal metabolic rate with protein catabolism, which places the patient at increased risk for infection and poor wound healing if appropriate caloric intake is not provided. Whenever possible, the enteral route is the preferred method for providing nutrition for the burn patient.[26] The current trend in most burn centers is to institute early enteral feedings and, whenever possible, to limit the use of parenteral nutrition. The reader is referred to chapter 14 for a full discussion of nutrition in the PICU patient.

Following the appropriate support of the cardiorespiratory system and the provision of resuscitation fluids, attention should be turned to wound management. Once the acute phase has passed, the ongoing risk to the burn patient is death from a burn-wound infection. The burn wound should be cleansed with saline, and blisters should be debrided. After a period of drying, a topical antimicrobial agent is applied to the wound, followed by a dressing. Several different topical antimicrobial agents are in common use.

The most commonly used is silver sulfadiazine, which is a broad-spectrum antibacterial agent that penetrates well into the eschar and is painless when applied. Silver sulfadiazine can cause sensitivity reactions due to the sulfonamide component and occasionally can result in a depression of the white blood cell count. It is generally applied twice daily, followed by a gauze dressing. Despite its broad-spectrum antibiotic coverage, several organisms including *Enterobacter cloacae, Staphylococcus aureus,* and occasionally *Pseudomonas aeruginosa* are resistant.

Alternatives to silver sulfadiazine include mafenide (Sulfamylon), silver nitrate, iodophors, and bacitracin cream. Mafenide cream has a broad spectrum of coverage, particularly against gram-positive organisms and clostridia species. Of all the topical antimicrobials in use, it provides the most rapid and effective penetration into the eschar. Due to its effective penetration into the eschar, it is frequently used on high-voltage electrical injuries, infected burns that have been neglected prior to transfer, and those on the face, ears, and nose, because secondary infection in these areas, especially the ears, can lead to infection of the cartilaginous supporting structures. Side effects of mafenide use include a metabolic acidosis related to its systemic absorption with the inhibition of the enzyme carbonic anhydrase, and pain with application.

Silver nitrate solution provides poor penetration of the eschar and can be associated with electrolyte disturbances including a hyponatremic, hypochloremic alkalosis due to the leakage of chloride into the dressings. Other topical antimicrobials such as iodophor preparations are seldom used in burn care due to their limited penetration into the eschar, staining of tissue, and absorption of iodine.

Burns are typically cleaned and debrided in a whirlpool and then dressed twice daily. Despite meticulous aseptic technique, the burn wound becomes colonized with airborne gram-positive and gram-negative organisms. An infected burn wound is characterized by a gray or dark appearance with a purulent discharge and, frequently, systemic signs of sepsis. The definitive diagnosis in most large burn centers in made by quantitative bacterial count with greater than 100 organisms/gram of tissue. When the diagnosis of burn-wound sepsis is entertained, broad-spectrum antibiotic coverage is started based on the most recent microbial isolates from the wound. If periodic cultures are not routinely obtained, broad-spectrum antibiotic coverage to include gram-positive cocci, including *Staphylococcus aureus,* and gram-negative organisms, including *Pseudomonas aeruginosa,* is provided. While the most likely etiology of fever in the pediatric burn patient is burn-wound sepsis, other sources of infection should be ruled out. These may include anything from routine infections such as otitis media to tracheitis or pneumonia in the intubated patient, central line-related bacteremia, and urinary tract infections.

Total excision and grafting is necessary for areas of deep, partial-thickness injury or full-thickness injury. The primary means of wound coverage is autografting from noninvolved donor sites. Recent developments in this area have provided techniques for culturing autologous and allogeneic epithelium for burn-wound coverage. These techniques are particularly useful when a large percentage of the surface area has been burned and only a small percentage is available for autologous grafting. Further future areas of research include synthetic and biosynthetic skin, which may eventually provide an abundant source of sterile coverage for burns.

Summary

Regardless of the mechanisms of injury, trauma remains a leading cause of morbidity and mortality in the pediatric population. A delay in instituting appropriate therapy for these patients can lead to significant morbidity and mortality. Regardless of the mechanism of injury, initial care provided to these patients should focus on control of the airway and resuscitation of the respiratory and cardiovascular systems. As is evident in this chapter, care of the pediatric trauma victim requires the cooperation of many subspecialists including emergency room physicians, anesthesiologists, critical care specialists, and surgical subspecialists. Providing effective care for these patients requires a broad understanding of the concepts of critical care medicine, as failure of any organ system may occur either as a result of the primary injury or as a secondary event.

References

1. Nakayama DK, Gardner MJ, Rowe MI. Emergency endotracheal intubation in pediatric trauma. *Ann Surg* 1990;211:218–223.
2. Davis JW, Phreaner DL, Hoyt DB, Mackersie RC. The etiology of missed cervical spine injuries. *J Trauma* 1993;34:342–346.
3. Bohlman HF. Acute fractures and dislocations of the cervical spine. *J Bone Joint Surg* 1979;61A:1119–1124.
4. Gerrelts BD, Petersen KU, Mabry J, Petersen SR. Delayed diagnosis of cervical spine injuries. *J Trauma* 1991;31:1622–1625.
5. Ross SE, Schwab CW, David ET, et al. Clearing the cervical spine: Initial radiographic evaluation. *J Trauma* 1987;27:1055–1058.
6. Fischer RP. Cervical radiographic evaluation of alert patients following blunt trauma. *Ann Emerg Med* 1984;13:905–909.
7. Shaffer MA, Doris PE. Limitation of the cross table lateral view in detecting cervical spine injuries: A retrospective analysis. *Ann Emerg Med* 1981;10:508–512.
8. Doris PE, Wilson RA. The next logical step in the emergency radiographic evaluation of cervical spine trauma: The five view trauma series. *J Emerg Med* 1985;3:371–375.
9. Apple DF, Anson CA, Hunter JD, Bell RB. Spinal cord injury in youth. *Clin Pediatr* 1995;34:90–95.
10. Pang D, Wilberger J. Spinal cord injury without radiographic abnormalities in children. *J Neurosurg* 1982;57:114–118.
11. Shoemaker WC, Hauser CJ. Critique of crystalloid versus colloid therapy in shock and shock lung. *Crit Care Med* 1979;7:117–121.
12. Skillman JJ. The role of albumin and oncotically active fluids in shock. *Crit Care Med* 1976;4:55–58.
13. Tullis JL. Albumen. *JAMA* 1977;237:355–362.
14. Rothschild MA, Bauman A, Yalow RS, Berson SA. Tissue distribution of I-131 labeled human serum albumin following intravenous administration. *J Clin Invest* 1955; 34:1354–1358.
15. Metcalf W, Papadopoulos A, Tufaro R, Barth A. A clinical physiologic study of hydroxyethyl starch. *Surg Gynecol Obstet* 1970;131: 255–259.
16. Wildenthal K, Mierzqiak DS, Mitchell JH. Acute effects of increased serum osmolarity on left ventricular performance. *Am J Physiol* 1969;216:898–904.
17. Rowe GG, Mckenna DH, Corliss RJ, et al. Hemodynamic effects of hypertonic sodium chloride. *J Appl Physiol* 1972;32:182–184.
18. Lundvall J, Mellander S, White T. Hyperosmolarity and vasodilation in human skeletal muscle. *Acta Physiol Scand* 1969;77:224–233.
19. Holcroft J, Vassar M, Perry C, et al. Use of a 7.5% NaCl/6% dextran 70 solution in the resuscitation of injured patients in the emergency room. *Prog Clin Biol Res* 1989;299:331–338.
20. Vassar M, Perry C, Holcroft J. Analysis of potential risks associated with 7.5% sodium chloride resuscitation of traumatic shock. *Arch Surg* 1990;125:1309–1315.
21. Holcroft J, Vassar M, Perry C, et al. 3% NaCl and 7.5%NaCl/dextran-70 in the resuscitation of severely injured patients. *Ann Surg* 1987;206:279–288.
22. Holcroft J, Vassar M, Perry C, et al. Perspectives on clinical trials for hypertonic saline/ dextran solutions for the treatment of traumatic shock. *Braz J Med Biol Res* 1989;22:291–293.
23. Demling RH. Burns. *N Engl J Med* 1985;313: 1389–1398.
24. Solomon JR. Pediatric burns. *Crit Care Clin* 1985;1:159–173.
25. Monafo WW, Halverson JD, Schectman K. The role of concentrated sodium solutions in the resuscitation of patients with severe burns. *Surgery* 1984;95:129.
26. Wolfe RR. Caloric requirements of the burned patient. *J Trauma* 1981;21:712–716.

Chapter 13

Fluid and Electrolyte Issues, Metabolic Disorders, Tumor Lysis Syndrome

Rosaleah V. Bernardo, MD,
Joseph E. Segeleon, MD, and Steven E. Haun, MD

Introduction

A basic understanding of the composition of body fluid compartments and the regulatory mechanisms that maintain their homeostasis is essential to the care of acutely ill children. This chapter reviews the anatomy of body fluid compartments, the regulation of water and sodium in the normal state and in specific diseases, and common electrolyte and acid-base abnormalities, and briefly discusses tumor lysis syndrome and hyperammonemia.

Body Fluid Compartments

Water is the most abundant component of the human body, constituting approximately 50% to 70% of body weight. Total body water (TBW) is largely distributed into two major compartments: extracellular fluid (ECF) and intracellular fluid (ICF). At birth, TBW, ECF, and ICF comprise approximately 79%, 45%, and 34% of body weight, respectively. By puberty, TBW, ECF, and ICF have reached their adult values of approximately 60%, 20%, and 40% of body weight, respectively.[1] The ICF comprises two thirds of the TBW, representing the sum of all the cellular fluid contents of the body. The ECF comprises one third of the TBW and is further subdivided into plasma (intravascular) and interstitial fluid, constituting 4% and 16% of body weight, respectively. Lymph is included in the interstitial fluid volume and comprises approximately 2% of body weight. A minor subdivision of the ECF compartment, known as the transcellular compartment, consists of cerebrospinal, pleural, pericardial, peritoneal, intraocular, synovial fluids, and gastrointestinal tract secretions. Under most circumstances, these volumes are small and do not contribute significantly to the maintenance of the total ECF volume.[2]

The distribution of the TBW into the ECF and ICF compartments is determined by the number of osmotically active particles (solute) in each compartment. In the ECF, sodium is the principal cation while chloride and bicarbonate are the major anions. These ions constitute more than 90% of the total solute of the ECF. Their concentrations in the plasma and interstitial fluid are quite similar because these compartments are separated only by the vascular endothelium, which is permeable to low molecular weight ions. Under normal circumstances, proteins, by virtue of their high molecular weight, are present predominantly in the plasma (intravascular) space.[2] In the ICF, potassium is the predominant cation, and magnesium is present in high concentrations as well. The major intracellular anions are phosphate, sulfate, and protein.[3]

Osmolality represents the number of osmoles (solutes) per kilogram of water (osm/kg water). A solution of higher osmolality will have more solute and less water per unit volume than a solution of lesser osmolality. Since sodium is the major extracellular solute, it accounts for the majority of the plasma osmolality, which in turn regulates the size of the ECF. During hyperosmolar states, water moves out of the ICF into the ECF to restore normal osmolality. Conversely, a decrease in plasma osmolality results in water movement out of the ECF into the ICF.

Solutes that exert an osmotic force across cell membranes and initiate water movement in and out of cells are called effective osmoles. In ECF and plasma, sodium, glucose, and urea (as measured by blood urea nitrogen [BUN]) are the major effective osmoles. In general, sodium and glucose, in the absence of insulin, are also called impermeable solutes because they are relatively confined to the ECF. In contrast, urea is a permeable solute and is distributed evenly between the ICF and ECF. Osmolality reflects the concentration of both permeable and impermeable solutes. Therefore, plasma osmolality can be estimated by the following formula:

$P_{osm} = 2$ (sodium [mmol/L]) + glucose (mg/dL)/18 + BUN (mg/dL)/2.8

The normal plasma osmolality ranges from 280 to 295 mOsm/kg H_2O.

Maintenance Requirements

Maintenance requirements of water and electrolytes are directly related to a child's metabolic rate. Metabolic rate or caloric expenditure in turn depends on the child's age, body weight, type of activity, temperature, and presence of illness.[4] Under normal conditions, maintenance requirements are calculated to replace water and electrolytes lost through the skin, lungs, and kidneys. Losses through the skin and the respiratory tract are called insensible or evaporative losses. Insensible losses account for one fourth to one third of the maintenance requirements, while urinary losses account for the remaining two thirds.[5]

From a series of formulas, Holliday and Segar[4] demonstrated that the rate of caloric expenditure of infants and children can be determined from body weight. For weights ranging from 0 to 10 kg, the caloric expenditure is 100 cal/kg/day; from 10 to 20 kg, the caloric expenditure is 1000 calories plus 50 cal/kg for each kilogram of body weight more than 10; and greater than 20 kg, the caloric expenditure is 1500 calories plus 20 cal/kg for each kilogram more than 20. Assuming normal renal function and under ordinary homeostatic conditions, an allowance of 50 mL/100 cal/day of water will replace insensible losses, and 66.7 mL/100 cal/day will replace the average urinary losses so that the total water requirement is 116.7 mL/100 cal/day. As the water of oxidation will supply approximately 16.7 mL/100 cal/day, the remaining 100 mL/100 cal/day must be supplied to replace renal and extrarenal water losses. In the same study, Holliday and Segar recommended approximate maintenance requirements for sodium, chloride, and potassium to be 3 mmol, 2 mmol, and 2 mmol, respectively, for every 100 calories expended or 100 mL of water replaced.[4] Table 1 summarizes water and electrolyte maintenance needs.

Maintenance fluid and electrolyte requirements are adjusted in the presence of disease states or abnormal conditions (eg, increased environmental temperature). For example, in the presence of fever, insensible losses are increased by 12.5% per degree of body temperature greater than 38° C.[5]

Table 1
Maintenance Requirements of Water and Electrolytes

Body Weight	Caloric Expenditure
1–10 kg	100 kcal/kg/24 h
10–20 kg	1000 kcal + 50 kcal/kg/24 h for wt >10 kg
>20	1500 kcal + 20 kcal/kg/24 h for wt >20 kg
Water	100 mL/100 kcal/24 h
Sodium	3 mmol/100 kcal/24 h
Potassium	2 mmol/100 kcal/24 h

From Reference 4.

Dehydration

Dehydration is generally defined as a loss of TBW from the normal values in the body. Deficits from dehydration may be classified as isotonic, hypotonic, or hypertonic. Since the serum sodium concentration largely determines the plasma effective osmolality (tonicity), dehydration may also be classified as isonatremic, hyponatremic, or hypernatremic.

In assessing a patient who is dehydrated, two factors must be considered: 1) the degree of dehydration, and 2) type of dehydration. As in most clinical situations, it is essential to obtain a good history, perform a thorough physical examination, and review the laboratory data. Historical data that can be useful are recent fluid intake, type and amount of ongoing losses, presence and duration of fever, and history of recent drug ingestion. In the physical examination, the most important and objective means of determining the degree or severity of dehydration is a change in the patient's weight. Other useful objective measurements are body temperature, blood pressure, presence of tachycardia, level of consciousness, and changes in the skin's elasticity and turgor. Clinical features that can be helpful in estimating the severity of dehydration are described in Table 2. Finally, laboratory studies should be based on the patient's clinical status.

When planning for replacement fluid and electrolyte therapy, careful attention to the volume and composition of ongoing losses via renal and extrarenal routes is essential. Table 3 lists several body fluids and

Table 2
Clinical Assessment of Degree of Dehydration

Signs and Symptoms	Mild	Moderate	Severe
Weight loss (%)	3–5	6–10	>10
Mental status	alert	irritable	lethargic, comatose
Heart rate	normal	tachycardia	tachycardia
Peripheral pulses	normal	diminished	very diminished or absent
Blood pressure	normal	orthostatic hypotension	hypotension
Mucous membranes	moist	dry	very dry
Tears	present	reduced	absent
Urine output	normal	oliguria	severe oliguria or anuria
Eyes	normal	sunken	very sunken
Anterior fontanelle	flat	slightly sunken	very sunken
Skin turgor	normal	mild tenting	pronounced tenting
Respirations	normal	deep	deep and rapid

Table 3
Composition of Body Fluids (mmol/L)

Fluid	Na⁺	K⁺	Cl⁻	HCO₃⁻
Gastric	60	20	100	0
Diarrhea	80	30	90	50
Jejunostomy	100	20	100	30
Ileostomy	130	20	120	20
Bile	140	10	100	40
Pancreatic	140	15	70	90

Table 4
Composition of Common Intravenous Solutions

Solution	Na⁺	Cl⁻	K⁺	Ca⁺⁺	Lactate	Glucose (g/L)
D5 0.2% NaCl	34	34	–	–	–	50
D5 0.45% NaCl	77	77	–	–	–	50
D5 0.9% NaCl	154	154	–	–	–	50
0.9% NaCl	154	154	–	–	–	–
Ringer's lactate	130	109	4	3	28	–
D5 Ringer's lactate	130	109	4	3	28	50
3% NaCl	513	513	–	–	–	–

Solute concentrations are expressed as mmol/L unless otherwise indicated.

their compositions, while Table 4 presents a number of commercially available intravenous fluids used for replacement therapy. Calculation of the maintenance and replacement therapy of fluids and electrolytes is outlined in the discussion of specific types of dehydration (see below). Patients presenting in shock from severe dehydration should be treated as a medical emergency. The goal of initial therapy is to rapidly expand the intravascular volume by intravenous administration of isotonic fluids such as normal saline or Ringer's lactate. Once intravascular volume is restored, therapy should be directed at further correction of water and electrolyte deficits and replacement of ongoing losses.

Disorders of Sodium Homeostasis

Hyponatremia

Hyponatremia is generally defined as a plasma sodium concentration ≤130 mmol/L. When assessing the child with hyponatremia, it is important to determine whether the low serum sodium is true or fictitious. It is also important to determine the patient's volume status (ie, euvolemia, hypovolemia, or hypervolemia). This allows the basic distinction between hyponatremia caused by sodium loss or hyponatremia caused by an increase in TBW, resulting in a relative dilution of the ECF compartment. The serum sodium cannot generally be used to estimate the patient's total body fluid status. A low serum sodium may occur in the presence of hypovolemia, hypervolemia, or euvolemia. Table 5 summarizes the causes of hyponatremia.

The severity of signs and symptoms of hyponatremia is dependent on the rapidity of its development and the degree of decline in plasma osmolality.[6] As the plasma osmolality decreases, an osmotic gradient across the blood-brain barrier develops which results in water movement into the brain. This cerebral overhydration is responsible for the majority of symptoms seen in hyponatremia. In general, neurologic manifestations do not occur until the serum sodium concentration is less than 125 mmol/L. However, patients with preexisting neuropathology may

Table 5

Etiology of Hyponatremia

Euvolemic hyponatremia
  fictitious hyponatremia
  pseudohyponatremia
  syndrome of inappropriate ADH
  adrenal insufficiency
  hypothyroidism
  excess free water intake: inappropriate free water administration to an infant, inappropriately mixing formula, iatrogenic administration of hypotonic fluids

Hypovolemic hyponatremia
  net loss of sodium in excess of water:
    GI: vomiting and diarrhea
    skin: sweat and burns
    CSF: ventriculostomy, CSF drains
    third space: pancreatitis, peritonitis, burns, and bowel obstruction
    renal: diuretics, recovery phase of acute renal failure, postobstructive, salt-losing nephropathy, diuretics, adrenal insufficiency, cerebral salt wasting
  inadequate salt intake: low-sodium diet
  redistribution: malnutrition

Hypervolemic hyponatremia
  edema-forming states: nephrotic syndrome, congestive heart failure, cirrhosis
  acute or chronic renal failure

ADH = antidiuretic hormone secretion; CSF = cerebrospinal fluid; GI = gastrointestinal.

exhibit symptoms at higher serum sodium levels. Signs and symptoms may include headache, agitation, disorientation, lethargy, nausea, vomiting, muscular cramps, decreased deep tendon reflexes, seizures, coma, pseudobulbar palsies, and signs of cerebral herniation.[7] The rapid development of hyponatremia (<24 hours) carries significant morbidity and mortality.

Within 24 hours, the brain cells partially adapt to the overhydration or hypoosmolality by gradually losing intracellular osmotically active solutes. Along with these solutes, water leaves the brain cells and partially reverses the cerebral edema. Therefore, patients whose hyponatremia developed over several days or weeks are less symptomatic than patients whose hyponatremia developed acutely.[6] These concepts are important to remember when correcting hyponatremia; this is discussed below.

Fictitious hyponatremia results from a redistribution of water between the ECF and ICF secondary to the addition of an impermeable solute such as mannitol or glucose.[8] In the presence of hyperglycemia, serum sodium can be estimated by adding 1.6 mmol/L to the measured serum sodium for every 100 mg/dL increase above the normal blood sugar, which is assumed to be 100 mg/dL. For example, if a patient's blood sugar is 600 mg/dL and the measured serum sodium is 130 mmol/L, then the true serum sodium will be 138 mmol/L ([1.6 mmol/L × 5] + 130 mmol/L).[9]

Other causes of a falsely low serum sodium are hyperlipidemia and hyperproteinemia. Sodium is dissolved in the percentage of serum that is water, and lipids and protein displace sodium and water from serum. Therefore, in the presence of severe hyperlipidemia, as seen in nephrotic syndrome, or of hyperproteinemia, lipids and protein may occupy a significant volume of serum. Consequently, the percentage of serum that is water is reduced, thereby resulting in a falsely low serum sodium concentration.[6]

The most common cause of euvolemic hyponatremia in the pediatric intensive care unit is the syndrome of inappropriate antidiuretic hormone secretion (SIADH). The most common cause of euvolemic hyponatremia in the postoperative patient is the administration of maintenance fluids that are inappropriately low in sodium. If solutions with sodium concentration of less than half normal saline are administered, the serum sodium level should be followed every 12 to 24 hours. During periods of stress related to acute illness or to surgical trauma, the body's response is to initiate a neurohormonal cascade to ensure the retention of free water. The latter can be provided at the expense of sodium if appropriate amounts of sodium are not administered.

There are several factors that affect ADH secretion, the most important of which is plasma osmolality.[10] Hyponatremia from SIADH occurs due to water retention secondary to a persistently elevated ADH level inappropriate to any osmotic stimuli that normally affect ADH secretion. The diagnosis of SIADH rests on the following criteria: 1) hyponatremia with corresponding plasma hypo-osmolality; 2) inappropriately elevated urine osmolality relative to plasma osmolality; 3) normal renal function; 4) normal adrenal and thyroid functions (particularly ruling out glucocorticoid deficiency and hypothyroidism); 5) high urine sodium excretion in the presence of normovolemia; 6) absence of clinical signs of hypovolemia and dehydration; 7) absence of edema-forming states or evidence of volume depletion; and 8) correction of hyponatremia and natriuresis by fluid restriction.[6,11,12] SIADH is commonly seen in the presence of disorders that affect the central nervous system, in the presence of pulmonary diseases, and with use of certain drugs. Conditions associated with SIADH are listed in Table 6.

Hypovolemic hyponatremia generally occurs in three clinical conditions: 1) net loss of sodium in excess of water; 2) inadequate sodium intake; and 3) movement of sodium into cells.[8] In the intensive care unit setting, inadequate sodium intake and sodium entry into cells are rare. Conversely, increased renal and extrarenal loss of solute-containing fluids that are replaced by water is a frequent occurrence. Conditions leading to hypovolemic hyponatremia are presented in Table 5.[8]

Hypervolemic hyponatremia occurs when the net water retention exceeds that of sodium. Clinically, it may be seen with: 1) edema-forming states such as congestive heart failure, cirrhosis, and nephrosis, and 2) acute or chronic renal failure.[8] Under normal conditions, an increase in sodium intake will result in sodium and water retention and an increase in intravascular volume. This increase in intravascular volume will in turn result in an increase in renal perfusion and in subsequent activation of the afferent and efferent mechanisms controlling renal sodium excretion. The net effect is an increase in renal sodium excretion in an attempt to return the intravascular volume to normal.[2] In the presence of disease states such as congestive heart failure, nephrotic syndrome, and cirrhosis, afferent and efferent mechanisms of sodium retention are activated. These mechanisms are summarized in Figure 1.

Regardless of the mechanism of hyponatremia, the therapy and rapidity of correction of hyponatremia depend on the eti-

Table 6

Disorders Associated with the Syndrome of Inappropriate Antidiuretic Hormone Secretion

CNS Disorders	**Malignancy**	**Medications**
Meningitis	Carcinomas	Vasopressin, oxytocin
Encephalitis	Thymoma	Antidepressants
Head trauma	Lymphoma	Antineoplastic agents
Brain tumor	Ewing's Sarcoma	Chlorpropamide
Brain abscess	**Pulmonary Disorders**	Thiazide diuretics
Hypoxic-ischemic brain injury	Pneumonia	Antipsychotic agents
Guillain-Barré syndrome	Tuberculosis	Monoamine oxidase inhibitors
Subarachnoid hemorrhage	Empyema	Carbamazepine
Hydrocephalus	Cystic fibrosis	Clofibrate
Cavernous sinus thrombosis	Mechanical ventilation	**Postoperative Period**
	Asthma	**Idiopathic**

CNS = central nervous system.

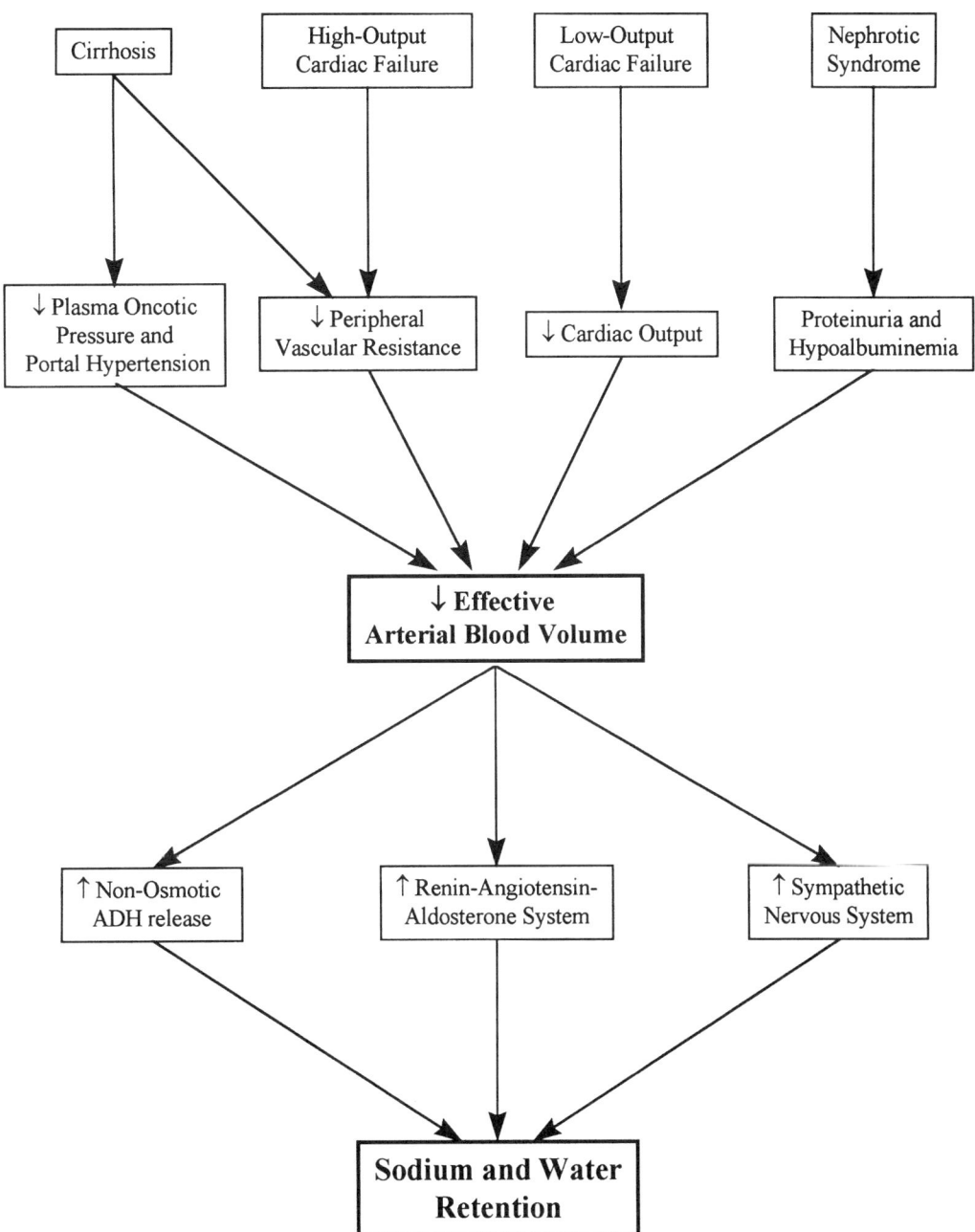

Figure 1. Mechanisms of sodium and water retention in cardiac failure, cirrhosis, and nephrotic syndrome.

ology and severity of clinical manifestations. Patients who present with severe neurologic symptoms (eg, seizures or coma) should be aggressively treated with hypertonic saline to rapidly raise their serum sodium concentration to 125 mmol/L. The sodium deficit may be estimated by the following formula:

TBW (L) = body weight (kg) × 0.6 (L/kg)
Sodium deficit (mmol) = TBW × [desired sodium − measured sodium (mmol/L)];
where the desired sodium is 125 mmol/L.

In patients with neurologic symptoms such as seizures, the amount of sodium required to raise the serum sodium to 125 to 130 mmol/L should be calculated using the above formula and administered over 10 to 15 minutes in the form of 3% hypertonic saline. If hypertonic saline is not readily available, sodium bicarbonate, standard adult strength which contains 1 mEq sodium/mL, can be used for the initial sodium replacement. The remainder is corrected over a 48-hour period. Asymptomatic patients are corrected by merely replacing the deficit plus maintenance and ongoing losses, correcting no faster than 25 mmol/L in the first 48 hours.[13,14] Rapid correction of hyponatremia can be associated with central pontine myelinolysis, a demyelinating disorder mainly restricted to the central pons. It is most commonly seen following rapid correction of chronic hyponatremia, and in patients with chronic debilitating illness, chronic alcoholism, or malnutrition. Symptomatic patients have findings of quadriplegia, pseudobulbar signs, and swallowing dysfunction.[15] Diagnosis can be confirmed by magnetic resonance imaging of the brain.[13]

Fluid restriction is the mainstay of therapy for SIADH. This may be accomplished by limiting fluid intake to 50% to 75% of maintenance.[16] However, in the presence of signs of severe water intoxication, more aggressive therapy is indicated. Infusion of 3% hypertonic saline (513 mmol/L) with or without administration of a potent diuretic (ie, furosemide at 1 to 2 mg/kg) may be used to induce ECF volume loss. Six milliliters of 3% saline per kilogram body weight will raise serum sodium level approximately 5 mmol/L.[17]

Patients with hypovolemic hyponatremia require sodium and volume replacement with sodium-containing solutions. Primary disturbances such as adrenal insufficiency, diabetic ketoacidosis, renal or cerebral salt wasting syndromes, and diuretic and mannitol use should be identified and appropriately treated. Hyponatremia associated with increased volume status usually requires both water and sodium restriction. Correction of underlying cardiac, hepatic, and renal dysfunction must also be addressed.

Hypernatremia

Hypernatremia is generally defined as a plasma sodium concentration greater than 150 mmol/L. As is true for hyponatremia, it is important to determine the status of the ECF space. This is useful for distinguishing hypernatremia secondary to excessive intake of sodium or failure to excrete sodium, from hypernatremia due to water loss in excess of sodium loss, or failure of water intake. In most cases, hypernatremia occurs because of a combination of sodium gain and water loss. The causes of hypernatremia are listed in Table 7.

Clinical signs and symptoms of hypernatremia with associated hypertonicity are directly related to cerebral cell dehydration resulting from water movement from the ICF to the ECF. Neurologic manifestations include varying degrees of depressed sensorium, ranging from lethargy to coma. The majority of patients exhibit marked irritability, a high-pitched cry, and seizure activity. Muscle tone may be normal or increased, and may be accompanied by hyperreflexia or twitching. Examination of the cerebrospinal fluid may show an elevated protein without pleocytosis. Some patients may also have hyperglycemia, hyperkalemia, hypocalcemia, and/or metabolic acidosis.[18,19] With extreme hypertonicity and resultant water movement from brain cells into ECF, the entire brain can shrink away from the cranium and produce rupture of cerebral vessels. Consequently, focal intracerebral and subdural hemorrhages and venous thrombosis may occur.[20]

Since the central nervous system is particularly vulnerable to hypertonicity, the brain cells adapt within hours by increasing intracellular osmolality with resultant movement of water back into the brain cells.

Table 7

Etiology of Hypernatremia

Euvolemic hypernatremia
  sodium bicarbonate administration
  formula errors
  use of high-sodium dialysate
  use of hypertonic saline

Hypovolemic hypernatremia
  net loss of water in excess of sodium
    GI: vomiting, diarrhea, and fistulas
    skin: sweat and burns
    lungs: hyperventilation
    renal: osmotic diuresis (mannitol, diabetes mellitus), postobstructive diuresis, diuretics, intrinsic renal disease, and diabetes insipidus

Hypervolemic hypernatremia
  sodium bicarbonate administration
  formula errors
  use of high-sodium dialysate
  use of hypertonic saline
  mineralocorticoid excess

GI = gastrointestinal

Glucose, myoinositol, taurine, and other amino acids may be the solutes (idiogenic osmoles) responsible for normalizing brain water content. If hypertonicity develops rapidly, idiogenic osmoles may not be generated fast enough to prevent brain cell shrinkage. Therefore, the severity of clinical manifestations of hypernatremia and associated hypertonicity is relative to its degree and rate of development.[6,21–23]

The mechanism of hypernatremia with normal volume status is excessive sodium intake. The majority of cases are iatrogenic, including the use of sodium bicarbonate, improperly diluted infant formula, or dialysis against a high-sodium solution.

In clinical medicine, the most common cause of hypernatremia is primary water deficit in excess of sodium, resulting in hypernatremia with decreased volume status. Water and sodium loss may occur via the extrarenal route or the renal route (Table 7). Included in this category are patients with diabetes insipidus (DI). DI is characterized by complete or partial failure of ADH secretion (central DI) or renal response to ADH (nephrogenic DI), resulting in excretion of hypotonic urine.[3] Central DI may be idiopathic, but the majority of affected patients have a history of head trauma, central nervous system infections, or tumors. Nephrogenic DI may be congenital or acquired, and results in hypernatremia usually associated with decreased water intake.

Hypervolemic hypernatremia results when sodium gain is greater than water intake. This may include administration of hypertonic saline in therapeutic abortion, sodium bicarbonate or hypertonic saline therapy, or dialysate errors. Hypernatremia with increased volume status may also be seen in patients with primary hyperaldosteronism or Cushing's syndrome because of sodium retention.[3]

Whenever possible, therapy should be directed at the underlying disease process (eg, administration of vasopressin analogues in DI). In the presence of shock or severe ECF volume contraction, restoration of the intravascular volume takes precedence over normalization of plasma osmolality. In this setting, isotonic solutions are the recommended fluid replacement to restore circulating blood volume.

The speed of correction of hypernatremia depends on the rate of its development and the accompanying clinical presentation. Correction of hypernatremia should be accomplished slowly, except in the setting of acute massive salt poisoning. Rapid lowering of serum sodium may result in water movement from the ECF into the brain cells, resulting in cerebral edema and possible herniation.[8,21,22] When serum sodium acutely exceeds 175 mmol/L (as in salt poisoning), dialysis may be performed to rapidly lower serum sodium.[24] Once serum sodium concentration is at 170 mmol/L, further reduction should be carried out over 48 hours, with the aim of lowering serum sodium no greater than 1 mmol/L/hour.[6,25]

Assuming no ongoing losses, the amount of water required in the therapeutic management of hypovolemic hypernatremia may be estimated using the following series of formulas:

$$TBW\ (L) = \text{body weight (kg)} \times 0.6\ (L/kg)$$

$$\text{Water required (L)} = \frac{\text{actual sodium} - \text{desired sodium (mmol/L)}}{\text{desired sodium (mmol/L)}} \times TBW$$

The desired sodium is assumed to be 140 mmol/L.

Serum sodium should be monitored closely to ensure that the rate of drop is not excessive.

Potassium

Hypokalemia

Hypokalemia is generally defined as a serum potassium level less than 3.5 mmol/L. Clinically, the etiology of hypokalemia can be divided into two broad categories: 1) reduction of total body potassium, and 2) redistribution into the intracellular space.[26–28] Total body potassium may be reduced secondary to inadequate dietary intake or increased potassium losses. In general, abnormal losses of potassium play a more significant etiologic role in hypokalemia than decreased intake. Table 8 outlines the etiologies of hypokalemia.

In general, signs and symptoms of hypokalemia are not exhibited unless the serum potassium level drops below 3 mmol/L. Clinical manifestations are a result of aberrations in membrane potential affecting the function of excitable tissues such as nerve and muscle. Neuromuscular findings may include weakness, fatigue, tetany, and cramps.

Muscle weakness resulting in respiratory insufficiency does not usually occur until the plasma potassium is less than 2.5 mmol/L.[27] Hypokalemia also affects gastrointestinal function by reducing motility, with symptoms ranging from constipation to ileus.

Clinically, the most significant manifestation of hypokalemia is its effect on the heart. Such effects may include arrhythmias and abnormal electrocardiographic findings. Decreased plasma potassium concentration sensitizes the heart and predisposes it to the development of ventricular ectopic activity. This is especially true for patients who have underlying cardiac disease and those taking digitalis compounds. Some of the arrhythmias that may be seen include premature atrial and ventricular beats, ventricular tachycardia, and ventricular fibrillation. The electrocardiographic changes that are produced with hypokalemia are primarily related to delayed ventricular repolarization. These findings include flattening of the T wave, ST segment depression, prominence of U waves, and prolongation of the QT interval. With more severe hypokalemia, the P wave becomes more prominent, the PR interval becomes prolonged, and the QRS complex widens.[26,27,29]

Potassium replacement is the mainstay of treatment for hypokalemia. Whenever possible, the oral route rather than the intravenous route should be used. The risk of inducing hyperkalemia must always be kept in mind when correcting hypokalemia; thus, it is generally prudent to replace deficits slowly. The oral dose of potassium is 2 to 4 mmol/kg/day in two to four divided doses. If the intravenous route must be used, potassium chloride may be given through a peripheral vein in concentrations not to exceed 40 mmol/L. If higher concentrations are required, a central vein should be used to avoid phlebitis. The risk of precipitating cardiac arrhythmias should always be kept in mind when administering potassium via a central venous line. The recommended rate of infusion ranges from 0.25 to 0.5 mmol/kg/h (maximum 10 to 20 mmol/h). Continuous electrocardiographic monitoring and frequent determinations of serum potassium levels are essential to avoid the risk of iatrogenic hyperkalemia.[26,27,30]

Table 8

Etiology of Hypokalemia

Reduction of total-body potassium
  inadequate intake
  increased losses
    GI: vomiting, diarrhea, biliary and pancreatic fistula secretions
    skin: sweat
    renal: volume expansion, diuretics, renal tubular acidosis, hypomagnesemia, alkalosis, mineralocorticoid excess, medications (Amphotericin B and Cis-platin)

Redistribution ECF → ICF
  alkalosis
  hyperinsulinism
  β_2-adrenergic agonists
  hypothermia

ECF = extracellular fluid; GI = gastrointestinal; ICF = intracellular fluid.

Hyperkalemia

Hyperkalemia is a life-threatening emergency. Patients' electrocardiograms (ECGs) should be continuously monitored and therapy should be initiated while ascertaining the etiology of the elevated serum potassium concentration. The first step in determining the cause of hyperkalemia is to rule out laboratory error. The most common cause of pseudohyperkalemia is hemolysis, resulting from the release of potassium from red blood cells. Hemolysis commonly results from heel stick and finger stick specimens. Other causes of spurious hyperkalemia are thrombocytosis (release of potassium from the platelets during clotting), leukocytosis (intracellular release when there is delay in separating the serum or plasma from the cellular elements), and an ischemic blood draw (potassium release from muscles after prolonged application of the tourniquet).

Once a true potassium level is established, the next step is to determine whether hyperkalemia results from redistribution, excessive potassium load, or inadequate excretion. In clinical practice, the majority of cases of hyperkalemia secondary to potassium retention are due to compromised renal function, or inability of the kidney to handle a substantial potassium load.[26,28] The causes of hyperkalemia are presented in Table 9.

As with hypokalemia, the most serious clinical manifestation of hyperkalemia results from aberrations in membrane polarization of cardiac tissue. Peaking or tenting of the T wave is the earliest ECG abnormality. As hyperkalemia progresses, there is flattening of the P wave, prolongation of the PR interval, widening of the QRS complex, development of a sine wave, and, ultimately, ventricular fibrillation or cardiac arrest (Fig. 2).[29] Acidosis, hyponatremia, and hypocalcemia potentiate the dangerous effects of hyperkalemia and must be corrected.

The first step in the treatment of hyperkalemia is to stop the administration of potassium-containing fluids and potassium-sparing diuretics. Therapeutic strategies are directed to counteract the cardiac toxicity, promote the intracellular movement of potassium, and remove excessive potassium from the body. Intravenous calcium chloride 10 to 25 mg/kg or calcium gluconate 50 to 100 mg/kg will antagonize the hyperkalemic effects on cardiac conduction but have no effect on the serum potassium concentration. Continuous cardiac monitoring is imperative during the treatment of hyperkalemia. Alkalinization (raising the pH) with sodium bicarbonate promotes movement of potassium into the cells in exchange for H$^+$ ion. Dosing of sodium bicarbonate starts with 1 to 2 mmol/kg intravenously over 10 minutes. Alternatively, alkaliniza-

Table 9
Etiology of Hyperkalemia

Pseudohyperkalemia
  RBC hemolysis
  thrombocytosis
  leukocytosis
  ischemic blood draw

Redistribution ICF → ECF
  acidosis
  succinylcholine
  insulin deficiency
  β-blockers
  cardiac glycosides
  hyperosmolality

Excessive potassium load
  tumor lysis syndrome
  intravenous potassium replacement

Inadequate potassium excretion
  renal insufficiency
  mineralocorticoid deficiency
  tubular defects in potassium excretion: renal transplants, systemic lupus erythematosus, obstructive uropathy, sickle cell disease, and potassium-sparing diuretics

tion can be induced by increasing the minute ventilation and lowering the partial pressure of arterial carbon dioxide (P_aCO_2). The latter is simple and quickly accomplished in patients who are receiving mechanical ventilation. Like bicarbonate, insulin also favors the cellular uptake of potassium. To prevent hypoglycemia, insulin (0.1 U/kg) is combined with glucose (0.5 g/kg). Sodium-postassium exchange resins (such as polystyrene sulfonate sodium [Kayexalate]) eliminate excess potassium in the gut in exchange for sodium ions. Kayexalate (1 to 2 g/kg) may be given orally or as a retention enema. It

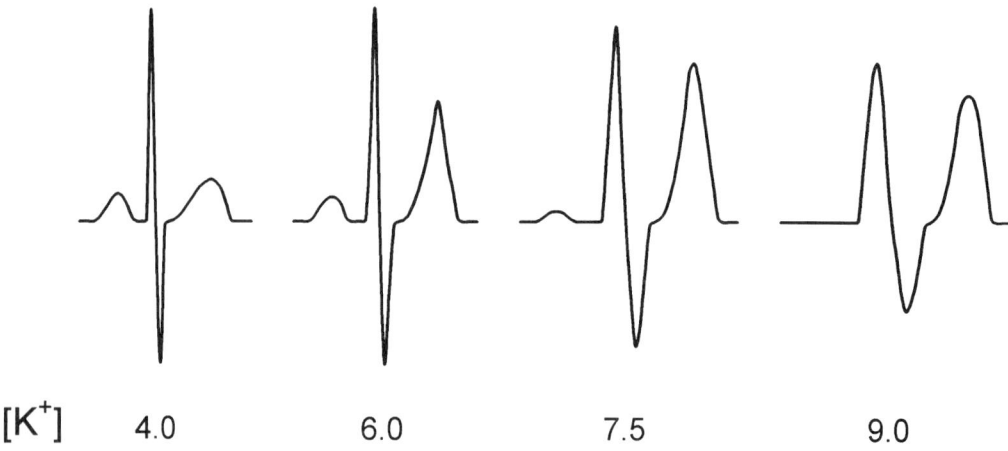

Figure 2. Electrocardiographic changes of hyperkalemia. Serum potassium concentration is expressed in mmol/L. At [K$^+$] ≥6.0, peaking or tenting of the T wave may be seen. At [K$^+$] ≥7.5, there may be flattening of the P wave, prolongation of the PR interval, and widening of the QRS complex. At [K$^+$] ≥9.0, there may be absence of the P wave, development of a sine wave QRS, and ultimately ventricular fibrillation.

should be kept in mind that Kayexalate also binds magnesium and calcium and, therefore, symptoms related to the deficiency of these ions must be addressed. Additionally, Kayexalate exchanges sodium for potassium and therefore hypernatremia and hypervolemia may develop. β-Adrenergic agonists such as epinephrine and isoproterenol also promote the intracellular movement of potassium, and their use has been suggested as a temporizing strategy for the treatment of hyperkalemia. In patients with intact renal function, loop diuretics with mannitol may increase potassium losses in the urine. Finally, in the setting of severe acute renal failure and worsening hyperkalemia, hemodialysis must be considered. Peritoneal dialysis is not as effective in quickly removing potassium. Table 10 summarizes the treatment of hyperkalemia.

Calcium

Calcium plays an integral role in membrane electrical conduction, muscle contraction, enzyme activity, and skeletal mineralization. In the serum, it consists of three fractions: 1) ionized or free calcium, accounting for 47% of total calcium; 2) protein-bound calcium, accounting for approximately 40%; and 3) calcium complexed with phosphate, citrate, or sulfate, accounting for the remaining 13%. Ionized calcium is the physiologically active portion. Aside from serum protein concentration (principally albumin), pH also influences protein binding of calcium and, thus, the ionized calcium level. When clinically available, the ionized calcium level should be followed.

Calcium homeostasis is maintained by effects of regulatory hormones in the bone, kidney, and intestine. In the bone, parathyroid hormone (PTH) promotes resorption and increases osteoclast population. It also enhances renal tubular reabsorption of calcium and stimulates 1,25-dihydroxyvitamin D synthesis in the kidney. 1,25-Dihydroxyvitamin D increases intestinal absorption of calcium and stimulates bone resorption. Calcitonin, by opposing PTH action, inhibits bone resorption and enhances renal tubular excretion. 24,25-Dihydroxyvitamin D stimulates bone synthesis. Therefore, the net effect of PTH and 1,25-dihydroxyvitamin D is to augment serum calcium level, whereas calcitonin and 24,25-dihydroxyvitamin D reduce serum calcium concentration. These regulatory mechanisms maintain ionized calcium level from 4 to 5 mg/dL (1 to 1.25 mmol/L), and the total calcium from 8.5 to 10.5 mg/dL (2.12 to 2.62 mmol/L).

Hypocalcemia

Hypocalcemia is generally defined as an ionized calcium level less than 4 mg/dL

Table 10

Treatment of Hyperkalemia

Stop exogenous administration of potassium and potassium-sparing diuretics.
For electrocardiographic changes:
   Calcium chloride 10–25 mg/kg i.v. or calcium gluconate 50–100 mg/kg i.v.
Increase intracellular movement of potassium:
   Raise pH:
      increase minute ventilation
      sodium bicarbonate 1–2 mmol/kg i.v.
   Insulin 0.1 unit/kg i.v. and glucose 0.5 g/kg i.v.
   β-adrenergic agonists
Increase potassium removal from the body:
   Kayexalate 1–2 g/kg PO or PR
   Furosemide 1 mg/kg i.v.: in patients with intact renal function
   Mannitol 0.5/kg i.v.: in patients with intact renal function
   Hemodialysis, continuous venous-venous or venous-arterial hemofiltration with dialysis,
     peritoneal dialysis

PO = by mouth; PR = per rectum.

(1 mmol/L). In many cases, it is a result of an inability to mobilize calcium from the skeletal system. This is secondary to decreased secretion of PTH (hypoparathyroidism and hypomagnesemia), impaired synthesis of 1,25-dihydroxyvitamin D (renal failure and vitamin D-dependent rickets), or inadequate responsiveness of target organs to PTH (pseudohypoparathyroidism, vitamin D deficiency, osteomalacia, renal failure, and hypomagnesemia). During critical illness, hypomagnesemia is an important cause of hypocalcemia, since low magnesium levels impair the body's regulatory response to low calcium concentrations. Hypocalcemia may also occur during administration of citrate-buffered blood products or plasma expanders due to free calcium binding with citrate and protein, respectively.

In general, the manifestations of hypocalcemia may be ascribed to increased neuromuscular excitability including numbness and tingling of lips, hands, and toes, to carpopedal spasms, irritability, laryngeal stridor, apnea, and generalized tonic clonic seizures. Trousseau's sign (tonic and clonic contractions of the hand muscles induced by decreasing blood flow to the extremity), and Chvostek's sign (spasm of the facial muscles evoked by tapping the facial nerve anterior to the ear) may be present. Decreases in cardiovascular contractility and systemic vascular resistance, as well as prolongation of the QT interval on ECG, may also be seen.

Severe, symptomatic hypocalcemia should be treated immediately. Calcium may be given intravenously as 10% calcium chloride (10 to 20 mg/kg/dose) or 10% calcium gluconate (50 to 100 mg/kg/dose) by slow infusion. The slow intravenous administration of calcium supplementation (10 to 15 minutes) and continuous ECG recording are critical to monitor for bradycardia or ventricular irritability. Intravenous access must be secure, as calcium infiltration can result in phlebitis and tissue necrosis. Except in the setting of life-threatening hypocalcemia, calcium salts are generally best administered into a central vein. Multiple doses must be guided by frequent ionized calcium determinations.

Hypercalcemia

In the pediatric intensive care unit setting, hypercalcemia is an infrequent occurrence. When seen, it is most frequently due to excessive PTH production (hyperparathyroidism), increased skeletal mobilization (neoplasms, thyrotoxicosis, and immobilization), increased intestinal absorption (vitamin D toxicity and milk-alkali syndrome), or increased release during chemotherapy (tumor lysis syndrome). Symptoms of hypercalcemia may be attributed to its depressive effects on the neuromuscular function. These include anorexia, nausea, vomiting, lethargy, muscular weakness, confusion, and stupor. With severe and longstanding hypercalcemia, renal parenchymal damage may ensue, and nephrolithiasis may develop. In the presence of hyperphosphatemia, soft tissue calcification may be seen in the cornea and blood vessels. Electrocardiographic changes (shortening of the QT interval) may also be exhibited.

The primary aim of therapy is to restrict calcium intake and promote calcium excretion. The underlying disorder must be identified and corrected. Nonspecific measures include: 1) hydration with normal saline to prevent tubular calcium reabsorption and ensure adequate urine output; 2) mobilization of the patient, whenever possible; 3) discontinuation of drugs that cause hypercalcemia; and 4) forced diuresis (furosemide 1 to 2 mg/kg/dose every 4 hours) to augment renal calcium excretion. Drugs that inhibit bone resorption such as mithramycin and calcitonin are therapeutic alternatives. If required, the dose of mithramycin is 25 µg/kg intravenously over 3 to 8 hours every 3 to 4 days, and the dose of calcitonin is 4 Medical Research Council (MRC) units per kg subcutaneously every 12 hours. Depending on the etiology, corticosteroids may be indicated. In life-threatening hypercalcemia, chelators such as orthophosphate and EDTA may be indicated. Their use, however, is discouraged because of the risk of soft tissue calcification and nephrotoxicity. Hemodialysis remains the most effective method for rapid removal of calcium, especially in the presence of renal failure.[31-33]

Phosphorus

Hypophosphatemia

Hypophosphatemia can result from redistribution or inadequate phosphate intake. Redistribution may occur in the settings of the following conditions: alkalosis and parenteral hyperalimentation. The latter, especially when initiated in patients with prior phosphate deficits, stimulates insulin secretion, which causes a phosphorus shift from the ECF to the ICF. Phosphate deficiency may result from gastrointestinal (vitamin D deficiency, malabsorption, and administration of phosphate binders), and renal losses (Fanconi syndrome, vitamin D-resistant rickets, and diuretics).

The manifestations of acute, life-threatening hypophosphatemia (serum level <1 mg/dL) are secondary to intracellular adenosine triphosphate (ATP) and/or erythrocyte 2,3-diphosphoglycerate deficiency. Clinically, it most often occurs when the serum phosphorus concentration precipitously drops after nutrient infusion (hyperalimentation). Symptoms of hypophosphatemia include neuropsychiatric disorders, disorientation, weakness, coma, seizures, acute circulatory collapse, rhabdomyolysis, hemolytic anemia, respiratory distress, and organ dysfunction secondary to tissue hypoxia.

Avoidance of phosphate depletion is the key to preventing hypophosphatemia. With the advent of parenteral nutrition solutions that contain phosphorus as either the sodium or the potassium salt, phosphate depletion resulting in hypophosphatemia has become less of a problem. Any underlying disorder should be identified and corrected. Whenever possible, the oral route should be used, and deficits should be slowly repleted. In the presence of symptomatic hypophosphatemia, phosphorus (2 mg/kg) can be administered intravenously as either the sodium or potassium salt every 6 hours. Frequent determinations of the serum phosphorus are mandatory, as well as serial monitoring of serum chemistries, blood pressure, and state of hydration. Phosphate salts should not be given in the presence of acute renal insufficiency, hypocalcemia, hypercalcemia, or hyperkalemia.[34]

Hyperphosphatemia

There are three possible mechanisms to explain the etiology of hyperphosphatemia: 1) redistribution of phosphate from the ICF to the ECF (severe hemolytic anemia, tumor lysis, hyperthyroidism, and rhabdomyolysis); 2) increased intake of phosphate; and 3) decreased renal phosphate excretion (hypoparathyroidism and renal failure). An intracellular phosphate shift to the ECF is the most common cause of severe hyperphosphatemia. Many of the clinical features of hyperphosphatemia may be attributed to the reciprocal decline in serum calcium concentration. Other manifestations may be explained by the association of hyperphosphatemia with acute renal failure and precipitation of Ca-PO$_4$ hydroxyapatite crystals in the cornea, lungs, kidney, blood vessels, and cardiac conduction system. This crystal formation is more likely to occur if the Ca-PO$_4$ product exceeds 60 to 75 mg/dL.[35]

Phosphate elimination via the gastrointestinal route or the renal route is the mainstay of therapy. Phosphate binders, when given with meals, are effective agents. The dose depends on the severity of hyperphosphatemia. The most commonly used orally administered phosphate binder is calcium carbonate. Aluminum hydroxide was formerly used; however, the long-term consequences of aluminum toxicity, including the exacerbation of renal osteodystrophy and its possible role in presenile dementia, have limited the use of aluminum hydroxide. More recently, sucralfate has been shown to effectively bind phosphate. In patients with normal renal function, maintenance of adequate intravascular volume and diuresis with sodium bicarbonate or acetazolamide may enhance phosphate excretion. In the setting of massive phosphate load and severe renal failure, dialysis, either peritoneal or hemodialysis, may be required.[34]

Magnesium

Hypomagnesemia

Magnesium deficiency usually results from intestinal losses or from renal wasting.

Examples of gastrointestinal diseases resulting in magnesium losses include malabsorption, short gut syndrome, steatorrhea, laxative abuse, and protein calorie malnutrition. Renal magnesium wasting may be congenital or acquired. In either form, the diagnosis is made by the presence of inappropriate renal excretion in the setting of hypomagnesemia. Drugs such as thiazide diuretics, aminoglycosides, amphotericin B, and cisplatin also cause excessive renal magnesium wasting.

Since magnesium plays a pivotal role in various ATP-dependent cellular processes, symptomatology from hypomagnesemia may be manifested by almost all organ systems. Furthermore, because of its close relationship with potassium and calcium, magnesium deficit parallels potassium and calcium deficiencies. The signs and symptoms of both hypokalemia and hypocalcemia are reviewed in their respective sections. The cardiac manifestations of hypomagnesemia include predisposition to digoxin-mediated arrhythmias, and other arrhythmias such as torsades de pointes, ventricular tachycardia, and ventricular fibrillation.

In the presence of severe, symptomatic hypomagnesemia, an intravenous infusion of $MgSO_4$ at a dose of 25 to 50 mg/kg/dose may be given over 15 to 30 minutes. Magnesium can be administered more slowly if the patient has mild symptoms or is asymptomatic. Close monitoring during intravenous administration is imperative, as hypotension, malignant dysrhythmias, and skeletal muscle weakness with respiratory failure have been reported. Calcium should be readily available as an antidote. Serial monitoring of serum magnesium levels is recommended as repeated doses may be required. Many intensive care units now have the capability to measure ionized magnesium levels. As with calcium, it is the ionized moiety that determines its clinical effects. Hypocalcemia and hypokalemia should be corrected separately. Extreme caution must be exercised when giving magnesium replacement to patients with renal insufficiency.[36–38]

Hypermagnesemia

Magnesium excess is usually secondary to excessive input or normal intake in the setting of renal impairment. The manifestations of hypermagnesemia include nausea, vomiting, muscle weakness, decreased deep tendon reflexes, coma, circulatory collapse, malignant dysrhythmias, bradycardia, and cardiopulmonary arrest. The initial goals of therapy are to discontinue intake and to enhance excretion. Calcium, by acting as a direct antagonist to magnesium, should be given in the setting of severe, life-threatening hypermagnesemia. The dose is calcium chloride 10 to 25 mg/kg or calcium gluconate 50 to 100 mg/kg given intravenously. In the presence of renal failure, peritoneal or hemodialysis may be necessary.[36]

Tumor Lysis Syndrome

Tumor lysis syndrome is a pattern of metabolic derangements due to massive neoplastic cell lysis with resultant release of potassium, phosphorus, and nucleic acids into the bloodstream. Consequently, hyperkalemia, hyperphosphatemia, hypocalcemia, hyperuricemia, and acute renal failure may ensue. The problems seen are associated with the Ps: potassium, phosphate, purines or uric acid, and proteins which can block renal tubules and lead to renal dysfunction. Dehydration, renal precipitation of calcium phosphate and urate, ureteral and venous obstruction from tumor compression, and tumor infiltration of the kidney, may exacerbate the primary metabolic abnormalities. Tumor lysis syndrome is most often seen in acute lymphocytic leukemia and Burkitt's lymphoma, both of which are associated with a large tumor burden and high responsivity to chemotherapy. Typically, tumor lysis syndrome occurs 24 to 48 hours after the onset of therapy. However, it may also be seen before or up to 5 days after induction of chemotherapy.

Ideally, the best treatment is prevention. Fluid loading, urine alkalinization, and blockade of uric production with allopurinol should be instituted prior to the start of chemotherapy. These measures reduce uric acid production and urate deposition in the kidney, and enhance phosphate, potassium, and urate clearance. Serial determinations of serum electrolytes, ionized calcium, phosphorus, uric acid, and pH levels are essential, especially in the first 24 hours after initiation of therapy. Conservative measures include vigorous hydration consisting of parenteral fluids at a rate of 3 to 6 L/m^2/day, maintaining urine output at or above 100 mL/m^2/h, and urine-specific gravity less than 1.010 with a pH of greater than 7.0. Recommended intravenous fluid is 2.5% to 5% dextrose in 0.25 normal saline with 50 to 100 mmol/L sodium bicarbonate, without potassium. Once hypovolemia is corrected, maintaining adequate urine flow may be accomplished by intravenous infusion of mannitol 0.5 g/kg every 6 hours. Urine alkalinization—achieving a urine pH between 6.5 and 7.5—decreases urate deposition and may be accomplished by incorporating sodium bicarbonate into the intravenous fluids, or by acetazolamide, 5 to 10 mg/kg every 6 hours. Overalkalinization should be avoided to prevent renal precipitation of xanthine, hypoxanthine, and phosphate. Allopurinol is used to reduce uric acid production. It is given at an oral or intravenous dose of 100 to 300 mg/m^2 every 8 hours. Oral aluminum hydroxide, 50 mg/kg every 8 hours, may be employed to act as phosphate binder. The risk of hyperkalemia is greatest in the first 24 hours after commencing chemotherapy. For therapy for hyperkalemia, please see the above section. Finally, if metabolic disturbances continue to worsen in spite of the above measures, dialysis may be required. The indications for hemodialysis are listed in Table 11.[39–41]

Table 11

Indications for Hemodialysis in Tumor Lysis Syndrome

Serum potassium ≥6.0 mmol/L
Volume overload
Symptomatic hypocalcemia
Serum phosphorus ≥10 mg/dL
Serum uric acid ≥10 mg/dL
Serum creatinine ≥10 mg/dL

From Reference 41.

Acid–Base Disturbances

Acid-base abnormalities are the result of primary changes in either P_aCO_2 or bicarbonate concentration. In general, increases or decreases in P_aCO_2 result in acid-base disturbances that are referred to as respiratory acidosis or respiratory alkalosis, respectively. Likewise, increases or decreases in bicarbonate concentration result in metabolic alkalosis or metabolic acidosis, respectively. In each of the four primary acid-base abnormalities, the initiating process not only changes the acid-base balance, but also triggers compensatory physiologic mechanisms to restore the HCO_3^-/P_aCO_2 ratio and eventually return the pH to normal.

Respiratory Acidosis/Alkalosis

Primary respiratory acidosis is the consequence of alveolar hypoventilation or excessive carbon dioxide production resulting in an inadequate ratio of carbon dioxide excretion relative to carbon dioxide production. The etiologies of respiratory acidosis are discussed in previous chapters. Signs and symptoms of respiratory acidosis depend on the duration and severity of the acidosis, the degree of compensation, and the patient's level of consciousness. Therapy should be directed at correction of the underlying problem.

Primary respiratory alkalosis is the consequence of alveolar hyperventilation which results in carbon dioxide excretion exceeding carbon dioxide production. The causes of respiratory alkalosis may be divided into two groups. The first group consists of disorders that stimulate the respiratory center (hysterical hyperventilation, central nervous system infections, salicylate poisoning, and gram-negative sepsis), while the second group comprises conditions that act on the pulmonary apparatus (pneumonia and iatrogenic mechanical overventilation). Again, therapy should address the underlying or initiating disturbance.

Metabolic Acidosis

The diagnostic approach to metabolic acidosis is remarkably simplified when examined in terms of the anion gap.[42] The anion gap is derived from the following formula: AG (mmol/L) = sodium − [Cl^- + HCO_3^-]. The normal range is 8 to 16 mmol/L (mean 12). In general, acidoses associated with an increased anion gap result from overproduction of endogenous acids (lactate and keto-anions), decreased excretion of fixed acids (renal failure), or toxic ingestions (salicylates, methanol, ethylene glycol). Normal anion gap acidoses can result from the net loss of base through the gut and kidney or from infusion of acidifying agents (Table 12). Many of the clinical manifestations of metabolic acidosis are nonspecific. Air hunger and tachypnea is a typical finding. Central nervous system depression, decreased peripheral vascular resistance, myocardial dysfunction, and lowered threshold for ventricular arrhythmias may be seen with worsening acidosis.

The main goals of therapy should be directed at correction of the underlying process, and maintenance of tissue perfusion and renal function by restoring adequate intravascular volume. In the presence of severe metabolic acidosis (pH <7.1), alkali therapy may be reasonable. However, the amount of sodium bicarbonate needed to achieve a pH greater than 7.1 is difficult to predict. Furthermore, sodium bicarbonate infusions may be fraught with theoretical adverse effects such as hyperosmolality, paradoxical intracellular and cerebrospinal fluid acidosis, and alkalemia resulting in increased affinity of hemoglobin for oxygen and consequent tissue hypoxia.[42-44]

Metabolic Alkalosis

The etiology of metabolic alkalosis may be classified based on the urinary chloride concentration and the response to chloride administration. The chloride-responsive group is usually associated with ECF volume contraction whereas the chloride-resistant group is associated with ECF volume excess (Table 13). The symptomatology of metabolic alkalosis may be the consequence of its effect on the neuromuscular system (confusion and muscle weakness), on cardiac conduction (refractory supraventricular and ventricular arrhythmias), and on oxygen delivery (tissue hypoxia secondary to shift of the oxygen-hemoglobin dissociation curve to the left).

Again, therapy should be directed at correcting the original disturbance. Many cases seen in the pediatric intensive care patient are the result of the aggressive use of loop diuretics which block the renal reabsorption of Cl^-. In response to this, the body reabsorbs HCO_3^- to maintain electrical neutrality. Administration of chloride in the form of sodium, potassium, or ammonium chloride salts may be justified in some cases. The latter agent is metabolized to NH_3, H^+, and Cl^-. An alternative approach is to administer the carbonic anhydrase inhibitors such as acetazolamide to block the renal re-

Table 12

Etiology of Metabolic Acidosis

Increased Anion Gap
  lactic acidosis
  ketoacidosis
  uremia
  poisoning: salicylates, methanol, and ethylene glycol

Normal Anion Gap
  bicarbonate loss
    gastrointestinal: diarrhea, pancreatic fistulas, biliary fistulas and urinary diversion procedures
    renal: renal tubular acidosis, renal insufficiency and medications (acetazolamide,
      amphotericin B, spironolactone)
  infusion of acidifying agents
    hydrochloric acid
    ammonion chloride
    arginine hydrochloride

Table 13

Etiology of Metabolic Alkalosis

Chloride-responsive
  gastrointestinal losses: vomiting, prolonged nasogastric drainage, congenital chloride diarrhea
  renal losses: thiazide and loop diuretics
  posthypercapnea

Chloride-resistant
  primary aldosteronism
  Cushing syndrome
  primary reninism
  mineralocorticoid excess: 11-hydroxylase and 17-hydroxylase deficiencies
  Bartter's syndrome
  chronic hypercalcemia
  massive citrated blood transfusion

---

absorption of HCO_3^-.[43,44] Most importantly, diuretic use should be restricted if possible.

Hyperammonemia

The inability to excrete waste nitrogen as urea results in the accumulation of ammonia and other nitrogenous compounds (see also chapter 21 for a discussion of hyperammonemia associated with hepatic failure). Hyperammonemia represents a metabolic emergency which relies on rapid recognition and prompt intervention to limit its neurologic sequelae. Transient hyperammonemia of the newborn, Reye's syndrome, hepatic failure, and inborn errors of metabolism comprise the bulk of etiologies of hyperammonemic syndromes. Transient hyperammonemia of the newborn is primarily a disease of the premature infant and usually presents within 48 hours of life. Its treatment is similar to that for those with inborn errors and is discussed in the following sections. Reye's syndrome occurs primarily in individuals older than 2 years, who were previously healthy, and is often preceded by an identified viral illness with salicylate exposure. Although hyperammonemia is a clinical characteristic of both Reye's syndrome and hepatic failure, there are unique aspects to their management and the reader is referred to the sections on encephalopathy and liver disease for further details. The remainder of this section concentrates on inborn errors of metabolism and the general principles applied to the management of hyperammonemia.

The typical patient with neonatal-onset hyperammonemia is well for 48 hours and presents in the first week of life with feeding intolerance, vomiting, lethargy, respiratory distress, seizures, and coma. The symptoms progress rapidly and are uniformly fatal without intervention. The majority of affected infants will have a urea cycle defect or an organic acidopathy (Fig. 3). Late-onset hyperammonemia may occur in infancy through adulthood and is often heralded by recurrent episodes of symptomatic hyperammonemia, triggered by concurrent illness or dietary intake of large protein loads. Late-onset hyperammonemia is particularly common in female carriers of ornithine transcarbamylase deficiency. Regardless of the etiology, efforts at stabilization, diagnosis, and prompt intervention to limit ammonia excess must be conducted in a timely fashion to optimize neurologic outcome.

Neonates may have clinical findings consistent with sepsis and cerebral catastrophes, potentially delaying the diagnosis of hyperammonemia. For older infants and children, historical data and associated findings will often aid in discerning underlying metabolic disorders from Reye's syndrome and hepatic pathology.[45] The symptom complex of vomiting, lethargy, seizures, and coma should alert the clinician to the possibility of hyperammonemia. The majority of infants with hyperammonemia will have an inherited urea cycle enzyme defi-

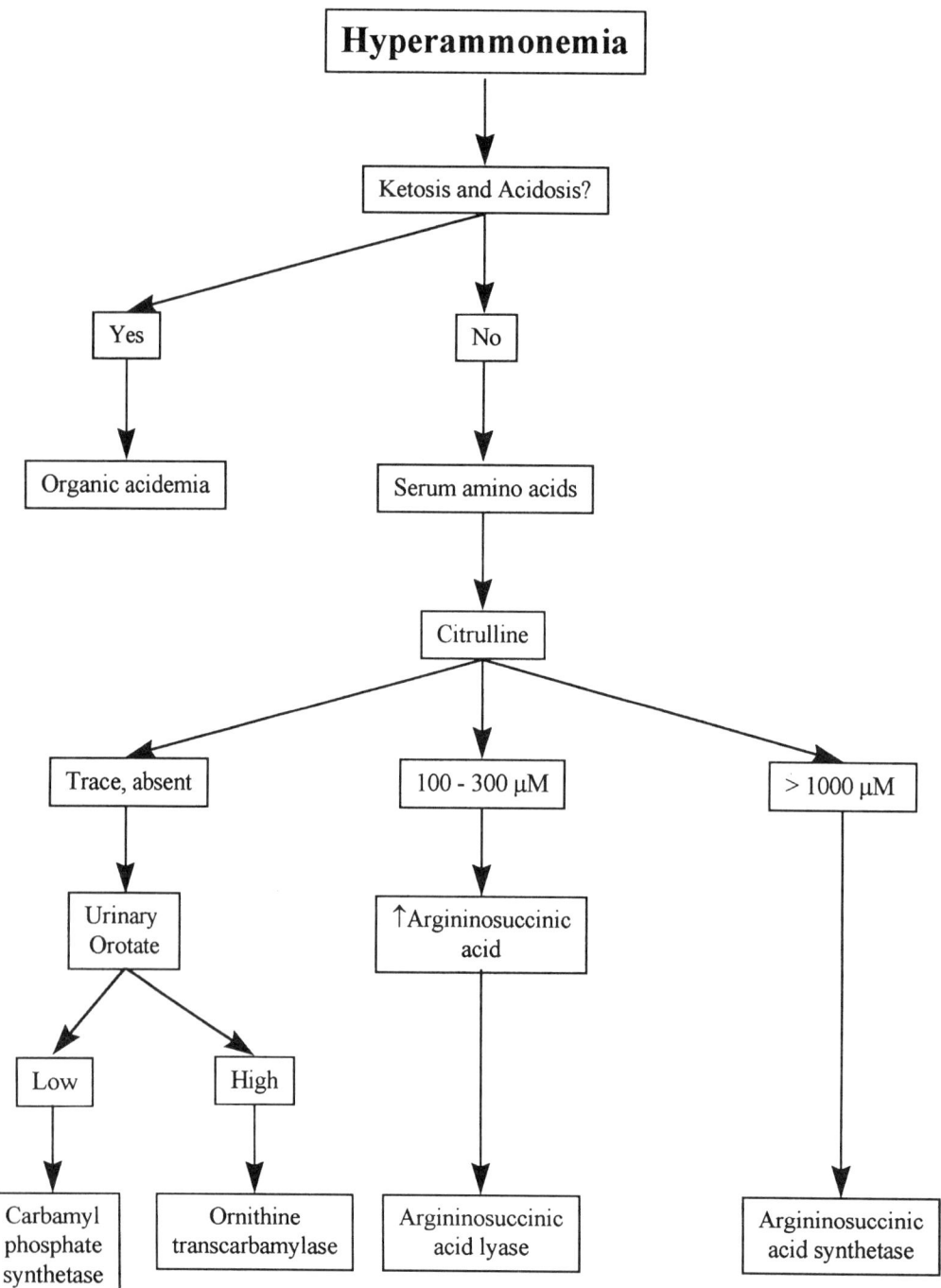

Figure 3. Algorithm for the diagnosis of neonatal hyperammonemia.

ciency. Along with the previously mentioned symptoms, neonates with urea cycle defects present with elevated ammonia, low arginine levels, and alkalosis. The presence of alkalosis may be useful in that other inborn errors of metabolism (organic acidopathies) are characterized by profound metabolic acidosis, and this distinction can be critical in elucidating the correct diagnosis. Figure 3 presents a scheme that may be useful for diagnosing enzyme defects that cause neonatal-onset hyperammonemia. In general, urinary orotic acid, serum amino acids, serum and urine organic acids, and liver function tests are useful initial tests. Often, specific enzyme deficiencies are later diagnosed by assays on fibroblasts or hepatic tissue. Patients with late-onset hyperammonemia may have a urea cycle defect, disorder of fatty acid metabolism, or an organic acidopathy. Regardless of the specific diagnosis, prompt intervention and initiation of ammonia reduction treatment is necessary in the symptomatic infant.

Acute hyperammonemia is a medical emergency. Plasma levels of ammonium that exceed three times the upper level of normal limits are considered toxic. Patients with this degree of hyperammonemia commonly present with coma. Neurologic outcome has been found to be directly related to the duration of hyperammonemic coma in infants with urea cycle defects.[46] Initial intervention should be directed toward the ABCs and cerebral edema as discussed in prior chapters. Additional therapies are directed toward protein restriction, provision of adequate substrate to avoid catabolism, elimination of ammonia and its precursors, and activation of alternate pathways to facilitate excretion.

Initially, all enteral and intravenous sources of nitrogen should be discontinued. Patients should receive intravenous dextrose of sufficient calories to prevent catabolism. Once ammonia and amino acid levels have stabilized, protein intake may be resumed. In fact, protein intake is ultimately necessary to prevent essential amino acid deficiency and to thwart catabolism. Comatose patients should undergo urgent dialysis to limit the extent of neurologic injury. Three techniques of dialysis are used in the pediatric intensive care unit: peritoneal dialysis, intermittent hemodialysis, and continuous arteriovenous or venovenous hemofiltration (CAVH-D, CVVH-D) dialysis. Hemodialysis rapidly lowers ammonium levels and is superior to peritoneal dialysis and exchange transfusion. Vascular access and potential for rebound hyperammonemia between runs of hemodialysis are possible complications. Peritoneal dialysis, though obviating the need for vascular access, is much less efficient with respect to ammonia clearance. CAVH-D and CVVH-D eliminate concerns for rebound hyperammonemia, and may be better tolerated hemodynamically than hemodialysis, though concerns exist regarding the efficiency of ammonia clearance as compared to hemodialysis.[47]

Alternate pathway therapy is an effective means of lowering ammonia, and is useful in neonates with urea cycle defects.[48] Sodium benzoate and sodium phenylacetate given intravenously combine with glycine and glutamine to produce hippurate and phenylacetylglutamine, respectively, which effectively remove nitrogen and are easily excreted.[49] Additionally, intravenous administration of arginine hydrochloride in neonates with urea cycle defects will prevent arginine deficiency and hasten the excretion of nitrogen in certain enzyme deficiencies. Table 14 provides specific dosages for alternate pathway agents. The extent of neurologic injury is directly related to the duration of hyperammonemic coma; thus, ammonia reduction is paramount. If alternate pathway therapy does not rapidly reduce ammonia levels (within 8 hours), dialysis should be instituted using either hemodialysis or CAVH-D (CVVH-D).

Specific therapies may be used once a definitive diagnosis is known. Unfortunately, most patients present without a family history of metabolic disease and treatment must proceed prior to diagnosis. Because urea cycle defects and organic acidopathies may present in similar fashion, it is appropriate to initiate therapeutic interventions directed at treatable defects. For example, the administration of biotin and hydroxycobalamin is appropriate in the event that an organic acidopathy exists which may respond to the administration of

Table 14

Dosing of Metabolic Agents for Hyperammonemia

Agent	Loading Dose	Maintenance Dose
Sodium benzoate	250 mg/kg i.v.	250–500 mg/kg/day continuous i.v. infusion
Arginine hydrochloride	800 mg/kg i.v.	200–800 mg/kg/day continuous i.v. infusion
Phenylacetate	250 mg/kg i.v.	250–500 mg/kg/day continuous i.v. infusion
Biotin		10–20 mg/day
Vitamin B_{12}		1–2 mg/day
Thiamine		5–20 mg/kg/day
Riboflavin		300 mg/day
Carnitine		100 mg/kg/day

certain cofactors and vitamins (Table 14). Additionally, sodium bicarbonate may be used for metabolic acidosis.

References

1. Friis-Hanson B. Body water compartments in children: Changes during growth and related changes in body composition. *Pediatrics* 1961;28:169–181.
2. McKeown JW. Disorders of total body sodium. In Kokko JP, Tannen RL (eds): *Fluids and Electrolytes*. Philadelphia: W.B. Saunders Company; 1986:63–117.
3. Saxton CR, Seldin DW. Clinical interpretation of laboratory values. In Kokko JP, Tannen RL (eds): *Fluids and Electrolytes*. Philadelphia: W.B. Saunders Company; 1986:3–62.
4. Holliday MA, Segar WE. The maintenance need for water in parenteral fluid therapy. *Pediatrics* 1957;19:823–832.
5. Siegel NJ, Carpenter T, Gaudio KM. The pathophysiology of body fluids. In Oski FA, DeAngelis CD, Feigin RD, et al (eds): *Principles and Practice of Pediatrics*. Philadelphia: J.B. Lippincott Company; 1994:60–79.
6. Humes DH. Disorders of water metabolism. In Kokko JP, Tannen RL (eds): *Fluids and Electrolytes*. Philadelphia: W.B. Saunders Company; 1986:118–149.
7. Arieff AI, Llach F, Massry SG. Neurological manifestations and morbidity of hyponatremia: Correlation with brain water and electrolytes. *Medicine* 1976;55:121–129.
8. Gruskin AB, Baluarte HJ, Prebis JW, et al. Serum sodium abnormalties in children. *Pediatr Clin North Am* 1982;29:907–932.
9. Katz MA. Hyperglycemia-induced hyponatremia-calculation of expected serum sodium depression. *N Engl J Med* 1973;289: 844–845.
10. Robertson G. The physiopathology of ADH secretion. In Tolis G (ed): *Clinical Neuroendocrinology: A Pathophysiological Approach*. New York: Raven Press; 1979:247–260.
11. Zebre R, Stropes L, Robertson G. Vasopressin function in the syndrome of inappropriate antidiuresis. *Ann Rev Med* 1980;31: 315–327.
12. Bartter FC, Schwartz WB. The syndrome of inappropriate secretion of antidiuretic hormone. *Am J Med* 1967;42:790–806.
13. Ayus JC, Krothapalli RK, Arieff AI. Treatment of symptomatic hyponatremia and its relation to brain damage. *N Engl J Med* 1987;317:1190–1194.
14. Arieff AI, Ayus JC. Treatment of symptomatic hyponatremia: Neither haste nor waste. *Crit Care Med* 1991;19:748–751.
15. Narins RG. Therapy of hyponatremia. *N Engl J Med* 1986;314:1573–1574.
16. Perkin RM, Levin DL. Common fluid and electrolyte problems in the pediatric intensive care unit. *Pediatr Clin North Am* 1980;27: 567–586.
17. Hantman D, Rossier B, Zohlman R, Schrier R. Rapid correction of hyponatremia in the syndrome of inappropriate secretion of antidiuretic hormone. *Ann Intern Med* 1973;78: 870–875.
18. Bruck E, Abal G, Aceto T. Pathogenesis and pathophysiology of hypertonic dehydration with diarrhea. *Am J Dis Child* 1968;115:122–144.
19. Finberg L, Harrison HE. Hypernatremia in infants. *Pediatrics* 1955;16:1–12.
20. Arieff AI, Guisado R. Effects of the central nervous system of hypernatremic and hyponatremic states. *Kidney Int* 1976;10:104–116.
21. Oh MS, Carroll HJ. Disorders of sodium metabolism: Hypernatremia and hyponatremia. *Crit Care Med* 1992;20:94–103.

22. Finberg L. Hypernatremic dehydration. In Finberg L, Kravath RE, Fleischman AR (eds): *Water and Electrolytes in Pediatrics*. Philadelphia: W.B. Saunders Company; 1982:78–89.
23. Lee JH, Arcinue E, Ross BD. Brief report: Organic osmolytes in the brain of an infant with hypernatremia. *N Engl J Med* 1994;331:439–442.
24. Miller NL, Finberg L. Peritoneal dialysis for salt poisoning. *N Engl J Med* 1960;263:1347–1350.
25. Finberg L. Therapeutic management of hypernatremic dehydration. In Finberg L, Kravath RE, Fleischman AR (eds): *Water and Electrolytes in Pediatrics*. Philadelphia: W.B. Saunders Company; 1982:129–135.
26. Tannen RL. Potassium disorders. In Kokko JP, Tannen RL (eds): *Fluids and Electrolytes*. Philadelphia: W.B. Saunders Company; 1986:150–228.
27. Linshaw MA. Potassium homeostasis and hypokalemia. *Pediatr Nephrol* 1987;34:649–681.
28. Moreno M, Murphy C, Goldsmith C. Increase in serum potassium resulting from the administration of hypertonic mannitol and other solutions. *J Lab Clin Med* 1969;73:291–298.
29. Surawicz B. Relationship between electrocardiogram and electrolytes. *Am Heart J* 1967;73:814–833.
30. Segar WE. Parenteral fluid therapy. *Curr Prob Pediatr* 1972;3:3–40.
31. Pak CYC. Calcium disorders: Hypercalcemia and hypocalcemia. In Kokko JP, Tannen RL (eds): *Fluids and Electrolytes*. Philadelphia: W.B. Saunders Company; 1986:472–501.
32. Khilnani P. Electrolyte abnormalties in critically ill children. *Crit Care Med* 1992;20:241–250.
33. Fleischman A. Calcium, phosphorus, and magnesium: Metabolism and regulation. In Finberg L, Kravath RE, Fleischman AR (eds): *Water and Electrolytes in Pediatrics*. Philadelphia: W.B. Saunders Company; 1982:62–70.
34. Lau K. Phosphate disorders. In Kokko JP, Tannen RL (eds): *Fluids and Electrolytes*. Philadelphia: W.B. Saunders Company; 1986:398–471.
35. Parfitt MA. Soft-tissue calcification in uremia. *Arch Intern Med* 1969;124:544–555.
36. Cronin RE. Magnesium disorders. In Kokko JP, Tannen RL (eds): *Fluids and Electrolytes*. Philadelphia: W.B. Saunders Company; 1986:502–512.
37. Berkelhammer C, Bear RA. A clinical approach to common electrolyte problems: Hypomagnesemia. *Can Med Assoc J* 1985;132:360–368.
38. Whang R. Magnesium deficiency: Pathogenesis, prevalence, and clinical implications. *Am J Med* 1987;82:24–29.
39. Kelly KM, Lange B. Oncologic emergencies. *Pediatr Oncol* 1997;44:809–830.
40. Stokes DN. Tumour lysis syndrome and the anaesthesiolgist: Intensive care aspects of pediatric oncology. *Semin Surg Oncol* 1990;6:156–161.
41. Cohen LF, Balow JE, Magrath IT, et al. Acute tumor lysis syndrome: A review of 37 patients with Burkitt's Lymphoma. *Am J Med* 1980;68:486–491.
42. Emmett M, Narins RG. Clinical use of the anion gap. *Medicine* 1977;56:38–53.
43. Kravath RE. Pathophysiology of hydrogen ion disturbance. In Finberg L, Fleischman AR (eds): *Water and Electrolytes in Pediatrics*. Philadelphia: W.B. Saunders Company; 1982:90–107.
44. Toto RD. Metabolic acid-base disorders. In Kokko JP, Tannen RL (eds): *Fluids and Electrolytes*. Philadelphia: W.B. Saunders Company; 1986:229–304.
45. Greene CL, Blitzer MG, Shapira E. Inborn errors of metabolism and Reye syndrome: Differential diagnosis. *J Pediatr* 1988;113:156–159.
46. Msall M, Batshaw ML, Suss R, et al. Neurologic outcome in children with inborn errors of urea synthesis. *N Engl J Med* 1984;310:1500–1505.
47. Rutledge SL, Havens PL, Haymond MW, et al. Clinical and laboratory observations: Neonatal hemodialysis: Effective therapy for the encephalopathy of inborn errors of metabolism. *J Pediatr* 1990;116:125–128.
48. Batshaw ML, Brusilow S, Waber L, et al. Treatment of inborn errors of urea synthesis. *N Engl J Med* 1982;306:1387–1392.
49. Brusilow SW, Danney M, Waber LJ, et al. Treatment of episodic hyperammonemia in children with inborn errors of urea synthesis. *N Engl J Med* 1984;310:1630–1634.

Chapter 14

Nutrition in the Pediatric Intensive Care Unit Patient

Adalberto Torres Jr., MD and Pat Wiggins, MS, RD, CS

Introduction

Nutritional support is an essential component of pediatric intensive care. Since malnutrition increases the risk of infection and mortality in critically ill children,[1,2] nutritional support is one of the therapies that should be administered early in the pediatric intensive care unit (PICU) stay. The prevalence of acute and chronic malnutrition in hospitalized children reported from one children's hospital in 1995 was approximately 24% and 27%, respectively.[3] Prevalence of acute and chronic protein-energy malnutrition in one tertiary care PICU was approximately 20%.[4,5] Children are at increased risk for malnutrition compared to adults because of increased energy requirements for growth and development and smaller lipid and glycogen reserves. Hospitalized children younger than 2 years of age and children with chronic diseases have a higher prevalence of malnutrition than do older, healthier children.[4-6]

In addition to the child's pre-illness nutritional status, the change in metabolic state associated with illness or injury and the anticipated length of inability to resume usual dietary intake factor into the child's risk of consequences of poor nutritional intake in the PICU. Certain illnesses and injuries, such as trauma, result in a hypermetabolic state in critically ill children,[7] whereas uncomplicated surgical procedures do not.[8,9] Although less than 25% of all children admitted to a PICU stay longer than 3 days, this subgroup of children is significantly younger, has a higher prevalence of chronic disease, has a higher severity of illness, requires more invasive monitoring, and consumes disproportionately more resources.[10,11] These characteristics make children with prolonged PICU stays more susceptible to complications related to poor nutritional status (eg, impaired immune function, delayed wound healing, etc.).

The goals of nutritional support in the PICU are to prevent loss of lean body mass and to avoid other consequences of stressed starvation, both of which can affect outcome. This chapter addresses the current recommendations for nutritional support and nutritional assessment in the critically ill child. To fill in the gaps in the pediatric literature, evidence supporting nutrition in the care of the critically ill adult is used to support some recommendations.

Enteral Nutrition

Despite differences in energy requirements based on differences in age, type and severity of illness, and preexisting nutritional status, most children admitted to the PICU should receive enteral nutrition (EN). In 1993, the American Society for Parenteral and Enteral Nutrition (ASPEN) published guidelines for the use of nutrition in adult and pediatric patients.[12] ASPEN and others[13] have recommended administration of EN as early as possible as the optimal approach to nutrition support of the critically ill child. EN is less expensive, less invasive, and more homeostatic than parenteral nutrition (PN). EN avoids central venous catheter (CVC)-associated sepsis and PN-associated liver disease. Theoretically, EN may also maintain the barrier function of the gastrointestinal mucosa and prevent bacterial translocation. This may be particularly relevant during prolonged PICU stays. A lack of enteral feedings results in atrophy of the villous line of the gastrointestinal tract and disruption of the normal barrier that prevents bacteria and endotoxin from gaining access to the circulation. When this barrier is not present, bacterial translocation can result, leading to nosocomial sepsis and multisystem organ failure. The latter is a primary factor in ICU morbidity and mortality.

Disadvantages of EN include exacerbation of gastroesophageal reflux and risk of pulmonary aspiration, bacterial overgrowth, and complications directly related to the feeding tube including nasal necrosis or bowel perforation. Malnourished children and children receiving no form of nutrition for greater than 7 days are at risk for the metabolic consequences of refeeding syndrome (eg, hyperglycemia, hypophosphatemia, hypomagnesemia, hypokalemia).[14] The low risk of these adverse consequences makes EN the optimal route of delivery.

Any child who is unable to consume adequate calories orally during his or her illness or injury should be considered a candidate for EN. Contraindications to EN include recent gastrointestinal surgery, severe gastrointestinal hemorrhage, intestinal obstruction, necrotizing enterocolitis, persistent emesis, or intractable diarrhea. PN administration should be considered for these patients.

EN has been well tolerated by children with no bowel sounds, those on vasoactive agents and/or neuromuscular blocking agents, and even children supported by extracorporeal membrane oxygenation.[15-17] However, tolerance of EN is dependent on the route of delivery and matching the conditional needs of the child. In children with absent bowel sounds, those receiving neuromuscular blockade, and/or those who have recently experienced a major insult (eg, head injury, surgery) when delayed gastric emptying is common,[18] nasoduodenal or transpyloric tube (TPT) feedings are the preferred method for delivery of EN. Nasogastric feedings are generally well tolerated by alert children recovering from illness or injury who require additional calories but are incapable of orally ingesting their daily requirements. Orogastric tube feedings should be considered in premature infants or infants with respiratory distress, to avoid partial obstruction of their obligate airway passages.

ASPEN recommends TPT feeding for critically ill infants or children (eg, mechanically ventilated, receiving vasoactive agents) since it theoretically reduces the risk of aspiration. However, strong evidence to validate this issue is lacking.[19] Sufficient evidence exists to support routinely starting enteral feeds within 24 hours of admission to the ICU.[15,19] Percutaneous endoscopic gastrostomy (PEG) is a viable option for providing EN to patients with extensive facial/skull trauma or surgery if a physician experienced in placement is available.[20]

TPT can be successfully placed at the bedside using a noninvasive approach.[21] Use of a nonweighted feeding tube with stylet is preferred, since this type of tube has better success of placement.[22] Use of the shorter length tube (56 cm, 6F; Corpack, Wheeling, IL) is recommended for infants less than 6 kg, while the longer tube (91 cm, 6F; Corpack) is of sufficient length for the majority of older children. Two marks, representing the distance from the nasal opening to the gastroesophageal junction and from the nasal opening to the pylorus, should be placed on the feeding tube with an indelible marker (Fig. 1). An intravenous dose of metoclopramide (0.1 mg/kg) should be administered immediately before starting to facilitate gastric emptying. If no intravenous access is present, a nasogastric dose of cisapride (0.2 mg/kg) may be administered 30 minutes prior to

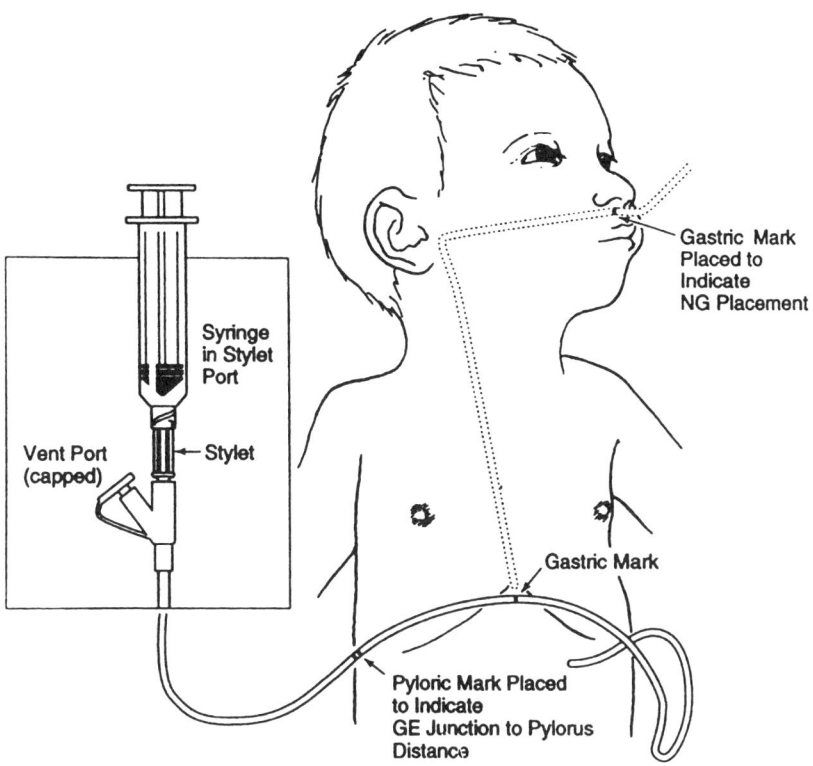

Figure 1. Marking nonweighted, bullet-tip feeding tube for transpyloric placement. Reproduced with permission, from Reference 21.

starting TPT placement.[23] The patient should be positioned in a supine or right lateral decubitus position. The head of the bed should be elevated 15 to 30°. If a nasogastric tube is present, the stomach must be decompressed of its contents prior to removal of the tube. After the ventilation port is capped, the tube should be lubricated with water. The tube is then inserted through a nostril in a position parallel to the palate (Fig. 1). When the gastric mark reaches the nostril, the stomach should be insufflated with 10 mL of air, using a Luer tip syringe without removing the stylet. Gastric position is confirmed by auscultation over the epigastrium followed by easy aspiration of the insufflated air. Cough, drop in pulse oximeter saturation, or resistance to tube advancement represent possible tracheal placement and, in such situations, the tube should be removed immediately. If possible, the patient should be placed in the right lateral decubitus position and the tube advanced 1 cm at a time to the pylorus mark, while gradually insufflating 10 mL of air. The sound of the insufflated air may change from low-pitched to higher pitched gurgles when the tube enters the pylorus. There may also be a sudden decrease in resistance when the tube enters the pylorus. An additional 10 mL of air should be insufflated. If less than 2 mL is aspirated, the tube is likely in the correct position. If fluid is aspirated, the pH should be tested at the bedside. A pH greater than 5 confirms transpyloric placement. Caution should be taken interpreting this result as positive if the patient is receiving an H_2-blocking agent. If insufflation of air is met with resistance, if the tube backs out when released, or if a noticeable increase in resistance occurs with advancement, there is reason to suspect that the tube has coiled or kinked in the esophagus or stomach. Once proper placement is confirmed, the tube should be advanced an additional 5 to 10 cm, to place the tip in the distal duodenum or proximal jejunum. An abdominal radiograph is then obtained to confirm tube placement. The feeding tube should course from left to right across the thoracolumbar spine and, in some instances, course back from right to left confirming placement in the distal duodenum or proximal jejunum (Fig. 2). Additional doses of metoclopramide and cisapride may be administered if the tip of the tube is not in the optimal position. A single dose of intravenous or oral erythromycin (3 mg/kg over 1 hour) will also facilitate propagation of the TPT tip into the small intestine if it is at the antrum of the pylorus prior to administration.[24] With this technique, radiographic assessment may not be necessary once placement of the TPT by experienced health care providers reaches a high level of confidence.[21] Feeding tubes with pH probes may require fewer radiographs for confirmation but may not be associated with fewer complications, placement time, or time to start feedings.[25]

Gastric feedings can be administered intermittently or continuously. The child who is unable to orally ingest sufficient calories may better tolerate continuous administration during nighttime feedings. Checking residual contents prior to the next intermittent feed or every 4 to 6 hours of continuous feeding assesses tolerance of nasogastric feedings. A volume of residual gastric content of greater than half an inter-

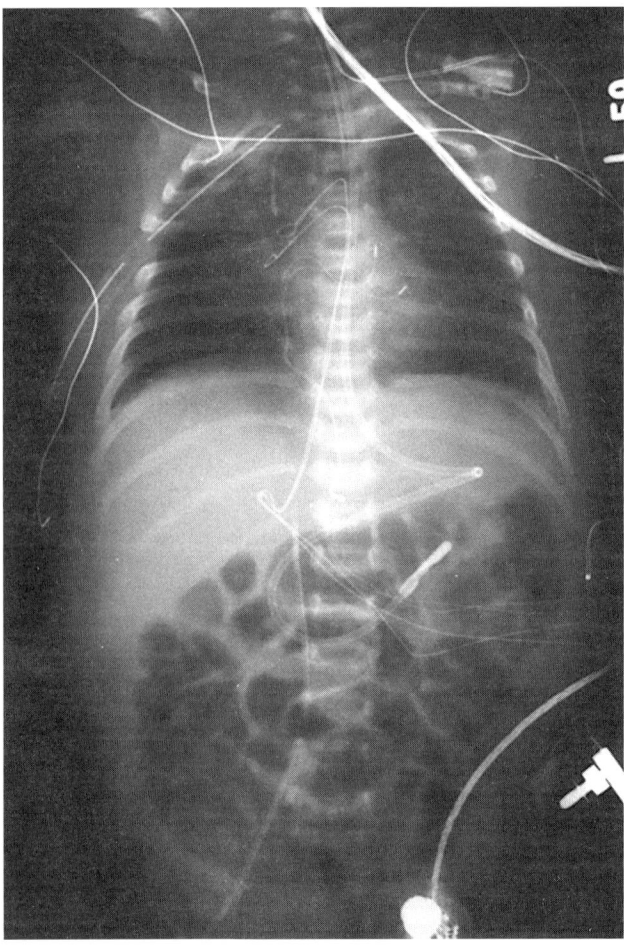

Figure 2. Abdominal radiograph demonstrating tip of feeding tube in distal duodenum/proximal jejunum.

mittent feed or greater than the volume infused over the previous 2 hours may represent intolerance. Feedings may be held for a short time and then restarted at the previous strength and rate. Administration of cisapride or metoclopramide should be considered at this time to facilitate gastric emptying. The volume and strength of formula to administer when feeds are started should vary depending on the prior condition of the child. Isotonic formulas started at full strength are usually well tolerated. High-density caloric formulas, often hypertonic, may not be tolerated initially and, even when diluted, can provide adequate calories. The child who does not eat or drink for more than 3 days might benefit from receiving formula initially diluted half to three-quarter strength.[26]

TPT feeds must be administered continuously. Intolerance of TPT feeds is suspected if the child develops abdominal distention, diarrhea, or constipation. Cisapride may improve gastrocecal transit time in children receiving opioids or inotropic agents.[27] Guidelines for initial volume administration and advancement of nasogastric and TPT feedings are shown in Table 1. To avoid problems with electrolyte imbalance and fluid overload, dilute formula should be concentrated to full strength prior to increasing to the goal volume.

Infants (<1 year) should receive breast milk or a standard infant formula. The infant's mother should be encouraged to express her milk regularly and to store it for administration when EN is started. Fortified human milk is recommended, since it results in better growth than unfortified milk and still provides the anti-infective benefits of human milk.[28] The formula should be chosen based on the child's age and gastrointestinal function (Table 2). The brand of formula received prior to PICU admission should be administered to the formula-fed infant. A pediatric dietitian may be consulted to discuss the various ways to increase the caloric density of formula administered without increasing the total volume (eg, adding a fat or carbohydrate supplement [Table 2] versus concentrating the formula).[26] A pediatric dietitian can also create a customized formula using substrate and vitamin supplements to better satisfy the individual needs of the patient.

Although ASPEN recommends that an elemental formula be used when EN is started, there is no evidence that elemental formulas are better tolerated than standard whey or soy protein formulas in children

Table 1

Enteral Nutrition Guidelines

Intermittent Nasogastric Feedings

Initiate at 2 to 5 mL/kg per feeding every 3 to 4 h.
Advance in increments of 2 to 5 mL/kg every two feedings to the goal as tolerated.
Check residuals before each feeding.
Hold feeding if the volume is greater than half the volume previously infused.
Restart feedings at previous rate and recheck for residual feeding.
Advance to goal volume gradually if residuals decrease.

Continuous Transpyloric or Nasogastric Feedings

Initiate with 1 to 2 mL/kg/h (60 mL maximum).
Advance slowly to goal rate by 1 to 2 mL/kg every 4 to 6 h as tolerated.
Adolescents can be started at 25 to 50 mL/h depending on expected tolerance.
Advance to goal rate in increments of 20 to 25 mL every 4 to 6 h as tolerated.
With nasogastric feeding, check residuals every 4 h.
Hold feedings if the residual volume is greater than the volume infused over the previous 2 hours.
Advance feedings to goal volume gradually if residuals decrease.
Advance dilute formula to full strength prior to advancing rate of infusion.
Monitor abdominal distention and stools to assess tolerance to small-bowel feedings.

Table 2
Infant and Pediatric Enteral Formulas

Infants (<1 Year Old)	Formula Characteristics	Formulas
Infant with normal GI function	60:40 whey/casein or casein	Human milk, Enfamil with Iron*, Similac with Iron†
Lactose intolerance or casein allergic	Lactose-free, soy protein	Prosobee*, Isomil†
Fat malabsorption or chylothorax	MCT oil (% of fat)	Portagen* (85%) Pregestimil* (55%) Alimentum† (50%)
Food allergies, protein or fat malabsorption:	Hypoallergenic hydrolyzed casein	For normal absorption: Nutramigen* For abnormal absorption: Alimentum†, Pregestimil*
	Free amino acids	Neocate‡
1 to 11 Years Old	**Formula Characteristics**	**Formulas**
Normal gastrointestinal function	Lactose free	Pediasure† Kindercal*
Fat malabsorption or chylothorax	MCT oil (% of fat)	Vivonex Pediatric§ (68%) Peptamen Junior‖ (60%)
Food allergies, protein or fat malabsorption:	Free amino acids	Neocate One Plus‡ Vivonex Pediatric§
> 11 Years Old	**Formula Characteristics**	**Formulas**
Normal gastrointestinal function	Casein protein + fiber	Jevity†
Fat malabsorption or chylothorax	MCT oil (% of fat)	Lipisorb* (85%)
Food allergies, protein or fat malabsorption:	Free amino acids	Vivonex TEN§ Tolerex§
Substrate Supplements		
Carbohydrate:	Polycose,† Moducal*	
Protein:	Promod,† Casec*	
Fat:	Microlipid,¶ MCT oil*	

*Mead Johnson Nutritionals, Evansville, IN; †Ross Laboratories Inc., Columbus, OH; ‡SHS North America, Gaithersburg, MD; §Sandoz Nutrition, Minneapolis, MN; ‖Clintec Nutrition, Deerfield, IL; ¶Sherwood Medical, St. Louis, MO; GI = gastrointestinal; MCT = medium chain triglyceride.

with no prior history of malabsorption.[19] One exception may be an infant or child without any enteral intake for greater than 5 to 7 days.

Children older than 1 year should receive a commercial formula designed to satisfy their caloric requirements and need for vitamins. Pediasure® (Ross Laboratories Inc., Columbus, OH) and Kindercal® (Mead Johnson Nutritionals, Evansville, IN) are the formulas of choice for children up to age 11 years. Children older than 11 years may receive one of the commercially available adult formulas. A formula high in fat (eg, Pulmocare® [Ross Products Division, Abbot Laboratories, Columbus, OH] or Respalor® [Mead-Johnson, Evansville, IL]) should be considered for the child with extremely poor ventilatory reserve (eg, bronchopulmonary dysplasia, acute respiratory distress syndrome). There is less carbon dioxide production associated with fat metabolism compared to carbohydrate metabolism, especially if there is conversion of carbohydrate to fat in the overfed patient. Other choices of formulas to be used during organ dysfunction or failure are discussed in the section on organ failure.

Mechanical, gastrointestinal, and metabolic complications result in discontinuation or interruption of feeds in approximately 10% of tube-fed children.[16] Position of tube markings should be checked every shift to ensure proper position. Regular irrigation of feeding tubes with normal saline, especially after enteral administration of medications, prevents tube occlusion. Tube occlusions can often be cleared with the infusion of a carbonated soft drink. Profuse diarrhea and dehydration may occur in children receiving concentrated or adult formulas secondary to the hyperosmolarity and the increased renal solute load of these formulas. Continuous delivery of nasogastric feedings with a mechanical enteral pump may resolve diarrhea in some patients.[29] Metabolic complications associated with refeeding syndrome may occur in children kept "nothing by mouth" (NPO) for a prolonged period of time; the actual incidence, however, is low. Intestinal perforations have been reported primarily in low birth weight infants.[30]

Infectious complications of EN are also secondary to mechanical cause. Sinusitis may occur from physical obstruction of the sinus tract opening. For decompression of the stomach, a nasogastric tube should be placed through the opposite nasal passage to avoid complete obstruction of the turbinates. Bacterial overgrowth with aspiration pneumonia is the most life-threatening complication of EN. Fortunately, aspiration pneumonia has not been noted with any significant frequency in reports of EN in critically ill children.[15,16]

EN, especially nasogastric feedings, is commonly interrupted for procedures or surgery. The TPT may need to be removed in young infants at the time of extubation, to remove any obstruction of the nasopharyngeal airway. However, TPTs should not be routinely removed from older infants and children so that feedings can be reinstituted if spontaneous oral intake is inadequate after extubation or if respiratory distress persists.

Parenteral Nutrition

PN has extended the lives of children who were unable to tolerate adequate amounts of nutrition enterally (eg, children with short bowel syndrome and extreme prematurity). PN can be administered to any child with venous access. PN can be administered into a peripheral vein (at lower caloric densities) or into a central vein via a CVC. PN can deliver an individualized assortment of solutes and nutrients on a daily basis for the patient in metabolic evolution during critical illness. PN administered soon after surgery (ie, postoperative day one) has been shown to blunt the catabolic response significantly in infants after cardiopulmonary bypass.[31] PN has been associated with a greater risk of nosocomial infection and metabolic disturbances (eg, hyperglycemia, hypertriglyceridemia) compared to EN. PN also requires serial laboratory monitoring, which further escalates its expense above that of EN.

PN is used in the PICU primarily for children who are unable to tolerate EN. Children presenting with a gastrointestinal disorder or some other reason why caloric needs cannot be met with EN (Table 3), should have PN administered early in their hospitalization. Because children have limited reserves, maximum time without administration of some form of nutritional support should be 3 days in patients from birth to 4 years of age, and 5 days for those 5 to 18 years of age.[32] Contraindications to PN include the decision not to continue or start aggressive supportive care, hypoten-

Table 3

Indications for Parenteral Nutrition

Gastrointestinal disorders
   malrotation with volvulus
   intestinal anomalies and atresia
   bowel ischemia
   pancreatitis
   intractable diarrhea
   persistent emesis
   short-bowel syndrome
   ileus and pseudo-obstruction
   gastrointestinal fistulas

Hypermetabolism
   severe trauma and burns

Malignancies/bone marrow transplants

Inflammatory bowel disease

Chylothorax if medium chain triglyceride oil-based formula fails

sion despite inotropic support, and a functional gut.[13]

Peripheral PN is best reserved for the child who requires minor caloric augmentation of EN or short-term support. Nutrient concentration is limited by the hypertonicity of elevated dextrose solutions. Dextrose concentrations greater than 10% to 12.5% cause a chemical phlebitis and tissue breakdown if the solution extravasates into the surrounding tissues. Intravenous administration of lipids into a peripheral vein has a venoprotective effect, is safe, and increases the nutritive value of peripheral PN. Peripheral PN administration with lipids also enables higher concentrations of dextrose to be infused more safely, due to its diluent effect.

Central venous access is necessary in order to provide hypertonic PN to the critically ill child. A CVC in a femoral, internal jugular, or subclavian vein can be used or placed for PN administration. Peripherally inserted central catheters (PICC) originating in a cephalic or basilic vein can be used to provide PN to the infant or child requiring central venous access for the sole purpose of full nutritional support. Long-term (ie, >1 month) central venous access can be accomplished with a permanent indwelling Broviac/Hickman type catheter or with a subcutaneous port. The choice of access depends on the individual patient's needs and the attending physician's preference.

Unlike the premature infant, the term infant or the child with normal hepatic and renal function can tolerate moderate quantities of carbohydrates, proteins, and lipids. A common approach to the rate of PN delivery of the three major energy substrates is to begin with a basal amount of each and increase each of them gradually on a daily basis (Table 4). However, any term infant or child tolerating a general diet for age within 48 to 72 hours of initiation of PN is capable of tolerating a more rapid increase in protein and lipids (eg, half the maximum g/kg on day one, maximum g/kg on day two) given normal renal and hepatic function continue. Carbohydrates should be increased more gradually to avoid major fluid shifts secondary to the hypertonicity of the fluid and hyperosmolarity caused by hyperglycemia. The degree of hypertriglyceridemia or azotemia present should result in a reduction or a temporary stall in the amount of lipid or protein administered (see organ failure section).

A general rule of thumb is that 10% of the total calories should be provided as amino acids. Specialized formulas for neonates (Aminosyn-PF®, Abbott Laboratories, Chicago, IL; Trophamine®, McGaw Inc., Irvine, CA), containing higher concen-

Table 4

Guidelines for Administration of Substrates in Parenteral Nutrition

Carbohydrate

	Initiation	Advancement	Maximum
Infants and children	5–10% dextrose	by 5% q d	30 g/kg/d
Adolescents	10% dextrose	by 5–10% q d	5 mg/kg/min

Protein

	Initiation	Advancement	
Infants and children	0.5–1.0 g/kg/d	0.5–1 g/kg/d	
Adolescents	1.0 g/kg/d	1.0 g/kg/d	

Lipid

	Initiation	Advancement	Maximum
Infants	0.5–1.0 g/kg/d	0.5–1.0 g/kg/d	3 g/kg/d
Children	1.0 g/kg/d	1.0 g/kg/d	10–20 kg: 2.5 g/kg/d
			20–30 kg: 2.0 g/kg/d
			>30 kg: 1.5 g/kg/d

trations of certain essential amino acids, are available. The division of the remaining 90% of the calories between lipid and carbohydrate is more controversial. Some authors recommend that 60% to 70% of the total calories be derived from carbohydrate administered as dextrose. Provision of 20% to 30 % of calories as lipid is generally well tolerated. However, the administration of lipid to the severely stressed patient remains controversial. The potentially detrimental effects of lipid administration (Table 5) must be taken into consideration on an individual basis. Essential fatty acid deficiency can be avoided by administering 0.5 g/kg of lipid two to three times per week. A step-by-step approach to prescribing PN during the first few days of nutritional support can be used for most children in the PICU (Table 6). An acceptable combination of carbohydrate, protein, and lipid administered results in a nonprotein calorie-to-nitrogen ratio of 150 to 200 calories to 1 gram of nitrogen (see Table 7 for calculations). A ratio of 240:1 to 350:1 has been suggested during periods of elevated stress (eg, systemic inflammatory response syndrome, trauma).

Electrolyte and mineral requirements vary from child to child according to intravascular volume status, medications administered (eg, diuretics), and renal function. Table 8 provides a range of daily maintenance requirements to use for the initial PN prescription. The concentrations of electrolytes are adjusted according to serum concentrations. It is important to remember to consider solutes delivered via arterial line catheter solutions and antibiotic salts (eg, penicillin G potassium) into the totals administered daily.[32]

Although some experts recommend administering vitamins and trace elements in excess of the National Research Council Recommended Daily Allowance (NRC-RDA),[33] most pediatric nutritionists administer the NRC-RDA of these essential micronutrients (Table 9).

Table 5

Potential Adverse Effects of Intravenous Lipid Administration

Increase in pulmonary artery pressure
Increase shunt fraction
Alternation in leukocyte function
Increase in production of leukotrienes and other arachadonic acid metabolites
Negative effect on microcirculation and platelet function

Table 6

Step-by-Step Approach to Prescribing Parenteral Nutrition

1. On day 1 of PN, begin with D% 5–10, 1/3 of amino acid goal, and 0.5–1.0 g lipid/kg/d. Administer entire solution over 24 h.
2. On day 2 of PN, administer D% 10–15, 2/3 of amino acid goal and advance lipid by 0.5–1.0 g/kg/d.
3. On day 3 of PN, administer D% 15–20, 100% amino acid goal and advance lipid by another 0.5–1.0 g/kg/d.
4. Continue to incrementally advance D% and lipid daily until goal achieved.
5. General guidelines for advancing PN daily:
    a. If serum glucose within normal limits or glucosuria absent, continue to increase D% incrementally. Consider maintaining or reducing D% administered if hyperglycemia or glucosuria present
    b. If serum triglyceride concentration <275 mg/dL, continue to next lipid step. If >275, consider decreasing amount administered or maintaining current dose until next serum triglyceride concentration checked.
    c. If BUN and creatinine are within normal limits and lipids are advanced, advance amino acids. If BUN and creatinine are abnormal, continue current dose or decrease dose of amino acids administered. Check nonprotein calorie to nitrogen ratio.
    d. If patient is being fluid restricted, D% may be advanced to 25%, 30% or even 35%.

PN = parenteral nutrition; D% = dextrose g/100 mL; BUN = blood urea nitrogen.

Table 7
Nonprotein Calories-to-Nitrogen Ratio Calculations

Dextrose volume/100	×	% dextrose	=	g dextrose
grams of dextrose	×	3.4 kcal/g	=	dextrose calories
10% lipid	=	1.1 kcal/mL	=	lipid calories
20% lipid	=	2.2 kcal/mL	=	lipid calories
[grams of amino acid	×	4.0 kcal/g	=	protein calories]*
Dextrose calories	+	lipid calories	=	nonprotein calories
grams of amino acids	÷	6.25	=	grams of nitrogen
Nonprotein calories	÷	g nitrogen	=	nonprotein calorie-to-nitrogen ratio
Goal: 150 to 200 nonprotein calories per g nitrogen				

*Protein calories are not taken into account by nutritionists when considering calories administered to the patient. However, consider protein calories into the total calories delivered until energy needs are met since protein administered during this period is being used for energy and not tissue growth and maintenance.

Table 8
Daily Electrolyte and Mineral Requirement

Solute	Suggested Initial Range*
Sodium	2.0–4.0 mEq/kg/d
Potassium	2.0–3.0 mEq/kg/d
Chloride	2.0–4.0 mEq/kg/d
Calcium	0.5–3.0 mEq/kg/d[†]
Magnesium	0.25–0.5 mEq/kg/d[‡]
Phosphorus	1.0–2.0 mM/kg/d[§]

*Recommended range based on normal serum concentrations and renal function.
[†]Administered as calcium gluconate to reduce risk of precipitation with phosphate; 18.75 mg = 1 mEq of calcium gluconate salt
[‡]125 mg = 1 mEq of magnesium sulfate salt
[§]Administer as potassium phosphate and adjust potassium chloride accordingly; 2 mEq $PO_4^=$ = 1mM $PO_4^=$; mM KPO_4 × 1.47 = __ mEq K^+.

Table 9
Vitamin and Trace Mineral Recommendations*

Pediatric multivitamins[†]
  indicated for infants and children <11 years of age
  dose: 2 mL/kg, 5 mL maximum
	Multivitamins[†]
	  indicated for children >11 yeas of age
	  dose: 10 mL/d

Pediatric trace elements[‡]
  indicated for newborn to 6 years of age
  dose: 0.2 mL/kg/d (3 mL/d maximum)
	Trace elements[‡]
	  indicated for children >6 years of age
	  dose: 1 mL/d[§]

*Based on specific brand; [†]Centeon L.L.C., Kankakee, IL; [‡]Fujisawa, USA, Inc., Deerfield, IL; [§]M.T.E.⁻4 Concentrate®.

Table 10

Metabolic Complications of Parenteral Nutrition

Congestive heart failure
Pulmonary edema
Hyperglycemia
Hypoglycemia
Azotemia
Electrolyte imbalance
Vitamin/mineral deficiencies
Essential fatty acid deficiency
Hyperlipidemia
Cholestasis
Rickets
Hepatomegaly
Hepatic fibrosis
Chronic liver dysfunction

Metabolic, infectious, and mechanical complications are associated with PN. Metabolic complications occur as a direct consequence of PN (Table 10), while infectious and mechanical complications are related in large part to the CVC. Sepsis, the most frequent serious complication of PN, may occur in as many of 15% of children receiving PN.[34] PN-related liver dysfunction is multifactorial and related to prematurity, low birth weight (<1000 g), and duration of PN administration (>14 days).[35] Serial laboratory monitoring (see below), introduction of small volume enteral feeding,[35,36] effective antiseptic protocols for insertion and handling of CVC,[37] personnel experienced in proper placement techniques of PICC and CVC, and discontinuation of PN as early as possible will reduce the rate of these complications.

Estimating Caloric Needs

Numerous predictive equations have been used to estimate caloric needs of the critically ill child.[7,38,39] The large intraindividual variability in energy expenditure makes it impossible to accurately predict with one equation.[39] Use of the NRC-RDA would substantially overestimate the caloric needs of most children admitted to the PICU.[40] The majority of studies measuring resting energy expenditure in infants and children admitted to the PICU have documented caloric needs to be approximately equivalent to basal metabolic rate (BMR).[8,41–44] For the majority of patients admitted to the PICU, BMR should be the caloric goal (Table 11). This approach avoids the complications of overfeeding. Two exceptions are acute trauma patients and patients with the systemic inflammatory response syndrome.[7,9,45] Children with two or more characteristic clinical findings of systemic inflammatory response syndrome including temperature greater than 38°C or less than 36°C rectal, tachycardia or tachypnea for age, white blood cell count greater than 12,000 cells/mm^3, less than 4000 cells/mm^3, or greater than 10% immature (band) forms, DAR93[46] or evidence of a stress response (eg, elevated acute phase reactant, CHW95[9]) should receive approximately 1.4 times their BMR to match their elevated needs. Children recovering from uncomplicated surgery do not have elevated needs beyond the first 24 postoperative hours.[8,42,47] Neuromuscular blockade does not cause a significant reduction in the caloric needs of intubated patients who are receiving adequate sedation and analgesia.[48] The basal calories should be increased by 10% to account for the thermic effect of enteral digestion. Calories provided to NRC-RDA should be increased once the patient is capable of performing routine daily living activities (eg, walking, eating without assistance).

An occasional patient may fail to grow even when provided with the appropriate calories, determined by using a predictive equation for caloric estimation. Resting energy expenditure (REE) measured with a metabolic cart provides the best approximation of caloric needs. However, meticulous attention to detail and the proper circumstances are required to obtain an acceptable measurement of REE.[49] Measurement of REE should be considered in the patient failing to grow with nutritional support or having difficulty weaning from mechanical ventilation.

Table 11

Basal Metabolic Rates of Children (Energy Requirements in kcal/day)

Body Weight (kg)	Male	Female	Body Weight (kg)	Male	Female
3.0	150	136	36.0	1270	1173
4.0	210	205	38.0	1305	1207
5.0	270	274	40.0	1340	1241
6.0	330	336	42.0	1370	1274
7.0	390	395	44.0	1400	1306
8.0	445	448	46.0	1430	1338
9.0	495	496	48.0	1460	1369
10.0	545	541	50.0	1485	1399
11.0	590	582	52.0	1505	1429
12.0	625	620	54.0	1555	1458
13.0	665	655	56.0	1580	1487
14.0	700	687	58.0	1600	1516
15.0	725	718	60.0	1630	1544
16.0	750	747	62.0	1660	1572
17.0	780	775	64.0	1690	1599
18.0	810	802	66.0	1725	1626
19.0	840	827	68.0	1765	1653
20.0	870	852	70.0	1785	1679
22.0	910	898	72.0	1815	1705
24.0	980	942	74.0	1845	1731
26.0	1070	984	76.0	1870	1756
28.0	1100	1025	78.0	1900	1781
30.0	1140	1063	80.0	1935	1805
32.0	1190	1101	82.0	1970	1830
34.0	1230	1137	84.0	2000	1855

With permission from Canate A, Duggan C. Nutritional support of the pediatric intensive care unit patient. *Curr Opin Pediatr* 1996;8:248–255.

Organ Failure

Renal Failure

Besides fluid and electrolyte imbalance and the accumulation of nitrogenous wastes, renal failure has many detrimental effects on the nutritional status of the critically ill child, including anorexia, growth failure, glucose intolerance, hypertriglyceridemia, and impaired protein synthesis and metabolism.[50] Therefore, the nutritional support provided to the child with renal failure will vary according to the severity of renal dysfunction and the effectiveness of renal replacement therapy. Adjustments in nutritional support must be individualized and discussed with the consulting nephrologist. EN is the preferred form of nutritional support. Specialized enteral products for patients with renal failure are readily available (Table 12). These formulas should be diluted to half strength when initiated, due to their hypertonicity and associated diarrhea. These formulas can be mixed together to deliver a more specific quantity of protein. Renal-failure–specific recommendations for PN are provided in Table 13.

Hepatic Failure

Critically ill patients with varying degrees of liver failure are often catabolic and malnourished.[51] Metabolic alterations are a result of impaired hepatic synthesis, impaired hepatic degradation, and malabsorption. Many experts prefer EN for

Table 12
Enteral Formulas for Children with Renal Failure**

Brand	Kcal/mL (per oz)	Protein g (% cal)	Carbohydrate g (% cal)	Fat g (% cal)	Na (mEq)	K (mEq)	Ca (mg)	P (mg)	Fe (mg)	Osmolality mOsm/kg Water	Indications
Suplena*	2 (60)	30 (6)	hydrolyzed corn starch (90%) sucrose (10%) 255 (51)	HO safflower oil (90%) soy oil (10%) 96 (43)	34	29	1385	728	19	600	patients NOT undergoing dialysis, or smaller patients
Nepro*	2 (60)	70 (14)	hydrolyzed corn starch (88%) sucrose (12%) 215 (43)	HO safflower oil (90%) soy oil (10%) 96 (43)	36	27	1373	686	19	635	patients undergoing dialysis, or larger patients

*Ross Laboratories, Inc., Columbus, OH; **concentrations of electrolytes, trace minerals, protein, fat, and carbohydrate are listed per liter of formula.

Table 13

Adjustments in Parenteral Nutrition for Renal Failure

Kilocalories*	no change
Protein†	no dialysis → BUN <60 mg/dL
	dialysis → BUN 60–100 mg/dL
Carbohydrate	no change (60%–70% of nonprotein calories)
	peritoneal dialysis → reduce by 10%‡
Lipids	advance slowly as tolerated§
Macrominerals‖	reduce calcium and avoid magnesium, phosphorus, and potassium
Vitamins	consider decreasing vitamin A supplementation
	dialysis → RDA + 0.5–1 mg/d folic acid, 5–10 mg/d pyridoxine, 75–100 mg/d vitamin C
Trace minerals	reduce by half

*Increase kilocalories provided for children with sepsis, multiple trauma, systemic inflammatory response syndrome (basal metabolic rate × 1.4).
†Attempt to administer optimal quantity of protein and maintain BUN within given range with renal replacement therapy.
‡Reduce to account for carbohydrate delivered through dialysate.
§Administer a minimum of 0.5 g/kg/d twice per week to avoid essential fatty acid deficiency; continue to increase if daily change in serum triglycerides <15%.
‖Supplement according to serum concentrations.
BUN = blood urea nitrogen; RDA = recommended dietary allowance

Table 14

Parenteral Vitamin Supplementation and Monitoring for Patients with Hepatic Failure

Vitamin	Deficiency	Drug	Daily Dose	Monitoring
Vitamin A	night blindness, degeneration of the retina, xerophthalmia, poor growth, and hyperkeratosis	emulsified vitamin A (may also require zinc)	5,000–15,000 IU	serum levels 400–500 μg/L
Vitamin D	rickets, osteroporosis, osteomalacia, cranial bossing, epiphyseal enlargement, persistently open anterior fontanel in infants	25–OH D	5–7 μg/kg/d	serum level 25 to 30 ng/mL (or higher), serum phosphate and parathyroid hormone
Vitamin E	peripheral neuropathy, ataxia, impaired intestinal absorption of vitamin E	generic	150–300 IU/kg/d	serum level >5 mg/L, vitamin E: total lipid ratio of 0.6 to 0.8 mg/g
Vitamin K	coagulopathy, hemorrhagic manifestations such as bruising	vitamin K_3	5–15 mg/d	prothrombin time, factor activities

With permission, from Carlin AC, Collier SB, Hendricks KM, et al. Pediatric disorders requiring specific nutrition management. In Hendricks KM, Walker WA (eds): *Manual of Pediatric Nutrition.* Toronto: BC Decker; 1990:251.

Table 15

Adjustments of Parenteral Nutrition for Hepatic Failure

Kilocalories	no change*
Protein	acute → restrict for hepatic encephalopathy†
	chronic → no change
Carbohydrate	no change (60% to 70% of nonprotein calories)
Lipids	advance as tolerated‡
Macrominerals	supplement according to serum concentrations
Vitamins§	may require greater than RDA supplementation
Trace minerals	monitor and supplement zinc; reduce or delete manganese or copper administration if obstructive jaundice present[13]

*Increase kilocalories provided for children with sepsis, multiple trauma, systemic inflammatory response syndrome (basal metabolic rate × 1.4).
†Nitrogen products should not be completely withheld except in child with overt hepatic coma.[51]
‡Patients with end-stage liver disease occasionally develop hypertriglyceridemia and may require partial fat restriction. Administer a minimum of 0.5 g/kg/d twice per week to avoid essential fatty acid deficiency; continue to increase if daily change in serum triglycerides <15%.
§Diminished bile salt production during hepatic failure may lead to fat-soluble vitamin deficiency.
RDA = recommended daily allowance.

patients with liver failure, but controversy exists as to which form of nutritional support is best for patients with hepatic encephalopathy. Medium-chain triglyceride (MCT)-based formulas such as Alimentum® (Ross Laboratories Inc.), Portagen® (Mead Johnson Nutritionals), and Pregestimil® (Mead Johnson Nutritionals) should be used to improve fat absorption in infants with hepatic failure. MCTs are absorbed directly into the portal venous system and, unlike other fats, do not require bile salts for absorption. MCT oil can be added to the foods or formulas of older children to increase fat and caloric intake. However, MCT oil does not increase absorption of fat-soluble vitamins, and parenteral administration of these vitamins may be necessary (Table 14). Malnourished patients awaiting liver transplantation who fail to grow with EN are most likely to benefit from PN.[12] Modifications in PN are based on the acuity and severity of the disease (Table 15). No data support the use of specialized nutrition (eg, high-branched chain, low aromatic amino acid preparations versus balanced amino acid preparations) to improve or abate the course of end-stage liver disease. Regardless of route chosen, early nutritional support should be the primary goal.

Intestinal Failure

Loss of intestinal function may be a primary process (eg, inflammatory bowel disease) or secondary to the underlying illness (eg, ileus associated with pancreatitis). PN is the nutritional support of choice for the small subgroup of affected children admitted to the PICU. Introduction of small volumes of enteral feedings as early as feasibly possible should be strongly considered. Partial EN may improve immune status and reduce the risk of infectious complications[36] and also delay the onset of or reverse PN-related liver dysfunction.[35]

Skin Failure

There is no other single organ failure that causes as great a hypermetabolic state with an accelerated loss of lean body mass as skin failure secondary to burns, severe atopic dermatitis, or Stephens-Johnson syndrome.[52] Factors that contribute to the increased metabolic rate seen in these patients include: increased circulating concentrations of counter-regulatory hormones (eg, cortisol, epinephrine, glucagon), increased insensible losses secondary to hyperthermia, a cool environment, extent and depth of wounds, and infectious complica-

Table 16
Nutritional Recommendations for Children with Skin Failure

Calories	BMR × 2 (see Table 11) *or* NRC-RDA (listed below):	
	Age (yr)	*Kcal/kg*
	birth–0.5	108
	0.5–1.0	98
	1–3	102
	4–6	90
	7–10	70
	males 11–14	55
	males 15–18	45
	females 11–14	47
	females 15–18	40
Protein*	<1 yr:	3–4 g/kg goal weight
	1–3 yr:	3 g/kg goal weight
	>3 yr:	1.5–2.5 g/kg goal weight
Carbohydrate	40%–50% of nonprotein calories	
Lipids	advance as tolerated	
Macrominerals[†]	supplement according to serum concentrations	
Vitamins[‡]	≤20% BSA:	RDA (1 multivitamin daily)
	>20% BSA:	1 multivitamin daily + supplemental
	vitamin C:	<3 yr: 250 mg daily
		≥3 yr: 500 mg daily
	vitamin A:	<3 yr: 5,000 IU daily
		≥3 yr: 10,000 IU daily
Trace minerals	supplement zinc:	<3 yr: 100 mg daily
		≥3 yr: 220 mg daily

*Consider increasing protein calories to 25% of total calories.[62]
[†]Serum phosphorus concentrations may become extremely low immediately after burn injury and during acute care.
BMR = basal metabolic rate; BSA = body surface area.

tions. However, there is sufficient evidence that supports the assertion that twice the BMR or NRC-RDA is sufficient caloric provision for good wound healing and growth.[52] Patients with burns of less than 20% of their body surface area (BSA) can often achieve adequate oral intake. For children who have greater than 20% BSA and/or are unable to achieve their predicted caloric goal, nighttime gastric or continuous TPT feeding should be strongly considered. Because of the very high risk of infectious complications in this subgroup of patients, PN should be strictly reserved for those patients who are totally unable to tolerate any appreciable amount of TPT feedings. See Table 16 for skin-failure–specific recommendations.

Nutritional Assessment and Monitoring

A multitude of techniques and approaches are available to evaluate the nutritional status and adequacy of nutritional support. There is no single assessment parameter that works in every patient under every circumstance. Therefore, the best approach is often a combination of various techniques that best suit the needs of the critically ill population (Table 17).

Anthropometric Measurements

Anthropometry, a population-based comparison of human body measurements, is the simplest class of nutritional assessment techniques. Anthropometry includes weight, height or length, skinfold thickness, and various extremity circumferences. Weight and height of all children should be recorded, preferably upon admission to the PICU prior to extensive fluid resuscitation. Electronic sling scales can be used to accurately measure the weight of children of all sizes. Recumbent length or height is measured using a certified measuring board placed directly under the child. Midarm circumference and skinfold thicknesses, estimators of total body fat and lean body mass, should be measured by the same individual(s) on all children, to reduce interobserver variability.

These measures have very limited use in assessing nutritional status in the critical

Table 17

Nutritional Assessment and Monitoring Recommendations

On admission:
  weight
  height (recumbent length)
  head circumference (children < 3 years of age)*
  serum electrolytes, blood urea nitrogen, creatinine, glucose

Enteral nutrition
  daily: electrolytes including magnesium, and phosphorus†
  triweekly: weight
  weekly: height (recumbent length), head circumference (children <3 years of age),* prealbumin ± orosomucoid‡

Parenteral nutrition
  daily: electrolytes including magnesium, and phosphorus, triglyceride§
  biweekly: total protein, bilirubin, transaminases, cholesterol
  triweekly: weight
  weekly: height (recumbent length), head circumference (children <3 years of age),* prealbumin ± orosomucoid‡

*Include midarm circumference and skinfold thickness if no evidence of edema and experienced technician available.
†Obtain daily for the first few days in patients not fed for 5 to 7 days or receiving dilute formula.
‡Consider measuring acute phase reactant in patient with fever, tachypnea, tachycardia, elevated white blood cells, etc.
§Check biweekly once parenteral nutrition delivered is unchanged for 2 to 3 days.

care setting. Monitoring daily weight reflects fluid status rather than nutritional status. Height, midarm circumference, and skinfold thickness do not change rapidly in response to nutritional support. Midarm circumference and skinfold thickness need to be measured early in the admission, since edema formation can cause tremendous error.

Weekly anthropometric measurements should be obtained, especially those of length and head circumference in children less than 3 years of age, plus weights three times per week in children cared for in the PICU for greater than 7 days. It is important to ensure that the measuring equipment is in good condition and calibrated regularly.

Biochemical Markers

Serum transport proteins including albumin, transferrin, and prealbumin have been used extensively for assessing nutritional status and response to nutritional support. Serum albumin is the least sensitive and the least specific of the three proteins for this purpose and is therefore no longer recommended. Reasons include decreased serum concentrations secondary to fluid redistribution following capillary injury and/or dilution due to increased plasma volume following aggressive fluid resuscitation, and its long half-life (15 to 20 days). Despite its relatively shorter half-life of 7 days, serum transferrin concentrations are no more useful than serum albumin concentrations. Serum transferrin concentrations may be increased by iron deficiency and hepatitis and decreased by rapid expansion of plasma volume and high-dose antibiotic therapy.[53] With a half-life of 2 to 3 days, thyroxine-binding prealbumin, or transthyretin works as a good marker for response to nutritional support rather than as an initial assessment of nutritional status. Retinol-binding protein has a half-life of only 24 hours, but concentrations are decreased with vitamin A or zinc deficiency and hyperthyroidism. Insulinlike growth factor-1 (IGF-1), a modulator of growth hormone, has the most promise as a nutritional marker because of its half-life of only a few hours and its excellent correlation with nitrogen balance.[54] However, IGF-1 is not readily available, is more costly, and is used mostly in research applications.

Regardless of the serum transport protein chosen as a marker for nutritional adequacy, all transport proteins produced by the liver are subject to decreased production or increased degradation for causes other than nutrition. Stress or injury resulting in a systemic inflammatory response result in a reprioritization by the liver to produce acute-phase reactants instead of transport proteins. It is strongly recommended that the clinician measure a C-reactive protein or α-1 antitrypsin (orosomucoid) concentration simultaneously when obtaining a transport protein concentration if a systemic inflammatory response is suspected.[55]

Enteral Nutrition Monitoring

Monitoring of EN includes anthropometric measurements, biochemical markers, and drug-nutrient interactions. Serum potassium, magnesium, and phosphorus should be monitored for the first few days after initiation of EN, to reduce the metabolic complications of refeeding syndrome.[14] Weekly prealbumin ± orosomucoid concentrations should be performed at least weekly to assess the nutritional adequacy of the nutritional support that is being provided. Serum phenytoin concentrations may decrease in patients receiving continuous EN with oral phenytoin and should therefore be monitored unless feedings are held 2 hours before and after phenytoin administration.[56]

Parenteral Nutrition Monitoring

Baseline laboratory tests should be obtained to assess glucose homeostasis, electrolyte and mineral balance, fluid status, hepatic and renal function, and triglyceride metabolism. Laboratory tests including serum electrolytes, blood urea nitrogen, glucose, and triglyceride concentrations should be checked daily while PN is being adjusted and then biweekly unless otherwise indicated medically (Table 17). Growth parameters and biochemical markers of nutritional adequacy for patients receiving PN should be assessed as they would be for patients receiving EN.

Future Directions

Many nutritional therapies and monitoring techniques are currently being investigated in both laboratory and clinical studies. Although most of these innovations will probably not be in routine use at the time of publication of this volume, the purpose of this section is to provide some initial exposure to those with the most promise.

The noninvasive technique for measuring fat-free or lean body mass that is attracting the most attention is bioelectrical impedance analysis (BIA). BIA measures lean body mass by determining differences in electrical conductivity between fat and fat-free mass. Besides being noninvasive, BIA is safe, inexpensive, and does not require patient cooperation. Body cell mass change measured with BIA has been correlated with energy and protein intakes in critically ill adults.[57] BIA may not be useful in patients with significant alterations in fluid and electrolyte status, since edema causes alterations in resistance measurements.[53]

Besides the evidence that early EN is beneficial in reducing infectious complications in critically ill adults, there is growing evidence that the various constituents of nutritional support provided may be beneficial as well. Glutamine (GLN), the most abundant amino acid in the human body, becomes essential during a critical illness secondary to increased depletion of intracellular stores in excess of GLN biosynthesis. Studies of GLN-supplemented PN and GLN-supplemented EN in premature infants have demonstrated its safety and potential for reducing morbidity and length of stay.[58,59] It has been suggested that supplementing the diets of critically ill patients with arginine, ω-3 fatty acids, and nucleotides may reverse the impaired immune response seen in severely stressed critically ill patients. Studies of early EN supplemented with GLN, arginine, ω-3 fatty acids, and nucleotides in critically ill adults have demonstrated a reduced infectious complication rate and shorter length of stay.[60,61] A multicenter, randomized, controlled trial with critically ill children is warranted.

Conclusion

Although the effects of illness on nutrition and metabolism are well known, the impact of nutritional support on outcome of the critically ill child is less clear. Despite the lack of overwhelming evidence supporting the role of nutritional support in the care of the critically ill child, most experts agree that nutritional support will remain an essential part of early intensive care management. Finally, one should never forget the old axiom, "if the gut works, use it."

References

1. Pollack MM, Ruttiman UE, Wiley JS. Nutritional depletions in critically ill children: Associations with physiologic instability and increased quantity of care. *J Parenter Enteral Nutr* 1985;9:309–313.
2. Leite HP, Isatugo MKI, Sawaki L, Fisberg M. Anthropometric nutritional assessment of critically ill hospitalized children. *Rev Paul Med* 1993;111:309–313.
3. Cameron JW, Rosenthal A, Olson AD. Malnutrition in hospitalized children with congenital heart disease. *Arch Pediatr Adolesc Med* 1995;149:1098–1102.
4. Pollack MM, Wiley JS, Holbrook PR. Early nutritional depletion in critically ill children. *Crit Care Med* 1981;9:580–583.
5. Pollack MM, Wiley JS, Kanter R, Holbrook PR. Malnutrition in critically ill infants and children. *J Parenter Enteral Nutr* 1982;6:20–24.
6. Hendricks KM, Duggan C, Gallagher L, et al. Malnutrition in hospitalized pediatric patients. *Arch Pediatr Adolesc Med* 1995;149: 1118–1122.
7. Tilden SJ, Watkins S, Tong TK, Jeevanandam M. Measured energy expenditure in pediatric intensive care patients. *Am J Dis Child* 1989;143:490–492.
8. Shanbhogue RLK, Lloyd DA. Absence of hypermetabolism after operation in the newborn infant. *J Parenter Enteral Nutr* 1992;16: 333–336.
9. Chwals WJ, Letton RW, Jamie A, Charles B. Stratification of injury severity using energy expenditure response in surgical infants. *J Pediatr Surg* 1995;30:1161–1164.

10. Pollack MM, Wilkinson JD, Glass NL. Long-stay pediatric intensive care unit patients: Outcome and resource utilization. *Crit Care Med* 1987;80:855–860.
11. Ruttiman UE, Pollack MM. Variability in duration of stay in pediatric intensive care units: A multiinstitutional study. *J Pediatr* 1996;128:35–44.
12. ASPEN Board of Directors. Guidelines for the use of parenteral and enteral nutrition in adult and pediatric patients. *J Parenter Enteral Nutr* 1993;17:1SA–28SA.
13. Marian M. Pediatric nutrition support. *Nutr Clin Pract* 1993;8:199–209.
14. Jolly AF, Blank R. Refeeding syndrome. In Zaloga GP (ed): *Nutrition in Critical Care.* St. Louis: Mosby; 1994:765–782.
15. Chellis MJ, Sanders SV, Webster H, et al. Early enteral feeding in the pediatric intensive care unit. *J Parenter Enteral Nutr* 1996;20:71–73.
16. Panadero E, Lopez-Herce J, Caro L, et al. Transpyloric enteral feeding in critically ill children. *J Pediatr Gastroenterol Nutr* 1998;26:43–48.
17. Pettignano R, Heard M, Davis R, et al. Total enteral nutrition versus total parenteral nutrition during pediatric extracorporeal membrane oxygenation. *Crit Care Med* 1998;26:358–363.
18. Ott L, Young B, Phillips R, et al. Altered gastric emptying in the head-injured patient: Relationship to feeding intolerance. *J Neurosurg* 1991;74:738–742.
19. Heyland DK, Cook DJ, Guyatt GH. Enteral nutrition in the critically ill patient: A critical review of the evidence. *Intensive Care Med* 1993;19:435–442.
20. De Vivo P, Mastronardi P, Ciritella P, et al. Early percutaneous endoscopic gastrostomy (PEG). A safe and effective enteral feeding technique in neurologic intensive care unit. *Minerva Anestesiol* 1996;62:197–201.
21. Harrison AM, Clay B, Grant MJC, et al. Nonradiographic assessment of enteral feeding tube position. *Crit Care Med* 1997;25:2055–2059.
22. Lord LM, Weiser-Maimone A, Pulhamus M, Sax HC. Comparison of weighted vs. unweighted enteral feeding tubes for efficacy of transpyloric intubation. *J Parenter Enteral Nutr* 1993;17:271–273.
23. Spagen HD, Duinslaeger L, Diltoer M, et al. Gastric emptying in critically ill patients is accelerated by adding cisapride to a standard enteral feeding protocol: Results of a prospective, randomized, controlled trial. *Crit Care Med* 1995;23:481–485.
24. Lorenzo CD, Lachman R, Hyman PE. Intravenous erythromycin for postpyloric intubation. *J Pediatr Gastroenterol* 1990;11:45–47.
25. Krafte-Jacobs B, Persinger M, Carver J, et al. Rapid placement of transpyloric feeding tubes: A comparison of pH-assisted and standard insertion techniques in children. *Pediatrics* 1996;98:242–248.
26. Warman KY. Enteral nutrition: Support of the pediatric patient. In Hendricks KM, Walker WA (eds): *Manual of Pediatric Nutrition.* 2nd ed. Toronto: BC Decker Inc.; 1990:72–109.
27. Bindl L, Buderus S, Ramirez M, et al. Cisapride reduces postoperative gastrocecal transit time after cardiac surgery in children. *Intensive Care Med* 1996;22:977–980.
28. Nutrition Committee CPS. Nutrient needs and feeding of premature infants. *Can Med Assoc J* 1995;152:1765–1785.
29. Cataldi-Betcher EL, Seltzer MH, Slocum BA, Jones KW. Complications occurring during enteral nutrition support: A prospective study. *J Parenter Enteral Nutr* 1983;7:546–552.
30. McAlister WH, Siegel MJ, Shackelford GD, et al. Intestinal perforations by tube feedings in small infants: Clinical and experimental studies. *AJR Am J Roentgenol* 1985;145:687–691.
31. Chaloupecky V, Huein B, Tlaskal T, et al. Nitrogen balance, 3-methylhistidine excretion, and plasma amino acid profile in infants after cardiac operations for congenital heart defects: The effect of early nutritional support. *J Thorac Cardiovasc Surg* 1997;114:1053–1060.
32. Wesley JR, Coran AG. Intravenous nutrition for the pediatric patient. *Semin Pediatr Surg* 1992;1:212–230.
33. Debiasse MA, Wilmore DW. What is optimal nutritional support? *New Horizons* 1994;2:122–130.
34. Yeung CY, Lee HC, Huang FY, Wang CS. Sepsis during total parenteral nutrition: Exploration of risk factors and determination of the effectiveness of peripherally inserted central venous catheters. *Pediatr Infect Dis J* 1998;17:135–142.
35. Kelly DA. Liver complications of pediatric parenteral nutrition-epidemiology. *Nutrition* 1998;14:153–157.
36. Okada Y, Klein N, Van Saene HKF, Pierro A. Small volumes of enteral feedings normalise immune function in infants receiving parenteral nutrition. *J Pediatr Surg* 1998;33:16–19.
37. Lange BJ, Weiman M, Feuer EJ, et al. Impact of changes in catheter management on infectious complications among children

with central venous catheters. *Infect Control Hosp Epidemiol* 1997;18:326–332.
38. El-Khatib MF, Rosolowski BJ. Prediction of the resting energy expenditure of mechanically ventilated patients in the pediatric intensive care unit. *Respir Care* 1996;41:191–196.
39. Selby AM, McCauley JC, Schell DN, et al. Indirect calorimetry in mechanically ventilated children: A new technique that overcomes the problem of endotracheal tube leak. *Crit Care Med* 1995;23:365–370.
40. Canete A, Duggan C. Nutritional support of the pediatric intensive care unit patient. *Curr Opin Pediatr* 1996;8:248–255.
41. Chwals WJ, Lally KP, Woolley MM, Mahour GH. Measured energy expenditure in critically ill infants and young children. *J Surg Res* 1988;44:467–472.
42. Groner JI, Brown MF, Stallings VA, et al. Resting energy expenditure in children following major operative procedures. *J Pediatr Surg* 1989;24:825–828.
43. Steinhorn DM, Green TP. Severity of illness correlates with alterations in energy metabolism in the pediatric intensive care unit. *Crit Care Med* 1991;19:1503–1509.
44. Gebara BM, Gelmini M, Sarniak A. Oxygen consumption, energy expenditure, and substrate utilization after cardiac surgery in children. *Crit Care Med* 1992;20:1550–1554.
45. Frankenfield DC, Wiles CE III, Bagley S, Siegel J. Relationships between resting and total energy expenditure in injured and septic patients. *Crit Care Med* 1994;22:1796–1804.
46. Darville T, Giroir B, Jacobs R. The systemic inflammatory response syndrome (SIRS): Immunology and potential immunotherapy. *Infection* 1993;21:279–290.
47. Jones MO, Pierro A HP, Lloyd DA. The metabolic response to operative stress in infants. *J Pediatr Surg* 1993;28:1258–1263.
48. Steinhorn DM. Neuromuscular blockade provides no benefit over adequate sedation in ventilated dogs. *J Crit Care* 1998;10:45–50.
49. Witte MK. Metabolic measurements during mechanical ventilation in the pediatric intensive care unit. *Respir Care Clin North Am* 1996;2:573–586.
50. Molina MF, Riella MC. Nutritional support in the patient with renal failure. *Crit Care Clin* 1995;11:685–704.
51. Gecelter GR, Comer GM. Nutritional support during liver failure. *Crit Care Clin* 1995;11:675–683.
52. Rodriguez DJ. Nutrition in patients with severe burns: State of the art. *J Burn Care Rehabil* 1996;17:62–70.
53. Charney P. Nutrition assessment in the 1990s: Where are we now? *Nutr Clin Pract* 1995;10:131–139.
54. Hawker FH, Stewart PM, Baxter RC, et al. Relationship of somatomedin-C/insulin-like growth factor I levels to conventional nutritional indices in critically ill patients. *Crit Care Med* 1987;15:732–736.
55. Kudlackova M, Andel M, Hajkova H, Novakova J. Acute phase proteins and prognostic inflammatory and nutritional index (PINI) in moderately burned children aged up to 3 years. *Burns* 1990;16:53–56.
56. Saklad JJ, Graves RH, Sharp WP. Interactions of oral phenytoin with enteral feedings. *J Parenter Enter Nutr* 1986;10:322–323.
57. Robert S, Zarowitz BJ, Eichenhorn M, et al. Bioelectrical impedance assessment of nutritional status in critically ill patients. *Am J Clin Nutr* 1993;57:840–844.
58. Neu J, Roig JC, Meetze WH, et al. Enteral glutamine supplementation for very low birth weight infants decreases morbidity. *J Pediatr* 1997;131:691–699.
59. Lacey JM, Crouch JB, Benfell K, et al. The effects of glutamine-supplemented parenteral nutrition in premature infants. *J Parenter Enteral Nutr* 1996;20:74–80.
60. Senkal M, Mumme A, Eickhoff U, et al. Early postoperative enteral immunonutrition: Clinical outcome and cost-comparison analysis in surgical patients. *Crit Care Med* 1997;25:1489–1496.
61. Bower RH, Cerra FB, Bershadsky B, et al. Early enteral administration of a formula (Impact) supplemented with arginine, nucleotides, and fish oil in intensive care unit patients: Results of a multicenter, prospective, randomized clinical trial. *Crit Care Med* 1995;23:436–449.

Chapter 15

Blood Product Administration and Coagulation Function

Joseph D. Tobias, MD

Introduction

Hematologic dysfunction is rarely the primary reason for admission to the pediatric intensive care unit (PICU). However, bone marrow dysfunction with alterations in the production of platelets, white blood cells (WBCs), and erythrocytes frequently occurs in patients with severe systemic disease processes. Coagulation function may be affected not only by decreased platelet production by the bone marrow, but also by increased peripheral consumption of platelets during disseminated intravascular coagulation (DIC). Likewise, coagulation function may be affected by decreased production of coagulation factors as well as increased consumption. Regardless of the underlying disease process, replacement of the various formed elements of the blood and coagulation factors may be required. This chapter reviews the basic approach to support of the hematologic and coagulation systems, including the transfusion of formed elements of the blood and support of the coagulation system.

Blood Component Therapy

Adverse Effects of Blood Product Administration

The major concern regarding the use of blood products is the risk of the transmission of infectious diseases. The current screening methods for donated blood and blood products have significantly decreased the risk of transmission of infectious agents. However, the risk of transmission is still present as individuals may donate blood during a time early in their infectious process when they are infectious and have not yet seroconverted. The current practice for screening of blood for infectious diseases in outlined in Table 1. Additionally, donated blood is screened by the measurement of alanine amino-transferase (ALT) as a marker of infection with non-A, non-B hepatitis. This test may identify a proportion of patients who are infected and yet have not had enough time to seroconvert. Recent estimates suggest that the cumula-

From: Tobias JD (ed): *Pediatric Critical Care: The Essentials.* ©Futura Publishing Co., Inc., Armonk, NY, 1999.

Table 1

Current Practice for Screening of Blood Products

Syphilis	serologic test for syphilis (STS)
Hepatitis	hepatitis B surface antigen
	antibody to hepatitis B core antigen
	antibody to hepatitis C virus
HIV	anti-HIV 1
	anti-HIV 2
	HIV p24 antigen
HTLV I/II	anti-HTLV I/II antibody

HIV = human immunodeficiency virus; HTLV = human T-cell lymphotrophic virus.

tive risk of transmission of an infectious agent (human immunodeficiency virus, human T-cell lymphotropic virus, hepatitis B, or hepatitis C) is 1 in 34,000 units.[1] The majority of cases (85% to 90%) are related to the transmission of hepatitis B or C.

Aside from infectious complications, other complications related to blood product administration include both hemolytic and nonhemolytic transfusion reactions. Hemolytic complications may be immune mediated or nonimmune mediated. The classic immune-mediated hemolytic transfusion reaction results from an incompatibility between the administered red cells and the patient. Most of these reactions result from the transfusion of incompatible red blood cells (RBCs), related to clerical errors. Its incidence is roughly 1 in 33,000 units, with a fatality of 1 patient for every 500,000 units.[2,3] The signs and symptoms of a hemolytic transfusion reaction are related to activation of the patient's humoral system by the fragmented RBCs. Signs and symptoms vary depending on the amount of incompatible blood that has been transfused. In a conscious, awake patient the signs and symptoms include chest pain, dyspnea, nausea/vomiting, fever, and chills. In anesthetized or unconscious patients, the only signs and symptoms may be hemoglobinuria, coagulopathy, or cardiovascular disturbances.

Treatment begins with immediate stopping of the transfusion. Serious sequelae of a transfusion reaction include hemoglobinuria with renal failure and activation of the coagulation cascade with DIC. Treatment includes maintenance of an alkaline diuresis with fluid administration, low-dose dopamine, loop diuretics, and mannitol. Cardiovascular instability is treated with fluid administration and direct-acting adrenergic agents as needed. Respiratory insufficiency related to acute respiratory distress syndrome may require endotracheal intubation and controlled ventilation. DIC and coagulation defects are treated as needed based on the platelet count, prothrombin time (PT), partial thromboplastin time (PTT), and fibrinogen level (see below). Documentation of the occurrence of a transfusion reaction is made by obtaining serum for free hemoglobin level and a direct Coombs' test.

Nonimmune hemolytic reactions result from external forces that damage the red cells prior to or during their administration. These problems can be prevented by appropriate handling and administration of blood products (see below). RBC lysis can be caused by exposure to hypertonic or hypotonic intravenous fluids, thermal injury during blood transport or storage, and inappropriate methods of warming the blood (eg, placing the blood in warm water). The signs and symptoms of nonimmune transfusion reactions are dependent on the quantity of hemolyzed blood that is administered. Treatment in severe cases is the same as that for immune-mediated hemolytic transfusion reactions.

One of the more commonly encountered problems occurring during the administration of blood products is fever (>1°C rise in core body temperature). The concern is that fever may be the first sign of an immune-mediated hemolytic transfusion reaction. When fever develops, the transfusion should be discontinued and the patient examined for other signs and symptoms of a hemolytic transfusion reaction. It is uncommon for fever to be the only sign of a transfusion reaction. Other possible causes of fever during transfusion include bacterial contamination of the blood product and a febrile, nonhemolytic transfusion reaction (FNHTR). The latter occurs most commonly in patients who receive numerous transfusions. Even if a hemolytic transfusion reaction is ruled out, there remains controversy over the advisability of resuming the transfusion. This decision is best made based on the hospital's transfusion policies and guidelines.

An FNHTR is the most common cause of fever during a transfusion. The diagnosis remains one of exclusion, by eliminating the possibility of a hemolytic transfusion reaction and bacterial contamination of the transfused blood product. The incidence of FNHTR is related to the patient's history of previous exposure to blood products and the specific component used (1% of packed RBCs [pRBCs] versus 20% to 30% of platelets). FNHTRs are immunologically mediated reactions related to the presence of antibodies in the recipient's plasma to WBC antigens. The antibody-antigen reaction leads to the release of endogenous pyrogens from the WBCs. The incidence and symptoms of FNHTRs can be decreased by decreasing the WBC content of RBCs by using filters that remove leukocytes from the blood, or by pretreating the patient with antihistamines and antipyretics. Other adverse consequences of blood transfusions, such as the metabolic consequences of massive transfusion, are discussed below.

Type and Screen Versus Type and Crossmatch

In an emergency situation, there may be inadequate time for either a type and screen or a type and crossmatch. In this rare instance, type O positive blood is administered to males and postmenopausal females, and type O negative blood is administered to females who are younger than or of childbearing age. Type O negative blood is preferred in females younger than or of childbearing age because of the risk of sensitizing them to the Rh antigen and setting them up for Rh problems with future pregnancies. Type O blood is referred to as the universal donor since it lacks antigens which may trigger a hemolytic transfusion reaction and can be administered to patients with type O, A, B, or AB blood. As there may be a significant quantity of anti-A or anti-B antibodies in type O blood, once a significant quantity of type O has been transfused (2 units in an adult or 15 to 20 mL/kg in a child), type O blood and not the patient's own blood type, once it is known, should be used for further transfusion therapy. In such patients, consultation with the pathologist in charge of blood banking or a hematologist may be helpful in determining when to switch back to using the patient's own blood type.

When more time is available, a type and screen or, in most cases, a type and crossmatch can be performed. A type and screen involves taking a sample of the patient's blood and determining its ABO and Rh type, in addition to screening the patient's serum for antibodies against the more common minor red cell antigens. The latter involves mixing the patient's serum with specific known red cell antigens and determining if there are antibodies to these antigens by using an indirect antiglobulin test. The type and screen involves the majority of red cell antigens that are capable of causing clinically significant hemolytic problems. The type and screen takes 45 to 60 minutes and, if negative, more than 99.99% of ABO-compatible blood units in stock will be compatible with the patient. In an emergency situation, if there is time to perform a type and screen, it is best to proceed with type-specific blood rather than type O blood. Additional testing, when time permits, involves the type and crossmatch. This involves mixing the patient's serum with blood from the actual unit that is to be used for transfusion. The full type and crossmatch is performed for the majority of transfusions that are performed, except in the rare emergency when blood is required immediately and time is limited.

Red Blood Cells

Much controversy surrounds the issue of the lowest tolerable hemoglobin and hematocrit. If intravascular volume is maintained, most patients tolerate an acute reduction of 15% to 30% of the circulating red cell mass. Patients without underlying end-organ disease processes are able to tolerate even further decreases of up to 30% to 40% in their red cell masses. Compensatory mechanisms, including increased cardiac output and a rightward shift of the oxyhemoglobin dissociation curve, maintain oxygen delivery to the tissues. Because of the interpatient variability, it is impossible to define the minimum hemoglobin for all patients. Rather, the criteria are based on the patient's previous medical history and current medical status. The transfusion of pRBCs is rarely indicated for patients with a hemoglobin greater than 10 g/dL.[4] The need for transfusion when the hemoglobin is between 6 and 10 gm/dL is based on the patient's ability to compensate for the decreased oxygen content of the blood.[4]

During collection of blood for transfusion, 450 mL are removed from the donor and added to roughly 50 mL of anticoagulant. The hematocrit of a unit of whole blood varies from 35% to 40% depending on the amount of anticoagulant added and the donor's hematocrit. The anticoagulant is CPD-A, containing "C" or citrate, which binds calcium and acts as the anticoagulant, "P" phosphate, "D" dextrose, and "A" adenine. The latter three compounds provide substrates for the metabolic processes of the RBCs and allow them to maintain viability for up to 35 days. The shelf life is regulated so that 75% of the transfused cells are viable at 24 hours following a transfusion. Prior to transfusion of a blood product, several steps are necessary to ensure that the correct unit is being used (Table 2). It should be kept in mind that the vast majority of serious transfusion problems are related to clerical errors resulting in the administration of an incompatible unit of blood.

Once whole blood is collected and added to the anticoagulation solution, it is further processed into pRBCs and the platelet-rich plasma. The latter is further processed into platelets, fresh frozen plasma (FFP), and cryoprecipitate (see below). The benefit of separating blood into specific components is that it ensures that there is an adequate supply of each component for patients who require them. There are few if any indications for the use of whole blood. One study has suggested that postoperative bleeding may be lessened following cardiac surgery in neonates and infants if fresh ($\leq$12 hours old) whole blood is used.[5] The term fresh whole blood is generally a misnomer, since once the blood is more than 24 to 48 hours old, there is little activity left in the platelets, and the concentration of labile coagulation factors (factors V and VIII) is inadequate to provide adequate hemostasis. Therefore, component therapy is used to provide the product needed based on the laboratory evaluation of the patient.

Packed RBCs contain a volume of 300 to 350 mL with a hematocrit of 75% to 80% when CPD-A is used as the anticoagulant. The addition of newer additive solutions (Adsol, Nutricel, Optisol) to the CPD-A solution is now common practice which results in a prolongation of the shelf life to 42 days, a decrease in the hematocrit to 60%, and, hence, a decrease in viscosity. This also results in a slightly larger volume for each unit of blood (350 to 400 mL). If there is a concern over the extra non-red-cell volume, the blood bank can centrifuge the blood and remove some of the fluid, resulting in a hematocrit of 80%. In children, the unit of pRBCs can be fractionated so that a transfusion can be administered and the remainder of the blood saved for use at a later date, thereby avoiding the need to expose the patient to another unit of blood. Transfusions are generally administered in aliquots of 10 to 15 mL/kg over 2 to 3 hours to raise the hematocrit to the desired level. One unit of pRBCs will raise the hematocrit by 3% to 4% in a 70-kg adult, while 10 mL/kg of pRBCs will raise the hematocrit by 8% to 10%.

When administering large volumes to patients, especially if administration is rapid, the blood product should be warmed to 37 to 38°C by use of a standardized blood warmer. Blood is routinely stored at 4°C and the administration of large volumes of blood products at this temperature can result in

Table 2

Suggested Procedures Prior to Blood Product Administration

1. The patient's name and hospital identification number should be verified from the patient's attached identification band or the anesthesia record and the form attached to the blood product to be transfused.
2. The unit identification number on the blood product should match the number on the form attached to the blood product.
3. The ABO and Rh type on the unit must agree with the form attached to the unit. The patient's blood type may not necessarily agree with the blood type on the unit and the form (see text for a description of the various blood products and the need for ABO and Rh compatibility).
4. The expiration date on the blood product should be acceptable.
5. Examine the unit for signs of bacterial contamination including clots, discoloration, or bubbles.

significant hypothermia. The rapid administration of blood and blood products for patients with massive hemorrhage can be accomplished with the use of blood pump tubing which contains a chamber that can be intermittently compressed to speed the administration of the unit of the blood. With large bore intravenous access, a unit of blood can be administered in 1 to 2 minutes. Alternatively, a pressure bag can be inflated over the unit, eliminating the need to occupy one person's time with intermittent compression of the chamber. All of these devices are most commonly used in the operating room by anesthesiologists for the rapid administration of blood and blood products. Ready access to such devices is suggested, to allow the rapid and efficient delivery of blood and blood products for the rapid resuscitation of patients with blood loss and other critical illnesses. In large tertiary centers that routinely care for trauma patients, mechanical rapid infuser systems are frequently used that allow the administration of units of blood and blood products within 1 minute. These devices use centrifugal roller pumps. Care must be taken with any of the previously mentioned techniques, as extravasation can occur with significant sequelae if the catheter becomes dislodged.

In addition to hypothermia, other complications of massive transfusion include metabolic alterations (hypocalcemia, acidosis, hyperkalemia) and coagulation disturbances. After 2 to 3 weeks of storage, potassium concentrations of pRBCs may reach levels of 20 to 30 mEq/L. Although there is a limited amount of plasma contained in pRBCs, its rapid administration (≥ 100 mL/min) can limit the time for potassium elimination and redistribution. The ECG should be monitored for signs of hyperkalemia during massive transfusions. The treatment of hyperkalemia is outlined in chapters 13 and 16. In patients with renal dysfunction or preexisting hyperkalemia, pRBCs can be washed (see below) prior to administration to remove the excess plasma and, hence, lower the potassium concentration. A second metabolic consequence of massive transfusion is hypocalcemia related to the binding of calcium by the citrate used in the pRBCs as an anticoagulant. Following the transfusion of 15 to 25 mL/kg of pRBCs, ionized calcium levels should be monitored and replacement therapy provided as needed. With a slower transfusion rate, the citrate is metabolized in the liver. Hepatic dysfunction may lead to a slower metabolism of citrate and thereby place the patient at greater risk of citrate toxicity. Signs and symptoms of hypocalcemia include a prolongation of the QT interval on the ECG, hypotension, and impaired myocardial contractility. These effects may be magnified by associated acidosis and hypothermia. In addition to binding calcium, citrate also binds magnesium, leading to hypomagnesemia.[6] The latter may impair the normal regulatory responses to hypocalcemia, including release of parathormone.

Packed RBCs also become more acidotic as time passes; this is related to the citrate used as an anticoagulant and the normal metabolic processes of the RBCs and the production of lactate. With the rapid administration of pRBCs, there may be inadequate time for the buffering of the acid load. Periodic measurement of arterial or venous blood gases and correction of the acidosis with sodium bicarbonate may be needed. The issues of hyperkalemia and acidosis have led the blood banking committees of some hospitals to institute protocols suggesting the use of relatively fresh blood (<7 to 10 days) in neonates and infants who may be less able to tolerate and compensate for the acid and potassium load.

Modifications and Treatment of Blood Products

In the majority of cases, standard pRBCs remain the component used to increase the patient's RBC mass. As mentioned previously, with pRBCs, a small amount of plasma is also transfused. If there is an issue regarding the patient's serum potassium concentration, it is possible to remove the plasma and, hence, the majority of the potassium load, which may be as high as 20 to 30 mEq/L after 2 to 3 weeks of storage. Washed pRBCs are prepared by centrifuging the cells with saline thereby removing the plasma, leukocytes, plasma proteins, and cytokines. Washing may be indicated for patients at risk for hyperkalemia and to prevent reactions related to the presence of white cell antigens (FNHTRs, see above) or immunoglobulin A (IgA). The latter is a problem only in patients with IgA deficiency in whom the presence of IgA in the donor blood can precipitate significant allergic/anaphylactic reactions.

Other patients may require that blood products be irradiated prior to their administration. The irradiation of blood products inactivates viable lymphocytes. Without such treatment, these lymphocytes can activate host defenses against the recipient, leading to graft-versus-host disease. This disease may occur in patients with altered cellular immunity related to congenital defects (DiGeorge syndrome) or chemotherapeutic and immunosuppressive regimens. Irradiation of blood products should also be considered for premature infants and even for term infants, as cellular immune function may be immature. Irradiation of blood products requires the appropriate equipment, which most blood banking facilities have, and can be accomplished in a matter of minutes. No significant alteration in the integrity or composition of the blood product occurs other than a slight increase in the potassium concentration.[7]

Glycerol can be used as an additive to RBCs to allow freezing at $-65°C$ for up to 10 years. Prior to administration, the glycerol is removed by washing the pRBCs (deglycerolized RBCs). This process is indicated only for the storage of very rare pRBCs for patients with antibodies to several RBC antigens or with rare phenotypes.

Blood/Hemoglobin Substitutes

Perfluorocarbons and stroma-free hemoglobin solutions are currently being investigated for assessment of their potential as blood substitutes, in order to eliminate the need for homologous transfusions of RBCs. These compounds can be considered clinically applicable if they efficiently transport and facilitate exchange of carbon dioxide and oxygen, provide buffering capabilities, and contribute to the maintenance of intravascular volume. The oxygen-carrying capacity of perfluorocarbons was first reported in 1969. The perfluorocarbon components carry oxygen dissolved in liquid, rather than being dependent on hemoglobin for the transport of oxygen. The volumes carried dissolved in solution are much greater than those carried by blood (40 to 50 mL of oxygen per 100 mL of liquid). A significant problem with these agents has been anaphylactic reactions related to Pluronic F-68, a surfactant.[8]

Tremper et al[9] evaluated the safety and efficacy of the perfluorocarbon emulsion, Fluosol, in severely anemic patients (hematocrit 14% to 16%) during administration of a low and high FiO_2. After the infusion of 20 mL/kg of Fluosol, the arterial oxygen content was significantly increased and the investigators noted increases in mixed venous oxygen tension and oxygen consumption. The solution carried 0.8% oxygen by volume, which accounted for $7\pm3\%$ of the patient's arterial content; however the oxygen consumption increased by 24±7%. The authors postulated that because the perfluorocarbons carry oxygen by direct solubility, at high PaO_2 values, the tissues will extract 75% to 80% of this dissolved oxygen before hemoglobin affinity is altered. They postulated that tissues preferentially extract oxygen from perfluorocarbons because oxygen is extracted at a higher partial pressure, and thus there is a greater partial pressure gradient for tissue diffusion. Additionally, the diameter of the perfluorocarbon particle is approximately 0.1 μm, which is 1/70 the size of an erythrocyte. This allows enhanced flow through small and constricted capillaries at a faster rate, which may also facilitate oxygen delivery. Despite such beneficial effects, in this initial study, no difference in eventual outcome (mortality) was noted between the patients who received Fluosol and controls.

Breuninger et al[10] demonstrated preservation of adequate oxygenation and acid-base status in newborn lambs undergoing isovolemic double volume exchange with FC-43, a more recently developed perfluorocarbon. Although hemodynamic stability, myocardial oxygenation, and cerebral oxygenation were well preserved, blood flow to the renal cortex significantly decreased. The authors were unable to explain the seemingly isolated decrease in blood flow to the renal cortex. Other studies have not been able to duplicate these findings. Additional laboratory investigations have demonstrated improvements in tissue oxygen delivery following perfluorocarbon administration in animal models of myocardial and cerebral ischemia.[11,12]

Further studies are needed to clearly define the adverse effect profile and role of perfluorocarbon emulsions as possible blood substitutes. The first generation agents such as Fluosol will have limited applications because of their adverse effect profile including anaphylactoid reactions, complement activation, short half-life, and the need for a high FiO_2. Second generation compounds with higher oxygen affinities, which may limit the FiO_2 requirements, are currently undergoing clinical trials.[13]

Another option is the use of exogenous, pure hemoglobin. Hemoglobin solutions have been available for research for more than 25 years. Options include both human hemoglobin or that produced through recombinant technology. Human hemoglobin has been synthesized in different bacteria including E. coli and S. cerevisiae. The use of the hemoglobin tetramer makes sense due to its natural property for binding, delivering, and releasing oxygen, as well as its high saturation and large carrying capacity at ambient oxygen pressures. Three hemoglobin-based strategies are currently under consideration: stroma-free hemoglobin, modified stroma-free hemoglobin, and liposome-encapsulated hemoglobin.[14] All three must still be considered extremely experimental with limited, if any, clinical applicability as of yet.

The rationale to use stroma-free hemoglobin (hemoglobin not encapsulated by the red cell membrane) is to avoid the antigens that are incorporated into the membrane, and therefore avoid the risks of mismatch and hemolytic transfusion reactions. However, problems arise when the hemoglobin is removed from the red cell membrane. Stroma-free hemoglobin has an increased oxygen affinity due to the loss of intracellular regulators of oxygen affinity such as 2,3-disphosphoglycerate. The altered affinity impairs oxygen release to the tissues. Additionally, the stroma-free hemoglobin has a significant osmotic effect that limits the amount that can be infused due to the risks of hypervolemia. Increases in mean arterial pressure are noted during infusion of these compounds. This effect is related to uptake of nitric oxide by the hemoglobin chains and an increase in the systemic vascular resistance, which may not be problematic in the hypotensive trauma patient but can cause significant increases in mean arterial pressure in patients who are normotensive prior to the infusion. The four globulin chains of stroma-free hemoglobin rapidly dissociate into dimers and monomers and thereby limit the effective duration of action. The globulin chains are cleared by the kidneys and can lead to nephrotoxicity.

Modification of the hemoglobin molecule has been attempted in order to eliminate some of these problems. The addition of pyridoxine 5-phosphate decreases the oxygen affinity of stroma-free hemoglobin to that of whole blood while various agents have been used to crosslink the globulin strands and prevent their dissociation. Looker et al[15] developed a recombinant hemoglobin in which the two globin units are fused thereby preventing in vivo dissociation and limiting its renal toxicity.

An additional modification is to encapsulate the hemoglobin in a nonantigenic, synthetic lipid envelope (liposome). Theoretically, this would allow the usual function of the hemoglobin while preventing the nephrotoxicity of the free product. Encapsulation within liposomes would also limit the osmotic effect of the product and allow for a higher plasma concentration.

While the availability of acceptable and safe hemoglobin or blood substitutes would eliminate the need for homologous transfusions, the use of such agents is still considered highly investigational. Concerns about their adverse effect profile may limit their clinical applications. Further refinements of these products is needed before they will be clinically available.

Blood Filters

Prior to administration, all blood products should be passed through a standard 170-μm filter to remove small clots and aggregates of cells that may develop during processing and storage. Additional microaggregates of platelets, leukocytes, and fibrin that can pass through standard 170-μm filters may also form. The administration of these microaggregates into the venous circulation has been suggested to be one of the factors responsible for the development of acute respiratory distress syndrome following massive transfusions. Microaggregate filters (20 to 40 μm) have been suggested as a means of removing these aggregates and preventing respiratory compromise. However, these microaggregate filters have not been shown to decrease the incidence of respiratory problems following massive transfusion[16] and are not routinely indicated. These filters are used to filter blood during cardiopulmonary bypass prior to its return via the aortic cannula to the systemic circulation.

Filters are also available to remove the majority of leukocytes (99.9%) from the blood product. These may be efficacious in patients with FNHTRs related to recipient antibodies directed against donor white cell antigens. The removal of leukocytes and lymphocytes may also be indicated for immunocompromised patients at risk for disease related to transmission of cytomegalovirus (CMV). If these patients have not been previously exposed to CMV as demonstrated by a lack of antibodies to the virus (CMV-negative), there is a significant risk that transmission of CMV infection via a blood product may develop into systemic disease. In such patients, the use of blood products from CMV-negative donors is the most prudent course of action; however, due to limitations in the donor blood supply, this may not always be possible. An alternative is to use leukocyte depletion filters to remove the majority of the lymphocytes/leukocytes and thereby lessen the risk of CMV transmission, since CMV resides within the WBCs. Leukocyte depletion filters are available for both pRBCs and platelet concentrates. Leukocyte depletion of blood products is not an alternative to irradiation. Even a few immunocompetent WBCs, which may elude removal by the filter, can cause graft-versus-host disease. These issues apply to RBC products and platelet concentrates which can contain significant numbers of WBCs. As plasma is relatively acellular, concerns of CMV transmission, graft-versus-host disease, and FNHTRs related to WBC antigens are not relevant to plasma administration (see below).

Fresh Frozen Plasma

Following the donation of a unit of blood, the whole blood is added to an anticoagulant and is separated into pRBCs and the platelet-rich plasma. The latter is centrifuged again to provide a unit of plasma and a unit of platelets. There is no standard specification as to the volume of plasma that is contained in a unit. The volume is dependent on the amount in the original donated unit as well as the amount removed by subsequent processing with the removal of the platelet unit. Most units of plasma contain 190 to 250 mL. Following processing, the plasma is frozen within 8 hours at −18°C to maintain the function of the labile coagulation factors. At this temperature, plasma or FFP can be stored for up to 1 year. Prior to its administration, FFP requires thawing for 30 to 60 minutes in a 37°C water bath.

FFP is indicated for the treatment of bleeding related to congenital or acquired deficiencies of coagulation factors that results in prolongation of PT or PTT to greater than 1.5 times control values.[4] FFP may also be indicated for the reversal of effects related to coumadin/warfarin derivatives in patients who require emergent surgical procedures or in those who develop excessive bleeding problems during therapy. If time permits, these effects can be reversed in 12 hours with the administration of exogenous vitamin K, thereby avoiding the infectious disease risks of FFP administration.

FFP is administered in an attempt to raise coagulation factor levels to 30% of normal. This should provide normal hemostatic function as well as result in normalization of the PT and PTT. One mL/kg of FFP will raise the coagulation factor level by 2%, thereby arriving at the usual recommendation for FFP administration of 10 to 15 mL/kg or 2 units of FFP in an adult. While such figures provide guidelines for FFP administration, subsequent doses of FFP should be guided by the frequent measurement of PT and PTT values. Additionally, fibrinogen levels should be followed, as cryoprecipitate may be required to replete fibrinogen levels and correct coagulation values (see below). Clinical experience suggests that the correction of PT and PTT values with FFP alone may be difficult in patients with low fibrinogen levels.

Many of the concerns of pRBC transfusions apply to the transfusion of FFP. A 170-μm filter should be used and, with large volumes of FFP, the products should be warmed to 37 to 38°C prior to their administration. Due to the presence of antibodies (anti-A or anti-B) in the plasma, ABO compatibility must be honored. However, since FFP is acellular, it is not mandatory to crossmatch for red cell antigen systems such as Rh. The presence of small amounts of anti-Rh antibodies in the donor plasma will not cause clinically significant hemolysis and, since the FFP is acellular, there is not a significant concern of stimulating production of anti-RH antibodies in the recipient. The latter can be problematic in premenopausal woman, as it may cause erythroblastosis fetalis in subsequent pregnancies. Rh compatibility is an issue in platelet concentrates (see below). FFP contains most of the anticoagulant that is added to a unit of blood, and therefore may result in citrate intoxication and hypocalcemia (see above) as well as hyperglycemia from the dextrose concentration when large volumes are infused.

Cryoprecipitate

Cryoprecipitate is the cold, insoluble, white precipitate that forms when a unit of FFP is thawed to 1 to 6°C. The precipitate is removed following centrifugation, and refrozen at −18°C. At this temperature, it is stable for up to 12 months. One unit of cryoprecipitate is the amount removed from one unit of FFP and generally consists of 10 to 20 mL. Cryoprecipitate contains significant quantities of factors I, VIII, XIII, fibronectin, and von Willebrand factor (vWF) (Table 3). Prior to the availability of factor VIII concentrate, cryoprecipitate was used as replacement therapy for patients with hemophilia. With the availability of factor VIII concentrates, cryoprecipitate is most commonly used as replacement therapy for patients with acquired bleeding disorders and low fibrinogen levels (≤100 to 150 mg/dL). One unit of fibrinogen per 10 kg body weight will increase the fibrinogen level by 50 mg/dL. As with the use of FFP, repeat dose of cryoprecipitate is best accomplished by periodic measurements of PT, PTT, and fibrinogen levels. Prior to its administration, cryoprecipitate is thawed and then should be administered within 4 hours. Due to the limited volume, ABO compatibility is not essential.

Platelet Concentrates

Two types of platelet concentrates are available from the blood bank. In the past, a unit of platelets referred to the platelets removed from a unit of blood. This process included the separation of the whole blood into pRBCs and platelet-rich plasma. The latter component was then separated into plasma and a unit of platelets. These are

Table 3

Composition of Cryoprecipitate

Factor VIII	100–200 units
Fibrinogen	150–250 mg
von Willebrand factor	40%–70% of original unit of FFP
Factor XIII	20%–30% of original unit of FFP
Fibronectin	15–30 mg
Total volume	10–20 mL

FFP = fresh frozen plasma.

now commonly referred to as random-donor platelets. Each unit contains approximately 5.5×10^{10} platelets in 50 to 75 mL of plasma. Following collection, platelets can be stored for 5 days. Storage requires constant agitation of the packs to prevent clumping of platelets and to facilitate gas exchange through the permeable plastic bag, which is important to prevent excessive decreases in the pH of the solution, as pH is a critical factor in platelet viability. One unit of platelets for every 10 kg body weight (0.1 U/kg) will raise the platelet count by roughly 20×10^9/L. This is sufficient to control bleeding related to thrombocytopenia, and results in the usual practice of administering 6 units ("a 6 pack") to adult patients.

More recently, platelets have also been provided by pheresis technology. During this process, a donor is attached to a pheresis machine and, over a 2-hour period, 200 to 300 mL of platelet-rich plasma is removed from the patient. This is referred to as a pheresis unit or a single-donor unit. Its composition is significantly different from that of a random-donor unit. A pheresis unit contains the equivalent of up to 6 to 10 units of random-donor platelets and yet exposes the patient to only a single donor. For pediatric patients, pheresis units can be divided in half or a quarter, and the remainder saved for use at a later time. As with random-donor platelets, pheresis units are viable for 5 days if kept at 22 to 24°C.

Platelet concentrates are indicated to correct bleeding related to qualitative or quantitative disorders of platelets. Due to the limited quantity of RBCs in the units, ABO compatibility is not essential. However, they can contain immunocompetent WBCs, and therefore irradiation of the blood product may be considered in specific patient populations (see above). Platelet concentrates are administered through standard 170-μm filters. Twenty- or 40-μm filters should not be used, as they can remove a significant number of the platelets.

Miscellaneous Plasma Derivatives

Other plasma derivatives available for clinical use include factor VIII concentrates, factor IX concentrates, factor IX complex, and antithrombin III (AT III). Factor VIII concentrate has replaced cryoprecipitate in the treatment of patients with hemophilia A. Recombinant technology has eliminated the need for factor VIII concentrates derived for plasma and has thereby eliminated the infectious disease risks of this product. Factor IX concentrate is indicated for the treatment of patients with hemophilia B or factor IX deficiency. As with factor VIII, factor IX concentrates can now be produced using recombinant technology, thereby eliminating the infectious disease risk. Another product that contains factor IX is known as factor IX, or prothrombin, complex. In addition to factor IX, it contains significant quantities of activated factors II, VII, and X. Besides being used to treat patients with hemophilia B, factor IX complex has also been used to treat patients with hemophilia A who have developed antibodies or inhibitors to factor VIII. The factor IX complex contains activated coagulation factors that activate the clotting cascade distal to the entry point of factor VIII and therefore is effective in controlling bleeding. However, the activation of the coagulation cascade has, at times, been excessive, and has resulted in thrombotic complications and DIC. Because of these issues, it is rarely used and certainly is used only under the guidance of a hematologist.

In recent years, problems with AT III deficiency have gained widespread clinical interest. Excessive thromboembolic events have been recognized as a consequence of acquired or congenital AT III deficiency. AT III is also necessary for heparin to provide its clinical anticoagulation effect. AT III concentrates are available for patients with congenital deficiencies with levels ≤50% normal, with a history of previous thromboembolic events or for those who are undergoing major surgical procedures that are associated with a significant risk of thromboembolic events. AT III concentrates are also used in AT III-deficient patients who require heparin therapy, such as during cardiopulmonary bypass.

Pharmacologic Modifiers of the Coagulation Cascade

Several pharmacologic agents have be used as adjunctive therapy to modify the coagulation cascade and control excessive bleeding. These agents include desmopressin, antifibrinolytic agents (ε-aminocaproic acid, tranexamic acid), and aprotinin. While the end result of these agents is the same, their mechanisms of action and their suggested clinical applications differ. Because of the limited number of pediatric patients that present each year with clinically relevant bleeding disorders, the efficacy of many of these agents has not been tested with large, multicenter studies. Their utility is further limited by the apparent contrasting findings of some of the studies.

Desmopressin

Desmopressin is a synthetic analogue of vasopressin that was initially used in the treatment of diabetes insipidus. Desmopressin was developed by the deamination of the hemi-cysteine at position 1 of the natural hormone, which protects the molecule from peptidase degradation. A second modification, D-arginine substituted for L-arginine at position 8, decreases its vasopressor activity.[17] These alterations have resulted in a more potent and prolonged antidiuretic effect with V_2 vasopressin receptor agonism and little or no activity at the V_1 vasopressin receptor. As a result, desmopressin has no effect on the smooth musculature of the uterus, the gastrointestinal tract, or the vascular system. The half-life in vivo is approximately 55 minutes. Desmopressin promotes hemostasis by promoting the release from the vascular endothelial cells of factor VIII and vWF. Factor VIII, a glycoprotein, accelerates the activation of factor X by factor IX. Hemostatic functions of vWF include an increase of platelet adherence to the vascular subendothelium, formation of molecular bridges between platelets to increase aggregation, protection of factor VIII in plasma from proteolytic enzymes, and stimulation of factor VIII synthesis. Desmopressin is not effective in patients with severe forms of hemophilia or von Willebrand disease. Patients with severe disease have little of either factor to release in response to desmopressin. Even in the normal host, tachyphylaxis may occur in response to desmopressin, due to depletion of vWF stores or impairment of the release mechanism caused by decreased receptor sensitivity.

The recommended dose of desmopressin is 0.15 to 0.3 µg/kg administered intravenously over 15 to 20 minutes. Factor VIII and vWF levels increase to three to five times that of baseline. Administration over 20 to 30 minutes avoids systemic hypotension, since the agent can cause systemic vasodilatation. Desmopressin may also be administered subcutaneously or intranasally. Both of these routes result in plasma levels of factor VIII and vWF that are equivalent to those seen with intravenous administration.[17]

Untoward effects of desmopressin include decreased free-water clearance due to its antidiuretic hormone activity, hypotension, and thrombotic events. Hyponatremia is uncommon following a single dose and is generally seen only when excessive free water is administered perioperatively or with repeated dosing. Hypotension results from endothelial cell release of prostacyclin when desmopressin is administered rapidly. This can be avoided by slow administration (15 minutes or longer). Although anecdotal reports of arterial thrombosis have occurred, prospective studies have indicated no difference in perioperative infarction rates between patients who received desmopressin and control groups.[18,19]

Desmopressin has been used for the treatment of von Willebrand disease and hemophilia A as well as for the correction of platelet dysfunction of various etiologies including uremia, cirrhosis, and aspirin therapy. It has also been suggested as a means of decreasing blood loss in major surgical procedures (spinal fusion, surgery for congenital cardiac defects) in patients with normal platelet function. Kobrinsky and Letts[20] evaluated the efficacy of the preoperative administration of desmopressin in patients with normal hemostatic function who are undergoing spinal fusion surgery. They found that desmopressin reduced blood loss by 32.5% and reduced the need for erythrocyte transfusion by 25.6%.

Because platelet dysfunction is the major hemostatic defect encountered in uremic patients, Mannucci et al[21] evaluated the effects of desmopressin in patients with renal failure. Decreases in the bleeding time and an elevation of the concentration of vWF were noted in all patients. Desmopressin has also been found to be effective in the treatment of prolonged bleeding times associated with cirrhosis.[22] Factors that contribute to abnormal hemostasis in patients with hepatic dysfunction include decreased hepatic synthesis of prekallikrein, decreased concentration of hepatic-dependent coagulation factors, molecular abnormalities in fibrinogen, thrombocytopenia secondary to splenomegaly and shortened survival time, fibrinolysis due to impaired clearance of tissue plasminogen activator, decreased α_2-antiplasmin, and decreased plasma concentrations of vWF. Mannucci et al[22] evaluated hemostatic function in patients with cirrhosis and a bleeding time greater than 16 seconds. They observed a significant decrease in the bleeding time following desmopressin administration. Although the hemostatic derangements that occur with cirrhosis are complex, the temporary improvement in primary hemostasis may be of benefit while other coagulation defects are being corrected.

ϵ-Aminocaproic Acid/Tranexamic Acid

ϵ-Aminocaproic acid (EACA) and tranexamic acid (TA) are γ-aminocarboxylic acid analogues of lysine. They are inhibitors of fibrinolysis that exert their effect by binding to plasminogen, preventing its conversion to plasmin, and protecting fibrinogen and fibrin from degradation. Fibrinogen is synthesized in the liver and has a half-life of 3 to 5 days. It contains six polypeptide chains which are cleaved by thrombin, to form fibrin monomers. These monomers then form fibrin strands which are crosslinked by factor XIII to form the fibrin mesh for clot stabilization. Plasminogen is also synthesized in the liver and circulates in the plasma, bound to fibrinogen via lysine-binding sites. Plasminogen is activated by tissue plasminogen activator or exogenous activator molecules (streptokinase, urokinase). After plasminogen is split to form plasmin, plasmin may cleave fibrin, preventing the formation of the fibrin mesh. This fibrinolytic system is a basic defense mechanism that prevents the excess deposition of fibrin following the activation of the coagulation cascade. Plasmin can also hydrolyze fibrinogen, factor V, and factor VIII. Plasmin that is released into the circulation is inactivated by α_2-antiplasmin.

EACA and TA bind to the lysine group that binds plasminogen and plasmin to fibrinogen, displacing these molecules from the fibrinogen surface and inhibiting fibrinolysis. EACA is administered as an intravenous loading dose of 100 to 150 mg/kg followed by an infusion of 10 to 15 mg/kg/h. Ninety percent is excreted in the urine within 4 to 6 hours of administration. TA is 7 to 10 times as potent as EACA and may be used at lower doses (a loading dose of 10 mg/kg followed by an infusion of 1 mg/kg/h). Ninety percent of TA is present in the urine after approximately 24 hours. Side effects may be related to the effect on coagulation and/or the route of excretion. Since these agents are cleared by the kidneys, thrombosis of the kidneys, ureters, or lower urinary tract may occur if urologic bleeding is present. Both EACA and TA may cause nausea, vomiting, diarrhea, and hypotension with rapid intravenous administration.

The benefits of both EACA and TA have been evaluated in various clinical scenarios associated with excessive activation of the fibrinolytic pathway (cardiac surgery, liver transplantation) and disorders or surgery of tissues with high levels of tissue plasminogen activator (gastric mucosa, salivary glands, brain, prostate gland). Some of the most convincing data concerning the efficacy of EACA are in regard to patients undergoing cardiac surgical procedures. Improved hemostasis, reduced blood loss, and decreased transfusion requirements have been demonstrated in patients receiving EACA or TA prior to the institution of cardiopulmonary bypass.[23,24] EACA and TA have also shown some clinical utility when used postoperatively in the form of a mouthwash by patients with hemophilia who are undergoing dental surgery.[25]

Aprotinin

Aprotinin is a naturally occurring serine protease inhibitor that was isolated from bovine lung in 1930. It is thought to act by forming a reversible enzyme-inhibitor complex which leads to the inhibition of trypsin, plasmin, and plasma kallikrein. This is especially important in the fibrinolytic system, since both plasmin and plasma kallikrein are key components of fibrinolysis. An additional mechanism may be the preservation of platelet adhesion by protecting membrane-bound glycoprotein receptors.

Aprotinin is administered intravenously and undergoes rapid redistribution into the extracellular fluid, followed by accumulation in renal tubular epithelium with subsequent lysosomal degradation. It undergoes a biphasic elimination with initial and terminal half-lives of 40 minutes and 7 hours, respectively. A constant infusion must be administered to maintain adequate plasma concentrations in light of its rapid renal accumulation and degradation. Adverse effects include allergic reactions and renal toxicity. Anaphylactoid reactions have been reported and are more frequent in patients who have been previously exposed to aprotinin. However, even with previous exposure, the incidence of anaphylaxis is low ($<0.1\%$). Adverse effects on renal function include decreases in renal plasma flow, glomerular filtration rate, and electrolyte excretion. These effects are thought to be the result of the inhibition of intrarenal kallikrein activation and decreased prostaglandin synthesis. The kallikrein-kinin system leads to renal afferent arteriolar dilatation, thereby regulating renal responses to hemodynamic, water, and electrolyte alterations. It has also been suggested that aprotinin may actually have a protective effect on renal function by reducing excretion of enzymes that induce renal injury, thereby enhancing glomerular filtration in models of renal ischemia.

During cardiopulmonary bypass, the dosing of heparin is controlled by measuring the activated clotting time (ACT). The ACT is a bedside test that is performed in the operating room and provides an immediate estimate of heparin's effect on the coagulation cascade. Aprotinin has been shown to artificially prolong the ACT measured with celite. In vitro studies have demonstrated that the increase in the ACT may be due to the use of celite as the surface activator, and that the ACT test should be measured using kaolin as the surface activator rather than celite. Both types of ACT tubes are commercially available. If only celite ACTs are available, then it is recommended to the keep the ACT longer than 750 seconds rather than the usual 400 seconds.

As with the other modifiers of the coagulation cascade including desmopressin, TA, and EACA, the studies concerning the use of aprotinin remain contradictory and its place in the management of the bleeding patient remains controversial.[26,27] Aprotinin may have some role in those surgical procedures that are associated with activation of the fibrinolytic cascade, including cardiopulmonary bypass. Careful clinical evaluation is necessary not only to confirm its efficacy, but also to evaluate its side effect profile, which may potentially include significant thrombotic events.

Summary

The bleeding patient poses significant problems, especially when the bleeding is associated with critical illnesses. Most important in the treatment of such patients is identification and, whenever possible, control of the precipitating factor. The use of red cell transfusions should be guided by the physician's judgment of the need to increase the patient's oxygen-carrying capacity. Many patients may tolerate a hemoglobin of 7 to 8 g/dL provided there is no other underlying end-organ dysfunction. Patients with cardiovascular or respiratory compromise may benefit from significantly higher hemoglobin concentrations. The use of blood products such as platelet transfusions, FFP, and cryoprecipitate should be guided by laboratory evaluation including the platelet count, PT, PTT, and fibrinogen levels. Use of adjuncts, such as desmopressin, EACA, TA, and aprotinin, to manipulate the coagulation cascade remain relatively anecdotal, especially in the pediatric population. Desmopressin may be helpful in patients with suspected platelet dysfunction related to uremia or hepatic failure.

References

1. Schreiber GB, Busch MP, Kleinman SH, et al. The risk of transfusion-transmitted viral infections. *N Engl J Med* 1996;334:1685–1690.
2. Linden JV, Kaplan HS. Transfusion errors: Cause and effects. *Trans Med Rev* 1994;8:169–183.
3. Linden JV, Tourault MA, Schribner CL. Decrease in frequency of transfusion fatalities. *Transfusion* 1997;37:243–244.
4. Practice guidelines for blood component therapy: A report by the American Society of Anesthesiologists Task force on Blood Component Therapy. *Anesthesiology* 1996;84:732–747.
5. Manno C, Hedberg KW, Kim HC, et al. Comparison of the hemostatic effects of fresh whole blood, stored whole blood, and components after open heart surgery in children. *Blood* 1991;77:930–936.
6. McLellan B, Reid R, Lane P. Massive blood transfusion causing hypomagnesemia. *Crit Care Med* 1984;12:146–147.
7. Rivet C, Baxter A, Rock G. Potassium levels in irradiated blood. *Transfusion* 1989;29:185–186.
8. Vercellotti GM, Hammerschmidt DE. Immunological biocompatibility in blood substitutes. *Int Anesthesiol Clin* 1985;23:47–62.
9. Tremper KK, Friedman HE, Levine EM, et al. The preoperative treatment of severely anemic patients with a perfluorochemical oxygen-transport fluid, Fluosol-DA. *N Engl J Med* 1982;307:277–283.
10. Breuninger HG, Rubenstein SD, Wolfson MR, Shaffer TH. Effect of exchange transfusion with a red blood cell substitute on neonatal hemodynamics and organ blood flows. *J Pediatr Surg* 1993;28:144–150.
11. Glogar DH, Kloner RA, Muller J, et al. Fluorocarbons reduce myocardial ischemic damage after coronary occlusion. *Science* 1981;211:1439–1441.
12. Peerless SJ, Ishikawa R, Hunter IG, Peerless MJ. Protective effect of Fluosol-DA in acute cerebral ischemia. *Stroke* 1981;12:558–563.
13. Dietz NM, Joyner MJ, Warner MA. Blood substitutes: Fluids, drugs, or miracle solutions? *Anesth Analg* 1996;82:390–405.
14. Rabiner SF, Helbert JR, Lopas H, Friedman LH. Evaluation of a stroma-free hemoglobin for use as a plasma expander. *J Exp Med* 1967;126:1127–1142.
15. Looker D, Abbott-Brown D, Cozart P, et al. A human recombinant haemoglobin designed for use as a blood substitute. *Nature* 1992;356:258–260.
16. Snyder EL, Bookbinder M. Role of microaggregate blood filtration in clinical medicine. *Transfusion* 1983;23:460–470.
17. Richardson DW, Robinson AG. Desmopressin. *Ann Intern Med* 1985;103:228–239.
18. Salzman EW, Weinstein MJ, Weintraub RM, et al. Treatment with desmopressin acetate to reduce blood loss after cardiac surgery: A double blinded, randomized trial. *N Engl J Med* 1986;314:1402–1406.
19. Czer LS, Bateman TM, Gray RJ, et al. Treatment of severe platelet dysfunction and hemorrhage after cardiopulmonary bypass: Reduction in blood product usage with desmopressin. *J Am Coll Cardiol* 1987;9:1139–1147.
20. Kobrinsky NL, Letts RM. 1-Deamino-8-D-Arginine vasopressin (desmopressin) decrease operative blood loss in patients having Harrington rod spinal fusion surgery. *Ann Intern Med* 1987;107:446–450.
21. Mannucci PM, Remuzzi G, Pusineri F, et al. Deamino-8-D-Arginine vasopressin shortens the bleeding time in uremia. *N Engl J Med* 1983;308:8–12.
22. Mannucci PM, Vicente V, Vianello L, et al. Controlled trial of desmopressin in liver cir-

rhosis and other conditions associated with a prolonged bleeding time. *Blood* 1986;67: 1148–1153.
23. DelRossi AJ, Cernaianu AC, Botros S, et al. Prophylactic treatment of postperfusion bleeding using EACA. *Chest* 1989;96:27–30.
24. Horrow JC, Hlavacek J, Strong MD, et al. Prophylactic tranexamic acid decreases bleeding after cardiac operations. *J Thorac Cardiovasc Surg* 1990;99:70–74.
25. Sindet-Pedersen S, Ramstron G, Bernvil S, et al. Hemostatic effect of tranexamic acid mouthwash in anticoagulant-treated patients undergoing oral surgery. *N Engl J Med* 1989;320:840–843.
26. Bidstrup BP, Harrison J, Royston D, et al. Aprotinin therapy in cardiac operations: A report on use in 41 cardiac centers in the United Kingdom. *Ann Thorac Surg* 1993;55: 971–976.
27. van Oeveren W, Jansen NJ, Bidstrup BP, et al. Effects of aprotinin on hemostatic mechanisms during cardiopulmonary bypass. *Ann Thorac Surg* 1987;44:640–645.

Chapter 16

Acute Renal Failure and Renal Replacement Therapy

R. Blaine Easley, MD and Ted Groshong, MD

Introduction

Acute renal failure (ARF) is the disruption of normal renal function resulting in the accumulation of nitrogenous waste products with fluid/electrolyte derangements. It can occur acutely in a previously normal kidney or in the setting of prior renal insufficiency. ARF accounts for approximately 5% of hospital admissions in adults and children and up to 30% of admissions to the intensive care unit.[1,2] ARF may present as either oligoanuric or nonoliguric failure. Oliguria is defined as urine output of less than 0.5 mL/kg/h (<200 to 300 mL/m²/day) in children or less than 1.0 mL/kg/h in infants. Anuria is the absence of urine production. Oligoanuric forms account for 25% to 30% of patients with ARF. Nonoliguric ARF is characterized by a rising blood urea nitrogen (BUN) and creatinine (Cr) in the presence of continued urine output greater than 1.0 mL/kg/h or 300 mL/m²/day. This type of ARF occurs in 60% to 75% of patients. Early recognition, supportive care, and treatment of the underlying causes of ARF are crucial for prevention of associated morbidity and mortality.

Epidemiology

The annual incidence of ARF is 3.7 per 100,000 children. Of these patients, greater than 50% will require admission and treatment in the pediatric intensive care unit. The incidence of ARF among neonates and infants is slightly higher, at 19.7 per 100,000. Initial reported mortality rates were as high as 50% in both infants and children. More recently, however, Moghal et al[3] demonstrated a mortality rate of 25%. This finding may reflect improved therapeutic and supportive modalities including peritoneal dialysis (PD), hemofiltration, and hemodialysis (HD). Associated conditions and etiologic factors can influence the overall mortality rate associated with ARF. Cardiac surgery in neonates and infants is identified with the highest mortality in association with ARF at 65% to 70%. Other etiologies of ARF in children can be associated with a lower incidence of mortality: hemolytic uremic syndrome (4% to 8%), acute tubular necrosis (ATN) (14%), and glomerulonephritis (22%).[4,5]

Risk factors for ARF include prematurity (in the neonatal period), sepsis, trauma, burns, congestive heart failure, surgery, anesthesia, various medications, hepatic failure, preexisting renal disease, and shock (all forms).[6] In neonates, ARF can occur secondary to perinatal events such as sepsis, hypoxia/asphyxia, and urinary tract anomalies. Outside of the neonatal period, 50% of cases are caused by two diseases: acute glomerulonephritis and hemolytic-uremic syndrome (HUS).[3,7]

From: Tobias JD (ed): *Pediatric Critical Care: The Essentials.* ©Futura Publishing Co., Inc., Armonk, NY, 1999.

If no preexisting renal disorder exists and ARF is treated aggressively, oligoanuric ARF will result in recovery of adequate renal function in the majority of patients. Nonoliguric ARF appears to have an even better prognosis for full recovery of renal function.[7,8] In the aforementioned study by Moghal et al,[3] only 11 of 227 patients studied progressed to chronic renal failure.

Pathophysiology and Common Causes

Renal function is dependent on four individual components: 1) renal vascular physiology; 2) nephron/renal tubular function; 3) filtrate collection/outflow; and 4) neural/humoral elements. Each kidney filters the blood through approximately 1 million nephrons. The filtration is controlled by interactions between renal blood flow (RBF) to the kidney and renal tubular function. The kidneys receive 20% to 25% of cardiac output. Blood enters the kidneys via the renal arteries. These larger vessels subdivide into progressively smaller vessels: interlobar to interlobular to afferent arterioles. Afferent arterioles bring blood into the glomerulus of the nephron, where glomerular filtration takes place. Efferent arterioles carry blood away from the glomerulus to the tubular capillaries. These vessels run adjacent to the renal tubules and descend into the renal medulla, creating the countercurrent capillary system which facilitates solute and water regulation. Ultimately blood enters progressively larger venous vessels and exits the kidneys via the renal veins.

Solute and water filtration from the blood into the renal tubule is called the glomerular filtration rate (GFR). GFR is controlled primarily by hydrostatic and oncotic pressures. Other contributing factors to filtration are the relative size and charge of the particles in the plasma, as the glomerular basement membrane possesses a strong negative charge. Normal adult GFR is approximately 120 mL/min in males and somewhat lower in females; it declines with age. In infants and children, GFR ranges from 40 to 130 mL/min/1.73 m². The lower range represents the normal GFR in neonates and infants; GFR increases to the higher range of normal adult values by 6 to 9 months of age. Hydrostatic pressure in the afferent arteriole is relatively higher than inside the renal tubule, and thus provides a driving force for the filtration of fluid and electrolytes into the tubule. Oncotic pressure also contributes to the filtration of plasma. It is determined by the size and number of unfiltered proteins (mainly albumin) that keeps fluid in the vascular space. As more fluid leaves the plasma and blood moves into the efferent arterioles, filtration slows as the oncotic pressure rises. This increased oncotic pressure facilitates resorption in the countercurrent capillary system (vasa recta).

The structure of the nephron or renal tubule includes the renal cortex, which contains Bowman's capsule and the proximal tubule, and the loop of Henle, which descends into the renal medulla and then ascends back to the renal cortex to become the distal tubule. Finally, multiple distal tubules coalesce into a common collecting duct. The sodium, chloride, glucose, amino acids and H_2O are reabsorbed in the proximal tubule through active, passive, and facilitated transport mechanisms. Then as the filtrate continues in the loop of Henle down into the renal medulla, countercurrent mechanisms between the capillary plexus and renal tubule allow for an equilibration of the solute. Potassium and waste products (such as urea) are excreted into the renal tubule and maintain the osmotic gradient in the loop of Henle and distal tubule. As the filtrate moves into the distal and convoluted tubule, regulatory mechanisms either increase H_2O resorption into the vasculature from the renal tubule (vasopressin) or decrease sodium, urea, and H_2O loss into the urine (aldosterone).

As mentioned earlier, ARF can be classified on the clinical basis of urine output, as oligoanuric ARF and nonoliguric ARF. These clinical descriptions have limited utility, as they give no indication of the underlying pathophysiology causing the renal failure. In addition, treatment modalities can cause oliguric failure to "convert" to nonoliguric failure without changing the underlying etiology of the ARF. For these reasons, it has become customary to catagorize ARF on the pathophysiologic basis of "where the lesion occurs." This method allows for the structuring of the differential diagnosis as well as treatment plans. Three categories are used: 1) prerenal ARF; 2) renal ARF (intrinsic or parenchymal); and 3) postrenal ARF (obstructive) (see Fig. 1 and Table 1).

Prerenal ARF represents a common and potentially correctable form of ARF (~50% to 60%). Prerenal ARF, or prerenal azotemia, results from hypoperfusion of the kidneys. If diagnosed and treated, this state is easily reversible by correcting volume deficits and/or improving cardiac output. Alterations in RBF result in autoregulatory mechanisms that compensate in an effort to maintain GFR. In the setting of volume depletion, vasodilatation of the afferent arteriole and vasoconstriction of the efferent arteriole occur to maintain glomerular perfusion and GFR. The intact humoral response of the kidney is to increase renin production which leads to increased angiotensin II and aldosterone production. Al-

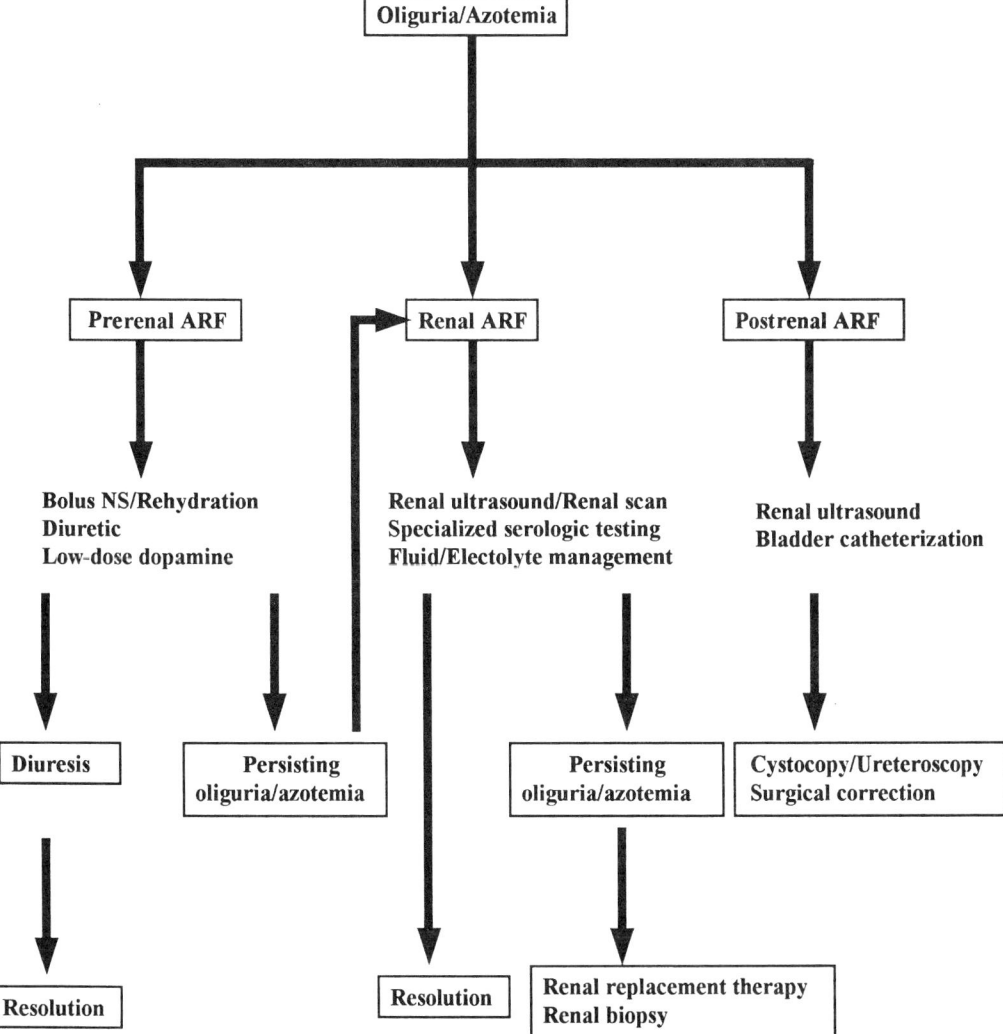

Figure 1. Outline of diagnostic approach to the patient with increasing blood urea nitrogen, creatinine, and oligoanuria.

Table 1

Common Etiologies of Acute Renal Failure in Children

Prerenal	Renal (Intrinsic)	Postrenal (Obstructive)
dehydration	acute tubular necrosis	congenital anomaly
hemorrhage	glomerulonephritis	papillary necrosis
shock	drugs	bladder dysfunction
burn	renal vein/artery thrombosis	intra-abdominal mass
cardiac failure	hemolytic uremic syndrome	retroperitoneal mass/fibrosis
surgery	vasculitis	
hepatorenal syndrome	pyleonephritis	

dosterone acts directly on the distal renal tubular to increase resorption of solutes, specifically sodium and urea. The posterior pituitary responds to the hypovolemia and increased serum osmolality by secreting vasopressin (antidiuretic hormone [ADH]). Vasopressin acts on the renal tubule, but increases water reabsorption from the collecting tubule. These two feedback mechanisms result in a more efficient resorption of sodium and water from the functional renal tubule. By these mechanisms, the kidneys attempt to increase intravascular volume. These compensatory mechanisms act to restore renal perfusion and maintain renal function. However, the failure to recognize and treat the problem may result in renal parenchymal injury from prolonged hypoperfusion.

Because of these appropriate response mechanisms to hypovolemia and the presence of an intact/functional renal tubule, the resultant laboratory findings of increased urine specific gravity, increased urine osmolality, decreased fractional excretion of sodium (FE_{Na}) of less than 1, and a renal failure index (RFI) of less than 1 are suggestive of prerenal ARF (Tables 2 and 3). The BUN/Cr ratio may be useful for making the diagnosis, as Cr is not reabsorbed but urea is actively reabsorbed by the renal tubules, resulting in azotemia and a high BUN/Cr ratio (>20). Restoration of the intravascular volume usually results in improved perfusion and enhanced GFR with a correction of the ARF, as discussed later in this chapter.

Many cases of ARF (∼40% to 60%) involve damage or injury to the renal tissues that leads to impaired renal function. These tissues can be vascular, glomerular, tubular, or interstitial. Incorrectly, many clinicians refer to intrinsic renal failure as ATN. However, ATN is a histopathologic diagnosis denoting renal tubular damage independent of renal vasculature or interstitial or glomerular dysfunction. ATN accounts for the majority of ARF cases in adults. In infants and children, it is less common and usually results from nephrotoxic agents or renal ischemia. Because of the increased metabolic demands of the renal tubule, it is especially susceptible to ischemic injury from hypoperfusion. Thus, prolonged prerenal ARF is a risk factor and can result in parenchymal injury and renal ARF (with or without true ATN). Many common causes of ARF in pediatric patients affect the renal vasculature, either through vasculitis and/or vaso-occlusive disease. In infants/neonates, renal vein thrombosis or renal artery thrombosis can present with anuria, hypertension, azotemia, and bilateral flank masses. Damage to the renal vasculature is also seen in HUS (see below). Alterations in the glomerular basement membrane from various disease processes can also result in ARF. Systemic lupus erythematosa, Alport's disease, IgA nephropathy, and post-streptococcal glomerulonephritis commonly cause glomerular injury and ARF.

In the preceding situations, the parenchyma of the kidney is damaged and normal regulatory mechanisms become impaired. Each of the aforementioned insults can disrupt normal renal feedback mechanisms. For example, vasculitis causes a decrease in GFR because of narrowing of the afferent and efferent arterioles and impaired arteriolar responsiveness to angiotensin II. Other disease processes may

Table 2

Laboratory Findings in Patients with Oliguria

Test	Prerenal	Renal	ADH Excess
Calculations			
FE_{Na}	<1 (<2.5)	>1 (>3.0)	~1
RFI	<1 (<3.0)	>1 (>3.0)	>1
plasma BUN/Cr ratio	>20	<10–15	>15
Urine laboratory tests			
sodium (mEq/L)	<10–20 (<40)	>20–40 (>40)	>40
specific gravity	>1.020 (>1.015)	<1.010 (<1.015)	>1.020
osmolality (mOsm/L)	>500 (>400)	<350 (<400)	>500
Urine/plasma ratios			
osmolality	>1.3	<1.3	>2
creatinine	>40 (>20)	<20 (<15)	>30
Urinalysis	hyaline casts	brownish red color, white cell casts, red cell casts, granular casts, eosinophils	nonspecific

Infant values are indicated between parentheses (.....). ADH = antidiuretic hormone; FE_{Na} = fractional excretion of sodium (see Table 3); RFI = renal failure index (see Table 3); BUN = blood urea nitrogen; Cr = creatinine.

directly damage the glomerular basement membrane and lessen the efficiency of the filtration of solute and proteins. In the setting of ATN, the renal tubule becomes "shocked," and active and passive transport mechanisms dependent on the renal tubular epithelium are lost or impaired, as is the renal tubular ability to respond to vasopressin and aldosterone. The singular or additive result of these processes is ineffective filtration and reabsorption of solutes and water. This results in an increased FE_{Na}, decreased urine osmolality, decreased Cr clearance (C_{Cr}), and increased RFI (Tables 2 and 3). In addition, urea is not reabsorbed as efficiently as it is in prerenal azotemia and this results in a lower BUN/Cr ratio (<10). The urinalysis usually shows an active sediment; this can assist the clinician in the diagnosis of a renal parenchymal etiology of ARF. Renal tubular epithelial cells are consistent with ATN. White blood cell casts

Table 3

Equations Used to Evaluate Renal Function

Fractional excretion of sodium (FE_{Na}) = $U_{Na}/P_{Na} \times P_{Cr}/U_{Cr} \times 100$

Renal failure index (RFI) = $(U_{Na} \times 100)/U_{Cr}P_{Cr}$

Creatinine clearance (C_{cr})/GFR = $k \times ht (cm)/P_{Cr}$

Serum osmolality (osm) = $2(Na^+) + BUN/2.8 + glucose/18$

k = 0.33 in low birth weight infants;
    0.45 in term infants;
    0.55 in toddlers, children, and adolescent girls;
    0.70 in adolescent boys.

FE_{Na} = fractional excretion of sodium; U_{Na} = measured urine sodium; P_{Na} = measured plasma sodium; GFR = glomerular filtration rate.

and/or red blood cell casts are more indicative of pyelonephritis/glomerulonephritis.

Obstructive ARF most commonly occurs in the newborn period secondary to congenital malformations of the urinary tract and kidneys (~5% to 10% of ARF). Outside the newborn period, obstructive lesions become more complicated and involve nephrolithiasis, tumors, bladder dysfunction, foreign bodies, etc. In situations where renal ARF is diagnosed and no obvious cause is found, some degree of long-term urinary tract obstruction and resultant intrinsic/parenchymal damage should be suspected. Ultrasound is essential in the diagnostic evaluation of ARF and can help identify many causes of urinary tract obstruction. The physical examination may reveal flank masses (unilateral or bilateral) or a distended bladder. In critically ill patients, something as simple as an obstructed urinary catheter could be the culprit. A urology consult may be necessary to help with the evaluation and/or to assist in relieving the obstruction. Urinary indices and calculations of renal function are usually nonspecific, but may "appear" more like renal ARF, especially in the presence of prolonged obstruction that has resulted in parenchymal damage.

Special Considerations/Etiologies in Children with Acute Renal Failure

Hepatorenal syndrome is a relatively rare condition in children, in which liver failure or dysfunction is followed by renal failure. It represents a form of prerenal ARF. Clinically, patients will have ascites, edema, jaundice, and other findings consistent with liver disease. Prior to the onset of renal failure, a precipitating event can usually be identified such as a gastrointestinal hemorrhage, overly aggressive diuresis, or sepsis. The "event" usually causes hypovolemia or poor renal perfusion. What follows is not clearly understood and remains controversial, but it is believed that there is a disproportionate amount of renal afferent and efferent arteriolar vasoconstriction. This creates a fall in GFR with preserved resorptive capacity of the renal tubule and other intact regulatory mechanisms. This results in a low urine sodium and increased urine specific gravity. Laboratory evaluation will often indicate a prerenal picture with an FE_{Na} less than 1 and a BUN/Cr greater than 20. Treatment is challenging because of the associated low serum oncotic pressure and loss of intravascular fluid to third spacing; the latter occurs in patients with hepatic dysfunction related to hypoalbuminemia. Patients who develop ARF in the setting of liver failure are resistant to treatment; in this group there is a high incidence of morbidity and a mortality that approaches 100%.[9]

HUS is the most common cause of intrinsic ARF in children older than 1 year. The history often includes a prior diarrheal illness (often bloody) with subsequent decreased urination and pallor. The usual etiology is a toxin (verotoxin) produced by certain bacterial organisms including *Shigella spp.*, *Salmonella spp.*, and *E. coli* O157:H7. Laboratory testing demonstrates the classic triad of thrombocytopenia, microangiopathic hemolytic anemia, and azotemia. Urinary indices are usually of little help. The incidence is 1 per 100,000 children with a distribution of typical (90%) and atypical (10%) occurrence.[10] Atypical HUS refers to onset of disease without the diarrheal prodrome and is usually sporadic. It is often associated with *Streptococcus pneumonia*. A peak incidence of typical HUS occurs between June and September, with males and females affected equally. The majority of etiologies are infectious. Other possible etiologic factors of HUS include hereditary forms, medication-induced, and viral.[11,12]

A large epidemic of HUS occurred in North America in 1992 and 1993 due to poorly cooked hamburger, contaminated with *E. coli* O157:H7. Mortality in that outbreak was 8%. Other studies have found the mortality to be 3% to 5% with an associated morbidity of 5% to 10%. Morbidity in most reports is based on cases that advanced to chronic renal failure. As noted by other authors, the overall morbidity may be up to 50% when other organ systems are included (neurologic, cardiac, pancreatic insufficiency, and renal impairment).[3,8,13] The pathophysiology is unknown, but the combined findings of hemolytic anemia, azotemia, and thrombocytopenia are thought to be related to a disseminated-intravascular-coagulation like phenomenon with the formation of microthrombi preferentially in the renal vasculature. In atypical HUS, Thomsen-Friedenreich antigen (T-antigen) is thought to facilitate immune-derived endothelial, glomerular, red cell, and platelet damage. Some authors recommend special precautions be taken to ensure that blood products administered to these patients do not contain anti–T-antigen antibody.[14,15]

Complications seen in HUS include central nervous system infarction, mesenteric artery thrombosis, myocardial infarction, hypertension, and chronic renal failure. Supportive care is the only treatment and includes careful monitoring of fluid and electrolyte status during the ARF. Fifty to sixty percent of children will require dialysis (either PD or HD). Experimental treatments involving toxin removal from the blood (plasmapheresis) and antitoxin strategies are being evaluated, but their utility in treating HUS has not been determined.

Myoglobinuria and/or hemoglobinuria can also result in intrinsic ARF. Both require aggressive hydration and alkaline diuresis to avoid their collection in and blockade of renal tubules. The history and physical examination may often give clues to the cause. Invariably, most patients report reddish/pink urine, and there is a strongly positive bedside dipstick urine test for blood and a negligible microscopic exam of the urine for red blood cells. Urine output is diminished. The history usually identifies a risk factor such as a recent blood transfusion, burns, crush injuries, trauma, rhabdomyolysis from an episode of malignant hyperthermia, or prolonged strenuous exercise. Laboratory findings are useful for discriminating between the two conditions. Microscopic examination of the blood for ongoing hemolytic processes should be performed. In the setting of myoglobinuria, serum aldolase and creatine phosphokinase will be elevated. Serum lactate dehydrogenase and free hemoglobin levels will be elevated in the setting of hemoglobinuria. Both require the same treatment with aggressive hydration and alkaline diuresis. Alkalinization of the urine raises the solubility constants of hemoglobin and myoglobin, thereby increasing the concentration that must be reached before they precipitate from solution. This can be accomplished with fluid boluses and infusions of normal saline along with diuretics (either furosemide or mannitol) to maintain a urine output of 2 to 3 mL/kg/h. Aggressive hydration followed by diuresis increases renal tubular filtrate flow and washes out obstruction caused by precipitated globin pigments.[16] Alkalinization with intravenous sodium bicarbonate or carbonic anhydrase inhibitors to achieve a urine pH of ≥7 has been recommended in the past, but its efficacy has recently been questioned.

Renal transplantation presents a group of unique concerns and problems in diagnosis and management when anuria/oliguria occurs. Risk factors in affected patients include use of immunosuppressive agents and nephrotoxic medications and unstable fluid balance. Complications encountered following renal transplantation include graft thrombosis, acute rejection, and serious infections.[17] Many children will require ongoing dialysis for fluid regulation and control of hyperkalemia until their graft is functioning sufficiently. All will require lifelong immunosuppressive therapy. In the initial postoperative period, children are at greatest risk for thrombosis of the graft. The national incidence for graft thrombosis in children is approximately 3% of renal transplants.[18] However, some centers report renal graft thrombosis rates that are much higher. Physical findings that suggest this complication are graft tenderness/swelling, anuria, and sometimes fever. The clinician must also watch for other possible complications including acute rejection, infection, or leak of the ureterovesicular anastomoses. Prompt imaging by ultrasound and renal radionucleotide scans can assess graft perfusion and assist in differentiating between thrombosis versus acute rejection. Early intervention is warranted if the graft is to be salvaged.

Acute rejection following induction therapy occurs in a majority (approximately

50%) of children undergoing renal transplantation.[19] Presenting features are fever, anuria/oliguria, and worsening signs of renal azotemia. Possible infection and/or graft thrombosis must be ruled out. Ultrasound and/or diethylenetriaminepentaacetic acid (DPTA) renal scans usually are nonspecific, but are useful in eliminating other causes. Renal biopsy of the graft provides a definitive diagnosis. Treatment often involves increased immunosupressive therapy combined with careful monitoring and supportive care until the episode resolves. Some patients will require temporary dialysis, while a subgroup will progress to chronic rejection and loss of the graft.[19–21]

Infections pose a special problem in all immunosupressed patients. However, renal transplant patients are at risk for urinary tract infections, in part due to an impaired immune system. Infectious complications include cytomegalovirus (70% of renal transplant patients become infected, either from the graft or from contaminated blood products), *Pneumocystis carinii*, *Candida* spp., and *Leptospira*. A complete evaluation including cultures, blood counts, and appropriate antibiotic coverage should be performed in transplant patients presenting with fever or other signs of a systemic illness.

Evaluation and Diagnosis of Acute Renal Failure

The diagnosis of ARF and its possible causes can usually be made by the history, physical examination, urinalysis, and minimal laboratory testing. The history is usually significant for decreased urine output or a precipitating event that started the child's current illness. The patient's fluid intake (type and amount), fluid losses/voiding patterns, and parental perception of weight loss or weight gain should be addressed. For example, the history of excessive vomiting, poor fluid intake, and weight loss suggests that dehydration is the cause of the child's rising BUN and poor urine output (prerenal ARF), while a combination of diarrhea, abdominal pain, and weight gain suggests that the rising BUN and poor urine output may involve renal impairment, as in HUS (renal ARF). During the interview, historical clues such as joint pain, headaches, rashes, and recent infections can be suggestive of systemic illnesses such as postinfectious glomerulonephritis, Henoch-Schonlein purpura, or other autoimmune process involving the renal parenchyma. Mental status changes can allude to metabolic problems, such as worsening uremia, or to accumulation of medications that are normally cleared by the kidney. Additionally, the history should always include medications, which may be a nephrotoxic source of ARF (antibiotics, diuretics, radiographic contrast, or recent chemotherapy). Finally, other circumstances such as surgery or trauma may point to the etiology of ARF.

The physical examination of the child, like the history, should assess for hydration status and signs of systemic illness. A dehydrated child may have findings of tenting skin, thready pulses, tachycardia, sunken eyes/fontanelle, mental status changes/irritability, and altered blood pressure. Alternatively, a child with renal ARF may present with signs of fluid excess such as hypertension, pink or red urine, and peripheral edema. Identification of joint involvement, skin changes, eye ground changes, fever patterns, and lymph node enlargement can aid in documenting systemic disease and can help in establishing the etiology of the ARF. Abdominal exam should include palpation of the kidneys and bladder. If the kidneys or bladder are readily palpable, urine outflow tract obstruction, either intrinsic (stone/clot) or extrinsic (neoplasm), must be suspected, and the diagnosis of postrenal ARF entertained.

Serum tests for urea and Cr, as well as sodium, potassium, bicarbonate, calcium, phosphate, and albumin, should be obtained at the time of initial assessment, along with a urinalysis and urine concentrations for sodium and Cr. Often, a rising BUN and Cr are the first indications of renal insufficiency, as up to 80% of children with ARF have the nonoliguric type. BUN rises approximately 10 to 20 mg/dL per day and Cr rises approximately 0.5 mg/dL per day in the setting of complete renal function loss. The BUN/Cr ratio and other calculations can be useful in determining the etiology of oliguria (Tables 2 and 3).

Additional calculations can assist in discriminating between prerenal and renal ARF. The FE_{Na} and RFI are used to determine the location of failure and to assess renal tubular function (see Tables 2 and 3). When clinical assessment and prior laboratory tests are inconclusive, additional tests such as calculated C_{Cr} can be useful for determining the source of the ARF.

Other laboratory tests are rarely needed to diagnose prerenal ARF. However, many of the causes of renal ARF have systemic symptoms, and other diagnostic tests may be needed. Serologic tests (eg, complement levels, erythrocyte sedimentation rate, antinuclear antibodies, or streptozyme) or cultures (eg, throat, stool, and urine) may be needed, depending on the specific clinical situation. If urine is being produced, a urinalysis can be obtained to search for hemoglobin, myoglobin, specific gravity, and pH. Microscopic evaluation includes searching for red cell casts, white cell casts, red blood cells, and crystals.

Finally, many clinicians obtain a renal ultrasound early in the management of ARF to rule out obstruction and structural abnormalities, and to evaluate the renal vasculature/blood flow by Doppler. Additional radiographic studies are rarely useful in the initial assessment and management of ARF. Contrast studies such as intravenous pyelography are relatively contraindicated in the setting of ARF because of the nephrotoxic nature of radiocontrast materials. Other imaging studies, such as dimercaptosuccinic acid (DMSA) or technetium 99m DPTA scans, can provide useful information on renal perfusion and renal tubular function following renal transplantation or in the setting of prolonged ARF.

Management and Treatment of Acute Renal Failure

Fluid management, nutritional support, and renal replacement therapy, when needed, are the keys to successful management of ARF. As a rule, early consultation with a pediatric nephrologist (and a urologist if necessary) can aid in more efficient and expeditious diagnosis and management of the condition. Daily physical assessment includes monitoring for evidence of worsening renal failure and for clues to underlying etiology, if unknown. Twice-daily weight measurements are essential, with additional weight measurements before and after dialysis therapy to assess fluid retention. Serum electrolytes are needed daily, and sometimes as frequent as every hour (eg, hyperkalemia). Blood pressure should be monitored frequently (every 4 hours).

Fluid and electrolyte management is an integral issue affecting all patients with ARF. Even if preliminary laboratory tests suggest "normal" values, ARF does not allow for adequate metabolic and electrolyte homeostasis. The most commonly seen abnormalities are hyperkalemia, hyponatremia, hypocalcemia, and hyperphosphatemia.

Potassium abnormalities are common in the setting of ARF and can be fatal. Hyperkalemia occurs in ARF because 90% of potassium elimination is via the kidney. In addition, metabolic acidosis causes an extracellular shift of potassium that contributes to the rise in serum potassium. It is extracellular potassium that is responsible for the clinical manifestations, including cardiac arrhythmias. If a rapid determination of serum potassium is unavailable, then a 12-lead electrocardiogram and ongoing cardiac monitoring may provide an assessment of the extracellular potassium concentration and its cardiac effects. Many authors recommend 24-hour cardiac monitoring in patients with ARF. If life-threatening hyperkalemia (>6.5 mEq/L) becomes a problem, acute hemodialysis is the therapy of choice. While arrangements are made for hemodialysis, temporizing measures should begin with removal of all potassium from intravenous fluids. While this may seem overly simplistic, exogenous sources of potassium administration are frequently overlooked in the patients with worsening hyperkalemia. Potassium replacement therapy is rarely, if ever, indicated in patients with ARF. Another measure to lower serum potassium concentrations is alkalinization to promote the intracellular movement of potassium. This may include the administration of sodium bicarbonate or airway control with modest hyperventilation in critically ill patients. Additional treatment options to reduce non–life-threatening hyperkalemia include oral/rectal polystyrene sulfonate sodium (Kayexalate), the administration of glucose and insulin, and attempts to increase urinary excretion in nonoliguric/anuric patients with loop diuretics/mannitol (see chapter 13). All of these therapies have their limitations and may cause significant adverse effects which include sodium and fluid overload with the administration of Kayexalate, as it is an exchange resin that exchanges potassium for sodium; hypernatremia and fluid retention with the administration of sodium bicarbonate; and hypoglycemia with insulin administration.

Another therapy for hyperkalemia is administration of low-dose adrenergic agonists including epinephrine or isoproterenol. These agents activate cell-surface adrenergic receptors and increase the extracellular-to-intracellular movement of potassium. While this type of therapy has been shown to lower serum potassium levels, significant adverse effects may occur. Electrocardiographic changes indicative of hyperkalemia are treated with intravenous calcium chloride or gluconate. Calcium salts do not alter the serum potassium concentration, but counteract potassium's effect on the myocardial membrane. While the above mentioned therapies serve to temporize and lower the serum potassium concentration, the only therapeutic modality is renal replacement therapy such as peritoneal or hemodialysis (Table 4).

Sodium abnormalities are also common. Most abnormalities are related to intravascular fluid volume. Hyponatremia is commonly seen and, in the setting of ARF and oliguria, is usually indicative of fluid overload. If hyponatremia is severe (<120 mEq/L or seizures), emergent hemodialysis is indicated. Other interventions for hyponatremia (primarily sodium administration) in the presence of fluid overload should be undertaken with the utmost caution, as they may precipitate congestive heart failure. Hypernatremia rarely occurs and, again, is probably best managed with dialysis.

Finally, calcium and phosphate abnormalities are commonly encountered in the setting of ARF. The typical derangement is hypocalcemia and hyperphosphatemia. The elevation of serum phosphate is caused by decreased excretion by the impaired kidney and increased production via catabolic processes of body tissues. In addition, calcium is lowered because of decreased absorption from the gut. Because of their inter-relationship, treatment of the two conditions becomes complex. If hypocalcemia results in seizures or tetany, acute hemodialysis may be indicated. Otherwise, treatment of hypocalcemia should comprise lowering the serum phosphate by decreasing phosphate intake and administering oral phosphate-binding agents such as calcium carbonate or calcium lactate. The overzealous correction of a metabolic acidosis can cause an abrupt drop in ionized calcium concentrations and can precipitate tetany or seizures.

Fluid management should focus on maintenance of a good fluid balance in the setting of diminished or absent urine output. Meticulous fluid regulation is the hallmark of therapy in ARF. In early ARF, if signs of hypovolemia are apparent, a bolus of isotonic crystalloid should be given (20 mL/kg/bolus) to replete the intravascular space and to restore adequate renal perfusion. Once the hypovolemia is corrected, or if the patient has fluid excess and renal impairment persists, additional fluid therapy must be limited to replacing insensible losses. Recommendations for replacement of insensible losses include 25% of standard maintenance fluids (300 to 400 mL/m^2/day or 25 to 50 mL/kg). It should include free water with limited added electrolytes. In addition to insensible losses, fluid replacement should return to the intravascular space the measured losses of the previous 24 hours, which may include urine output, nasogastric drainage, excessive stool losses, and third-space losses. It is also necessary to take into account the composition of the fluids lost (eg, urine, gastric secretions, diarrhea) when deciding on the fluid to be used for replacement therapy. The latter may include isotonic fluids for third-space losses and more hypotonic fluids for urinary and gastrointestinal losses. Analysis of urine

Table 4

Treatment Strategies for Hyperkalemia

1. Stop exogenous sources of potassium administration and potassium-sparing diuretics.
2. Renal replacement therapies:
    hemodialysis
    peritoneal dialysis
    hemofiltration
3. Alkalinization:
    administration of sodium bicarbonate
    hyperventilation
4. Glucose + insulin
5. Kayexalate
6. Low-dose adrenergic agonist
7. Loop diuretics/mannitol
8. Calcium for ECG changes

and other bodily fluid output can be used to determine the appropriate fluid for replacement therapy. It is also important to provide nutritional support in a hypercatabolic state (see below). Commonly encountered problems are fluid excess leading to hypertension and congestive heart failure, which would precipitate the need for dialysis.

Diuretic therapy in the setting of ARF is based on two principles: 1) the conversion of oliguric ARF to nonoliguric ARF results in a better prognosis, and 2) diagnostically, the response to diuretic therapy implies an intact renal tubule and glomerulus, supporting a prerenal etiology for the ARF. Furosemide is the most commonly used diuretic in the setting of prerenal ARF or in fluid overload in renal ARF. The loop diuretics (such as furosemide and bumetanide) are thought to act as vasodilators of the renal and systemic vasculature, in addition to their naturetic effects on the ascending loop of Henle. Increased GFR combined with increased sodium and H_2O excretion increases renal tubular filtrate flow and urine output. Because of these effects, some authors prefer continuous furosemide infusion (3 to 5 mg/kg/day), rather than intermittent boluses (1 to 2 mg/kg/dose).[22,23] Loop diuretics may be used in conjunction with mannitol. The combination of mannitol and furosemide has been shown to shorten the oliguric phase of ARF in some patients and promote conversion to nonoliguric failure, theoretically improving prognosis.[24]

The benefits of mannitol are distinct from those of the loop diuretics. Many clinicians use a "mannitol test" dose (0.5 g/kg) in prerenal ARF and observe for increased urine output. A response of increased urine output following: 1) a bolus of fluid, and 2) the "test" mannitol dose is thought to be suggestive of prerenal ARF. Some researchers feel that mannitol diminishes ischemic tubular damage in renal and prerenal ARF by acting as an oxygen free radical scavenger, vasodilating the vasculature of the postischemic kidney, diminishing proximal tubular swelling, and, like other diuretics, increasing filtrate flow in the renal tubule.[24] However, caution should be given to the increases in serum osmolality that can result from repetitive dosing of mannitol, as well as to problems with fluid shifts. Some evidence indicates that mannitol administration may lead to congestive heart failure in fluid overloaded patients with ARF.

Low-dose dopamine (1 to 3 µg/kg/min) may be beneficial the treatment of ARF, by promoting vasodilatation and improving RBF, GFR, and urine output.[25] The direct diuretic effect of dopamine occurs due to increased sodium excretion into the loop of Henle. This probably facilitates diuresis, independent of the vasodilatation and increased GFR. There is some controversy over the benefit of low-dose dopamine either alone or in combination with diuretic therapy, as neither has demonstrated a clear benefit. Of concern are the vasoconstrictive effects of dopamine at higher doses.

Other pharmacotherapies are directed

at improving renal recovery following toxic or ischemic injury. These experimental therapies mostly apply in the setting of renal ARF from ischemia, and only limited information is available regarding the use of these methods in children. Vasoactive agents such as theophylline, atrial-naturetic peptide, and antiendothelin antibodies are thought to increase RBF and reduce ischemia.[26-28] After early experience in adults with these agents, their use has not gained acceptance for routine management.

Nutritional management of the patient during ARF focuses on providing maintenance metabolic needs to avoid catabolizing the body's stores of fat and protein. Routine nutrition can be calculated per the Holliday-Segar method or body surface area method (see chapter 14). If a child is able to eat, his or her caloric needs may be provided orally, with a focus on fluid and electrolyte restriction. In this situation, orders must be written that specify a daily fluid limit and a diet that is low phosphate, low sodium, and without potassium. As a rule, infants, children, and adolescents should not be protein restricted. Exceptions do exist. But unlike adults, who are routinely protein restricted, the pediatric population in ARF often has increased metabolic needs that mandate adequate nutrition and even additional protein supplementation if dietary sources are insufficient. Protein at 2 g/100 kcal/day is needed to give the 8% of total daily calories required, without causing a nitrogen imbalance.

If the patient is unable to tolerate enteral nutrition, parenteral nutrition should be instituted early in the management of an ARF patient. Dextrose solution (minimum of 10%), lipid preparations, and amino acid solutions can also be used as a supplement for daily nutritional needs.

Renal Replacement Therapy

Renal replacement therapy is essential in the management of children with ARF when conservative methods fail. Over the last 10 years, several modalities have become available for children. Traditional methods of PD and HD are the mainstay of therapy, and their availability is essential for the adequate management of ARF. Newer treatments such as hemofiltration, with and without dialysis, have received increased usage in children with fewer complications.[29] The indications for renal replacement therapy are listed in Table 5. Common toxic compounds that can be removed from the body by hemodialysis, hemofiltration, and/or hemoperfusion (HP) methods are listed in Table 6.

HD offers the distinct advantage of rapid correction of metabolic and fluid deficits. The indications for HD are the same as for any replacement therapy (Table 5). Acute poisonings, and life-threatening electrolyte abnormalities with an anticipated short-term need for dialysis are reasons to consider HD. In HD, clearance depends on the permeability and surface area of the dialyzer membrane and the flow rates of blood and dialysate fluid. Filtration is limited to particles whose molecular weight (MW) is less than 500 d. The exact mechanisms for removal are diffusion and convection. A contraindication to HD has historically been insufficient vascular access; however, modern catheters and techniques exist that permit dialysis to be performed through a single-lumen, 7F-diameter catheter. The preferred locations for catheter insertion are the right internal jugular, left subclavian, and femoral veins. Complications of HD include hypotension, bleeding, muscle cramps, embolism, disequilibrium syndrome, catheter infections, and complement activation. Hypotension occurs from the rapid removal of fluid (ultrafiltrate) and resultant intravascular deficit which may necessitate slowing the dialysis rate. Disequilibrium syndrome is thought to occur from osmotic shifts. By definition, this syndrome comprises a "mixture" of symptoms including, nausea, vomiting, headache, and hypertension brought on by aggressive solute clearance. Children are more predisposed to this phenomenon than adults. Risk factors are patient size and the relative severity of uremia. This phenomenon can be prevented or limited by reducing HD blood flow to 5 to 7 mL/kg/min, and slowing solute removal.

PD can be used in patients of all ages, from infants to adults. This is a popular

Table 5

Indications for Renal Replacement Therapy

1. Dialyzable toxin or poison
2. BUN >150 mg/dL; Creatinine >8 mg/dL
3. Metabolic acidosis: pH <7.2 or serum HCO_3 <10 mEq/L
4. Hyperkalemia: >6.5 mEq/L or electrocardiographic changes
5. Volume overload with evidence of pulmonary edema, hypertension, hyponatremia
6. Calcium and phosphorus imbalance
7. Neurologic symptoms secondary to uremia, hyperammonemia, or electrolyte imbalance

BUN = blood urea nitrogen.

Table 6

Common Toxins and Their Removal with Renal Replacement Therapies

Drug/Toxin	Modality
Analgesics	
acetaminophen	HD; HP
salicylate	HD
Anticonvulsants	
carbamazepine	HP
barbiturates	HD; HP
phenytoin	HP
Antidepressants	
amphetamine	HD; HP
amitriptyline	HP
imipramine	HP
Alcohols	
ethanol	HD
ethylene glycol	HD
methanol	HD
Sedatives and hypnotics	
glutethimide	HP
methaqualone	HP
ethchlorvynol	HP
methyprylon	HP
chloral hydrate	HP; HD
Miscellaneous	
atenolol	HD; HP
digoxin	HP
diphenhydramine	HP; HD
lithium	HD
mushroom toxins	HP; HD
paraquat	HD; HP
theophylline	HP; HD

The preferred or more efficient method of removal is listed first.
HD = hemodialysis; HP = charcoal hemoperfusion.

means of dialyzing patients, especially children. The indications for PD are the same as those for HD and are as listed in Table 4. PD does not provide the immediate and rapid intervention capabilities of HD in the settings of acute poisonings or life-threatening metabolic disturbances such as hyperkalemia. Circumstances under which PD may be favored over HD are hemodynamic instability, difficult vascular access, and coagulopathy. Plasma components with a MW less than 500 d are removed by PD. An intact peritoneal membrane is required. The mechanism for dialysis in PD uses the peritoneal membrane as the semipermeable membrane across which H_2O and solutes equilibrate. A dialysis solution is infused into the peritoneal space via a catheter. A "cycle" in PD refers to the infusion, time the solution is left in the peritoneal space, and removal of the fluid. The time the dialysis solution is left in the peritoneal space is the dwell time. Solute removal is regulated by adjusting the composition of dialysate fluid, the volume used, the length of dwell time, and the frequency of cycles. The amount of fluid removed is generally regulated by increasing the glucose concentration of the dialysis fluid. If more fluid needs to be removed, the glucose concentration of the fluid is increased to increase the osmotic gradient from the blood to the dialysis fluid. As there is some absorption of the glucose, the patient's blood glucose concentration should be monitored. The removal of other solutes and electrolytes is regulated by adjusting their concentration in the dialysis fluid. The dialysis fluid generally contains a normal physiologic amount of sodium and other essential electrolytes. Initially, no potassium is added to the dialysis fluid. As potassium is removed, small amounts (2 to 3 mEq/L) are added to the dialysis solution. With an intact and functioning peritoneal membrane, the concentrations of solutes and electrolytes in the dialysis fluid will equal those in the plasma.

Because the surface area of the peritoneal membrane in comparison to body mass is greater in infants and children than in adults, efficiency of dialysis via PD approaches 50% (versus 20% in adults) when compared to HD. "Efficiency" refers to the amount of solute load that can be removed over a given amount of time (ie, if a method removes more urea in the same amount of dialysis time, it is more efficient.) Recent abdominal surgery, including insertion of the PD catheter, is a relative contraindication to this method of dialysis, as the efficiency of the peritoneal membrane is greatly reduced until it has healed. Complications experienced during PD include leakage around the peritoneal catheter site, peritonitis, blockage of the catheter, leakage across the diaphragm to the pleural space, and gastrointestinal perforation. Cell counts, gram stains, and cultures are obtained if the patient develops systemic signs of infection or if the fluid becomes cloudy. Most infectious problems can be treated by adding antibiotics to the dialysate without removing the PD catheter. Benefits of PD are increased hemodynamic stability and slower electrolyte/volume equilibration. Fluid leaks can be managed with smaller volumes and more frequent cycles.[30,31] Benefits of PD over HD include improved hemodynamic stability and a slower electrolyte/volume equilibration.

Continuous hemofiltration and hemofiltration with dialysis are alternatives for patients who are not good candidates for HD or PD, and are a means of providing a slow and steady removal of fluid, electrolytes, and toxins from the body.[32,33] Another benefit is that these techniques can remove much larger molecules, depending on the filter, with MW up to 40,000 d. The major indications for this form of therapy are the need for fluid or for fluid and solute removal with cardiovascular stability. Contraindications are related to vascular accessibility. Complications are also similar to those seen with HD with the exception of hypotension (which is less often seen in this therapy). The general concept is that blood is filtered through a hemofiltration cartridge. Solutes, fluid, and toxins are removed from the blood across the semipermeable membrane of the cartridges' microfiber system, and are eliminated in the ultrafiltrate. Solute clearance can be greatly enhanced by countercurrent dialysate flow through the microfibers of the cartridge. Continuous heparinization is necessary to maintain patency of the circuit and prevent clot formation, as in HD. In arterial-venous forms of hemofiltration, flow through the filter and filtration are driven by the patient's arterial pressure. This form requires arterial and venous access. Drawbacks to this form of hemofiltration are the difficulties of arterial access and the fluctuating flow and filtration provided by arterial pressure. Use of this modality has decreased markedly in recent years in favor of venous-venous hemofiltration.

In venous-venous forms of hemofiltration (continuous venovenous hemofiltration [CVVH]), flow and filtration are driven by an in-circuit roller pump. Because of problems with obtaining larger bore arterial access and the inherently low mean arterial pressure in infants and young children, CVVH is now more commonly used in children. This form of hemofiltration provides the benefits of consistent flow and ultrafiltrate formation and easier vascular access. This access can be accomplished through a double-lumen catheter, or dual venous access can be obtained with separate single-lumen catheters. The only complication that is unique to this system is that air bubble detectors, or bubble traps, are needed in the circuit because of the in-line roller pumps. If not appropriately monitored, the roller pumps can entrain air, resulting in an air embolism. Pressure gauges are used before and after the filter, along with pre- and post-filter roller pumps to maintain flow and identify problems of clotting in the circuit.

The use of replacement fluid prefiltration and/or postfiltration varies by author, institution, and clinical scenario. The initial electrolyte content of replacement fluids should closely approximate serum electrolyte concentrations of the patient, with the exception of those targeted electrolytes being removed by the hemofiltration process. For instance, if the indication for hemofiltration is an elevated serum potassium, then the replacement fluids should contain a significantly lower amount of potassium. The amount of replacement fluid to be added is based on the amount of fluid one wants to remove from the patient per hour and the amount of fluid that is already being delivered. No single fluid can be used to provide replacement fluid. Although lactated Ringer's comes relatively close to providing an appropriate amount of the necessary solutes, its calcium concentration may be inadequate. Another option is to alternate replacement fluids on an hourly basis with normal saline plus physiologic amounts of calcium chloride and one-half normal saline with 20 to 40 mEq/L of sodium bicarbonate. It may be necessary to add potassium and phosphate after 12 to 36 hours due to the efficiency of their removal with CVVH. Alternations in the replacement fluid content should be guided by frequent measurements of serum electrolytes.

The benefit of a prefiltration replacement fluid is that it increases the movement of urea and other metabolic waste from inside the red blood cells into the plasma, thus increasing the gradient of those solutes and driving them into the ultrafiltrate. Another benefit is that it dilutes the blood and decreases the episodes of filter clotting. A disadvantage of prefiltration fluid is that, with its use, some plasma electrolytes become diluted, and the diffusion gradient to the dialysate may be lessened, thus reducing the efficacy of plasma solute removal. Postfilter replacement fluids have been reported to replenish plasma volume and electrolytes, correct acid-base abnormalities, and correct inborn errors of metabolism.[34,35] The various types or setups for hemofiltration, including continuous arteriovenous hemofiltration (CAVH), continuous arteriovenous hemofiltration with dialysis (CAVH-D), CVVH, continuous venovenous hemofiltration with dialysis (CVVH-D), and HP, are outlined in Figure 2.

HP is not a true form of renal replacement therapy but an adjuvant therapy for elimination of toxins and other protein-bound materials from the blood. The patient undergoing HP requires heparinization and vascular access. Relative contraindications to HP are hypotension, poor vascular access, and poor cardiac output. HP works best for toxins and chemicals that bind well with activated charcoal or that are highly protein-bound. Venous or arterial blood passes freely over a cartridge of activated charcoal or carbon with a relatively large surface area and then returns to the venous pool of the patient. Over time, the efficiency of toxin removal decreases as serum proteins, cellular debris, and toxin are bound; the average cartridge life is 4 hours. As with continuous hemofiltration, flow through the HP filter can be efficiently regulated by use of a roller pump. The use of a roller pump also avoids the need for arterial access. Complications are similar to those of HD, with added problems of thrombocytopenia, leukopenia, and hypocalcemia.[36]

Continuous arteriovenous hemofiltration (CAVH)

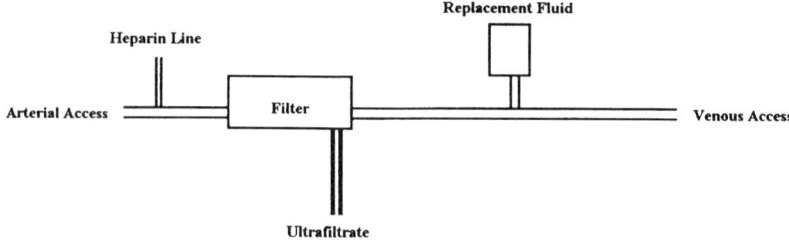

Continuous arteriovenous hemofiltration with dialysis (CAVH-D)

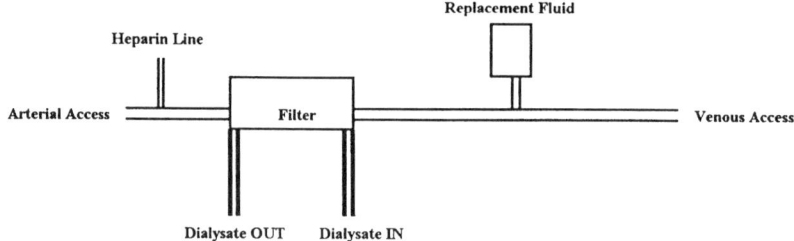

Continuous venovenous hemofiltration (CVVH)

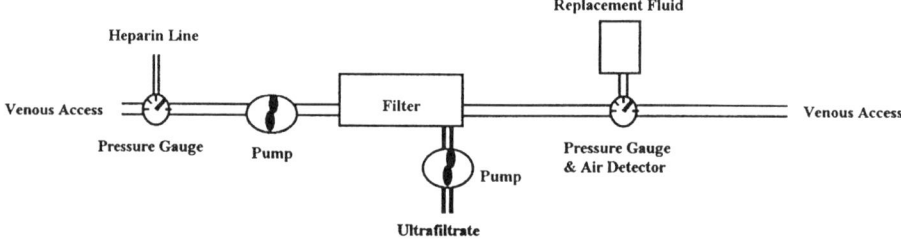

Continuous venovenous hemofiltration with dialysis (CVVH-D)

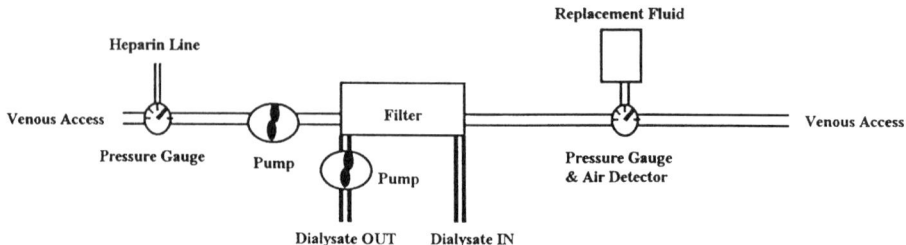

Hemoperfusion (HP)

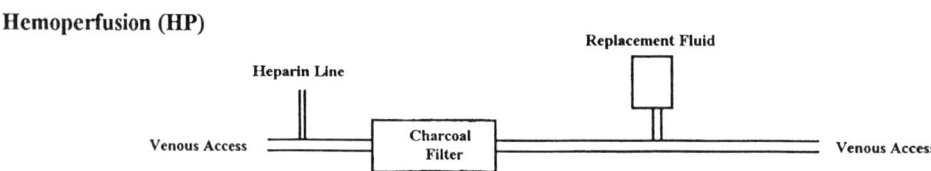

Figure 2. Schematic representation of forms of renal replacement therapy including continuous arteriovenous hemofiltration (CAVH), continuous arteriovenous hemofiltration with dialysis (CAVH-D), continuous venovenous hemofiltration (CVVH), continuous venovenous hemofiltration with dialysis (CVVH-D), and hemoperfusion (HP).

Complications

ARF presents foreseeable problems, and efforts should be made to monitor for, identify, and treat these problems. Complications in the setting of ARF may be related to the underlying disease that resulted in ARF, ARF itself, or therapies aimed at correcting the consequences of ARF. In all forms of ARF, fluid retention, coagulopathy and infections can occur. Fluid and electrolyte management is crucial in order to avoid problems of hypertension and electrolyte disturbances. Increased fluid retention in the setting of ARF is common and can develop over days in spite of appropriate medical therapy. Hypertension, as a consequence of fluid retention, may mandate antihypertensive therapy with calcium channel blockers or vasodilators (see also chapter 18). A coagulopathy can result from uremia-mediated platelet and factor VIII dysfunction. Desmopressin acetate dosed at 0.2 to 0.4 μg/kg/dose has been used to correct bleeding times in uremic patients.[37] Because of the uremia, metabolic acidosis, and underlying diseases that are common in ARF along with the use of urinary catheters and intravenous catheters that is characteristic in the setting of ARF, patients with ARF are at a greater risk for infections. Commonly identified infections include urinary tract infections, pneumonia, sepsis, and line infections. Because of these risks, the duration of use of indwelling lines and Foley catheters should be kept to a minimum. In addition, it is necessary to evaluate fevers by obtaining appropriate cultures from all available sites, including peritoneal fluid in patients receiving PD and vascular catheters in other forms of renal replacement therapy. To date, no specific therapy exists to reverse renal dysfunction; however, with supportive care, many of the disease processes that cause ARF in children are reversible and may not require life-long renal replacement therapy.

References

1. Hou SH, Bushinsky DA, Wish JB, et al. Hospital acquired renal insufficiency: A prospective study. *Am J Med* 1983;74:243–248.
2. Stewart CL, Barnett R. Acute renal failure in infants, children and adults. *Crit Care Clin* 1997;13:575–590.
3. Moghal NE, Brocklebank JT, Meadow SR. A review of acute renal failure in children: Incidence, etiology, and outcome. *Clin Nephrol* 1998;49:91–95.
4. Van der Merwe WM, Collins JF. Acute renal failure in a critical care unit. *N Z Med J* 1989;102:96–98.
5. Hodson EM, Kjellstrand CM, Mauer SM. Acute renal failure in infants and children: Outcome of 53 patients requiring hemodialysis treatment. *J Pediatr* 1978;93:756–761.
6. Gaudio KM, Siegel SJ. Pathogenesis and treatment of renal failure. *Pediatr Clin North Am* 1987;34:771–787.
7. Arora P, Kher V, Rai PK, et al. Prognosis of acute renal failure in children: A multivariate analysis. *Pediatr Nephrol* 1997;11:153–155.
8. Dixon BS, Anderson RJ. Nonoliguric acute renal failure. *Am J Kidney Dis* 1985;6:71–80.
9. Epstein M. Hepatorenal syndrome: Emerging perspectives of pathophysiology and therapy. *J Am Soc Nephrol* 1994;4:1735–1753.
10. Siegler RL. The hemolytic uremic syndrome. *Pediatr Clin North Am* 1995;42:1505–1529.
11. Siegler RL. Atypical hemolytic uremic syndrome: A comparison with post-diarrheal disease. *J Pediatr* 1996;128:505–511.
12. Kaplan BS. Hemolytic uremic syndrome with recurrent episodes: An important subset. *Clin Nephrol* 1977;8:495–498.
13. Brandt JR, Fouser LS, Warkins SL, et al. Escherichia coli O157:H7-associated hemolytic-uremic syndrome after ingestion of contaminated hamburgers. *J Pediatr* 1994;125:519–526.
14. McGraw ME, Lendon M, Stevens RF, et al. Haemolytic uraemic syndrome and the Thomsen Friedenreich antigen. *Pediatr Nephrol* 1989;3:135–139.
15. Erickson LC, Smith WS, Biswas AK, et al. Streptococcus pnuemonia-induced hemolytic uremic syndrome: A case for early diagnosis. *Pediatr Nephrol* 1994;8:211–213.
16. Eneas JF, Schoenfeld PY, Humphreys MH. The effect of infusion of mannitol-sodium bicarbonate on the clinical course of myoglobinuria. *Arch Intern Med* 1979;139:801–805.
17. Neu AM, Warady BA. Dialysis and renal transplantation in infants with irreversible renal failure. *Adv Renal Replace Ther* 1996;3:48–59.
18. Harmon WE, Stablein D, Alexander SR, et al. Graft thrombosis in pediatric renal transplant recipients. A report of the North American Pediatric Renal Transplant Cooperative Study. *Transplantation* 1991;51:406–412.
19. Tejani A, Stablein D, Alexander S, et al. Analysis of rejection outcomes and implications—a report of the North American Pedi-

atric Renal Transplant Cooperative Study. *Transplantation* 1995;59:500–504.
20. Muller T, Sikora P, Offner G, et al. Recurrence of renal disease after kidney transplantation in children: 24 years of experience in a single center. *Clin Nephrol* 1998;49: 82–90.
21. Warady BA. Treatment of infants with end-stage renal disease. *Curr Opin Pediatr* 1992;4:264–268.
22. Brown CB, Ogg CS, Cameron JS. High dose furosemide in acute renal failure. A controlled trial. *Clin Nephrol* 1986;15:90–96.
23. Brezis M, Rosen S. Hypoxia of the renal medulla—its implications for disease. *N Engl J Med* 1995;332:647–655.
24. Zager RA, Mahan J, Merola AJ. Effects of mannitol on the post ischemic kidney. *Lab Invest* 1985;53:433–442.
25. Flancbaum L, Choban PS, Dasta JF. Quantitative effects of low-dose dopamine on urine output in oliguric surgical intensive care unit patients. *Crit Care Med* 1994;22:61–68.
26. Thadhani R, Pascual M, Bonventre JV. Medical progress: Acute renal failure. *New Engl J Med* 1996;334:1448–1460.
27. Gellai M, Jugus M, Fletcher T, et al. Reversal of post ischemic acute renal failure with a selective endothelin A receptor antagonist in the rat. *J Clin Invest* 1994;93:900–906.
28. Gaudio KM, Siegel NJ. New approaches to the treatment of acute renal failure. *Pediatr Nephrol* 1987;1:339–347.
29. Evans ED, Greenbaum, LA, Ettenger RB. Principles of renal replacement therapy in children. *Pediatr Clin North Am* 1995;42: 1579–1602.
30. Reznik VM, Griswold WR, Perterson BM, et al. Peritoneal dialysis for acute renal failure in children. *Pediatr Nephrol* 1991;5:715–717.
31. Werner HA, Wensley DF, Lirenman DS, LeBlanc JG. Peritoneal dialysis in children after cardiopulmonary bypass. *J Thorac Cardiovasc Surg* 1997;113:64–70.
32. Ronco C, Bellomo R, Wratten ML, Tetta C. Today's technology for continuous renal replacement therapies. *Clin Intensive Care* 1996; 7:198–205.
33. Kaplan AA. Continuous renal replacement therapy (CRRT) in the intensive care unit. *J Intensive Care Med* 1998;13:85–105.
34. Bunchman TE, Donckerwolcke RA. Continuous arterial-venous diahemofiltration and continuous veno-venous diahemofiltration in infants and children. *Pediatr Nephrol* 1994; 8:96–102.
35. Thompson GN, Butt W, Shann FA, et al. Continuous venovenous hemofiltration in the management of acute decompensation in inborn errors of metabolism. *J Pediatr* 1991;118:879–884.
36. Pond S, Rosenberg J, Benowitz NL, et al. Pharmacokinetics of haemoperfusion for drug overdose. *Clin Pharmacokinet* 1979;4: 329–354.
37. Mannucci PM, Remuzzi G, Pusineri F, et al. Deamino-8-D-arginine vasopressin shortens the bleeding time in uremia. *N Engl J Med* 1983;308:8–12.

Chapter 17

Diabetic Ketoacidosis

Jessica Klekamp, MD and Kevin B. Churchwell, MD

Introduction

Diabetic ketoacidosis (DKA) is one of the most frequently occurring medical conditions that requires admission to the pediatric intensive care unit (PICU). With current clinical management, the mortality from DKA has fallen to 2% to 5%.[1-3] The morbidity and mortality seen in this disease clearly indicate that although insulin deficiency is the primary derangement, the sequelae of this deficiency can result in multiorgan system dysfunction.

This chapter outlines the initial assessment and therapy of DKA, describes the ongoing management of DKA in the PICU, and addresses the treatment of the potentially serious complications that may arise during therapy for DKA.

Pathophysiology

As this chapter is intended to focus on the clinical management of the pediatric patient with DKA, only a short review of the pathogenesis of DKA is included. DKA develops secondary to a deficiency of insulin, either absolute or relative. The major functions of insulin include glucose uptake into the liver with stimulation of glycogen synthesis, glucose utilization in skeletal muscle for protein synthesis, and stimulation of both glucose and lipoprotein uptake in fat cells driving lipogenesis. In the setting of insulin deficiency, glycogenolysis and gluconeogenesis result in hyperglycemia, proteolysis, and lipolysis. These unopposed processes lead to increased amino acids and free fatty acids in the blood, which cause formation of ketone bodies and a metabolic acidosis.

In addition, the actions of glucagon, catecholamines, cortisol, and growth hormone, which usually function in a counterregulatory role, are unopposed. This activity leads to marked imbalances in the metabolism of carbohydrates, proteins, and lipids. Release of glucagon worsens hyperglycemia and acidosis by increasing hepatic glycogenolysis and stimulating lipolysis, without any concurrent increase in glucose utilization. Acidosis stimulates release of the catecholamines epinephrine and norepinephrine, which in turn increase hepatic glucose production and mobilization of fatty acid stores, worsening hyperglycemia and acidosis. Cortisol excess decreases peripheral glucose utilization, further exacerbating the pathologic state.

As these processes lead to DKA and hyperglycemia, the patient develops an osmotic diuresis caused by massive excretion of glucose in the urine. This leads to a severe loss of free water, as well as sodium, chloride, magnesium, and potassium. The osmotic diuresis causes hypovolemia, resulting in tissue hypoperfusion, an increase in

From: Tobias JD (ed): *Pediatric Critical Care: The Essentials.* ©Futura Publishing Co., Inc., Armonk, NY, 1999.

anaerobic glycolysis, and production of lactic acid, worsening the metabolic acidosis. The combination of insulin deficiency, unopposed counter-regulatory hormone secretion, and the development of an osmotic diuresis secondary to glucosuria leads to the clinical presentation of hyperglycemia, metabolic acidosis, dehydration, and multiple electrolyte disturbances.

Clinical Presentation

Up to one quarter of cases of DKA occur as the initial presentation of insulin-dependent diabetes mellitus (IDDM).[2] The clinical appearance of the child in DKA can be quite variable, and the diagnosis may not be immediately clear in patients who do not have a previous history of diabetes. The usual acute clinical presentation is of a child with moderate to severe dehydration. Many patients present with a history of nausea and vomiting or abdominal pain simulating acute intra-abdominal surgical conditions such as appendicitis. Signs that indicate dehydration include poor skin turgor, dry mucous membranes, skeletal muscle weakness, tachycardia, and hypotension with orthostatic blood pressure changes. Clinical findings that are also frequently present include depressed level of consciousness to frank lethargy or obtundation, hyperventilation (Kussmaul's respirations), and a fruity odor of the breath. Any combination of these findings, together with a history of polydipsia, polyuria, and weight loss, should prompt the physician to rapidly obtain initial laboratory studies (serum glucose, urine for glucose and ketones) to confirm the diagnosis of DKA. Hyperglycemia, metabolic acidosis with arterial pH ≤7.3 and serum bicarbonate ≤15, and ketonuria confirm the diagnosis of DKA.

Occasionally patients with new-onset diabetes and DKA will present with profound shock and early multiorgan system failure. In this situation, management of the ABCs (airway, breathing, and circulation) is obviously critical, but persistently elevated blood glucose levels in the patient with profound acidosis and shock that appears refractory to fluid replacement may signal DKA. In these patients, it may be difficult to manage their shock and organ failure until the DKA is treated and the acidosis begins to resolve.

Initial Assessment and Management

The primary goal of management during the first few hours is to establish hydration and restore cardiovascular stability (Fig. 1). The degree of dehydration can be approximated with the physical examination and measurement of blood pressure, heart rate, skin temperature, color, capillary refill time, and quality of the peripheral pulses. Most of the pediatric patients presenting in DKA will be 5% to 10% dehydrated. Those with more significant losses will be more symptomatic with hypotension, orthostatic blood pressure changes, tachycardia, lethargy, etc., and will show definite signs of shock. Placement of at least two large bore intravenous cannulae is recommended. With intravenous access, blood samples can be obtained for serial measurements of serum glucose, electrolytes, blood urea nitrogen, creatinine, and venous pH.

Fluid therapy is aimed at reestablishing adequate tissue perfusion. It is possible, however, that overly aggressive hydration in pediatric patients with DKA may lead to profound complications (Table 1), one of the most serious being cerebral edema.[4,5] In order to avoid this complication, a few general rules and concepts should be kept in mind:

1. Patients who are less than 10% dehydrated are usually hemodynamically stable.
2. Gradual rehydration with an isotonic fluid over 24 to 36 hours is usually sufficient.
3. An hourly fluid rate is calculated by determining the patient's deficit and correcting the deficit over 24 to 36 hours by adding that volume to the patient's hourly maintenance rate.
4. The total hourly volume should not exceed twice the maintenance rate.

Hemodynamic instability in a child with DKA is a medical emergency. Patients

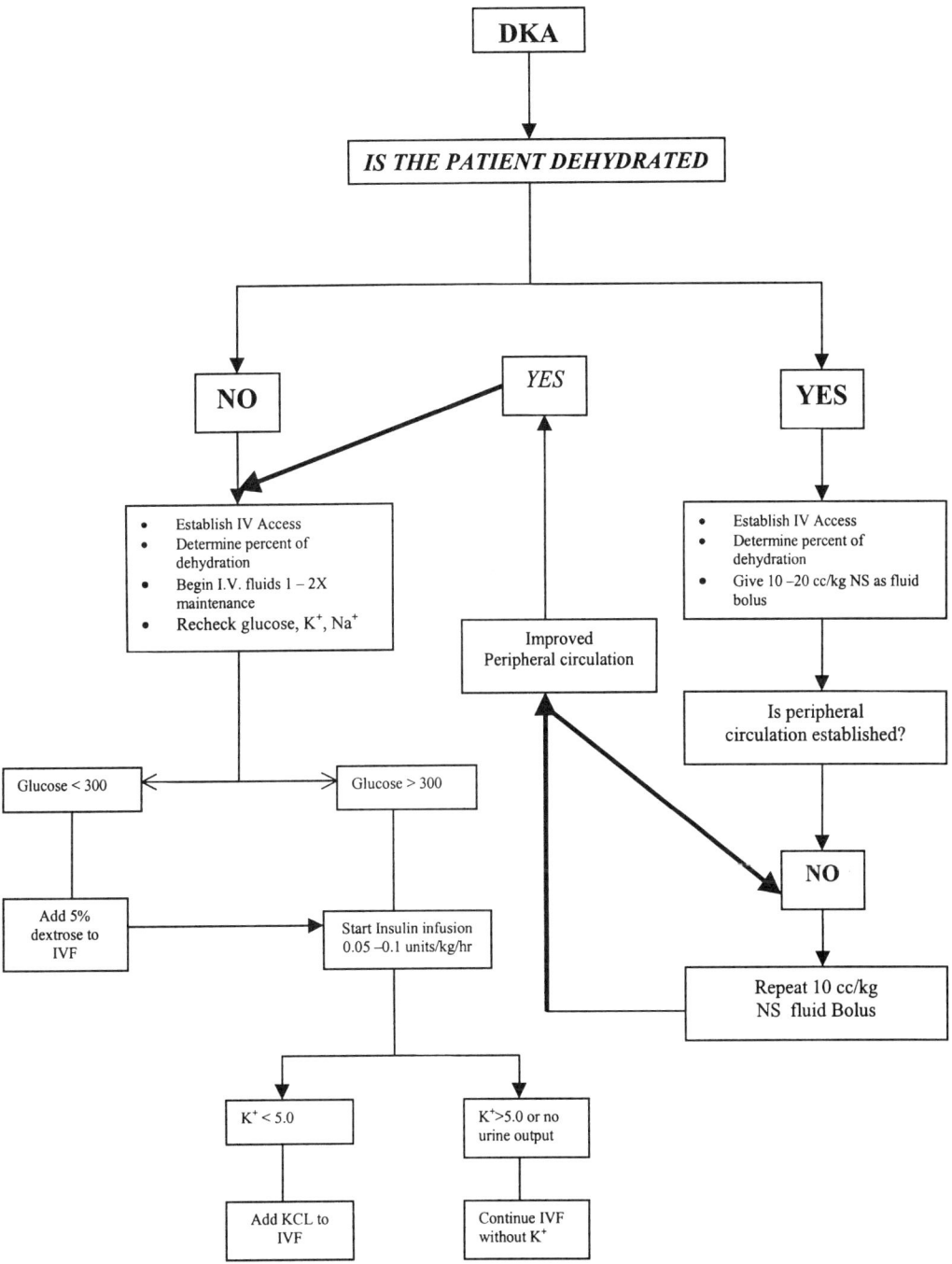

Figure 1. Algorithm for the management of diabetic ketoacidosis (DKA). IV = intravenous; IVF = intravenous fluids; UOP = urine output.

Table 1

Complications of Diabetic Ketoacidosis

Complication	Etiology	Treatment
Hyperkalemia	acidosis, insulin deficiency, decreased renal tubular secretion, iatrogenic	insulin/glucose, $CaCl_2$, $NaHCO_3$
Hypokalemia	K^+ loss	KCL 10–40 mEq/L added to i.v. fluids
Hypoglycemia	too much insulin	1–3 mL/kg D_{25} i.v.
Cerebral edema	unknown, multifactorial	mannitol 0.25–1 g/kg i.v., endotracheal intubation, hyperventilation
Pulmonary edema	low oncotic pressure, increased capillary permeability, neurogenic	supplemental O_2, airway control, positive end-expiratory pressure, diuresis
Cardiac arrhythmias	electrolyte abnormalities	supplementation of low calcium, potassium, or magnesium

who are 10% to 20% dehydrated will often show signs of cardiovascular instability. A fluid bolus of 5 to 20 mL/kg of an isotonic fluid (normal saline or lactated Ringer's) followed by gradual rehydration, as described above, once peripheral circulation is reestablished is appropriate. Patients with more than 20% dehydration will show overt signs of shock. Fluid management in these patients involves rapid isotonic fluid boluses in 10- to 20-mL/kg aliquots until cardiovascular stability is reestablished. Subsequent rehydration therapy is as described above.

In general, cautious administration of fluid boluses using only isotonic fluids should be used to correct peripheral circulation, and should be followed by calculated fluid rehydration over 24 to 36 hours. A safe rule during rehydration is that no patient should receive fluid at a rate greater than twice their maintenance requirements after the initial management of shock. The choice of fluid for the patients ongoing rehydration is also of significant importance, as these fluids will often run at two times the normal maintenance rate. During the early stages of therapy, when the serum glucose remains ≥300 mg/dL, we recommend using either normal saline or lactated Ringer's, with potassium added as described below. It is imperative that isotonic fluids are used not only for boluses, but for ongoing replacement, as there has been a clear correlation of the use of hypotonic fluids and the development of cerebral edema in an animal model of DKA.[6] After serum glucose level falls below 300 mg/dL, maintenance fluids can be switched to D_5NS $D_5\frac{1}{2}NS$ with the appropriate amount of potassium. Even in the setting of significant hypernatremia, ¼NS **would not be an appropriate choice of fluid.** The high serum sodium may be beneficial in that it provides a high extracellular/intravascular osmotic load and thus prevents the intracellular movement of free water and, perhaps, lessens the incidence of cerebral edema. The concomitant rapid decrease in extracellular serum glucose and serum sodium can result in an extracellular-to-intracellular osmotic gradient favoring the intracellular movement of free water.

After cardiovascular stability has been established, a directed history must be obtained from the patient or from the patient's caregivers in order to determine precipitating factors. The most common initiating events are: 1) presenting signs of IDDM; 2) noncompliance with insulin regimen; 3) infection (bacteremia, urinary tract infection, pneumonia); 4) systemic stress (surgery, antecedent viral illness); and 5) pregnancy.[3] If infection is suspected after a careful history and physical examination, further laboratory studies including a complete blood count, cultures, and chest x-ray may be warranted. Although an invasive infection is uncommon in pediatric patients in DKA, when present, it can be devastating and must be aggressively searched for and treated with an appropriate antibiotic regimen based on the patient's age and the suspected source of infection (see also chapter 19). Although unlikely, specific drug ingestions such as acetylsalicylic acid can masquerade as DKA. If the diagnosis is suspect, toxicologic screening is indicated.

After the patient's hemodynamic status and the etiology of DKA have been addressed, any abnormal electrolyte values can be addressed during the first hours of therapy. The initial potassium concentration may range from normal to significantly elevated, despite the probable existence of total-body potassium depletion. The etiology of hyperkalemia in DKA is multifactorial. In part, the initial hyperkalemia is secondary to a shift of potassium from intracellular to extracellular in the presence of profound acidosis. Causes of hyperkalemia also include serum hyperosmolality, low insulin levels, and decreased renal tubular potassium secretion.[7] The elevated potassium levels observed do not correlate well with either the severity of lactic acidosis or ketoacidosis. Disturbed potassium homeostasis is a distinct entity and, thus, an independent phenomenon in DKA which may result in its own sequelae and morbidity.

With correction of systemic acidosis and rehydration, a rapid drop in serum potassium usually occurs. Specific treatment for hyperkalemia should be reserved for those patients who are symptomatic, specifically those with evidence of abnormal ECG findings such as peaked T waves or a wide QRS complex. Initial treatment involves the administration of sodium bicarbonate (1 to 2 mEq/kg) administered intravenously over 10 to 15 minutes, the administration of calcium (either 0.1 mL/kg of calcium chloride or 0.3 mL/kg of calcium gluconate), and the administration of insulin as described below (Table 1).

The majority of patients in DKA with any significant degree of hyperglycemia will also have hyponatremia at the time of admission. Serum sodium is decreased because hypertonicity of the serum moves water into the extracellular space, diluting the sodium concentration. With the use of isotonic fluid during rehydration, serum glucose levels fall while the serum sodium concentration rises to a more appropriate level for the amount of free water loss. Several recent retrospective analyses have pointed to the trend of declining serum sodium in the patient who is being treated for DKA as a concerning sign for the development of cerebral edema,[5,8-10] although, as it occurs in a significant number of patients who develop no complications, the positive predictive value of this finding is in question.

After fluid therapy is started, the next major decision concerns the initiation of insulin therapy. Every patient with DKA will need insulin to reverse the major metabolic abnormalities of the disorder. Large doses of insulin are not required. The initial therapy is aimed at reversing hypovolemia and end-organ hypoperfusion. Low doses of insulin will reverse or stop the ongoing metabolic derangements, including lipolysis and the production of keto acids. The standard approach has consisted of an initial bolus dose followed by an infusion of insulin. However, the majority of patients may not require a bolus dose of insulin, as fluid administration generally causes a significant reduction in the serum glucose. Thus, many patients do well with only insulin by infusion. We have found the following protocol to be safe and effective (Table 2): Serum glucose is obtained before and after any fluid boluses are administered. If the serum glucose remains ≥700 mg/dL after fluid bolus, or if an insulin infusion cannot be readily obtained or safely delivered, a bolus of 0.05 to 0.1 U/kg of regular insulin may be given intravenously followed by an insulin infusion with an initial dosing rate of 0.1 U/kg/h. In most patients, the lower insulin bolus (0.05 U/kg) is appropriate, as larger doses result in a more rapid than desired drop in the serum glucose (>50 to 100 mg/dL/h). If the serum glucose is ≥300 mg/dL but ≤700 mg/dL, no bolus of insulin is administered and the insulin infusion is started at 0.1 U/kg/h. Bolus doses of insulin should never be administered subcutaneously during the initial treatment of DKA. Inadequate tissue perfusion can result in erratic absorption from the subcutaneous space.

If the serum glucose is ≤300 mg/dL, no bolus of insulin is given. The insulin infusion is started at 0.05 U/kg/h and 5% dex-

Table 2
Insulin Therapy in Diabetic Ketoacidosis

Serum Glucose (mg/dL)	Insulin Bolus (U/kg)	Insulin Infusion (U/kg/h)	Intravenous Fluids
≥700	0.05–0.1	0.05–0.1	normal saline
300–700	none	0.05–0.1	normal saline
≤300	none	0.05	D_5 NS or D_3 1/2 NS

NS = normal saline.

trose should be added to the rehydration fluids. The insulin infusion rate is adjusted to maintain a decrease in serum glucose no faster than 50 to 100 mg/dL/h. When the serum glucose approaches 300 mg/dL, intravenous fluids with 5% dextrose are added to maintain the glucose in the 150- to 250-mg/dL range throughout the correction of ketoacidosis. The insulin infusion should also be maintained at no less than 0.03 to 0.05 U/kg/h during this period. Some patients will require increased amounts of glucose ($D_{7.5}$ or D_{10}) in their rehydration fluids to maintain their serum glucose with this insulin infusion rate. This requirement is seen in many new-onset diabetics who are particularly sensitive to the effects of exogenous insulin.

Along with hyperglycemia, metabolic acidosis is a hallmark of DKA. Treatment for the metabolic acidosis involves recognition of its etiology. The acidosis is caused by the low insulin state, and results in the production of serum ketone bodies (β-hydroxybutyric acid and aceto-acetic acid) and the volume-contracted state produced by the osmotic diuresis. Therapy therefore should be directed toward correction of these abnormalities. The administration of $NaHCO_3$ should only be used in children with DKA for the treatment of symptomatic hyperkalemia or in patients presenting with complete cardiovascular collapse. In these situations, patients should receive 1 to 2 mEq/kg of $NaHCO_3$ over 10 to 15 minutes, in addition to rapid isotonic volume boluses for reestablishment of peripheral circulation. In these patients, invasive hemodynamic monitoring should be considered to guide fluid therapy appropriately. Patients with severe cardiovascular collapse may require large volumes of isotonic fluids to restore intravascular volume and tissue perfusion. When large volumes of fluids are administered, fluids should be appropriately warmed to 37 to 40°C with fluid warmers prior to their administration to prevent inadvertent hypothermia.

All patients should receive no oral intake throughout the period of initial evaluation and stabilization. After initial stabilization, pediatric patients should be allowed small volumes of fluid by mouth during the first several hours. Although these patients tend to be very thirsty, despite their declining mental status, any degree of oral intake may induce further nausea and vomiting. In the face of significant systemic acidosis, excessive free water intake without adequate electrolytes may only complicate gradual rehydration.

Ongoing management of patients in DKA includes frequent neurologic examinations with documented Glasgow Coma scales and checks of pupillary function on at least an hourly basis throughout the first 12 to 24 hours. The development of cerebral edema can be rapid in onset and fatal (see below). The patient will also require frequent reassessment of acid-base status with venous pH measurements, as well as measurements of glucose, sodium, and potassium levels. Urine samples should be intermittently checked for ketones to ensure that the degree of ketonuria is diminishing. The insulin infusion should be continued until the systemic acidosis is corrected.

Once the serum pH is normal and the patient's metabolic acidosis has resolved, it is safe to switch over to an intermittent subcutaneous insulin regimen. The first dose may be administered to coincide with the morning or evening meal and the infusion may be discontinued approximately 1 hour after the first subcutaneous dose. The amount of subcutaneous insulin administered to new-onset diabetics varies between patients, but ranges between 0.5 and 1.0 U/kg/day depending upon the severity of presentation, including length of symptoms prior to diagnosis, the degree of weight loss, and the endogenous reserves for insulin production. Once a total daily dose has been selected, it should be divided, with two thirds of the total daily dose administered in the morning and one third in the evening. The morning dose should again be divided as two thirds neutral protein Hagedorn (NPH) insulin and one third regular insulin. The evening dose may be similarly divided, however some advocate the use of ultralente insulin, rather than NPH, at night. Another approach to switching from continuous intravenous insulin to subcutaneous delivery involves using a sliding scale with regular insulin for 24 hours, and then totaling the amount required to determine the patient's total daily dose.

Complications of Diabetic Ketoacidosis

Cerebral Edema

Cerebral edema and other intracranial complications account for a significant percentage of the mortality associated with DKA. Cerebral edema generally manifests suddenly and may progress rapidly to brain herniation even if recognized and treated aggressively. Cerebral edema often becomes clinically apparent several hours into therapy for DKA at a time when serum acidosis, dehydration, and hyperglycemia are all improving. However, it can also occur very early in the course, even as a presenting symptom. A review of all of the available literature[5,6,8,9] indicates that the pathogenesis of cerebral edema in DKA is multifactorial, a fact that contributes to the difficulty of establishing preventive treatment strategies.

Initially, the development of cerebral edema was almost uniformly fatal. However, outcomes have improved with rapid and aggressive intervention (Table 3) as well as early identification. These findings underline two important points in the treatment of cerebral edema associated with DKA: first, the importance of frequent neurologic evaluation especially in the lethargic patient, and second the importance of readily available treatment in the event of a rapid neurologic change.

The patient who complains of a headache followed by decreased mental status or unresponsiveness should receive 0.25 to 1.0 g/kg of intravenous mannitol. Other signs that may occur include relative bradycardia and hypertension. In the event of true unresponsiveness consistent with impending herniation, or for the patient who does not rapidly improve with intravenous mannitol, mannitol administration should be followed by endotracheal intubation and hyperventilation. Endotracheal intubation in these patients must be performed with attention to increased intracranial pressure (ICP) when selecting appropriate sedative and neuromuscular blocking agents (see also chapter 1 for a full discussion of airway management in the patient with increased ICP). In the patient who has remained NPO prior to the development of cerebral edema, use of the technique of modified rapid sequence intubation, which involves short-term bag-valve mask ventilation prior to intubation, may allow for a decrease in the partial pressure of arterial carbon dioxide and, thus, the ICP, prior to direct laryngoscopy. Patients should receive lidocaine 1 mg/kg to blunt the reflexive rise in ICP with direct laryngoscopy, in addition to a sedative and neuromuscular blocking agent. For the patient who has been normotensive and has had adequately repleted intravascular volume, sodium pentothal (2 to 5 mg/kg) can be used to provide effective sedation and amnesia for the procedure while decreasing the cerebral metabolic rate for oxygen and thus decreasing ICP. In some patients with a rapid decline in the level of consciousness, mannitol will effect a rapid improvement and obviate the need for endotracheal intubation. Close observation of these patients is mandatory because mannitol may need to be redosed after several hours.

After successful endotracheal intuba-

Table 3
Treatment of Cerebral Edema Associated with Diabetic Ketoacidosis

Level of Consciousness	Intervention
Somnolent, but arouses to stimuli	continue hourly neuro checks
Obtunded, responds only to painful stimuli	mannitol 0.25–1.0 g/kg endotracheal intubation and hyperventilation if no prompt improvement

Obtunded, unresponsive or posturing, pupillary changes	mannitol 0.25–1.0 g/kg
	edotracheal intubation/hyperventilation:
	  atropine 10 μg/kg
	  lidocaine 1 mg/kg
	  sedative/NMBA

NMBA = neuromuscular blocking agent.

tion and delivery of mannitol, computed-tomography (CT) scan of the head is indicated. Although the majority of patients with DKA who develop coma during the course of their therapy will demonstrate diffuse cerebral edema on CT scan, there have been a handful of cases demonstrating development of obstructive hydrocephalus or intracranial bleeding in this setting.[11] Such complications may require neurosurgical intervention or placement of a ventricular drain. Ongoing management of patients with cerebral edema includes placement of a device to monitor ICP and ongoing treatment of cerebral edema (see also chapter 10 for a discussion of management of increased ICP and ICP monitoring).

Hypoglycemia

More common complications during the therapy for DKA include hypoglycemia and electrolyte abnormalities. Many patients will have a very rapid decline in their glucose level, especially if given a bolus of insulin following a fluid bolus. It may be prudent to withhold an insulin bolus in the patient who is going to be transported some distance to a PICU if adequate glucose monitoring en route is not possible. Any patient with symptomatic hypoglycemia or glucose less than 60 mg/dL should receive 1 to 3 mL/kg of a 25% dextrose solution if still acidotic and not ready to take oral glucose-containing fluids. In the majority of patients receiving a continuous insulin infusion, if glucose levels are checked hourly, a falling glucose will be noted before it reaches a dangerously low level, and dextrose may be added to fluids or the concentration of dextrose increased.

Hypokalemia

Hypokalemia should be anticipated as acidosis resolves and rehydration progresses. The clinician will need to add potassium to rehydration fluids as soon as the serum level reaches ≤5.0 mEq/dL in patients who have urine output. While an initial addition of 20 mEq/L of potassium may be adequate, continued close monitoring will indicate those patients who need increased infusion rates. Many new-onset diabetics who have been symptomatic for prolonged periods of time prior to diagnosis will require potassium supplementation.

Other electrolyte abnormalities have been observed during therapy for DKA, including hypophosphatemia, hypomagnesemia, and hypocalcemia. These abnormalities are related to both ion shifts due to hyperglycemia and insulin infusions with correction of acidosis in addition to total-body depletion from the prolonged prehospital osmotic diuresis. Studies have shown no substantial benefit from replacement of these electrolytes early in the course of therapy. While some clinicians have suggested early replacement of phosphate by the inclusion of potassium phosphate as half of the potassium in intravenous fluids, this is not our current practice and, to date, no studies have demonstrated a significant benefit in patients with DKA. Rapid correction of pH may result in a precipitous drop in the ionized calcium and the development of tetany due to increased protein binding of the calcium cation.

Pulmonary Edema

An unusual complication reported in DKA is the development of pulmonary edema. Various theories have been suggested to explain the increased oxygen requirement with or without radiographic changes consistent with pulmonary edema seen in patients with DKA. Possible etiologies include low plasma oncotic pressure,[12] increased pulmonary capillary permeability,[13,14] and neurogenic pulmonary edema from increased ICP. Treatment involves supplemental oxygen, correction of the underlying metabolic derangements, continued diuresis, and endotracheal intubation with mechanical ventilation for severe cases. If neurogenic in origin, control of the airway with endotracheal intubation should be established to treat both the increase in ICP and the pulmonary edema.[15]

Cardiac Arrhythmias

Although rare, life-threatening arrhythmias do occur in DKA. The etiology is usually an electrolyte imbalance such as hyperkalemia, hypokalemia, hypomagnesemia, or hypocalcemia. Treatment of the cardiac arrhythmia involves identifying the electrolyte abnormality and correction for hypokalemia, hypomagnesemia, or hypocalcemia. Treatment for hyperkalemia has been addressed elsewhere in this chapter (see Table 1).

Conclusion

Treatment of the pediatric patient with DKA can be an extremely rewarding clinical experience. It encompasses much of the pathophysiology and thought processes involved in the treatment of critically ill children. Despite the remarkable improvement in outcome after DKA with the advent of insulin therapy, there is still a significant and perhaps excessive mortality in childhood-onset IDDM.[16] As research continues to look at the causes and treatment of diabetes and DKA, therapy directed toward treatment or, more importantly, prevention of complications such as cerebral edema hopefully will be developed and will continue to improve the outcome for those pediatric patients afflicted with this disease.

References

1. Krane EJ. Diabetic ketoacidosis: Biochemistry, physiology, treatment, and prevention. *Pediatr Clin North Am* 1987;34:935–960.
2. Lebovitz HE. Diabetic ketoacidosis. *Lancet* 1995;345:767–772.
3. Kitabchi AE, Wall BM. Diabetic ketoacidosis. *Med Clin North Am* 1995;79:9–37.
4. Harris GD, Fiordalisi I. Physiologic management of diabetic ketoacidemia. *Arch Pediatr Adolesc Med* 1994;148:1046–1052.
5. Harris GD, Fiordalisi I, Harris WL, et al. Minimizing the risk of brain herniation during treatment of diabetic ketoacidemia: A retrospective and prospective study. *J Pediatr* 1990;117:22–31.
6. Silver SM, Clark EC, Schroeder BM, Sterns RH. Pathogenesis of cerebral edema after treatment of diabetic ketoacidosis. *Kidney Int* 1997;51:1237–1244.
7. Fulop M. Hyperkalemia in diabetic ketoacidosis. *Am J Med Sci* 1990;299:164–169.
8. Hale PM, Rezvani I, Braunstein AW, et al. Factors predicting cerebral edema in young children with diabetic ketoacidosis and new onset type I diabetes. *Acta Paediatr* 1997;86: 26–631.
9. Duck SC, Wyatt DT. Factors associated with brain herniation in the treatment of diabetic ketoacidosis. *J Pediatr* 1988;113:10–14.
10. Rosenbloom AL. Intracerebral crises during the treatment of diabetic ketoacidosis. *Diabetes Care* 1990;13:22–33.
11. Eskandar EM, Weller SJ, Frim DM. Hydrocephalus requiring urgent external ventricular drainage in a patient with diabetic ketoacidosis and cerebral edema: Case report. *Neurosurgery* 1997;40:836–839.
12. Sprung C, Rackow E, Fein I. Pulmonary edema: A complication of diabetic ketoacidosis. *Chest* 1980;77:687–689.
13. Brun-Buisson C, Bonnet F, Bergeret S. Recurrent high permeability pulmonary edema

associated with diabetic ketoacidosis. *Crit Care Med* 1985;13:55–57.
14. Powner D, Snyder J, Grenvik A. Altered pulmonary capillary permeability complicating recovery from diabetic ketoacidosis. *Chest* 1975;68:253–256.
15. Young MC. Simultaneous acute cerebral and pulmonary edema complicating diabetic ketoacidosis. *Diabetes Care* 1995;18:1288–1290.
16. Sartor G, Dahlquist G. Short-term mortality in childhood onset insulin-dependent diabetes mellitus: A high frequency of unexpected deaths in bed. *Diabetes Med* 1995;12:607–611.

Chapter 18

Hypertensive Emergencies in the Pediatric Intensive Care Unit Patient

Ted D. Groshong, MD

Introduction

Hypertensive emergencies are highly unusual in patients at any age, particularly those patients in the pediatric age range.[1] Unless one commonly deals with patients who have chronic renal disease or other conditions likely to result in severe hypertension, one may practice medicine for an entire lifetime without caring for a patient with a hypertensive emergency. However, when children present with profound hypertension, prompt and effective therapy is mandatory in order to prevent severe morbidity, permanent neurologic sequelae, and even mortality.

It is necessary to differentiate between hypertensive emergencies and hypertensive urgencies.[2] By definition, the former requires clear evidence of end-organ damage, the direct result of elevated blood pressure. The latter is simply the recording of a very high blood pressure without the presence of symptoms.[3] A hypertensive emergency requires immediate therapy in a controlled and carefully monitored setting. A hypertensive urgency does not require immediate treatment; in this situation, reduction of blood pressure may occur over 24 to 48 hours or longer, often in an ambulatory setting.

Presentation

As noted previously, by definition a hypertensive emergency is characterized by evidence of end-organ damage. Consequently, the presenting symptoms will reflect the involvement of those organs most susceptible to damage from hypertension (Table 1). In general, the most prominent findings in children are associated with neurologic disease, with cardiac and hematologic symptoms occurring somewhat less frequently.[4,5]

Hypertensive encephalopathy, resulting from diffuse or localized edema of the brain, may present with seizures, focal neurologic findings, visual loss, or, in severe cases, loss of consciousness. It may be difficult to differentiate in the patient presenting with seizures and hypertension whether the seizures are responsible for the hypertension, or the converse.[6] Headaches may be the initial presenting complaint. Characteristically, headaches resulting from hypertension are either occipital or parietal. Physical findings will often include evidence of retinopathy, including papilledema, retinal hemorrhages, and exudates. Ocular lesions may not be apparent in patients with visual loss, as these patients may experience loss of vision due to ischemia or necrosis within the

From: Tobias JD (ed): *Pediatric Critical Care: The Essentials.* ©Futura Publishing Co., Inc., Armonk, NY, 1999.

Table 1

Signs and Symptoms of Severe Hypertension in Children

Seizures
Visual changes
Retinopathy
Altered mental status
Hemiplegia
Facial palsy
Headache
Vomiting
Papilledema
Left heart failure

---

central nervous system and the retina.[7] Focal neurologic lesions may or may not be present, depending on the location and degree of brain edema.[8,9]

Reduced cardiac output, particularly in patients with longstanding hypertension, may be the cause of initial clinical symptoms.[10] Patients may present with dyspnea on exertion, or other symptoms of congestive heart failure. Such a presentation is most common with severe hypertension in early infancy. Cardiac manifestations may be the primary presenting complaint in these patients. Careful measurement of blood pressure is suggested in neonates and infants presenting with poor growth, poor feeding, dyspnea, or other respiratory symptoms.

Malignant hypertension involving acute renal failure and hematologic dysfunction is an unusual manifestation of hypertensive emergency.[7] Patients present in a similar fashion to those with hemolytic-uremic syndrome, but without preexisting bloody diarrhea. Thrombocytopenia and microangiopathic hemolytic anemia, with neurologic symptoms and acute renal failure, are characteristic.

Finally, symptoms may occur from the specific diseases that are also responsible for the hypertension. Patients with catecholamine-producing tumors may have a history of episodic weakness with tremor. It is generally said that such children are quite thin; however, that is not an invariable finding. Weakness, lethargy, poor appetite, and poor growth in this, as in other causes of hypertensive emergency, are characteristic.

Signs and symptoms related to hypokalemia, the result of chronic hyperaldosteronism, may occur in children with longstanding renal artery stenosis or with primary aldosteronism.

Pathogenesis

Hypertension in children is ordinarily tolerated well, even when the blood pressure values are very high. It may be difficult to determine the exact extent of the hypertension, since some patients may not present until there is end-organ dysfunction. End-organ damage due to hypertensive crisis appears to result from severe vasoconstriction resulting from release of vasoconstricting agents.[3] These agents include angiotensin, norepinephrine, and vasopressin.[7] Endothelial damage occurs with the development of fibrinoid necrosis. Histologically there may be partial or complete occlusion of small arterioles, particularly in the kidneys. This renal ischemia results in further output of vasoconstricting agents, in particular angiotensin II, causing still further vasoconstriction. Cortical and subcapsular hemorrhages are noted in the kidney. The medulla is usually hyperemic.[7] Proliferative endarteritis of the small vessels is noted, with later development of epithelial crescents in the glomeruli.

Histologically, in the brain, similar lesions can be identified. Grossly, microinfarctions and petechial hemorrhages are noted with histologic evidence of fibrinoid necrosis of cerebral arterioles with disruption of the blood-brain barrier and cerebral edema. Autoregulation of cerebral blood flow is seriously impaired.[7]

Etiology

While the frequency of hypertensive crisis is much lower in the pediatric population, children who present to an emergency room with hypertension are more likely to require emergency treatment. Only 1% of hypertensive adults presenting to an emergency department require immediate treatment in contrast to 24% of children.[1] While in theory any cause of hypertension in children may lead to malignant or accelerated disease, in practice hypertensive emergencies complicate only a limited number of diseases (Table 2).

The condition may be acute or chronic. In any series, renal disease tends to predominate as a cause of severe hypertension,[10] and is also the primary etiology of secondary nonemergent hypertension. In one large series,[5] acute renal disease was far less common than chronic renal disease as the etiology of severe hypertension. Among these etiologies, acute poststreptococcal glomerulonephritis, hemolytic-uremic syndrome, and systemic lupus erythematous are the most notorious for causing severe increases in blood pressure.

Vascular disease, particularly that involving the kidneys, is frequently responsible for emergent hypertension. Renal artery stenosis[11,12] resulting from fibromuscular dysplasia or, in some nations, aortoarteritis,[13] is one of the most prominent causes. Polyarteritis nodosa is a known cause of hypertension, although the pathogenesis may be more closely related to renal damage and subsequent volume expansion than to vascular disease.

Several renal tumors, including Wilm's tumor, mesoblastic nephroma,[14] and juxtaglomerular cell tumor[15] may present with or lead to hypertensive emergencies. Extrarenal causes include pheochromocytoma and catecholamine-producing neuroblastoma.[5]

Patient Evaluation

Often, the underlying disease that is causing the hypertensive emergency will be known to the patients' physician. Chronic renal failure or diseases of the urinary tract known to predispose to hypertension will often have been previously identified in children. In a substantial portion of cases, however, hypertension has not been suspected and is the presenting symptom of the patient's disease process. This is especially true of patients with rapid-onset diseases such as hemolytic-uremic syndrome, acute poststreptococcal glomerulonephritis, or conditions that have resulted in a subtle, progressive course (renal artery stenosis).

With hypertensive emergencies, as with almost all other pediatric illnesses, the most powerful diagnostic tools are the history and physical examination. A careful history is often adequate to make the diagnosis. For example, the presence of gross hematuria following a recent episode of sore throat or impetigo should lead to the tentative diagnosis of acute poststreptococcal glomerulonephritis. Similarly, bloody diarrhea prior to onset of symptoms of hypertension would indicate a high probability of hemolytic-uremic syndrome. The presence of symptoms such as headache, dyspnea, nocturia, edema, abdominal pain, polydipsia, and polyuria are important to consider in the determination of specific diagnoses. Many of the conditions to be considered when evaluating hypertensive emergencies, however, may present with a history that is somewhat more subtle. Children with pheochromocytoma may present with episodes of flushing attacks, palpitations, irritability, and diaphoresis. Alternatively, they may present simply with prolonged and progressive weakness and lack of stamina with extreme irritability. Children with chronic renal failure frequently have polyuria including nocturia, but little else besides poor growth.

Poor growth and failure to thrive are

Table 2

Etiology of Hypertensive Emergencies in Children

Renal
  hypoplastic/dysplastic renal disease
  renal artery stenosis
  polycystic kidney disease
  systemic lupus erythematous
  polyarteritis nodosa
  hemolytic-uremic syndrome
  renal transplant rejection
  Wilms' tumor
  glomerulonephritis
  juxtaglomerular cell tumor
  chronic renal failure

Extrarenal
  neuroblastoma
  pheochromocytoma
  intracranial bleed or other cause of ICP
  drug ingestion

ICP = intracranial pressure.

useful clues when found in association with severe hypertension, ordinarily indicating a chronic condition. A history of normal growth would lead one, conversely, to the diagnosis of an acute disease.

The family history is an important means of identifying a variety of conditions. Neurofibromatosis, polycystic kidney disease of either autosomal dominant or autosomal recessive transmission, pseudoxanthoma elasticum,[16] and a variety of other familial diseases[5] are among a large number of genetic conditions leading to possible hypertensive emergency. Stroke occurring at a young age, or early-onset myocardial infarction, may also be important clues in the family history.[17] Finally, a drug history is critical. This is true of all ages, but particularly in adolescents, as many recreational drugs including cocaine and amphetamines can lead to hypertensive crisis.

A careful physical examination is mandatory for the identification of the severity of hypertension and to guide the clinician to the correct etiology. A rapid physical examination should be performed. Pulse and blood pressures should be obtained in all four extremities. Although uncommon, coarctation of the aorta may be missed until the patient presents with hypertension and/or cardiac failure. It may occur at any age from infancy through adulthood. Careful attention to appropriateness of cuff size and normal blood pressure values for age is essential.[18] Examination should include a careful funduscopic inspection for evidence of vasculopathy and/or papilledema. Exudates can be seen in children as they are in adults. A full neurologic examination is useful as well, because of the high frequency of neurologic signs as part of the presentation of hypertensive emergency. Similarly, careful palpation of the abdomen for masses or tenderness in the flanks may be extremely helpful in diagnosing polycystic kidney disease, cystic dysplasia, or tumors involving the kidney or adrenal gland. The rare patient with hypertensive emergency secondary to hydronephrosis or renal vein thrombosis may also be identified in this way. If the child is quiet, auscultation for abdominal bruits may be productive in directing one toward renal artery stenosis. Skin striae and café-au-lait spots may be useful in directing the clinician's attention to Cushing's syndrome and neurofibromatosis, respectively.

Laboratory studies are important, initially, to gauge the presence of coexisting disease as well as to alert the clinician to a possible etiology. Abnormal blood count with indication of microangiopathic hemolytic anemia and thrombocytopenia suggests a diagnosis of hemolytic-uremic syndrome. More subtly, however, the presence of normocytic, normochromic anemia could indicate the present of chronic renal failure. Elevated blood urea nitrogen and serum creatinine are obviously of importance. The presence of hyperphosphatemia, particularly with hypocalcemia, is highly suggestive of renal failure that has been present for at least 1 to 2 weeks. Conversely, hypokalemia with an elevated serum bicarbonate is helpful in alerting one to the possibility of a renal artery stenosis, as chronic release of angiotensin results in hyperaldosteronism or, less likely, a primary aldosterone-producing tumor.

A renal ultrasound can usually be obtained expeditiously, and is perhaps the most useful radiologic investigation. A rapid diagnosis of urinary obstruction or polycystic kidney disease is therefore possible. Small contracted kidneys which are hyperechoic will generally indicate the presence of chronic renal failure. Conversely, normal or enlarged kidneys which are hypoechoic, indicating the presence of edema, alert the clinician to a high probability of acute renal disease. While a Doppler study of the renal arteries is not definitive, an abnormal examination may play a powerful roll in directing the clinician's attention toward the presence of renal artery stenosis.[12]

Electrocardiogram and echocardiogram are important, in that they aid the physician in determining cardiac status at the time of the hypertensive crisis, and they may uncover evidence of longstanding hypertension. Characteristically, left posterior wall and septal hypertrophy are indicative of hypertension that has been present for at least 6 months.

In general, treatment of the hypertensive emergency should take precedence over, or at least be performed at the same time as, treatment for the underlying condition. With a few exceptions, decisions regarding the type of therapy chosen and the aggressiveness of therapy may be made regardless of the etiology. This means that diagnostic maneuvers may often be performed in a safer, more leisurely atmosphere. One obvious exception to this rule is when the hypertension has occurred from a catecholamine-producing tumor, particularly a pheochromocytoma. Treatment of this condition is specific, and alternatives are potentially dangerous. The use of β-adrenergic blockade, for example, while perhaps helpful in hypertensive crises of other etiologies, may very likely exacerbate the hypertension in a patient with a pheochromocytoma and lead to an intracranial catastrophe. With pheochromocytoma, α-adrenergic blockade or, if a positive diagnosis has not been made, calcium channel blockers or direct-acting vasodilators may be used to gently lower blood pressure while further diagnostic tests are performed. Similarly, a patient with severe renal artery stenosis should be treated cautiously with angiotensin-converting enzyme (ACE) inhibitors, as aggressive treatment may result not only in too rapid a lowering of blood pressure, but ischemia of the affected kidney, with consequent renal failure. This is particularly likely when the renal artery stenosis involves a renal transplant. With the exception of the above, diagnostic maneuvers are not critical. Studies that should be performed at the time of presentation are outlined in Table 3.

A complete listing of diagnostic studies that are appropriate for evaluation of hypertension in children is beyond the scope of this chapter. Suffice it to say that a definitive examination is best left to circumstances in which the child is stabilized, the blood pressure is reduced to an acceptable level, and the immediate danger has been removed. The studies outlined in Table 3 should adequately provide enough information in almost all circumstances to proceed with treatment. Table 4 provides a brief summary of appropriate diagnostic studies, other than those listed above, that may be performed more leisurely and applied to conditions that are likely to result in hypertensive emergency.

Table 3

Initial Evaluation of Patients with Hypertensive Crisis

Complete blood count with platelet count
Examination of the peripheral blood smear
Serum chemistries, including:
   electrolytes
   blood urea nitrogen, serum creatinine
   calcium, phosphate, alkaline phosphatase
   albumin
Urinalysis
Renal ultrasound with Doppler examination
Electrocardiogram, echocardiogram

Table 4

Definitive Diagnostic Maneuvers

Chronic renal failure:
   24-hour urine for creatinine and protein (to determine the degree of renal damage)
   serum C3, C4 complement (for diagnosis of systemic lupus erythematosus, acute postinfectious glomerulonephritis, membranoproliferative glomerulonephritis)
   renal biopsy (whenever the etiology is unknown)
   radionuclide scan (to determine relative dysfunction)

Pheochromocytoma:
   24 hour urinary collection for VMA, HVA, catecholamine, and metanephrine
   serum catecholamines
   radionuclide examination

Renal artery stenosis:
   renal scan with ACE inhibitor
   digital subtraction arteriography

ACE = angiotensin-converting enzyme; HVA = homovanillic acid; VMA = vanillylmandelic acid.

Management: General Principles

The key to treating children who present with hypertensive crises is the placement of the patient into a controlled and monitored environment. Prompt admission to a pediatric intensive care unit is crucial. Only in such an environment can there be careful monitoring of the patients' condition. A quiet, calm environment is often very helpful, not only for reducing anxiety on the part of the child and family, but for mild reduction of blood pressure. Continuous monitoring of vital signs is mandatory. Careful measurement of fluid and electrolyte intake and urinary output is critical, as are frequent weight measurements. This is particularly true under circumstances in which hypertension is associated with impairment of renal function. Many experts routinely place intra-arterial catheters for continuous blood pressure measurement.[19] These devices have the advantage of permitting continuous, accurate evaluation of blood pressure, unaffected by the patients' movement, which is common in the pediatric population. Careful attention must be paid, however, to ensure that monitoring is carried out with a consistent relationship between the arterial line and the level of the heart at the right atrium. Discrepancies between the transducer height and the heart can result in erroneous blood pressure measurements, as can dampening of the waveform from partial catheter occlusion.

The immediate goal for control of hypertensive emergencies is the prompt, controlled reduction of blood pressure to safe levels. Unfortunately, precise definition of "safe" has not been established. Various recommendations have been made, essentially all resulting from experience with adult patients. It is advised that mean arterial pressure be lowered no more than 20% to 25% or not to below 100 mm Hg. One study[5] in children demonstrated conclusively that patients whose blood pressure is reduced by one third, toward the eventual desired level, experience significantly fewer adverse effects than those in whom blood pressure was returned to "normal" in the first 24 hours. Of particular significance was an increased frequency of transient and even permanent visual loss in patients whose blood pressures were returned to normal too rapidly. Similarly, too rapid a drop in blood pressure may result in acute renal failure.[20] In general, these authors have found it safe to lower mean arterial pressure below 120 mm Hg in patients whose mean blood pressure was much higher. In most circumstances, it may be lowered to a mean arterial pressure of 100 mm Hg.

Pharmacologic Therapy

There are a variety of agents available for the treatment of hypertensive emergen-

Table 5

Drugs for Hypertensive Emergencies in Children

Intravenous Medications	Dose
Nicardipine	infusion: 1–5 μg/kg/min
	bolus: 0.03 mg/kg
Sodium nitroprusside	0.5–8 μg/kg/min
Labetalol	infusion: 1–3 mg/kg/h
	bolus: 0.2–1 mg/kg
Diazoxide	1–3 mg/kg/dose
Enalaprilat	5–10 μg/kg (intravenous)
Oral Medications	*Dose*
Nifedipine	0.15–0.25 mg/kg/dose
Minoxidil	0.05–0.2 mg/kg/day
Clonidine	0.005–0.01 mg/kg/dose
Isradipine	0.1 mg/kg/dose (BID or TID)
Enalapril	0.01–0.05 mg/kg/dose (BID, TID)

BID = twice daily; TID = three times daily.

cies in children. Unfortunately, for many of these agents there is only limited published experience, especially in the pediatric age range. The classes of hypertensive agents that are most useful include: the dihydropyridine calcium channel blockers, direct-acting vasodilators, ACE inhibitors, and, to a lesser extent, α- and β-adrenergic blocking agents. Table 5 lists these medications and recommended dosing guidelines for children.

Nicardipine

This calcium channel blocker has been extremely effective for the controlled reduction of blood pressure in children.[21,22] Nicardipine, like nifedipine (see below), is a dihydrophyridine derivation, but it is available for intravenous administration. The usual starting dose is 5 μg/kg/min. When adequate control of blood pressure is achieved, the dose is reduced; most children are maintained on 1 to 3 μg/kg/min. As with other calcium channel blockers, the effectiveness of this drug results from its ability to prevent the movement of calcium from the sarcoplasmic reticulum into the intracellular space, thus blocking contraction of smooth muscle. It therefore reduces blood pressure by selectively dilating peripheral arteries. The result is a prompt reduction in peripheral vascular resistance. As with other dihydropyridines, nicardipine reduces peripheral vascular resistance with minimal effects on myocardial contractility and therefore does not reduce cardiac output.

When administered intravenously, nicardipine has a rapid onset of action (1 to 2 minutes) with a half-life of approximately 40 minutes. Blood pressure control is even, and excessive hypotension is unusual. Should an excessive drop in blood pressure occur, it can be reversed rapidly by the administration of fluid or calcium. Due to the limited incidence of excessive hypotension, this agent can be used without the need for invasive intra-arterial monitoring of blood pressure. Unlike other vasodilators such as sodium nitroprusside (SNP) (see below), a significant compensatory increase in heart rate does not occur; thus there is a limited need to add a β-adrenergic blocking agent to control heart rate. Limitations of this agent are those common to other vasodilators, and it must be used with caution in patients with space-occupying intracranial lesions or other conditions affecting intracranial compliance, as it may increase intracranial pressure. As a direct vasodilator, nicardipine may inhibit hypoxic pulmonary vasoconstriction, increase ventilation-perfusion mismatch/shunt fraction, and decrease oxygenation in patients with atelectasis or pulmonary parenchymal disease.

Sodium Nitroprusside

Precise control of blood pressure is also possible with intravenous SNP. With continuous infusion of this agent, by taking advantage of SNP's very short half-life, blood pressure can be titrated rapidly to the desired level. Onset of action is virtually instantaneous. Discontinuation of the drug results in a return to previous blood pressure levels within 30 to 60 seconds. As photodegradation may occur, the solution must be wrapped, most commonly in aluminum foil.

The mechanism of action of nitroprusside is by metabolism to nitric oxide, stimulating the guanylate cyclase system with an increase in intracellular cyclic guanosine monophosphate and peripheral vasodilatation. Unlike nicardipine, this agent dilates both arteries and veins, resulting in reduction of preload and afterload. Due to the drop in systemic vascular resistance, a reflex stimulation of the sympathetic nervous system occurs, leading to tachycardia. Control of the increase in heart rate may require the addition of a β-adrenergic blocking agent such as propranolol or esmolol. As with nicardipine, this agent should be used with caution in patients who have increased intracranial pressure or pulmonary diseases.

Nitroprusside is metabolized initially to cyanide, which is transported to the liver and metabolized to thiocyanate via the hepatic rhodanase system. Thiocyanate is then excreted by the kidneys.[23] Toxicity related to these two compounds may occur with prolonged use or high infusion rates. Neurologic symptoms including vomiting, nausea, disorientation, hallucination, and anorexia may result from the accumulation of thiocyanate. This problem occurs more commonly in patients with renal failure.

Cyanide toxicity inhibits oxidative phosphorylation at the cellular level, resulting in a metabolic acidosis. Cyanide also increases the response of smooth muscle to norepinephrine, thereby increasing blood pressure and necessitating an increased dose of SNP. With prolonged infusions, cyanide and thiocyanate levels should be monitored.

Labetalol

This agent may be administered either intravenously (bolus or continuous infusion) or orally. When administered by bolus infusion, effects may be seen within 5 to 10 minutes. More prolonged control of blood pressure can be achieved by following the bolus with a continuous infusion. An initial dose of 0.2 to 1 mg/kg may be given safely to most patients. Continuous infusion dosage ranges from 1 to 3 mg/kg/h.

Labetalol works primarily through β-adrenergic blockade, with approximately 10% to 15% α-adrenergic blockade. It also has selective β_2-agonist activity in the peripheral vasculature. As a result, while the primary mechanism of action is the reduction of cardiac output, there is some peripheral vasodilation. While this drug is very useful for the treatment of hypertensive emergencies, it is somewhat less potent than nicardipine and SNP. A significant limiting factor is its potential for inducing bronchospasm in patients who have asthma, or worsening cardiac failure in patients with diminished left ventricular function. However, labetalol is relatively safe for patients with renal disease, as it is metabolized entirely in the liver. Additionally, unlike the direct-acting vasodilators, labetalol does not increase intracranial pressure or interfere with hypoxic pulmonary vasoconstriction.

Diazoxide

There is an abundance of experience with the use of this vasodilator in children. Diazoxode is effective with a prompt clinical response. Onset of action is within 1 to 5 minutes with a duration of response as long as 12 hours. Diazoxide is a potent peripheral vasodilator. However, because of its somewhat unpredictable influence on blood pressure, with a propensity to cause hypotension and a relatively long duration of action, it has generally been replaced by other agents, particularly nicardipine and SNP. Additional limitations to its use include inhibition of insulin release leading to hyperglycemia and fluid retention as seen with other vasodilators. Following initial use of diazoxide, a potent diuretic agent, preferably a loop diuretic, is recommended.

Enalapril

Enalapril is an ACE inhibitor. Agents in this group may be useful for controlling hypertension that is suspected to result from high levels of renin. Following oral administration, enalapril is converted to its active form, enalaprilat. The latter agent, or prodrug, is also available for intravenous administration.

Children most likely to respond to enalapril are those with renal artery stenosis or a mass lesion of the kidney, which reduces perfusion to a portion of the organ. Renin may play a major role in malignant hypertension following a renal transplant. Unfortunately, the use of this agent poses a significant risk because many patients with hypertensive emergencies are also volume-contracted. In such patients, a sudden, unexpected drop in blood pressure may occur.

In patients experiencing reduced perfusion to the kidney, enalapril can reduce perfusion even further. For example, if hypertension is secondary to a stenotic anastomosis in a renal transplant patient, the ACE inhibitors may precipitate acute renal failure. The ACE inhibitors preferentially dilate the efferent arteriole of the glomerulus and thereby can reduce perfusion pressure and glomerular filtration if there is disease in the vascular system proximal to the glomerulus (the afferent arteriole). In this setting, the preferential dilation of the efferent arteriole reduces the glomerular filtration pressure. Because of these problems and a somewhat prolonged onset time of 30 to 60 minutes, even with intravenous administration, enalapril is not commonly used for hypertensive emergencies.

Fenoldopam

This agent is the most recently released (spring 1998) intravenous agent for the control of blood pressure.[24] It is a selective, postsynaptic dopamine$_1$ receptor agonist with minimal or no effects on the α-/β-adrenergic and the dopamine$_2$ receptors. As such, it acts as a peripheral vasodilator. Its advantages include the fact that it has no toxic metabolites, and that it produces beneficial effects on renal blood flow, glomerular filtration rate, and cardiac output. Unlike SNP, there is no associated increase in heart rate. Although there is some clinical information available concerning its use in adults, to date there are limited data concerning its use in children. In the adult population, onset times have varied from 10 to 15 minutes with infusion rates of 0.05 to 0.3 µg/kg/min. Based on its pharmacologic effects, it appears that fenoldopam may be a useful agent for the pediatric population, especially for those with underlying renal dysfunction for whom the increase in renal blood flow may be particularly beneficial.

Nifedipine

This oral antihypertensive agent is frequently recommended for the treatment of hypertensive emergencies in children. Like nicardipine, it is a dihydropyridine derivative. Onset is quite rapid for an oral drug, at 20 to 30 minutes. While some have recommended sublingual administration of this agent by drawing out the liquid from the capsule, there is little evidence that the drug is absorbed across the mucus membrane. This agent is frequently used for treating hypertension in asymptomatic children who can take oral medication. As its duration of action is fairly short (3 to 4 hours), repeated doses may be necessary. As a result, there may be considerable fluctuation of blood pressures. Absorption is best when the drug is not administered with food. Like nicardipine, the primary effect of nifedipine is from a reduction in peripheral vascular resistance. There is a modest increase in cardiac output. Occasional patients will complain of headache and some may develop pedal edema. Unfortunately, nifedipine has a predilection to reduce blood pressure very rapidly. It may, in fact, reduce blood pressure to normal values in a very short period of time, resulting in adverse effects (see above). As a result, it has recently been recommended that nifedipine not be used for hypertensive crises.[25]

Isradipine

Like nifedipine, isradipine is a dihydropyridine calcium channel antagonist. In contrast to nifedipine, its therapeutic effect is substantially longer following oral administration, lasting 8 to 12 hours. Consequently, a more even control of blood pressure may be achieved with isradipine than with nifedipine. An additional advantage is increased dosing flexibility. Immediate-release nifedipine is available as a liquid-containing capsule. The dosage can be controlled in small children by aspirating the liquid from the capsules. However, this is difficult for parents and hospital personnel. Fortunately, isradipine is also commercially available in 2.5- and 5-mg powder-filled capsules. This powder may be placed in a stable suspension,[26] providing substantial convenience in administration and allowing the administration of precise doses based on the patient's weight. The therapeutic indication and limitations are similar to those of other dihydropyridine calcium channel blockers.

Minoxidil

This vasodilator has been used for many years in children who are able to take oral medications. Onset of action is within 30 minutes with a duration of 1 to 2 days. For a variety of reasons the response is somewhat less predictable than that of intravenous agents. Reflex tachycardia and fluid retention are major limiting side effects. It is generally recommended that β-adrenergic antagonists and loop diuretics be given simultaneously with minoxidil. Reflex tachycardia is routinely seen and this limits minoxidil's effectiveness in the absence of β-adrenergic blockade. Marked fluid retention may result in edema while hirsutism is a cosmetic concern.

Miscellaneous Agents

There are several other drugs that have been previously advocated for hypertensive emergencies. Agents such as trimethaphan (a ganglionic-blocking agent) and phentolamine or phenoxybenzamine (peripheral α-adrenergic antagonists) are rarely, if ever, indicated in children. These agents are useful only when there is known catecholamine excess, as from a pheochromocytoma. Agents such as reserpine and hydralazine have similarly been superseded by newer agents. The latter is no longer routinely available for intravenous use.

While some have advocated the use of central-acting α-agonists such as clonidine and α-methyl-dopa, it would appear that these drugs have been superseded by the more effective recently introduced agents. Advantages of the central-acting agents include a lack of rebound tachycardia and limited effects on intracranial pressure and hypoxic pulmonary vasoconstriction. Clonidine is relatively inexpensive and has a relatively rapid onset of action, but is somewhat difficult to control. Of particular concern with this agent, is its propensity for rebound hypertension following discontinuation. However, clonidine does offer options for the route of dosing, with both oral and transdermal preparations and the recent release of an intravenous preparation. The latter preparation has not been marketed for control of blood pressure, but rather as an analgesic agent for use in epidural anesthesia.

Summary

Hypertensive emergencies are uncommon, but when identified require careful and knowledgeable management. Prompt institution of treatment should take priority over investigative work-up. A carefully controlled intensive care environment is of major importance for the management of this condition. A variety of pharmacologic agents are available for control of blood pressure. Regardless of the agent chosen, blood pressure reduction should be controlled carefully. A partial lowering of blood pressure is essential. A rapid return to a normal blood pressure should be avoided.

References

1. Sanders AB. Hypertensive emergencies. *Am Fam Physician* 1991;44:1767–1774.
2. Sinaiko AR. Treatment of hypertension in children. *Pediatr Nephrol* 1994;8:603–609.
3. Tepel M, Zidek W. Hypertensive crisis: Pathophysiology, treatment and handling of complications. *Kidney Int* 1998;64:S2–S5.
4. Ingerfinger JR. Hypertension. In *Pediatric Kidney Disease*. 2nd ed. Boston: Little Brown and Company; 1978:1899–1900.
5. Deal JE, Barratt TM, Dillon NJ. Management of hypertensive emergencies. *Arch Dis Child* 1992;67:1089–1092.
6. Proulx F, Lacroix J, Farrell CA, Gauthier M. Convulsions and hypertension in children: Differentiating cause from effect. *Crit Care Med* 1993;21:1541–1546.
7. Kitiyakara C, Guzmann N. Malignant hypertension and hypertensive emergencies. *J Am Soc Nephrol* 1998;9:133–142.
8. Jones BV, Egelhoff JC, Patterson RJ. Hypertension encephalopathy in children. *Am J Neuroradiol* 1997;18:101–106.
9. Wright RR, Matthews KD. Hypertension encephalopathy in childhood. *J Child Neurol* 1996;11:193–196.
10. Sulochanal A, Asirvadam C, et al. Hypertension in childhood. *Ann Acad Med India* 1981;10:485–493.
11. Wells TG, Belsha CW. Pediatric renovascular hypertension. *Curr Opin Pediatr* 1996;8:128–134.
12. Stanley JC, Zelenock GB, Messina LM, Wakefield TW. Pediatric renal vascular hypertension: A 30 year experience of operative treatment. *J Vasc Surg* 1995;21:212–226.
13. Koumar P, Arora P, Kher V, et al. Malignant hypertension in children in India. *Nephrol Dial Transplant* 1996;11:1261–1266.
14. Miles J, Groshong T, Hakami N, et al. Congenital mesoblastic nephroma with hypertension, hypokalemia, and hyperreninemia. *J Pediatr* 1977;91:837–839.
15. McVicar M, Carman C, Chandra M, et al. Hypertension secondary to renin-secreting juxtaglomerular jell tumor: Case report and review of thirty eight cases. *Pediatr Nephrol* 1993;7:404–412.
16. Ekim M, Tumer N, Atmaca L, et al. Pseudoxanthoma elasticum: A rare cause of hypertension in children. *Pediatr Nephrol* 1998;12:183–185.
17. Faulkner B. The hypertensive adolescent. *Pediatr Ann* 1989;18:570–577.
18. Update on the 1987 Task Force Report on

High Blood Pressure in Children and Adolescents: A Working Group Report from the National High Blood Pressure Education Program, National High Blood Education Program Working Group on Hypertension Control in Children and Adolescence. *Pediatrics* 1996;88:649–658.
19. Prisant LM, Carr AA, Hawkins DW. Treating hypertensive emergencies. *Postgrad Med* 1993;93:92–110.
20. Greene TP, Nevins TE, Houser MT, et al. Renal failure as a complication of acute hypertensive therapy. *Pediatrics* 1981;67:850–854.
21. Tobias JD. Nicardipine: Applications in anesthesia practice. *J Clin Anesth* 1995;7:1–9.
22. Michael J, Groshong T, Tobias JD. Nicardipine for hypertensive emergencies in children with renal disease. *Pediatr Nephrol* 1998; 12: 40–42.
23. Sinako AR. Pharmacologic management of childhood hypertension. *Pediatr Clin North Am* 1993;40:195–212.
24. Post JB, Frishman WH. Fenoldopam: A new dopamine agonist for the treatment of hypertensive urgencies and emergencies. *J Clin Pharmacol* 1998;38:2–13.
25. Truttmann AC, Zehnder-Schlapbach RK, Bianchetti MG. A moratorium should be placed on the use of short-acting nifedipine for hypertensive crisis. *Pediatr Nephrol* 1998; 12:259–261.
26. MacDonald JL, Johnson CE, Jacobson P. Stability of isradipine in extemporaneously compounded oral liquid. *Am J Hosp Pharmacol* 1994;51:2409–2411.

Chapter 19

Infectious Disease Issues in the Pediatric Intensive Care Unit Patient

Sayonara Pérez Mato, MD and Sara S. Viessman, MD

Introduction

Infectious disease remains a primary cause of morbidity and mortality for patients in the pediatric intensive care unit (PICU). Infectious disease may be the primary disease process necessitating admission to the PICU, or it may arise as a nosocomial problem in patients admitted for other reasons. Regardless of the scenario, prompt recognition, identification of the source of the infection, and the institution of appropriate antibiotic therapy are mandatory to prevent severe sequelae or mortality. This chapter presents some of the more common primary and secondary infections encountered in the PICU, and provides suggestions for the initial work-up and antibiotic therapy.

Sepsis/Septic Shock

Sepsis refers to the clinical presentation of the systemic inflammatory response syndrome that occurs as a response to invasion of the host by infectious agents or to the presence of endotoxin lipopolysaccharide in the bloodstream. The signs and symptoms of the systemic inflammatory response syndrome are listed in Table 1. Early recognition is critical, as classic signs and symptoms may be absent or delayed due to compensatory mechanisms. Unrecognized or untreated sepsis may progress to septic shock. In turn, sepsis-induced hypotension and tissue hypoperfusion may lead to cellular hypoxia and lactic acidosis. As a result, multiorgan dysfunction syndrome may ensue, despite successful microbial eradication. In addition, septic shock frequently is associated with disseminated intravascular coagulopathy because of widespread activation of the coagulation pathways. Early recognition and optimal treatment of sepsis is mandatory to prevent irreversible cellular damage.

The morbidity and mortality of septic shock in infants and children vary with age, inoculum size and virulence of the specific infecting microorganisms, immunologic status and magnitude of the inflammatory host response, presence or absence of underlying diseases, and the timing of optimal antimicrobial and intensive care therapies.

Isolation of the organism responsible for sepsis is essential for providing optimal antimicrobial therapy. Initial work-up includes the following:

Complete blood count with manual white blood cell (WBC) differential, and platelet counts.

Blood cultures, prior to initiating antibiotic therapy, whenever possible.

Table 1

Signs and Symptoms of Sepsis/Septic Shock

Signs	Symptoms
Early	poor feeding
tachycardia	altered consciousness:
tachypnea	lethargy or irritability
hyperthermia or hypothermia	confusion
leukocytosis or leukopenia + bandemia	combativeness
Late	
respiratory distress/apnea	
decreased peripheral perfusion:	
mottled skin	
cool extremities	
weak peripheral pulses	
increased capillary refill time >2 seconds	
decreased urine output <1 mL/kg/h	
hypotension	
disseminated intravascular coagulopathy (DIC)	

Anaerobic cultures when an intra-abdominal source of infection is suspected.

Urine for urinalysis, microscopic examination, and culture.

Cerebrospinal fluid (CSF), if the patient's condition allows, for cell count, gram stain, glucose, protein and culture. (Hold any additional CSF for future tests.)

Serum electrolytes, glucose, blood urea nitrogen (BUN), creatinine, ionized calcium and magnesium, lactate, arterial blood gases/venous blood gases (ABG/VBG). Hepatic transaminases, prothrombin time (PT), partial thromboplastin time (PTT), fibrinogen, and d-dimer, if appropriate.

Chest radiograph. Echocardiogram, if indicated.

If central lines are in place, blood cultures should be obtained through the catheters and from a peripheral site if possible. The presence of persistently positive cultures may require line removal. Changing the central line over a wire remains controversial, but if done, the tip of the central line should be cultured.

Prompt institution of empiric antimicrobial therapy.

Antibiotics should be administered as soon as a diagnosis of septic shock is suspected. Appropriately obtained cultures and susceptibility testing will assist in adjusting empiric coverage to optimize therapy. When venous access cannot be established immediately, antibiotics may be administered via an intraosseous needle. The etiologic agents vary according to age, immune status, and place of microbial acquisition (community-acquired versus nosocomially acquired) as depicted in Table 2.

Early-onset neonatal sepsis presents during the first week of life and is related to maternal risk factors such as prolonged rupture of membranes, premature labor, chorioamnionitis, and presence of maternal fever in the immediate postpartum period. It has a high mortality (5% to 20%), and is frequently associated with pneumonia. Late-onset neonatal sepsis occurs after 1 week of age. As with early-onset neonatal sepsis, the infecting organisms are those that colonize the mother. Although late-onset disease is associated with a lower risk of mortality (2% to 6%), a higher percentage (30%) of the affected neonates has associated meningitis.[1] Therefore, in this age group, the antimicrobial regimen should provide adequate coverage for meningitis until the diagnosis of meningitis has been excluded.

Table 2

Microorganisms Responsible for Sepsis in Infants and Children

Age Group or Clinical Status	Likely Pathogens
0–1 Month (neonates)	group B streptococcus (GBS) gram-negative enteric bacilli *Listeria monocytogenes* Enterococcus spp. gram-negative enteric bacilli *Staphylococcus aureus, epidermidis* *Candida* spp.
1–2 Months	includes pathogens from both neonates and 2-months to 12-year-old age groups
2 Months to 12 years	Streptococcus pneumoniae Staphylococcus aureus Neisseria meningitidis group A β-hemolytic streptococcus (GABHS) *Haemophilus influenzae* type b (Hib) gram-negative bacilli
>12 Years	*Streptococcus pneumoniae* *Staphylococcus aureus* GABHS *Neisseria meningitidis* gram-negative bacilli
Immunosuppression or nosocomial infection	*S. pneumoniae, H. influenzae* type b (Hib), *S. aureus*, gram-negative enteric bacilli, *Salmonella* spp., *Candida* spp., *Pseudomonas aeruginosa, Staphylococcus epidermidis*

Table 3 outlines the current recommendations for empiric antibiotic therapy for suspected sepsis and septic shock in the pediatric population.[2,3] Table 4 outlines suggested dosing regimens. The initial antibiotic therapy of the sick neonate includes ampicillin and gentamicin. This combination provides not only effective broad coverage for most pathogens encountered in this age group, but also synergistic bactericidal activity against group B streptococci. A suitable alternative therapeutic regimen would be ampicillin plus cefotaxime, especially if an aminoglycoside-resistant nosocomial organism is suspected. The use of cefotaxime is preferred over ceftriaxone in neonates because ceftriaxone can displace bilirubin from albumin-binding sites, thus potentially increasing the risk for hyperbilirubinemia. An antimicrobial agent such as clindamycin or metronidazole with broad anaerobic coverage should be added when an intra-abdominal infection is suspected.[2] Methicillin-resistant *Staphylococcus epidermidis* is a leading isolate among neonatal intensive care unit patients. Therefore, the addition of vancomycin to the empiric antimicrobial therapy should be considered for neonates who have a history of a central venous catheter or a recent stay in the neonatal intensive care unit, and who are toxic.

In the older infant and child, empiric therapy for serious nosocomial infection is based on the current prevalence and susceptibility pattern of resistant isolates within the hospital or in the community. In general, a combination of a semisynthetic antistaphylococcal penicillin (eg, nafcillin/oxacillin) or vancomycin if a central line is present, and

Table 3

Initial Empiric Antimicrobial Therapy for Infants and Children with Suspected Sepsis

Age Group or Clinical Status	First-Line Agents	Alternative Agents
0–1 Month	ampicillin + gentamicin	ampicillin + cefotaxime
nosocomial	vancomycin + cefotaxime (plus Amphotericin B, if indicated)	
1–2 Months	ampicillin + cefotaxime (plus vancomycin, if indicated)*	ampicillin + ceftriaxone (plus vancomycin, if indicated)*
2 Months to 12 Years	cefotaxime or ceftriaxone (plus vancomycin, if indicated)*	—
>12 Years	cefotaxime or ceftriaxone (plus vancomycin, if indicated)*	—
Immunosuppression or nosocomial infection	vancomycin + ceftazidime (plus amphotericin B, if indicated)	—

*Vancomycin should be added to the initial empiric regimen in any infant/child *suspected* of having pneumococcal meningitis, methicillin-resistant *Staphylococcus aureus* (MRSA) sepsis, methicillin-resistant *Staphylococcus epidermidis* (MRSE) sepsis, ampicillin-resistant Enterococcus spp. sepsis, and for critically ill children, including those with myopericarditis or severe multilobar pneumonia with hypoxia, or hypotension. Vancomycin should be discontinued as soon as clinically appropriate. Must reevaluate need for continuing vancomycin therapy beyond 72 hours when isolate(s) antibiotic-susceptibility testing is available.

an aminoglycoside (eg, gentamicin) or an extended-spectrum penicillin (eg, ticarcillin) is administered initially until a specific pathogen(s) is isolated. Coverage is adjusted according to susceptibility testing, normally within 72 hours after initiation of empiric therapy.

Broad-spectrum penicillins and aminoglycosides are frequently synergistic against gram-negative organisms, especially *Pseudomonas aeruginosa*. Ticarcillin and clavulanate potassium (Timentin®), an extended-spectrum penicillin with additional β-lactamase inhibitor activity to include *Staphylococcus aureus* and *Haemophilus influenzae* type b (Hib), represents a useful alternative agent in this setting.[1,4] In the clinically stable patient without central venous access, this agent can be used as initial empiric one-drug therapy until culture results are available.

In the United States and throughout the world, the prevalence of antibiotic-resistant *Streptococcus pneumococcus* is rapidly increasing. In some communities, as many as 30% of pneumococcal isolates are penicillin-nonsusceptible, 20% are resistant to penicillin, and 25% are nonsusceptible to third-generation cephalosporins such as cefotaxime or ceftriaxone.[5,6] The resistance of pneumococci to penicillins is not mediated by the production of β-lactamase. Instead, it is the result of multiple alterations in the affinity of the penicillin-binding proteins of the organism. These multiple changes in the penicillin-binding proteins account for the variation in the resistance of different strains of pneumococci to β-lactam antibiotics, including cefotaxime and ceftriaxone. Once the antibiotic cannot bind to the penicillin-binding protein of the bacteria, it is rendered ineffective to disrupt cell wall synthesis and unable to kill the organism. Resistant strains are increasingly being represented in invasive pneumococcal infections. Therefore, vancomycin is considered the drug of choice as empiric therapy for suspected invasive pneumococ-

Table 4

Initial Parenteral Dosages of Antimicrobial Agents in Suspected Sepsis

Antimicrobial Agent	Dosage*	Interval	Maximum Daily Dosage
Amphotericin B,† Fungizone®	1 mg/kg/day or	q24h	
	1.5 mg/kg/dose	qod	
cholesteryl sulfate (Amphotec®)	3–6 mg/kg/day	q24h	
liposomal (Abelcet®)	5 mg/kg/day	q24h	
Ampicillin‡	200–300 mg/kg/day	q6h	10–12 grams
Cefotaxime	150–300 mg/kg/day	q6–8h	10–12 grams
Ceftazidime	100–150 mg/kg/day	q8h	6 grams
Ceftriaxone	100 mg/kg/day	q12–24h	2–4 grams
Chloramphenicol§	75–100 mg/kg/day	q6h	3 grams
Clindamycin	20–40 mg/kg/day	q6–8h	2–4 grams
Doxycycline¶	2–5 mg/kg/day	q12–24h	200 mg
Gentamicin**	2.5 mg/kg/dose	q8–12h	500 mg
Meropenem	60–120 mg/kg/day	q8h	4 grams
Metronidazole	30 mg/kg/day	q6h	2–4 grams
Nafcillin	150–200 mg/kg/day	q6h	10–12 grams
Oxacillin	150–200 mg/kg/day	q6h	10–12 grams
Penicillin G	250–400,000 U/kg/day	q4–6h	20 million units
Tetracycline¶	20 mg/kg/day	q6h	2 grams
Ticarcillin	200–300 mg/kg/day	q4–6h	18–24 grams
Timentin® (ticarcillin/clavulanate)	200–300 mg/kg/day	q4–6h	18–24 grams
Vancomycin††	15 mg/kg/dose	q6–8h	2 grams

*Higher end of dosage range is indicated when meningitis is suspected.

†For treatment of systemic fungal infections, especially in immunocompromised patients. Impairment of renal function and bone marrow suppression are the best recognized complications of prolonged amphotericin B therapy. Lipid-based amphotericin B is associated with decreased renal toxicity and adverse effects. Potential neurologic toxicity exists with all formulations.

‡Neonatal dosing interval > 35 wk, q8h.

§Though chloramphenicol should not be used in neonates, and it is not commonly used since the introduction of third-generation cephalosporins, it is listed for those rare occasions when it will be used. Follow hematologic status for dose-related or idiosyncratic bone marrow suppression, rarely irreversible aplastic anemia. Drug interactions with phenytoin, phenobarbital, and rifampin. Therapeutic serum drug concentrations: *trough:* 5–15 mg/L for meningitis and 5–10 mg/L for other infections; *peak:* 15–25 mg/L for meningitis and 10–20 mg/L for other infections. Serum drug concentrations above 50–80 mg/L have been associated with "gray baby" syndrome and impaired myocardial contractility. Consider only for patients with life-threatening allergic response after administration of β-lactam antibiotics.

¶May cause tooth enamel hypoplasia and discoloration in children <7 years of age. However, in the case of life-threatening infections, the benefits outweigh the risks.

**May cause nephrotoxicity and ototoxicity with high serum drug concentrations. The loop diuretics potentiate the ototoxicity of aminoglycosides. Adjust dose and/or dosing interval in patients with renal failure. Therapeutic drug concentrations (gentamicin); *trough:* <1.5 mg/L; *peak:* 6–8 mg/L.

††Neonatal dosing interval >35 wk, q12h. May cause nephrotoxicity and ototoxicity with high serum drug concentrations, and allergy from histamine release. "Red man syndrome" associated with rapid i.v. infusion (<60 minutes). Use diphenhydramine to reverse red man syndrome and lengthen i.v. infusion time to 120 minutes. Adjust dose and/or dosing interval in patients with renal failure. Therapeutic drug concentrations; *trough:* 5–10 mg/L; *peak:* 25–35 mg/L. Obtain urinalysis, serum BUN and creatinine when therapy is started and follow at regular intervals.

cal infection in geographic areas where resistant pneumococci are common. Alternative antibiotics such as imipenem-cilastatin are indicated if vancomycin administration does not result in clinical improvement or cure. Meropenem, another carbapenem, may represent an useful alternate drug for these severe infections, as it lacks the epileptogenic properties of imipenem-cilastatin.

Optimal management of infants and children with sepsis is twofold and includes the following: 1) stabilization of cardiorespiratory status and tissue oxygen delivery by airway management and cardiovascular resuscitation including the administration of parenteral isotonic fluids, inotropic agents, oxygen, and mechanical ventilatory support, as required, and 2) prompt administration of effective antimicrobial agents with draining or early removal of infected foci, when indicated. The eventual clinical application of potential adjunctive immunomodulating agents, currently being developed, could improve the outcome for these patients in the future.[4] To date, the benefits of high-dose corticosteroid therapy in the treatment of endotoxin shock remain unproven. The general supportive care of the patient with septic shock includes attention to nutritional and metabolic requirements as well.

Several less common diseases can present with severe fulminant systemic illness. Early recognition and prompt treatment may improve the child's outcome. Clinically, the majority of these diseases present as toxic shock syndromes defined as acute, febrile, exanthematous illnesses with multisystem involvement and organ dysfunction (cardiovascular collapse, renal failure, myocardial dysfunction, hepatic insufficiency, adult respiratory distress syndrome, encephalopathy, and disseminated intravascular coagulation). The severity of associated multisystem organ dysfunction is directly related to the degree of loss of intravascular volume and hypotension secondary to the extensive capillary inflammation and leakage of fluid from the intravascular space caused by inflammatory mediators. Thus, supportive care of the patient cannot be overemphasized. Most patients improve rapidly when aggressive fluid management (plasma expansion), optimal antimicrobial treatment, and management of focal infection are instituted early. To date, the benefits of high-dose corticosteroid therapy in the treatment of endotoxin-related shock remain unproven.[7] Therefore, short courses of methylprednisolone or dexamethasone should be restricted to the hypotensive patient who is unresponsive to conventional forms of therapy. Likewise, intravenous immunoglobulin use to provide antitoxin antibodies should probably be reserved for patients with either streptococcal or staphylococcal toxic shock syndrome who continue to deteriorate despite adequate fluid administration, cardiovascular support, and the institution of appropriate antimicrobial therapy. The potential risks and benefits of either form of therapy must be considered for each patient.

In the evaluation of the severely ill child who has a rash, other aspects of the illness (eg, exposure, season, incubation period, geographic location, patient age, associated signs and symptoms) may be more important in the determination of the underlying etiologic agent than the cutaneous manifestations alone. The differential diagnosis of diseases presenting with the triad of fever, erythematous exanthem and shock is outlined in Table 5.

Invasive meningococcal disease deserves special consideration, as it can be fulminant in 10% to 20% of all cases. Morbidity consists of neurologic disability, limb loss, and/or need for skin grafting. Therapy must be specific, appropriate, and administered without delay, especially in those patients meeting three or more of the poor prognostic features outlined in Table 6, as their mortality approaches 85%.[8,9] With the identification of this group of patients, invasive monitoring techniques and rapid therapeutic action are likely to be instituted early, in anticipation of potential acute deterioration due to severe cardiovascular collapse secondary to high levels of circulating endotoxin.

These poor prognostic factors relate both to the virulence of the organism and to host resistance factors. It is thought that they are present in those patients whose neutrophils have failed to adequately mount an appropriate response or to localize the infection. Purpura fulminans and shock are uniformly poor prognostic signs. Death from invasive

Table 5
Differential Diagnosis of Fever + Exanthem + Hypotension

Disease Process	Exanthem Type	Initial Empiric Parenteral Antibiotic Therapy
Pneumococcal septicemia	macular → maculopapular → petechial	cefotaxime or ceftriaxone *plus* vancomycin*
Staphylococcal toxic shock/exfoliative syndromes	erythroderma maculopapular desquamation	nafcillin or oxacillin or vancomycin (*if MRSA is suspected*) *plus* clindamycin
Severe invasive GABHS infections: severe scarlet fever streptococcal toxic-like syndrome	macular maculopapular → petechial	nafcillin or oxacillin or cefotaxime/ceftriaxone *plus* clindamycin†
necrotizing cellulitis fasciitis‡	maculopapular, bullous, petechial/purpuric, *painful*	nafcillin or oxacillin or ceftriaxone or cefotaxime *plus* gentamicin *plus* clindamycin†
Acute meningococcemia	maculopapular → petechial → purpuric	cefotaxime or ceftriaxone (*pending sensitivity testing*)§
Rickettsial diseases: Rocky Mountain spotted fever (RMSF)	maculopapular → petechial	doxycycline or tetracycline or chloramphenicol
human ehrlichiosis	maculopapular → petechial	doxycycline or tetracycline
Leptospirosis	macular	high-dose penicillin G or doxycycline or tetracycline
Viral hemorrhagic shock	macular → maculopapular → petechial	none¶
Stevens-Johnson syndrome (erythema multiforme exudativum major)	ulcerative enanthem; maculopapular → bullous	none
Severe measles	maculopapular	none
Atypical measles	maculopapular → petechial	none
Drug reactions	maculopapular	none

(Must reevaluate need for continuing vancomycin therapy beyond 72 hours when isolate(s) antibiotic-susceptibility testing becomes available

†The coadministration of a protein synthesis inhibitor (ie, clindamycin, gentamicin) is indicated to inhibit toxin production by the organism.

‡Suspicion of necrotizing fasciitis warrants immediate surgical consultation for early extensive debridement of necrotic tissue. Initial empiric therapy should provide coverage for mixed aerobic and anaerobic infection until culture results are available.

§For penicillin-susceptible meningococcemia or meningitis, high-dose intravenous penicillin G is effective. Chloramphenicol is an alternative drug for patients with penicillin and cephalosporin allergies.

¶Antibiotic therapy is not indicated unless secondary bacterial (streptococcal/staphylococcal) infection of skin lesions is present.

GABHS = group A β-hemolytic streptococcus; MRSA = methicillin-resistant *Staphylococcus aureus*.

Table 6

Unfavorable Prognostic Factors in Meningococcal Disease

Petechiae present <12 hours before admission (rapidly progressive purpuric rash).
Presence of shock: SBP <70 mm Hg, age <4 years
　　　　　　　　　SBP <85 mm Hg, age ≥4 years
Absence of meningitis: <20 WBC/mm^3 CSF, infants and children
　　　　　　　　　　　<50 WBC/mm^3 CSF, neonates
Absence of leukocytosis: <10,000 WBC/mm^3 blood
Thrombocytopenia: <100,000 platelets/mm^3 blood
Base deficit >8

CSF = cerebrospinal fluid; SBP = systolic blood pressure; WBC = white blood cells.
From Stiehm ER, Damrosch DS. Factors in the prognosis of meningococcal infection. *J Pediatr* 1966;68:457–467; Niklasson PM, Lundbergh P, Strandell T. Prognostic factors in meningococcal disease. *Scand J Infect Dis* 1971;3:17–25; and Algren JT, Lal S, Cutliff SA, Richman BJ. Predictors of outcome in acute meningococcal infection in children. *Crit Care Med* 1993;21:447–452.

---

meningococcal disease is generally due to intractable shock. Disseminated intravascular coagulopathy can progress rapidly despite prompt and appropriate intervention. It should be treated with blood product replacement, as follows:

Fresh frozen plasma at 20 cc/kg/dose when PT and/or PTT values are prolonged, d-dimer is increased, or the patient is actively bleeding.
Cryoprecipitate if the serum fibrinogen concentration is less than 100 mg/dL.
Vitamin K for elevated PT.
Platelet transfusion for a platelet count less than 20,000/mm^3, a rapidly declining platelet count, or if the patient is actively bleeding.
Packed red blood cell transfusions as indicated to maintain an adequate hematocrit for oxygen delivery.

With all cases of meningococcal disease, eradicating nasopharyngeal colonization of the index case is important. The usual drug used for this purpose is rifampin. If the patient has been treated for meningococcal disease with cefotaxime or ceftriaxone, additional prophylactic therapy is not necessary. Chemoprophylaxis is recommended for household contacts of the index patient, young day care center contacts, and health care workers who have had direct exposure to index patient's nasopharyngeal secretions (eg, mouth-to-mouth resuscitation or unprotected contact during endotracheal intubation) (Table 7). Ill contacts should be evaluated immediately with a high suspicion for

Table 7

Meningitis Prophylaxis

Drug	Age Group	Dose	Duration
Rifampin*	≤1 month	5 mg/kg/dose PO q12h	4 doses
	>1 month	10 mg/kg/dose PO q12h	4 doses
	adults	600 mg PO q12h	4 doses
Ciprofloxacin†	adults	500 mg PO	single dose
Ceftriaxone‡	≤12 years	125 mg IM	single dose
	>12 years	250 mg IM	single dose

*Warn patients of side effects: orange staining of urine, sweat and tears (contact lenses), stimulation of liver microsomal enzymes, and reduction in levels of other concurrent medications (eg, oral contraceptives, anticoagulants, digoxin, phenytoin). Contraindicated in pregnancy.
†Not recommended for use in children due to evidence of cartilage damage in juvenile beagles. Contraindicated in pregnancy.
‡Drug of choice for pregnant contacts. May be indicated in children due to greater compliance
IM = intramuscular; PO = by mouth.

meningococcal disease, since chemoprophylaxis is not 100% effective.

Corticosteroid administration in invasive meningococcal disease is somewhat controversial. Clearly, corticosteroid treatment is indicated for patients with associated Waterhouse-Friderichsen syndrome (adrenal hemorrhage) and/or adrenal insufficiency. This group of patients usually presents with persistent hypotension despite aggressive volume resuscitation and inotropic support.

Meningitis

Meningitis is an inflammatory process of the meninges and usually is a result of viral or bacterial infection Approximately two thirds of diagnosed cases are viral and one third are bacterial. The most common viral agents are the nonpolio enteroviruses (coxsackieviruses A and B, enteroviruses, and echoviruses) and herpes simplex virus (HSV-1 and HSV-2). In the neonatal period, the three most common microorganisms that cause hematogenously acquired acute bacterial meningitis are group B streptococcus, gram-negative enteric bacilli, and *Listeria monocytogenes*. Beyond the neonatal period, *Streptococcus pneumoniae*, *Neisseria meningitidis*, and Hib predominate. Specific risk factors or patient conditions may predispose to meningitis with specific infectious agents (Table 8).

The prevalence of infection with penicillin- and cephalosporin-nonsusceptible strains of *S. pneumoniae* has increased worldwide in the past decade (see above). Invasive Hib among US children 4 years and younger has become rare as a result of widespread immunization of infants with Hib conjugate vaccines since 1990.

The route of infection in bacterial meningitis most commonly is hematogenous dissemination of organisms from a distant site of infection, often from the respiratory tract. Meningeal seeding with microorganisms follows the bacteremic period. Direct bacterial invasion of the meninges may occur from a contiguous focus of infection, as well. Once the microorganisms reach the CSF, they multiply rapidly and liberate cell wall or membrane components (endotoxin, teichoic acid, peptidoglycans) because of insufficient opsonic and phagocytic activity found within normal CSF. Neuropathologic changes (ie, injured vascular endothelium, augmented vascular permeability of the blood-brain barrier, vasogenic edema, cytotoxic edema, and interstitial edema, activation of the coagulation cascade, and neuronal damage) result from the bacterial products and the inflammatory response of the host to those products. The cytokines trigger increased cerebral blood flow and further edema formation, leading to increased intracranial pressure. The vasculitis and the increased intracranial pressure lead

Table 8

Risk Factors and Microorganisms Associated with Bacterial Meningitis

Risk Factor	Likely Microorganism
CSF leak (otorrhea, rhinorrhea)	S. pneumoniae, H. influenzae type b
Mastoiditis/sinusitis	S. pneumoniae, H. influenzae type b
Dermoid sinus tracts/meningomyelocele	Staphylococci, gram-negative enteric bacilli
Ventriculoperitoneal shunt, skull-orbital-sinus trauma	S. pneumoniae, N. meningitidis, H. influenzae type b (hematogenous); staphylococci, diphtheroids (contaminated VP shunt)
Osteomyelitis of the axial skeleton	S. aureus, group A streptococci, S. pneumoniae, H. influenzae type b
Asplenia (anatomic or functional)	S.pneumoniae, N. meningitidis, Salmonella spp.
Sickle-cell disease/hemoglobinopathies	S. pneumoniae, H. influenzae type b, Salmonella spp.
Terminal complement deficiencies (C5–C8)	N. meningitidis
Antibody deficiency states (including HIV)	S. pneumoniae, N. meningitidis, H influenzae type b
Impaired cellular immunity	L. monocytogenes, gram-negative bacilli

CSF = cerebrospinal fluid; HIV = human immunodeficiency virus; VP = ventriculoperitoneal.

to a subsequent decrease in cerebral blood flow. Venous and microvascular thrombosis may ensue due to activation of the coagulation cascade. The foramina of Magendie and Luschka can be obstructed by a purulent subarachnoid exudate that consists primarily of neutrophils, resulting in obstructive hydrocephalus. Meningitis can be associated with the release of antidiuretic hormone, causing water retention and a relative loss of sodium by the kidney, leading to further increases in intracranial pressure if excessive free water is administered during therapy.

Papilledema is uncommon in uncomplicated meningitis. When present, other diagnoses (brain abscess, epidural/subdural empyema) or a complication of meningitis (venous sinus thrombosis) should be sought. Deafness or disturbances in vestibular function are relatively common. Subdural effusions are also common during the acute illness. Several factors that have been associated with a poor prognosis (defined as neurologic sequelae, developmental delay, mental retardation, behavioral/learning problems, and permanent seizure disorder on long-term follow-up) include:

Coma at the time of admission.
Focal neurologic signs at the time of admission.
Focal seizures or seizures that are difficult to control.
Seizures that persist beyond the fourth hospital day.
Seizures that present late in the hospital course.
Purpura, shock, or hypothermia.

Clinical manifestations are often nonspecific and include irritability, poor feeding, and fever (Table 9). Nonspecific symptoms are especially common in neonates and infants. A lumbar puncture (LP) to obtain CSF (Table 10) should be done as soon as the possibility of meningitis is raised, unless there are specific contraindications to this procedure, such as:

Clinical signs of increased intracranial pressure in a patient with a closed fontanelle and closed sutures, or focal neurologic deficit. A cranial imaging study should be performed prior to LP to exclude intracranial space-occupying lesion.
Cardiovascular instability and respiratory insufficiency. In this setting, positioning for the LP can cause significant cardiorespiratory compromise, and it should be deferred until the patient is stable.
Thrombocytopenia (<50,000/mm3) or coagulation disorders.
Pyoderma/cellulitis overlying the lumbar vertebrae.

If the decision is made to delay LP, antibiotic therapy should be instituted immediately. If possible, blood can be obtained for culture and antibiotics can be administered. Examination of the CSF can be performed, and the diagnosis of meningitis can be made on other criteria including CSF cell count, gram stain, or latex agglutination studies that identify bacterial antigens in the CSF.

The remainder of the initial work-up includes:

Complete blood count with manual WBC differential, and platelets.
Blood cultures, prior to initiating antibiotic therapy, if possible.
Serum electrolytes, glucose, BUN, creatinine, ionized calcium and magnesium, lactate, ABG/VBG as indicated. Hepatic transaminases, PT, PTT, fibrinogen, and d-dimer, if appropriate.
Urine: microscopy, culture, specific gravity, electrolytes, osmolality (if inappropriate antidiuretic hormone secretion [SIADH] is suspected).
Rectal and nasopharyngeal swabs for viral cultures in those patients suspected of having viral meningitis.
Tuberculin skin test (PPD) in those patients suspected of having tuberculous meningitis.
Aspiration of joint effusion, abscess, paranasal sinus, mastoid bone, purpuric lesion, or purulent middle ear effusion, if appropriate (for gram stain, culture and susceptibility testing) to maximize identification of infecting organism.
Cranial imaging studies (computed tomography [CT] or magnetic reso-

Table 9

Clinical Manifestations in Infants and Children with Acute Bacterial Meningitis

Infants	Children
±Fever	Fever
Altered mental status:	Altered mental status:
irritability, restlessness	confusion, disorientation
decreased interaction	behavioral abnormalities
poor feeding	obtundation
lethargy	stupor
coma	coma
seizures	seizures
Meningeal irritation/increased ICP:	Meningeal irritation/increased ICP:
full/bulging fontanelle	nuchal rigidity
increased head circumference	positive Kernig + Brudzinski signs
diastasis of cranial sutures	headache, photophobia
cranial nerve abnormalities	cranial nerve abnormalities
irregular respiratory pattern + ↓ HR + ↑ BP	irregular respiratory pattern + ↓ HR + ↑ BP

Infants and Children

Respiratory: cough, coryza, sore throat, tachypnea, respiratory distress, apnea
Gastrointestinal: vomiting, anorexia, diarrhea, abdominal pain ± distention, heme-positive stools
Skin: maculopapular rash, petechial/purpuric rash
Musculoskeletal: arthralgia/myalgia
Hematological: DIC
Shock: mottled skin, slow capillary refill, tachycardia, hypotension

BP = blood pressure; DIC = disseminated intravascular coagulation; HR = heart rate; ICP = intracranial pressure.

Table 10

Cerebrospinal Fluid Findings in Acute Meningitis

CSF Finding	Aseptic/Viral	Bacterial	Partially Treated
Opening pressure* (mm H_2O)	normal	usually elevated (average, 300)	usually elevated
Cell count/mm†	usually 100–500	usually 500 to >1000	200–500
Predominant WBC	early PMNs late lymphocytes	PMNs (>50%)	PMNs or mononuclears
Gram stain smear‡	negative	usually positive	may be negative
Protein (mg/dL)	usually mildly elevated (50–100)	elevated (100–500)	normal or elevated
Glucose (mg/dL)	normal	low (<40)	low or normal
Bacterial culture	negative	usually positive (>90%)	often negative
Antigen-detection tests§	negative	positive	positive

CSF = cerebrospinal fluid; PMN = polymorphonuclear; WBC = white blood cell.

*Normal value: ≤180 mm H_2O. For the neonate, normal range: 90–110 mm H_2O. An opening pressure >200 mm H_2O warrants neurosurgical consultation for continuous ICP monitoring.
†After the neonatal period, a normal CSF should have ≤10 WBC/mm³ and *no* PMN leukocytes.
‡Gram stain is positive in 85% to 99% of patients without pretreatment with antibiotics and in 79% of pretreated patients with culture-proven bacterial meningitis.
§Detection of polysaccharide antigen by latex agglutination is most reliable for H. influenzae type b (85%–95%), followed by S. pneumoniae (50%–75%) and N. meningitidis (33%–50%).

nance imaging) prior to performing LP when an intracranial space-occupying lesion must be ruled out in the presence of signs of increased intracranial pressure or focal neurologic signs.

Chest radiograph may be helpful in disclosing a focus of infection.

Surgical drainage of wound infections following trauma or neurosurgery.

Removal of contaminated devices including ventriculoperitoneal shunts and central venous catheters.

Optimal antibiotic treatment requires that the drug have a bactericidal effect for sterilization of the CSF. Prompt institution of antimicrobial therapy is needed, given the potential for neurologic morbidity and mortality. Table 11 shows the current recommendations for initial empiric therapy for suspected acute bacterial meningitis in the pediatric population. As in sepsis, initial antibiotic therapy is based on the age of the patient and thereby the presumed infecting organism. In the neonatal period, ampicillin is needed to cover *Listeria monocytogenes* and enterococci. Cefotaxime is added to broaden coverage for resistant Hib. Therapy is modified to the most appropriate agent(s) following organism identification and antibiotic susceptibility testing. For dosages of specific antimicrobial agents refer to Table 4.

In the setting of suspected bacterial meningitis, vancomycin is added to a third-generation cephalosporin in patients 1 month of age and older (due to the increased prevalence of penicillin-resistant, cefotaxime-resistant, and ceftriaxone-resistant *S. pneumoniae* strains) in immunocompromised children or critically ill children; especially if gram-positive diplococci are seen on the CSF gram stain. If nonsusceptibility (intermediate level of resistance) to penicillin (minimum inhibitory concentration [MIC] 0.1 to 1.0 µg/mL) and cephalosporins (MIC 1 µg/mL for ceftriaxone or cefotaxime) is documented, treatment is continued with vancomycin, and rifampin is added to the regimen (Table 12).[10]

Vancomycin should not be administered alone, as CSF bactericidal concentrations are difficult to sustain, and it has a narrow therapeutic index and variable CSF penetration.[11] Rifampin also should not be given as monotherapy because resistance may develop during therapy.

For penicillin-allergic patients (history of anaphylaxis, urticaria, exfoliative dermatitis, or respiratory distress due to penicillin or other β-lactam antibiotics), agents that can be

Table 11

Initial Empiric Antimicrobial Therapy for Infants and Children with Suspected Bacterial Meningitis

Age Group or Clinical Status	Antimicrobial Agent
0–1 Month	ampicillin + cefotaxime
1–2 Months	vancomycin* + cefotaxime
2 Months to 12 Years	vancomycin* + cefotaxime or ceftriaxone
>12 Years	vancomycin* + cefotaxime or ceftriaxone
Impaired cellular immunity	ampicillin + ceftazidime
Immunosuppression or nosocomial infection	vancomycin* + ceftazidime
Head trauma, neurosurgery, or ventriculoperitoneal shunt	vancomycin* + ceftazidime

*Reevaluate need for continuing vancomycin therapy beyond 72 hours when isolate(s)' antibiotic-susceptibility testing becomes available.

Table 12

Modification of Antimicrobial Therapy for Bacterial Meningitis Caused by S. Pneumoniae Based on Quantitative Susceptibility Testing

S. Pneumoniae Susceptibility Testing	Antibiotic Management
Susceptible to PNC	D/C vancomycin start PNC *or* continue cefotaxime/ceftriaxone alone
Nonsusceptible to PNC *and* susceptible to cefotaxime/ceftriaxone	D/C vancomycin continue cefotaxime/ceftriaxone alone
Nonsusceptible to PNC *and* nonsusceptible to cefotaxime/ceftriaxone	Continue vancomycin + cefotaxime/ceftriaxone and add rifampin*

*Rifampin is added to the vancomycin and cefotaxime/ceftriaxone combination particularly if there is a delay in the expected clinical and/or bacteriologic response (lack of CSF sterilization).
CSF = cerebrospinal fluid; PNC = penicillin.

substituted for the penicillins and cephalosporins include chloramphenicol, vancomycin with rifampin, and meropenem. A cross-reactivity of approximately 10% to 15% has been noted for cephalosporins in penicillin-allergic patients. For meropenem-susceptible isolates, meropenem alone or in combination with other drugs may provide a satisfactory alternative for children older than 3 months who do not tolerate vancomycin. Cefuroxime should *not* be used to treat bacterial meningitis in children, due to delayed sterilization of the CSF, higher relapse during or after treatment, and more frequent sensorineural hearing loss demonstrated in clinical studies.

It is recommended that the duration of antibiotic therapy be tailored to the individual patient on the basis of the clinical (eg, patient afebrile for 5 days) and microbiologic (no organisms on CSF gram stain, sterile CSF cultures, and CSF WBC count ≤30% polymorphonucleocytes) evidence. Generally 10 days of treatment for uncomplicated pneumococcal and Hib meningitis, and 7 days for uncomplicated *N. meningitidis* meningitis. A repeat LP is indicated if there is no clinical improvement after 24 to 48 hours of therapy, particularly in patients with pneumococcal infection, to document a sterile culture and negative gram stain.

Approximately 40% of children with bacterial meningitis receive oral antibiotics prior to diagnosis because of presumed respiratory infection or possible occult bacteremia. As a rule, prior oral therapy usually does not markedly alter cell count or glucose and protein concentrations of the CSF (Table 10). However, children may present with different clinical findings compared with those without prior therapy including lesser fever, improved mental status, and a longer duration of symptoms before diagnosis.[12,13] Neither clinical course nor outcome is improved by prior treatment with oral antibiotics. In this era of increasing prevalence of multidrug-nonsusceptible strains of pneumococci, careful follow-up of infants and young children who are placed on oral antibiotics to treat respiratory infections including acute otitis media is mandatory. Those who fail to improve clinically may become bacteremic and subsequently develop sepsis and/or meningitis.[14,15]

The administration of anti-inflammatory agents such as dexamethasone (0.15 mg/kg/dose intravenously every 6 hours) for the first 2 days of antibiotic therapy, to be given shortly before or at the time of the first dose of intravenous antibiotics, appears to reduce the incidence of sensorineural hearing loss without increasing mortality or other complications in Hib meningitis. It is thought that by reducing inflammation, especially that which occurs after the initiation of therapy with β-lactam antibiotics, the incidence of adverse outcomes can be decreased. However, corticosteroid-mediated reduction in inflammation may potentially compromise the entry of antimicrobial agents into the CSF to the site of infection.

Dexamethasone has not shown a beneficial effect in either pneumococcal or meningococcal meningitis. It should not be used in infants younger than 6 weeks of age or in aseptic or "partially treated" meningitis.[16,17] The anti-inflammatory effects of dexamethasone might interfere with the clinical interpretation of signs and symptoms usually present in conditions that fail to respond to antibiotic therapy such as resistant *S. pneumoniae*, brain abscess, and mycobacterial or fungal infection. The decision to use dexamethasone in children with bacterial meningitis should be individualized. If it is used, careful and frequent observation of the patient is indicated. Gastrointestinal prophylaxis should always be used when corticosteroids are administered, to reduce the risk of gastrointestinal hemorrhage.

During the summer and fall, management of children with suspected aseptic meningitis does not need to include antibiotics based on the child's clinical appearance and the results of CSF cell count and chemistries. Repeat LP may be indicated in patients who appear clinically well and yet have a predominance of polymorphonuclear leucokytes on the initial LP. Repeat LP 8 to 12 hours later may show the shift to lymphocytes and thereby eliminate the need for hospitalization and antibiotic administration until cultures are negative. Based on the clinical presentation, some patients will be treated with cefotaxime/ceftriaxone until the CSF and blood cultures are negative. Vancomycin should *not* be used under these circumstances unless the child appears toxic and/or is hypotensive. Other forms of aseptic meningitis that require immediate therapy, such as tuberculous and herpes meningitis, may present initially with a clinical and CSF picture resembling that of viral meningitis. These entities must be kept in mind and appropriate therapy must be initiated early on if there are signs or symptoms suggestive of these processes.

Tuberculous Meningitis

Tuberculosis has reasserted its importance as a cause of morbidity among urban, minority, and foreign-born children in the United States. Nationally reported tuberculosis cases among children younger than 15 years of age increased 24% from 1985 through 1995.[18] Furthermore, tuberculosis in infants and children younger than 4 years of age is much more likely to disseminate. Eighty percent of the meningeal and 71% of the miliary disease occurs in young children. Tuberculous meningitis complicates approximately 0.5% of untreated primary tuberculosis infections in children, and it is still an important cause of death or significant neurologic disability.

Vigorous therapy for CNS tuberculosis should be initiated early whenever an increased index of suspicion is present, even in a child with a negative PPD skin reaction and a normal chest radiograph. Pulmonary or hilar disease will be evident on the chest x-rays in about 50% of the cases of tuberculous meningitis. Therefore, *when chest radiography findings are present in aseptic meningitis, the diagnosis of tuberculous meningitis should be considered*. The Mantoux skin test (PPD) is positive in less than 50% of cases of tuberculous meningitis.

Typically, the CSF findings in tuberculous meningitis are: increased opening pressure, low glucose (<50% of the serum concentration), raised protein concentration, and pleocytosis with greater than 500 WBC/mm^3. Early polymorphonuclear predominance is seen followed by lymphocytic predominance after 48 hours. Gram stain is negative. CSF should be sent for Mycobacterium tuberculosis PCR (the most sensitive method for the laboratory diagnosis of tuberculous meningitis),[19] acid-fast bacilli (AFB) culture, and AFB stain microscopy. Likewise, serial gastric aspirate and respiratory tract infections should be sent for AFB culture and AFB stain microscopy.

The recommended regimen for drug-susceptible tuberculosis meningitis in childhood (pending microbiologic diagnosis and drug-susceptibility testing on the isolate) includes four drugs: isoniazid (INH), rifampin, pyrazinamide (PZA), and either ethambutol or streptomycin, given once a day for the initial 2 months of directly observed therapy (DOT), followed by 10 months of INH and rifampin once a day or twice a week (12 months total).[20]

Provided antituberculosis therapy is adequate, high-dose corticosteroid treatment should be considered for all children with tuberculous meningitis. It has shown to improve neurological and intellectual outcomes and to decrease mortality, especially when administered early in the course of the disease. Also, enhanced resolution of the basal exudate and tuberculomas by steroids has been shown by serial head CT scanning.[21] The recommended dosage of prednisolone is 1 to 2 mg/kg/day for 4 to 6 weeks, followed by tapering over the next 2 to 3 weeks. Rifampin decreases the bioavailability of corticosteroids by as much as 66% and increases plasma clearance of the drug by 45%.[22] Therefore, when used in conjunction with rifampin, the dose of prednisolone should be increased to 2 to 4 mg/kg/day.

Adjunctive Care for Meningitis

Neuroimaging (CT) should be performed at regular intervals to demonstrate the various aspects of cranial tuberculosis on initial presentation and to monitor the evolution of disease and response to therapy.

For the initial 24 to 48 hours, careful and continuous monitoring of the critically ill child with bacterial meningitis is essential, to achieve early and timely intervention for optimal outcome. Oxygenation, ventilation, and maintenance of cerebral perfusion pressure are the mainstays of therapy. Sedation, analgesia, and seizure control may help to prevent an elevated cerebral metabolic rate and secondary brain injury. Supportive care includes:

- Airway maintenance, including optimal ventilation/oxygenation status.
- Maintenance of hemodynamic stability with adequate fluid resuscitation ± inotropic support.
- Fluid restriction (restriction of free water) after restoration of intravascular space.
- Recognition of seizure activity and aggressive seizure control.
- Early detection and management of increased intracranial pressure.
- Monitoring of urine output, specific gravity, and osmolality; serum sodium and osmolality to identify hyponatremia and hypo-osmolality associated with SIADH.

Persistent fever or recurrence of fever (beyond 8 or 9 days) may indicate the development of suppurative complications such as subdural or pleural empyema, septic arthritis, pneumonia, pericarditis, and brain abscess. Nosocomial intercurrent infection and poor therapeutic response should be included in the differential diagnosis for prolonged fever. The mortality rate and incidence of neurologic sequelae are greatest with pneumococcal meningitis. The most common neurologic sequela following meningitis is sensorineural hearing loss, which occurs in approximately 30% of children after *S. pneumoniae* meningitis, and in 5% to 10% of children after Hib or *N. meningitidis* meningitis.

Rifampin prophylaxis is needed in the settings of invasive Hib disease and *N. meningitidis* infection. Prophylaxis for patients and closed contacts is outlined in Table 7. In order to eradicate nasopharyngeal carriage of Hib and decrease the risk of secondary invasive Hib disease in exposed household contacts of the index patient, rifampin should be administered to *all* household contacts, regardless of age, in those households with at least one contact younger than 4 years of age whose immunization status against Hib is incomplete. In the setting of child care, rifampin is indicated to all attendees and supervisory personnel *only* if 2 or more cases of Hib invasive disease have occurred within 2 months, and if unvaccinated or incompletely vaccinated children attend the facility. The dose of Hib rifampin prophylaxis is 20 mg/kg/dose by mouth once a day (maximum dose, 600 mg/day) for 4 days. For a listing of side effects and contraindications see the footnote of Table 7.

Encephalitis

Encephalitis, or infection of the brain, is most often viral in origin. The incidence peaks at 17 per 100,000 child-years during the second year of life and declines to 1 per 100,000 child-years by the sixteenth year of life.[23] Encephalitis is often classified as primary, or para- or postinfectious. When encephalitis is the major manifestation, it is classified as primary. In this case, infectious agents directly invade and replicate in the central nervous system (CNS), leading to clinical manifestations of cerebral or cerebellar dysfunction. Postinfectious or parainfectious encephalitis occurs in conjunction with or following infections or illnesses or vaccine administration, and is thought primarily to be immune mediated.

In 60% to 70% of all cases of encephalitis, an infectious etiologic agent cannot be identified. The most common identifiable etiologic agent of severe primary encephalitis in neonates, infants, and children is HSV. HSV-2 causes most cases of neonatal disease while HSV-1 is the most common cause of severe disease in older infants and children. Encephalitis with HSV-1 can result from primary (30%) or recurrent (70%) infection. Other common causes of encephalitis in children include enteroviruses and some arthropod-borne viruses (arboviruses). In contrast to HSV, which shows no preference for seasons, enteroviruses, arboviruses, and tick-borne infectious agents have distinct seasonal preferences of late summer and fall. Outside of the newborn period, enteroviral encephalitis typically is less severe than disease with HSV. For a more detailed list of etiologic agents and diagnostic methods, the reader is referred to Table 13.

As in the settings of most viral illnesses, the clinical presentation of encephalitis is a continuum. The severity of illness is related to the characteristics of the etiologic agent and the immune stability of the host. Neonates with encephalitis generally show signs of severe systemic disease. Infants and children may present with signs and symptoms of meningitis (such as fever, headache, irritability, and poor feeding) along with signs and symptoms of more severe CNS involvement (altered behavior, seizures, personality changes, lethargy). Meningismus is an uncommon finding in encephalitis unless there is an accompanying meningitis. The specific area of the brain parenchyma involved will determine the neurologic findings. Of those children diagnosed with HSV-1 encephalitis, more than half will present with the following: alteration of consciousness, fever, personality changes, seizures, dysphagia, and autonomic dysfunction.

The CSF findings may include pleocytosis with 50 to 2000 WBCs per mm^3, usually with a lymphocytic predominance. (Neutrophils may be the predominant cells early in the infection.) Most patients who have encephalitis with HSV will have elevated red blood cell count and protein concentration in the CSF. In general, the abnormalities of the CSF do not correlate with the severity of the disease. The CSF will be normal in less than 5% of the patients. Polymerase chain reaction of the CSF is the quickest and most definitive way to diagnose disease due to HSV. The sensitivities for diagnosing infection with HSV are 60% for CT, 80% for magnetic resonance imaging, and 80% for electroencephalogram. Temporal and frontal abnormalities are suggestive of HSV infection. The routine use of brain biopsy to establish the diagnosis in the case of a negative polymerase chain reaction for HSV remains controversial. A careful history may reveal epidemiologic or clinical clues to begin diagnostic testing for other potential causes (Table 13). HSV rarely grows from CSF, and isolation of HSV from other sources does not confirm it as the etiologic agent in encephalitis. Enteroviruses, however, can often be isolated from the CSF. Nasopharyngeal and rectal swabs are good additional sites for specimen collection for viral cultures. In encephalitic patients with seizures that are prolonged and refractory to the usual anticonvulsants, cat scratch disease should be a strong consideration.

Infants and children with encephalitis should be monitored in the PICU. They require aggressive flied management (watching for SIADH and increased intracranial pressure) and intense monitoring of the progression of their neurologic disease. They may require assisted ventilation or intracranial pressure monitoring. Because of the focal and often hemorrhagic process, seizures may be prolonged and difficult to control. Although acyclovir and vidarabine are equally effective in treating neonatal HSV encephalitis, acyclovir is the treatment of choice for HSV encephalitis in infants and older children, as its toxicity is less; vidarabine is relatively insoluble and requires dilution in a relatively large amount of free water (Table 14).

Table 13

Diagnostic Studies to Consider in Acute Encephalitis

Neonates	Infants and Children

CSF
  routine analysis, gram stain and culture
  viral culture
  herpes simplex virus (HSV) PCR
  enteroviruses PCR
 	
Nasopharyngeal & rectal swabs
  viral culture
 	
Blood
  bacterial culture
  buffy coat viral culture
  Serologies: RPR, VDRL
    toxoplasma gondii
    rubella virus
 	
Urine
  bacterial culture
  culture for cytomegalovirus (CMV)
	CSF
	  routine analysis, gram stain and culture
	  viral culture, India ink stain
	  herpes simplex virus (HSV) PCR
	  enteroviruses PCR
	  mycobacterium tuberculosis PCR
	  AFB smear and culture
	
	Nasopharygeal & rectal swabs
	  viral culture
	
	Nasopharyngeal washing
	  rapid antigen by immunofluorescence
	  (influenza virus A & B)
	
	Gastric aspirates*
	  AFB smear and culture
	
	Blood
	  bacterial culture
	  buffy coat viral culture
	  serologies: arboviruses panel
	    Epstein-Barr virus (EBV)
	    Mycoplasma pneumoniae
	    Borrelia burgdorferi
	    Rickettsia rickettsii
	    Ehrlichia chaffeensis
	    Bartonella henselae
	Urine
	  bacterial culture

*Collect sample in early a.m. (before child gets up and has anything to drink or eat for breakfast). Gastric aspirates of 3 consecutive days are needed. Specimen must be received in TB lab within 2–3 hours since gastric acid kills *Mycobacterium tuberculosis* resulting in negative cultures. Collect sample in sterile water to prevent bacteriostatic effect of saline solution.

CSF = cerebrospinal fluid; PCR = polymerase chain reaction; RPR = rapid plasma reagin; VDRL = Venereal Disease Research Laboratory.

Table 14

Therapy of Herpes Simplex Encephalitis

Neonates	Older Infants and Children

acyclovir (intravenous)
  30–45 mg/kg/day in 3 divided doses
vidarabine (intravenous)
  30 mg/kg/day in 1 dose (12-hour infusion)
	acyclovir (intravenous)
	  30 mg/kg/day in 3 divided doses

Serious Respiratory Infections

Pneumonia

Most childhood cases of pneumonia are a result of infection with the respiratory viruses or *Mycoplasma pneumoniae*. Bacterial pneumonia accounts for 10% to 15% of all pneumonias, has a seasonal preference for winter and spring, and occurs in males twice as frequently as in females. In the critically ill child with pneumonia, empiric antibiotic therapy is indicated. The antibiotic choices should provide coverage based on the clinical picture, the patient's age, and general underlying status. Common pathogens include *Streptococcus pneumoniae*, influenza, respiratory syncytial virus, *Mycoplasma pneumoniae*, and *Chlamydia*. *Hemophilus influenzae*, *Staphylococcus aureus*, and *Legionella pneumophilia* occur less commonly. *Pneumocystis carinii* should be considered a potential pathogen in immunocompromised children, especially those with AIDS, leukemia (AML), lymphoma, and specific T-cell defects. In general, cefuroxime or ceftriaxone plus azithromycin would offer coverage of the most common bacterial pathogens. Compared to erythromycin, azithromycin offers the convenience of once-a-day dosing, and has a smaller incidence of thrombophlebitis, with administration through a peripheral intravenous site. Unlike erythromycin, azithromycin has limited interactions with medications metabolized by the hepatic P450 system. Vancomycin may be necessary for coverage of resistant pneumococci.

For patients with underlying systemic illnesses or for those who are at risk for aspiration, empiric anaerobic therapy may be indicated. In such patients, the addition of penicillin or clindamycin should be considered. Alternatively, a semisynthetic penicillin such as ticarcillin or piperacillin can be used in place of the third-generation cephalosporin. Ticarcillin and piperacillin both provide acceptable coverage of usual pathogens covered by the cepahlosporins, in addition to anaerobic coverage.

Acute Epiglottitis

Acute epiglottitis is an acute, life-threatening, and rapidly progressive bacterial infection of the entire supraglottic region. It leads to symptoms of obstruction related to both the airway and the digestive tract. The typical patient is a child between the ages of 2 and 4 years who was completely well 24 hours prior to presentation. Patients present with symptoms of progressive obstruction of the subglottic region which include sore throat, dysphagia, stridor, fever, and, often, panic. They typically are drooling, refusing to swallow their saliva, refusing oral fluids, and may even be positioning themselves leaning forward on their hands (tripod position) or with their chin up (sniffing position).

Ever since the development and implementation of hemophilus vaccines, the predominant etiologic organism remains Hib. Other isolated agents include *Staphylococcus aureus*, *Streptococcus pneumoniae*, *Klebsiella*, and *Candida albicans*.[24]

There are two important steps for treating the pediatric patient suspected of having epiglottitis. First, *do not aggravate or irritate the patient until the airway is secure*. Do not remove the child from the parent's lap (unless of course the patient is developing respiratory failure or is obtunded). Do not attempt to look at the oropharynx. Second, *quickly assemble the physicians and the space for evaluating and securing the airway*. Each child should have a direct laryngoscopy and, if positive, intubation in the operating room with appropriate personnel assembled, including anesthesiologists and pediatric surgeons or otolaryngologists. If epiglottitis exists, the child should remain tracheally intubated for 24 to 48 hours after antibiotic therapy is initiated. Ideally, the treatment of the child suspected of having epiglottis should be a collaborative effort and should include physicians who are expert in pediatric airway management and are capable of performing an emergency tracheostomy should that become necessary. It is most appropriate to have a specific protocol in place for dealing with such patients.

Bacterial cultures of blood and of the surface of the epiglottis should be obtained. The patient should be started on an intravenous antibiotic that would cover the common etiologic agents. Intravenous cefuroxime at 150 mg/kg/day divided into three doses is an appropriate choice. If a gram stain reveals gram-negative rods, third-generation cephalosporins (cefotaxime, ceftazidime, or ceftriaxone) are among the alternative choices. The condition should be managed in the PICU with sedation and, if possible, without neuromuscular block, until there is resolution of the supraglottic edema. If the infectious agent is *Haemophilus influenzae*, prophylaxis of family members or day care attendees may be necessary.

Laryngotracheobronchitis

Laryngotracheobronchitis, sometimes referred to as croup, is an inflammation of the larynx and trachea. It usually is viral in origin, with parainfluenza being most common. It must be distinguished from epiglottitis, retropharyngeal abscess, and bacterial tracheitis. This most often is evident by the history and physical examination. Children with croup commonly are 6 to 36 months of age and have preceding signs of an upper respiratory tract infection with coryza, rhinorrhea, and cough. They develop a cough that is barking in nature and can be accompanied by retractions and inspiratory stridor. Unlike children with epiglottitis, those with laryngotracheitis usually will drink until the respiratory distress is severe.

Therapy for laryngotracheitis is primarily supportive. Children should be closely monitored with little disruption. Cool mist is indicated but occasionally the anxiety of the patient about the mist tent overrides the potential therapeutic benefits. Nebulized racemic epinephrine has short-term beneficial use. It should not be used in the outpatient setting. Corticosteroid therapy with dexamethasone may hasten the resolution of symptoms and at times prevent the need for hospital admission or return visits to the emergency department. Oxygen therapy is necessary only for those children with hypoxemia. Antibiotics are rarely indicated.

Bacterial Tracheitis

Occasionally, a child with laryngotracheitis will suddenly worsen and develop a high fever with progressive respiratory difficulty. A secondary bacterial infection of the trachea should be suspected, and the clinician should be prepared to intubate the airway and provide assisted ventilation if the symptoms warrant. The progression of airway obstruction can be rapid. An x-ray of the lateral neck may reveal subglottic haziness, a tracheal intraluminal mass, or pseudomembrane. The most common organisms isolated are *Staphylococcus aureus, Streptococcus pyogenes, Streptococcus pneumoniae,* and *Haemophilus influenzae.* Intravenous antibiotic should be initiated.

The Immunocompromised Patient

Fever and Neutropenia

The infant or older child undergoing treatment of cancer who develops neutropenia and fever should receive special attention via history, physical evaluation, laboratory studies, and empiric intravenous antibiotic therapy. The physical examination should include a careful evaluation of the oral cavity, skin (including periungual areas and line sites), and perirectal area for mild signs of inflammation. The clinician should be aware of the prevalence of seasonal pathogens in the patient's environment. Necessary laboratory studies include, but are not limited to, the following:

blood cultures (peripheral and through each port of central intravenous and all intra-arterial lines);
urinalysis and urine culture;
chest x-ray or rapid antigen tests for seasonal pathogens if abnormal respiratory signs or symptoms exist, or if it is respiratory season and the patient had potential contacts, tracheal aspirates for gram stain and culture if the patient is intubated.

The most common isolates are gram-positive organisms including *Staphylococcus aureus,* coagulase-negative *Staphylococcus,* and α-hemolytic streptococci followed by gram-negative organisms such as *Escherichia coli, Klebsiella,* and *Pseudomonas.*[25] Empiric antibiotic regimens should include ceftazidime alone or in combination with an antistaphylococcal drug such as nafcillin or oxacillin. Alternatively, nafcillin or oxacillin can be combined with another antipseudomonas β-lactam. Vancomycin should be initiated instead of oxacillin or nafcillin if the patient is toxic and a gram-positive organism is suspected. If there is no clinical response within 5 to 7 days and no pathogen has been identified, empiric antifungal therapy with amphotericin B should be considered.

Sickle Cell Disease

Patients with sickle cell disease (SCD) have an increased risk of invasive infections with encapsulated bacteria (*Streptococcus pneumoniae, Haemophilus influenzae,* and *Salmonella* spp.), as well as influenza virus and *Mycoplasma* spp. Penicillin prophylaxis, pneumococcal vaccine, and influenza vaccine have decreased morbidity and mortality. Still, the mortality rate of children under 3 years of age who have SCD and invasive pneumococcal disease is 15%. Children with SCD and fever should be promptly evaluated. If there are physical signs or laboratory findings suggestive of bacterial infection, immediate antibiotic therapy is indicated.

Pneumonia is referred to as acute chest syndrome (ACS) in the SCD population because it has been recognized that pneumonia in this population is vastly different from pneumonia in the general population. ACS is the leading cause of death in patients with SCD. *Mycoplasma pneumoniae, Chlamydia pneumoniae,* and parvovirus B19 have been implicated in the etiology of ACS.[26] Without appropriate therapy including partial exchange transfusion based on the patient's respiratory status, progressive respiratory failure and death may occur. The pathogenesis of ACS remains controversial. It may reflect a primary infection with secondary vaso-occlusive phenomena in the lungs or a primary vaso-occlusive event.

Human Immunodeficiency Virus Infection

Children with human immunodeficiency viral infection are at risk for serious desease with common pathogens. When they present with signs of sepsis, antibiotics, as discussed previously, based on the patient's age and condition are indicated. If the patient's condition is deteriorating or if the patient fails to respond to initial antibiotic therapy, less common pathogens should be considered and antibiotic choices rethought.

Nosocomial Infections

Nosocomial infections include all infections that occur during a patient's hospital course that were not present or incubating on admission. Although pediatric services tend to have lower rates of nosocomial infections than adult services, the percentage of infections with secondary bacteremias (12%) is highest among pediatric large teaching hospitals. Researchers have noted that length of stay greater than 1 week and very young age of the patient are predictive of patients with increased risk of nosocomial infection.[27] Infections that occur following a surgical procedure in the same anatomic area as the procedure are termed surgically related infections. Nosocomial infections represent a significant cause of morbidity and even mortality for the PICU patient. Some patients will survive their acute life-threatening illness only to die from a secondary, nosocomial infection.

In the PICU or in any hospital setting, the normal flora of the host is altered by diet, foreign devices, other exposures, and medications. Patients are colonized with organisms that live on or in their body or bodily fluids without evidence of adverse effects. The presence of an organism in or on the body, with local or systemic adverse effects, is an infection. Inflammation can develop due to infection or in response to a foreign or irritating material. The distinction between a patient who is *colonized* with *Candida albicans* and one who is *infected* with *Candida albicans* is very important in terms of treatment and prognosis. However, in the PICU patient, making this distinction may be difficult.

A common problematic scenario is that of evaluating tracheal aspirate gram stain results and making the distinction between colonization and infection. The decision is made by combining the clinical course, ventilator requirements, x-ray findings, and tracheal aspirate gram stain results. In general, unless the patient is neutropenic, when there is infection there are white cells. Therefore, a gram stain with moderate gram-negative rods and no white cells may represent colonization. But if that same gram stain is accompanied by significant increases in ventilator requirements or if there are many WBCs on the gram stain, it may be interpreted as an infection. The tracheal aspirate for examination, when possible, should be obtained without adding saline prior to suctioning and obtaining the culture. The addition of saline may dilute the sample and interfere with bacterial growth. Many WBCs but no organisms on a tracheal aspirate gram stain may represent a viral process.

Pneumonia accounts for approximately 15% of all nosocomial infections. Gram-negative bacilli are the most common bacterial pathogens. Many of these are resistant to first-line antibiotics. When the patient is tracheally intubated, the tracheal aspirate gram stains and cultures should guide antibiotic choices. If gram-negative organisms are suspected, an extended-spectrum penicillin (ticarcillin, mezocillin, or piperacillin), with or without an aminoglycoside, would be appropriate initial therapy.

Central Line Infections

Central catheters can also become colonized with bacteria which can, given the right circumstances, cause bacteremia or sepsis. The rate of line-associated infections is particularly high among patients receiving total parenteral nutrition (TPN) with intralipid. These TPN-related infections can be drastically reduced with use of protocols for catheter insertion methods, prohibition of stopcocks and piggyback infusions through TPN catheters, avoidance of blood drawing through the TPN line, and limitation of catheter manipulation and care to the specialized TPN team. While these are practical ways of limiting the incidence of central line infections, they may not always be practical in the critically ill PICU patient with limited intravenous access. However, when possible and clinically practical, these guidelines are suggested.

Organisms that cause infection and are isolated from central lines most often include the gram-positive organisms (*Staphylococcus* spp), but also include gram-negative organisms and *Candida* spp. When an infection develops related to a central line, it is logical that the line should be removed. This, however, is not always necessary or possible. In general, central lines should be immediately removed if the patient's condition is rapidly deteriorating (in which case a replacement line will likely be crucial), if a tunnel infection exists, or if the infectious agent is a *Candida* spp.

Fungal Infections

The diagnosis of a fungal infection can be difficult. In general, any PICU patient with a gradual deterioration and no other explanation could have a systemic fungal infection. Predisposing factors include neutropenia, malnutrition, high-dose corticosteroid therapy, prolonged antibiotic use, and the presence of central venous catheters. Patients with T cell defects or dysfunction also have an increased incidence of fungal infections. Many PICU patients will be colonized with *Candida* spp. and, commonly, the dilemma will arise: are they now infected with *Candida*? Unfortunately, blood cultures remain negative in over 50% of those patients who have serious disseminated fungal infections. Any patient who is immunocompromised and develops CNS symptoms should be thoroughly evaluated for CNS fungal disease. CT scans of the chest and abdomen may be useful in identifying fungal infiltrates or abscesses. Bone marrow aspirates may increase the yield.

Once the decision has been made to presumptively treat the patient for disseminated fungal infection, intravenous amphotericin B (AMB) should be initiated. To exclude the possibility of a major allergic reaction, a test dose of 1 mg is given intravenously. Then full maintenance therapy can be initiated (0.5 to 1.0 mg/kg/day administered slowly over 1 to 6 hours). A common reaction to AMB is rigors and chills. These may be controlled with premedication (meperidine 0.5 mg/kg i.v., diphenhydramine 0.5 mg/kg i.v., and/or acetaminophen 10 to 15 mg/kg by mouth). Sometimes, the addition of low-dose corticosteroids may be necessary to control rigors and chills. Nephrotoxicity and potassium wasting should be closely monitored. The incidence of nephrotoxicity may be decreased by avoiding the concomitant use of other nephrotoxic agents and provision of optimal intravascular status and renal blood flow. Most patients will develop an increase in the BUN after 2 to 3 days of therapy. As the BUN and creatinine rise, it may be appropriate to switch to alternative-day therapy. Lipid-encased/enclosed/bound AMB can be given in larger aggregate doses before nephrotoxicity develops. Because it is significantly more expensive, this form should be reserved for patients who have significant renal disease at the onset of therapy.

Summary

Infectious disease represents a significant risk to the PICU patient as an initial cause for his or her admission to the PICU as well as when nosocomial infections develop. A high index of suspicion is required when caring for the PICU patient, to allow for early identification of nosocomial infections. Subtle signs such as a rising WBC count, modest increase in oxygen requirement, or temperature instability may be early signs of infection. Immediate investigation with culture of all available bodily fluids and institution of appropriate antibiotic therapy is indicated. As important as early and aggressive antibiotic therapy, is the discontinuation of antibiotics when cultures prove negative.

References

1. Baker CJ. Infections in perinatology: Group B streptococcal infections. *Clin Perinatol* 1997;24:59–70.
2. Sotiropoulos SV. Medical emergencies I. Antibiotic choices: The critical first hour. *Pediatr Ann* 1996;25:345–350.
3. Jacobs RF, Stimson JM. Presumptive antibiotic therapy for hospitalized children with sepsis and meningitis: Cost-effective analysis and antibiotic restriction guidelines. *Pediatr Ann* 1996;25:631–638.
4. Zeni F, Freeman B, Natanson C. Anti-inflammatory therapies to treat sepsis and septic shock: A reassessment. *Crit Care Med* 1997;25:1095–1100.
5. Schreiber JR, Jacobs MR. Antimicrobial resistance in pediatrics: Antibiotic-resistant pneumococci. *Pediatr Clin North Am* 1995;42:519–537.
6. Committee on Infectious Diseases, American Academy of Pediatrics. Therapy for children with invasive pneumococcal infections. *Pediatrics* 1997;99:289–299.
7. Todd JK, Ressman M, Caston SA, et al. Corticosteroid therapy for patients with toxic shock syndrome. *JAMA* 1984;252:3399–3402.
8. Kirsch EA, Barton RP, Kitchen L, et al. Pathophysiology, treatment and outcome of meningococcemia: A review and recent experience. *Pediatr Infect Dis J* 1996;15:967–979.
9. Tesoro LJ, Selbst SM. Factors affecting outcome in meningococcal infections. *Am J Dis Child* 1991;145:218–220.
10. Quagliarello VJ, Scheld WM. Treatment of bacterial meningitis. *N Engl J Med* 1997;336:708–716.
11. Ahmed A. A critical evaluation of vancomycin for treatment of bacterial meningitis. *Pediatr Infect Dis J* 1997;16:895–903.
12. Rothrock SG, Green SM, Wren J, et al. Pediatric bacterial meningitis: Is prior antibiotic therapy associated with an altered clinical presentation? *Ann Emerg Med* 1992;21:146–152.
13. Kaplan SL, Smith EO, Wills C, et al. Association between preadmission oral antibiotic therapy and cerebrospinal fluid findings and sequelae caused by Haemophilus influenzae type b meningitis. *Pediatr Infect Dis J* 1986;5:626–632.
14. Reid R Jr, Bradley JS, Hindler J. Pneumococcal meningitis during therapy of otitis media with clarithromycin. *Pediatr Infect Dis J* 1995;14:1104–1105.
15. Jackson MA, Burry VF, Olson LC, et al. Breakthrough sepsis in macrolide-resistant pneumococcal infection. *Pediatr Infect Dis J* 1996;15:1049–1050.
16. Wald ER, Kaplan SL, Mason EO, et al. Dexamethasone therapy for children with bacterial meningitis. *Pediatrics* 1995;95:21–28.
17. Prober CG. The role of steroids in the management of children with bacterial meningitis. *Pediatrics* 1995;95:29–31.
18. Ussery X, Valway SE, McKenna M, et al. The epidemiology of tuberculosis among children in the United States: 1985–1994. *Pediatr Infect Dis* 1996;15(8):697–704.
19. Bonington A, Strang JI, Klapper PE, et al. Use of Roche AMPLICOR myobacterium tuberculosis PCR in early diagnosis of tuberculous meningitis. *J Clin Microbiol* 1998;35(5):1251–1254.
20. American Thoracic Society and the Centers of Disease Control and Prevention. Treatment of tuberculosis and tuberculosis infection in adults and children. *Am J Respir Crit Care Med* 1994;149:1359–1374.
21. Schocman JF, Van Zyl LE, Laubscher JA, et al. Effect of corticosteroids on intracranial pressure, computed tomographic findings, and clinical outcome in young children

with tuberculous meningitis. *Pediatrics* 1997;99:226–231.
22. McAllaister WAC, Thompson PJ, Al-Habet SM. Rifampin reduces effectiveness and bioavailability of prednisolone. *Br Med J* 1983;286:923–925.
23. Koskiniemi M, Rautonen J, Lehtokoski-Lehtiniemi E, et al. Epidemiology of encephalitis in children: a 20 year survey. *Ann Neurol* 1991;29:492–495.
24. Valdepena H, Wald E, Rose E, et al. Epiglottitis and Haemophilus influenza immunization: The Pittsburgh experience-a five year review. *Pediatrics* 1995;96:424–427.
25. Sotiropoulos S, Jackson M, Woods G, et al. Alpha-streptococcal septicemia in leukemic children treated with continuous or large dosage intermittent cytosine arabinoside. *Pediatr Infect Dis J* 1989;8:755–758.
26. Vichinsky E, Styles L, Colangely L, et al. Cooperative Study of Sickle Cell Disease: Acute chest syndrome in sickle cell disease: Clinical presentation and course. *Blood* 1997;89:1787–1792.
27. Pollock E, Ford-Jones EL, Corey M, et al. Use of the pediatric mortality score to predict nosocomial infection in a pediatric intensive care unit. *Crit Care Med* 1991;19:185S-191S.

Chapter 20

Poisonings and Toxic Ingestions

R. Blaine Easley, MD and Joseph D. Tobias, MD

"It is more important to treat the patient than the poison"

S. Locket[1]

Introduction

Poisonings and toxic ingestions are a common occurrence in children and adolescents; there are approximately one million cases reported each year.[2] The majority (85% to 90%) of pediatric intensive care unit admissions for toxic ingestions involve children less than 5 years of age. In this age group, poisonings are usually unintentional, involving a single agent. Adolescents represent a smaller percentage of pediatric intensive care unit admissions for ingestions, and differ from younger children in that their intoxications are often intentional, involving multiple agents. The prognosis for recovery following toxic ingestions is generally good, but depends largely on the supportive care and the particular toxic agent ingested.[3]

Initial Evaluation and Stabilization

The care of children with toxic ingestions starts with suspecting and identifying the ingestion. The ingestion is readily apparent when the caretakers provide the appropriate history; however, the possibility of ingestion must always be considered in patients with altered mental status, cardiorespiratory insufficiency, hypertension, arrhythmias, or a new-onset seizure disorder. In the situation of a diagnostic dilemma, the possible role of toxins must always be considered. In children suspected of a toxic ingestion or poisoning, the initial evaluation should focus on stabilization of the airway, breathing, and cardiovascular system (ABCs). The majority of life-threatening complications seen with acute intoxication are related to airway obstruction, respiratory failure, hypotension, cardiac arrhythmias, and seizures. The issues of stabilization of the airway and support of the cardiorespiratory system must be addressed before any treatment is undertaken (eg, the administration of antidote, gastric lavage, etc.). Once the patient has been stabilized and the appropriate interventions have occurred (eg, intubation of the trachea to protect the airway), additional history can be obtained, a physical examination performed, and diagnostic tests ordered.

Identification of the toxic agent depends greatly on the initial history and physical examination. Fazen et al[4] reported, in a prospective study, that up to 90% of ingested substances can be accurately diagnosed by history alone. The history should focus on the circumstances surrounding the toxic ingestion/exposure, and should answer the ques-

From: Tobias JD (ed): *Pediatric Critical Care: The Essentials.* ©Futura Publishing Co., Inc., Armonk, NY, 1999.

tions outlined in Table 1. Past medical history should seek prior hospitalization or family history of psychological problems, as these can effect long-term treatment goals or give clues as to whether the possibility of a suicide attempt is present. Always ask to see all available containers of medications, remaining substances, and other accessible medications/drugs in the household for evaluation by you and your pharmacist or toxicologist. Ingested substances can include both prescription and over-the-counter medications. This fact mandates a thorough questioning regarding the medications that are present in the household and in other households visited by the child.

Physical examination should look closely at vital signs, general appearance, odor, pupil size, skin, and mental status. Patterns of the physical findings, known as toxidromes, may be useful in identifying particular groups of toxic agents (Fig. 1, Table 2). When determining the toxic agent ingested and deciding on interventions and additional stabilizing measures, the history and physical examination often prove more useful than most drug screens.

Laboratory tests can offer useful clues in the diagnosis and care of children suffering from poisoning. Serum electrolytes, specifically glucose and calcium, the anion gap, serum osmolality, and urinalysis can be used to confirm clinical suspicions of ingestion (Table 3). Several ingestions, including the alcohols, can cause profound depression of the serum glucose that must be identified and treated early to prevent irreversible central nervous system (CNS) dam-

Table 1

Questions of Possible Toxic Ingestions in the History

Who	. . . was supervising the child?
	. . . was around when this event happened?
	. . . was notified/called when this occurred?
	. . . witnessed the event/ingestion? Family, other chidren, neighbors, etc.?
	. . . do the medications/drugs belong to?
	. . . told you the child took the medications/drugs?
What	. . . medications/drugs were ingested or thought to be ingested?
	. . . behaviors did the child have prior to and following the event?
	. . . medications/drugs are the child or others taking at that location (ie, siblings, parents, or grandparents, etc.)?
	. . . appeared different or appears different now about the child?
	. . . quantity of medications/drugs was ingested?
	. . . history of substance abuse or depression does the child or family have?
	. . . peculiar odors or smells did the family or others notice?
	. . . medications/drugs were found around the patient?
When	. . . did this ingestion/exposure happen?
	. . . did you first notice symptoms?
	. . . did you find out about the ingestion?
Why	. . . do you think the child took the medications/drugs? Has he/she done this before?
	. . . did you see (or not see) the child take the medication?
Where	. . . are the rest of the medicine/drugs now?
	. . . did the ingestion/exposure occur?
How	. . . did the child look when you found him or her?
	. . . did the family respond?
	. . . was the medicine/drugs made accessible to the child?
	. . . did you determine the child took the medications/drugs? Were there pill fragments, empty containers, etc.?
	. . . many others are having symptoms or showing signs of intoxication?
	. . . many times has this happened before to this child or other family members or friends?
	. . . many/much of the medication was there before the child took it? And how much after?

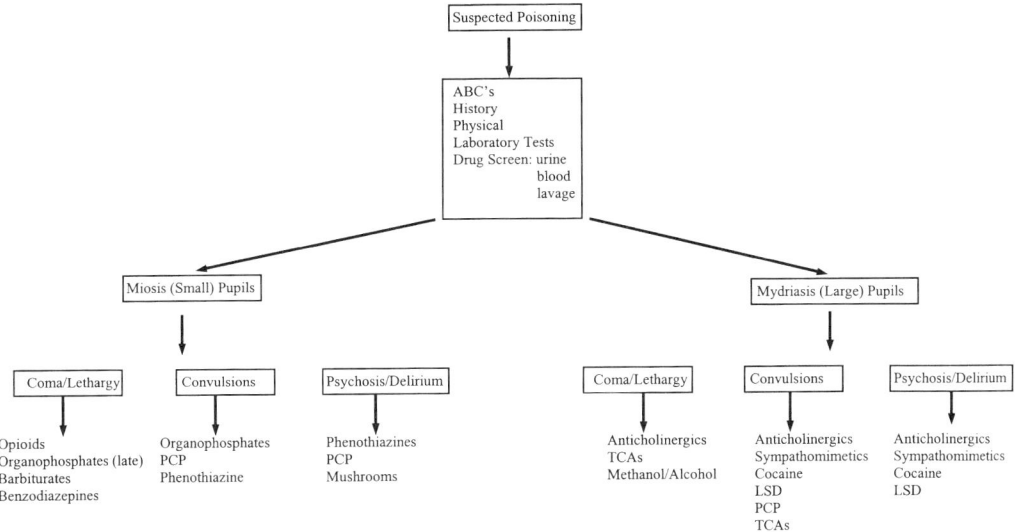

Figure 1. Suggested algorithm for the initial treatment of the child with a toxic ingestion and the subsequent identification of the agent based on the pupil size and CNS findings.

age. The basic calculations for anion gap, serum osmolality, and osmolar gap are outlined in Table 4. The differential diagnosis for the metabolic/toxic causes of an increased anion gap can be remembered by using the acronym MUD PILES: methanol, uremia, diabetic ketoacidosis, paraldehyde, iron, isoniazid, isovaleric acid, lactic acidosis, ethanol/ethylene glycol, salicylates. Causes of an increased osmolar gap include mannitol, ethylene glycol, and the alcohols: ethanol, methanol, and isopropyl alcohol.[5]

Drug screens are important for documentation and confirmation of the presence of a toxic compound and for detection of other possible etiologies (ie, multiple agents), especially if the patient's clinical course is unstable or atypical. Gastric lavage fluid, emesis, blood, and urine should be collected and sent for toxicologic evaluation. The emesis or gastric lavage fluid should be sent for toxicology evaluation even if it does not contain obvious pill fragments.[6] Toxicology screens vary from hospital to hospital and it is therefore important to know the compounds tested for by your institution's emergency and comprehensive toxicology screens. Usually, "emergency screens" will analyze blood and urine but look for a very limited number of agents (4 to 10 compounds) with a relatively rapid return of results, usually available in 3 to 5 hours. The more comprehensive screens institute more sophisticated techniques for compound detection (liquid and gas chromatography and mass spectrometry) and can identify panels of 100 plus substances. These larger panels are usually available at larger referral centers and laboratories and may not be available for up to 24 to 48 hours after admission. A physician should always list the suspected agents when ordering the drug screen, to help the laboratory to identify the offending agent. In many hospitals specific assays are available for many therapeutic agents, such as salicylates, acetaminophen, digoxin, theophylline, and anticonvulsants. If ingestion of one of these agents is suspected, a serum level should be obtained, in addition to the drug screens. The former may be available more quickly than the drug screens.

Finally, the local poison control agency should be notified in the case of all poisonings/ingestions. Often, they are familiar with the patient and may have even referred them to the local emergency department for evaluation. They will provide useful, up-to-date information on the management of all suspected and confirmed agents requested of them. In addition, they can assist in interpreting unusual physical findings, labora-

Table 2
Identification of the Toxic Agent Based on Findings Noted in Initial Physical Examination

Toxidromes	Eyes	Skin	Cardiovascular	Respirations	Neurologic	Other Sx	Common Agents
Anticholinergic	dilated	flushed dry skin and mucous membranes	tachycardia	increased	agitated/hallucinations	urinary retention, fever	atropine, anithistamines, jimson weed
Cholinergic	pinpoint lacrimation		bradycardia	increased, wheezing	coma, fasciculations	incontinence salivation	organophosphates, insecticide, nicotine
Hemoglo-binopathy		cyanosis (MetHb), cutaneous bullae, "cherry red" lips (COHb)	tachycardia	dyspnea, tachypnea	disoriented, headache, coma, syncope, convulsions	gastroenteritis	carbon monoxide, methemoglobin, sulfhemoglobin
Opioid	pinpoint	tracks (rare)	hypotension	decreased	coma/sedate	hypothermia	narcotics, lomotil, darvon
Phenothiazine	pinpoint		cardiac arrhythmias, orthostatic hypotension	decreased	coma, extrapyramidal signs, rigidity		phenothiazine
Salicylates		diaphoretic		increased	tinnitus, agitation, coma	fever, alkalosis (early), acidosis (late)	aspirin, Oil of Wintergreen, Pepto Bismol
Sedative/hypnotic	dilated		cardiac arrhythmias, hypotension QT prolongation	decreased	coma, convulsions, early agitation, myoclonus, hyperreflexia		benzodiazepines, barbiturates
Sympatho-mimetic	dilated	diaphoretic	tachycardia	increased	agitated, hallucinations, convulsions, tremor, hyperreflexia	fever	cocaine, theophylline, amphetamines, caffeine
Tricyclic anti-depressants	dilated		cardiac arrhythmias widened QRS prolonged QT	decreased	seizures, myoclonus, hyperrelexia, coma	emesis	amitryptilline, nortryptilline, imipramine, dimepramine

Table 3

Interpretation of Laboratory Data in the Setting of Acute Poisoning

Laboratory Abnormality	Possible Agents
Low anion gap	lithium, iodine, bromide
Elevated anion gap (metabolic acidosis)	alcohols, salicylates, isoniazid, iron
Elevated osmolar gap	alcohols
Hyperkalemia	potassium, digoxin, lithium, fluoride
Hypokalemia	theophylline, barium, caffeine, diuretics
Hyperglycemia	salicylates, theophylline, caffeine, iron
Hypoglycemia	alcohols, insulin, salicylates, sulfonylureas, propranolol
Urinalysis:	
oxalic acid crystalluria	ethylene glycol
ketonuria	salicylates, ethanol, isopropanol

Table 4

Calculations Commonly used in Acute Poisonings

Anion gap = $(Na^+ + K^+) - (Cl^- + HCO_3^-)$; normal = 7 ± 4 mEq/L
Calculated serum osmolarity (mOsm) = $2(Na^+) + BUN/2.8 + glucose/18$; normal = 285 to 295 mOsm/L
Osmolar gap* = calculated serum mOsm − measured serum mOsm; normal = <10 mOsm

Na^+ = serum sodium; K^+ = serum potassium; Cl^- = serum chloride; HCO_3^- = serum bicarbonate; BUN = serum blood urea nitrogen; glucose = serum glucose.
*This calculation is only accurate with serum osmolarity measured by the freezing point depression method.

tory data, or the utility of certain therapeutic interventions.

Local poison control phone number: (_ _ _) _ _ _- _ _ _ _.

Management

After the airway is secure, cardiorespiratory function stable, and ongoing monitoring established, the focus can then turn to the management and treatment of the specific ingestion. The principles of poisoning management are: 1) decontamination; 2) decrease of further absorption; 3) enhancement of elimination; and 4) administration of an antidote, if available. At all times during this phase of treatment, ongoing monitoring and assessment of the patient is mandatory, as the vital signs and the patient's status may change rapidly. Ongoing monitoring may include continuous pulse oximetry and electrocardiography with intermittent assessment of respiratory rate, blood pressure, and temperature.

Induced Emesis, Gastric Lavage, Activated Charcoal, Whole-Bowel Irrigation

Decontamination involves removal of any remaining poison from the patient. In most poisonings, this is by gastric lavage or by induced emesis. However, in contact poisonings, including pesticides such as organophosphates, this may involve removing the clothing and thoroughly washing the skin. Induced emesis remains the treatment of choice for gastric emptying. Most pediatricians will include a brief discussion and education of poisoning when children reach the toddler stage. This involves instructing the parents to keep a bottle of ipecac at home. The poison control center or the pediatrician will often have parents administer this in the home prior to driving to the hospital. It has been demonstrated that up to 80% of the stomach contents can be evacuated by this method[7]. Syrup of ipecac is the most common agent used for inducing emesis. The dose is: 10 mL for infants ≥6 months, 15 mL for toddlers and children, and 30 mL for adolescents and adults, given orally, followed by a glass of water. The onset of action can be immediate or delayed up to 30 minutes. A second dose can be administered if emesis has not occurred after 30 minutes. The duration of action is 30 to 45 minutes, during which time activated charcoal or the oral antidote should not be administered. Ipecac acts as a local gastrointestinal (GI) irritant and stimulates the chemoreceptor trigger zone in the area postrema of the medulla. Adverse effects of ipecac, occurring almost exclusively with toxic doses, include arrhythmias, hypotension, and altered mental status. Contraindications to induced emesis in the setting of a toxic ingestion include age less than 6 months, possible oral antidote usage, and the "5 C's": coma, caustic ingestion, hydrocarbon ingestion, convulsions, or coagulopathy. The issue of whether ipecac should be administered if there is an oral antidote that can be given is somewhat controversial. The theory is that the emesis will be protracted and interfere with the ability to give the oral antidote. Due to its short effective half-life of 30 to 45 minutes, this is generally not a true issue. Additionally, ipecac is very effective in eliminating a significant amount of the toxin from the body, thereby decreasing the total dose absorbed and the likelihood of significant sequelae.[8]

Apomorphine, which can be given intravascularly or subcutaneously (0.06 mg/kg/dose to a maximum of 6 mg/dose in adults), is a second choice. It can be used in children who are candidates for induced emesis, but who refuse ipecac. It has a rapid onset of action 6 to 10 minutes, acting on the same chemoreceptor trigger zone in the area postrema of the medulla.

Gastric lavage is indicated when induced emesis is contraindicated, when there is insufficient gastric emptying by induced emesis, when or an ingestion has occurred with an agent that results in the rapid loss of consciousness (eg, tricyclic antidepressants [TCADs]).[9] In the latter situation, the fear is that loss of consciousness will occur after the ipecac has been administered but before the emesis has occurred. Contraindications to gastric lavage include caustic materials and an unprotected airway. Prior to gastric lavage, the airway should be protected by endotracheal intubation if there is any concern regarding the patient's level of consciousness or ability to protect the airway. The technique involves positioning the patient with his or her left side down with the head slightly lower than the body, inserting a large-bore orogastric tube into the stomach, and performing repeated lavage with small volumes of fluid. Verification of tube placement can be done clinically if good return of gastric contents and auscultation is demonstrated; a radiograph is not required unless a question exists. Once placement is confirmed, irrigation of the stomach begins with normal saline via the orogastric tube. Orogastric tube size should be 16F for neonates, 22F for toddlers, 28F for children, and 36 to 40F for adolescents/adults. Lavage is performed with aliquots of 4 to 5 mL/kg of normal saline until either the fluid is clear or the maximum volume is reached (maximum volume: 40 to 50 mL/kg). Ideally, lavage should be performed within 1 to 2 hours following the ingestion. However, many of the toxic ingestions (eg, TCADs, carbamazepine) result in slowing of GI motility, so that induced emesis or lavage should be considered even if the ingestion is reported to have occurred hours earlier.

Prevention of further absorption involves binding the ingested toxin in the GI tract or speeding its transit along the GI tract to prevent further absorption. Activated charcoal, cathartics, and whole-bowel irrigation (WBI) are commonly used means of preventing further toxin absorption. These compounds remove the drug from the gut by diluting the drug, reducing bioavailability, increasing bowel motility, and increasing transit time thereby limiting further absorption of the ingested substance into the bloodstream. In specific circumstances, the addition of various agents to the lavage fluid may be used to bind the ingested agent in the GI tract, making it unable to be absorbed. Examples of this technique include the addition of sodium bicarbonate or deferoxamine to the gastric lavage fluid to bind the iron in the GI tract.

The administration of activated charcoal

should be considered for all toxic ingestions. Some authors indicate that a single dose of activated charcoal is more effective than gastric lavage or induced emesis at preventing substance absorption.[7] However, the use of induced emesis or lavage followed by the dose of activated charcoal is the most common practice. The initial dose is 1 g/kg orally or per nasogastric tube with 70% sorbitol. The 70% sorbitol is used as an osmotic agent to counteract the constipating effects of charcoal. Repeat dosing of activated charcoal with 0.5 g/kg administered every 2 to 4 hours, also known as GI dialysis, is indicated in specific ingestions in which there is a significant enterohepatic circulation. These include phenobarbital, theophylline, and carbamazepine. With these ingestions, the compounds are excreted compounded by glucoronyl transferase. If not bound in the GI tract, the glucuronide can be cleaved and the medication or toxin reabsorbed. Therapy with repeated doses of activated charcoal is stopped when symptoms of intoxication cease and blood levels have returned to nontoxic ranges. Contraindications to activated charcoal are ileus, hydrocarbon ingestion, and an unprotected airway. It is important to reevaluate the child prior to each charcoal dose and to hold administration if bowel sounds are absent or there is significant increase in abdominal girth. Complications of activated charcoal treatment include pulmonary aspiration and mechanical small bowel obstruction.[10]

Cathartic agents such as sorbitol and magnesium citrate are frequently used to treat toxic ingestions.[11] They reduce drug absorption by increasing GI transit time thereby limiting the time for absorption of the toxin. Sorbitol in a 70% solution is dosed at 0.5 g/kg orally or per orogastric tube with or without activated charcoal. Magnesium citrate is administered in a dose of 4 mL/kg to a maximum of 250 mL. Either agent can be administered every 4 to 6 hours, with activated charcoal every 4 hours, as long as stool output is not excessive. Contraindications to cathartics include age less than 1 year, ileus, diarrhea, or recent abdominal surgery/trauma. Magnesium citrate should be avoided in all patients with acute renal failure, as a significant amount of the magnesium cation can be absorbed, resulting in hypermagnesemia. Overaggressive multiple dosing of cathartics, especially sorbitol in children, has been associated with metabolic abnormalities due to electrolyte loss in the stool.[12,13] However, there are no reported significant adverse effects from one to two appropriate doses of a cathartic in a previously healthy child.

WBI has been suggested for treatment of ingestions of agents that are poorly bound by activated charcoal, such as lithium, iron, ampicillin, and enteric coated aspirin. The theory of action for WBI is similar to that of bowel preparation for surgery. Isotonic polyethylene glycol is infused into the stomach via a well placed orogastric or nasogastric tube at a rate in children of 0.5 L/h, and in adolescents/adults at a rate 1 to 2 L/h. Therapy is continued for 4 to 6 hours or until stool output is clear without pill fragments. Contraindications to this therapy include the recent administration of ipecac, altered mental status in the absence of appropriate airway protection, and GI bleeding or obstruction.[14]

Enhanced Elimination of Poison/Toxin

Techniques for eliminating toxic compounds from the body should be considered in the setting of life-threatening poisonings. Many of the indications are controversial, but generally involve a lethal ingestion, severe/irreversible symptoms (eg, refractory status epilepticus or cardiovascular depression), or impairment of the normal route of elimination (eg, acute renal or hepatic failure). The most commonly used methods are: diuresis (with or without acidification/alkalinization of the urine), hemodialysis, and charcoal hemoperfusion. Hemodialysis and hemoperfusion for toxic compounds are discussed in chapter 16. Additional techniques, the values of which remain untested in randomized prospective studies, include exchange transfusion and plasmapheresis. The latter should be considered in the setting of severe compromise from poisonings with highly protein-bound drugs. The technique of "GI dialysis," with the increase in elimination of specific drugs provided by repetitive dosing of activated charcoal, has already been discussed. This process produces a gradient to remove toxins from the enterohepatic circulation and by increased excretion through the bowel wall and into the bowel lumen where they are bound by the charcoal (see section on activated charcoal).

Diuresis for the elimination of poisons from the body is routinely practiced in conjunction with the other techniques for decontamination and decreasing absorption.[15] Forced diuresis can be obtained using increased intravenous infusion of fluids at 1.5 to 2 times maintenance. The addition of diuretics such as mannitol or furosemide has been used, but is often unnecessary in the absence of nephrotoxicity. The goal is to maintain a urine output of 2 to 5 mL/kg/h. Alkalinization or acidification of the urine can assist in the elimination of certain compounds by preventing reabsorption from the renal tubule. Only unionized compounds are reabsorbed by the distal tubules. Alteration of the charge of specific compounds leads to ion trapping and decreases reabsorption by the renal tubules. Alkalinization of the urine to a pH ≥ 7.0 is accomplished by adding sodium bicarbonate (50 to 75 mEq/L) to the infusing fluids. Adverse effects include hypernatremia, hypokalemia, and fluid overload. Indications for alkalinization include ingestion of isoniazid, phenobarbital, and salicylate. Acetazolamide (5 mg/kg every 8 hours) can be added to sodium bicarbonate therapy to maintain an alkaline urine and to limit the adverse effects of sodium bicarbonate. Excessive dosing of acetazolamide can result in hypokalemia and metabolic acidosis.

Acidification of the urine to a pH ≤ 6.5 can be achieved by oral or intravenous ammonium chloride, intravenous hydrochloric acid, or oral ascorbic acid. Urinary acidification can increase the urinary excretion of quinidine, phencyclidine (PCP), fenfluramine, and amphetamine. The adverse effects of acidification, such as hyperkalemia, limit the applicability of this therapy.

Antidotes

Antidotes are pharmacologic agents that can be administered to reduce, limit, or prevent toxicity of a particular agent.[16] Their mechanism of action may be antagonistic (naloxone for opioids), to act as a chelating agent (deferoxamine for iron), or to reduce the bioavailability of the drug (digoxin antibodies for digoxin). Unfortunately, antidotes are available for only a minority of poisonings. Their administration should neither precede nor replace appropriate supportive care of the patient. Table 5 lists some of the commonly ingested agents and their respective antidotes.

Table 5

Antidotes for Common Poisonings

Drug or Toxin	Antidote
Acetaminophen	N-acetylcystiene
Benzodiazepines	flumazenil
β-adrenergic antagonists	glucagon
Carbon monoxide	oxygen
Cyanide	amyl nitrate
Digoxin	FAB fragments (digoxin antibody)
Ethylene glycol	ethanol, fomepizole (alcohol dehydrogenase inhibitor)
Iron	deferoxamine
Methanol	ethanol
Methemoglobin	methylene blue
Opioids	naloxone
Organophosphates	atropine, pralidoxime

Common Agents in Childhood Poisonings

Acetaminophen

Sources of Exposure

Acetaminophen remains one of the most common causes of toxicity in children and adolescents. Unintentional poisonings can occur from inaccurate dosing or accidental ingestion, and represent the usual causes of acetaminophen intoxication in younger children. Inadvertent overdoses may occur when patients do not realize that the products they are using, which may be prescription pain medications or over-the-counter cold medications, contain acetaminophen, and therefore ingest these agents in addition to standard doses of acetaminophen. Intentional poisonings (ie, suicide) are the typical experience of acetaminophen toxicity in adolescents. Intoxications in both settings usually result from over-the-counter preparations of acetaminophen.[17]

Mechanism of Action

The severity of acetaminophen toxicity is related to the amount ingested. Acetaminophen is metabolized by the liver via conjugation with sulfate and glucuronate. A small amount is conjugated via the cytochrome P450 with glutathione to make mercapturic acid. The combined accumulation of toxic metabolic products with the depletion of hepatocellular glutathione produces hepatic necrosis.

Toxic Signs and Symptoms

Nausea, vomiting, and malaise are the most prominent features. These will usually resolve in 24 to 48 hours. However, the absence and/or resolution of these symptoms does not determine the severity of ingestion. Patients suspected of ingesting greater than 150 mg/kg should be evaluated and treated because of an increased risk for fulminant liver necrosis.

Special Considerations in Treatment

In suicidal patients, coingestion of another drug should be considered. Children who have ingested less than 150 mg/kg can probably be monitored at home following induced emesis provided their 4-hour postingestion level falls in the nontoxic range on the nomogram (Fig 2). Those children and adolescents who have ingested over 150 mg/kg of acetaminophen should be evaluated and should undergo induced emesis and gastric lavage. A 4-hour postingestion serum acetaminophen level should be obtained and plotted on the acetaminophen toxicity nomogram.[18] The resulting level and its place on the nomogram determines the therapeutic plan. The nomogram was developed for immediate-release preparations of acetaminophen. There is limited information concerning the toxic levels with extended-release preparations. In the case of such ingestions, treatment options must be individualized, and repeated measurements of the serum acetaminophen level may be indicated. Certain underlying conditions increase the risk of toxicity and, therefore, treatment may be indicated with lower levels even if they fall in the nontoxic range on the nomogram. Such conditions include AIDS, alcohol abuse, chronic acetaminophen usage, preexisting liver disease, and use of medications that induce the P450 system (carbamazepine, phenytoin, and barbiturates) and increase the production of toxic metabolites. In patients who have ingested greater than 200 mg/kg and/or have a serum acetaminophen level at 4 hours that plots in the toxic range, N-acetylcysteine therapy is indicated. N-acetylcysteine should be administered orally; intravenous preparations are not yet in widespread clinical use. The optimal time for dosing is less than 16 hours from ingestion; however, patients with late presentation (≥16 hours) should still be treated with N-acetylcysteine if a hepatotoxic ingestion is suspected. Oral dosing begins with 140 mg/kg administered orally in a carbonated beverage or by nasogastric tube, followed by 70 mg/kg every 4 hours for 17 doses. The exact mechanism of N-acetylcysteine is unknown, but metabolism of this compound is thought to increase intracellular concentrations of glutathione, which binds toxic intermediate metabolites of acetaminophen or prevents their toxic effects on the hepatocytes. Due to its unpalatable nature, emesis may occur following N-acetylcysteine. If this

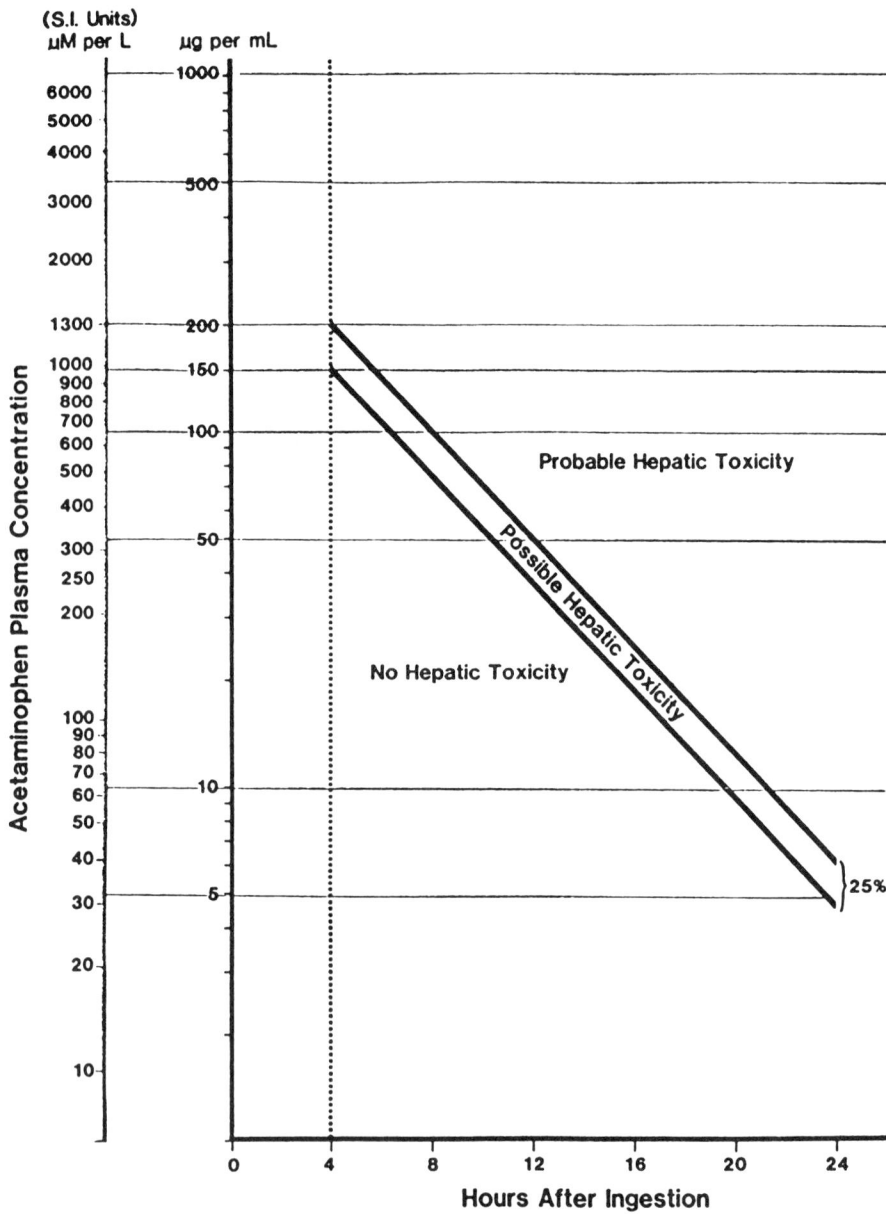

**RUMACK – MATTHEW NOMOGRAM
FOR ACETAMINOPHEN POISONING**

Figure 2. Rumack-Matthew nomogram for estimating the possibility of hepatotoxicity following acetaminophen ingestion. The acetaminophen plasma concentration obtained at least 4 hours after ingestion is listed on the y axis, while the time after ingestion is listed on the x axis. Values that fall above the line require therapy with N-acetylcysteine. The nomogram is valid only for immediate-release acetaminophen preparations and has not been validated for sustained release preparations. Additionally, the nomogram should not be used in patients with conditions that increase the likelihood of acetaminophen hepatotoxicity including AIDS, alcohol abuse, chronic acetaminophen usage, pre-existing liver disease, and medications that induce the P450 system (carbamazepine, phenytoin, and barbiturates) and increase the production of toxic metabolites. Reproduced by permission of *Pediatrics* vol. 55, pp 871–876, 1975.

occurs within 1 hour of the dose, the dose should be repeated. Emesis may be prevented by slow administration of the dose or by the prophylactic administration of antiemetics such as ondansetron.[19]

Alcohols: Ethanol, Methanol, Ethylene Glycol, Isopropyl Alcohol

Sources of Exposure

Alcohol ingestions are a common occurrence in children. Ethanol is in most liqueurs/liquors, and is present in much higher concentrations in aftershave lotions, mouth washes, and colognes. Isopropanol (isopropyl alcohol) is in rubbing alcohol, hair tonics, and skin lotions. Methanol is present in model airplane fuel and paint remover. Ethylene glycol is present in antifreeze and in automobile wiper fluids.[20]

Mechanism of Action

All alcohol/glycol compounds have rapid absorption and rapid onset of toxicity. All are metabolized by alcohol dehydrogenase with varying degrees of toxicity based on their metabolites. Methanol is metabolized in the liver to formaldehyde by alcohol dehydrogenase, and then to formic acid by aldehyde dehydrogenase. The metabolism of ethylene glycol is complex. The initial metabolic step involves formation of glycolaldehyde by alcohol dehydrogenase. Subsequent metabolic steps lead to multiple toxic metabolites, including oxalic acid, leading to metabolic disturbances (hypocalcemia) and increased calcium oxalate crystal formation in multiple tissues (the renal tubules and brain). The presence of oxalate crystals in the urine can be used diagnostically. Isopropyl alcohol is metabolized by alcohol dehydrogenase with less toxic metabolites than methanol or ethylene glycol. An additional metabolic complication is an excess of nicotinamide adenine dinucleotide phosphate (NADPH) produced by the metabolism of all of these alcohols by alcohol dehydrogenase. This leads to inhibition of the Krebs cycle and increased lactic acid formation and decreased gluconeogenesis leading to hypoglycemia.[21]

Toxic Signs and Symptoms

Alcohols cause depressed sensorium with respiratory depression, hypoglycemia, depression of cardiovascular function, metabolic acidosis, and widened anion and osmolar gaps. The more toxic alcohols, methanol and ethylene glycol, have more severe systemic manifestations. Methanol can lead to blindness due to the toxic effects of formic acid on the retina. Ethylene glycol ingestion can result in renal failure, from the production of toxic metabolites as well as the accumulation of calcium oxalate in the renal tissue.

Special Considerations in Treatment

Initial therapy for all alcohol ingestions focuses on supportive care and resuscitation of the cardiorespiratory system. Early investigation into the possibility of and treatment for hypoglycemia is indicated. Ethanol has been the "classic" antidote for alcohol/ethylene glycol poisoning because it competes with the other alcohols for alcohol dehydrogenase, thereby decreasing or slowing the metabolism of the other, more toxic, alcohols. Ethanol infusions can be complimented with hemodialysis or hemofiltration for methanol and ethylene glycol ingestions. The loading dose for ethanol is 0.7 g/kg followed by an infusion rate of 125 mg/kg/h, to maintain a blood ethanol level of 100 mg/mL. Fomepizole, an antidote for ethylene glycol poisonings, has recently become available. The latter agent also inhibits the activity of alcohol dehydrogenase and lacks the adverse effects associated with ethanol therapy. Recommended dosing includes an initial intravenous loading dose of 15 mg/kg followed by 10 mg/kg every 12 hours for four doses, then increased to 15 mg/kg every 12 hours until the serum ethylene glycol concentration is less than 20 mg/dL. Since fomepizole acts as an inhibitor of alcohol dehydrogenase, the elimination of ethylene glycol from the body still depends on filtration by the kidneys or by dialysis.[22]

Anticholinergic Syndromes

Sources of Exposure

Agents that are commonly associated with anticholinergic toxidromes are diphenhydramine, TCAD, phenothiazines, antiparkinsonian drugs, belladonna alkaloids, antispasmodics, jimson weed, nightshade, and mushrooms.

Mechanism of Action

Acetylcholine is a neurotransmitter that functions at muscarinic and nicotinic receptors. Nicotinic receptors are located in parasympathetic and sympathetic ganglion, as well as in the neuromuscular junction. Muscarinic receptors are located at the nerve endings of parasympathetic and sympathetic nerves. "Anticholinergic" drugs block the effects of acetylcholine by competitive inhibition at the muscarinic receptors peripherally, and in the brain, creating the clinical signs and symptoms of anticholinergic intoxication.

Toxic Signs and Symptoms

The classic anticholinergic symptoms can be recalled by the mnemonic: "red as a beet, mad as a hatter, hot as a hare, blind as a bat, dry as a bone." Additional clinical manifestations of anticholinergic intoxication include bradycardia, hypertension, decreased GI motility, altered mental status, and convulsions. If TCADs are the causative agent of the anticholinergic syndrome, arrhythmias are a major concern.

Special Considerations in Treatment

Supportive care is the mainstay of therapy. Because TCADs can have significant effects on the cardiac conduction system, an electrocardiogram (ECG) should be obtained to evaluate any abnormalities in the QT or QRS intervals (see below for a full discussion of TCAD ingestion). The use of physostigmine, a centrally acting inhibitor of acetylcholinesterase, remains controversial. Recommended dosing for physostigmine in adults is 0.5 mg every 5 to 10 minutes until a total of 2.0 mg has been administered or symptoms are reversed. Structurally, physostigmine resembles two joined molecules of acetylcholine and binds competitively to acetylcholinesterase. This effectively increases acetylcholine in the synapse and can reverse anticholinergic symptoms. Adverse effects of physostigmine include precipitation of convulsions, bradyarrhythmias, asystole, or cholinergic crisis.[23]

Calcium Channel Blockers, β-Adrenergic Antagonists, Clonidine

Sources of Exposure

Because of the increased use of antihypertensive agents in adults, many children ingest these agents unintentionally in settings inside their own home and while visiting relatives. Additionally, the indications and applications of clonidine continue to increase with its suggested efficacy in various behavioral disorders. The most common classes of antihypertensive agents seen in poisoning include the calcium channel blockers, β-adrenergic antagonists, and clonidine.[24] Common calcium channel blockers include diltiazem, nifedipine, nicardipine, and verapamil. Commonly prescribed β-adrenergic antagonists include propranolol, nadolol, labetalol, and metoprolol. Although clonidine is the prototype for the central acting α-adrenergic agonists, similar agents are found in many over-the-counter nasal sprays and ophthalmic solutions. Ingestions of these compounds can also result in significant toxicity.[25]

Mechanism of Action

Calcium channel blockers are a common class of medications used to treat hypertension, ischemic heart disease, arrhythmias, and migraine headaches. There are a variety of cardiovascular effects related to the primary mechanism of action of calcium channel blockers, which is to reduce entry of calcium into myocardial and vascular smooth muscle cells. The primary cardiovascular effects of calcium channel blockers include decreased myocardial contractility, vasodilation, and decreased chronotropic/

dromotropic function of the cardiac conducting tissue. The cardiovascular effects of the β-adrenergic antagonists are similar, and include a decreased force of contraction, vasodilation, and decreased chronotropic and dromotropic function of the conduction system. Clonidine is an α_2-adrenergic agonist that decreases central sympathetic output.

Toxic Signs and Symptoms

All of these agents cause hypotension and, to a more variable degree, bradycardia and decreased dromotropic function when ingested in toxic doses. Significant ingestions can result in prolongation of the PR interval or in complete heart block. All of these agents can produce CNS and respiratory depression, which are particularly common with α_2-agonists such as clonidine. Calcium channel blockers and β-adrenergic antagonists, in toxic doses, can cause seizure activity. Additional adverse effects include bronchospasm and hypoglycemia with β-adrenergic antagonists, and hypothermia with clonidine.

Special Considerations in Treatment

Management of the toxic ingestion of all of these agents begins with cardiorespiratory support followed by gastric lavage and activated charcoal. Induced emesis can be undertaken, but is relatively contraindicated in the setting of clonidine poisoning, due to the rapid onset of CNS depression. Hypotension should be treated with the administration of isotonic fluids and a direct-acting adrenergic agent such as epinephrine, starting at 0.1 μg/kg/min and increased as needed to maintain an adequate mean arterial pressure and heart rate. In the case of calcium channel blocker ingestions, calcium chloride (0.1 to 0.2 mL/kg of a 10% solution intravenously) or calcium gluconate (0.2 to 0.4 mL/kg of a 10% solution intravenously) are effective adjuncts in the treatment of the arrhythmias and hypotension. Bradycardia that is unresponsive to atropine or epinephrine should be treated with transcutaneous or intravenous pacing. Glucagon, an inotropic agent that bypasses the adrenergic receptor, may be particularly effective in the treatment of hypotension and bradycardia seen with β-adrenergic antagonist ingestion. Dosing for glucagon includes 0.05 mg/kg intravenously followed by an infusion of 0.07 mg/kg/h. For clonidine ingestions, large doses of naloxone (0.1 mg/kg) may help to reverse CNS and cardiovascular depression.

Caustic Agents: Acid and Alkali Ingestions

Sources of Exposure

Alkaline caustic materials are present in a variety of materials, such as lye (sodium hydroxide), ammonia cleaners, chemical drain openers, mildew removers, and button batteries. Acidic products include rust removers, cement cleaners, metal cleaners, toilet bowl cleaners, oven cleaners, and automobile batteries.[26]

Mechanism of Action

Caustic materials differ in their potency and degree of injury to the mucosa, depending on their concentration, pH, and the duration of exposure/contact. Ingestion of caustic materials, both alkali and acids, results in two types of injury: liquefactive necrosis and coagulation necrosis. Ingestion of alkali materials usually results in the saponification of cellular fats, protein degradation, and deep-tissue injury to the mouth and proximal esophagus. Acidic ingestion results in the production of heat and extensive burns from the mouth, along the esophagus, and into the stomach.

Toxic Signs and Symptoms

Ingestion of these agents results in mucosal and dermal injury from contact. Problems of aspiration pneumonitis have also been reported. Severe intoxication is characterized by throat pain, refusal to eat or drink, dysphagia, nausea, vomiting, and mouth sores. Additional findings may include fever, acidosis (with acid ingestion), respiratory distress, and cardiovascular instability. The physical examination should be performed with an emphasis on the identification of subcutaneous air and crepitus, as well as pneumoperitoneum, pneumothorax, or pneumomediastinum, which indicate possible esophageal or tracheal perforation.

Special Considerations in Treatment

Initial evaluation of the airway and breathing are important for the assessment of any compromise in the airway. The patient whose airway is compromised should be taken quickly to the operating room. These patients should be cared for with use of the same protocols as for other causes of upper airway obstruction (eg, epiglottitis and foreign bodies). Injury to the laryngeal structure may result in edema and the rapid onset of upper-airway edema, making routine airway management difficult (see chapter 3 for a full discussion of management of the patient with upper airway obstruction). If stable, decontamination of the skin and mucous membranes should occur by washing with water and wiping debris from the skin and mouth.

Swallowed button batteries should be evaluated with chest x-ray and abdominal radiograph. If they are located in the esophagus, they should be removed. If they are below the lower esophageal sphincter they can be watched for passage in the stool. Administration of a cathartic agent is a consideration.[27]

If the patient has ingested liquid agents and has extensive oral and esophageal burns, administration of oral materials, induced emesis, and placement of an orogastric tube are contraindicated. Endoscopic evaluation should be undertaken in the first 24 hours because of the increased risk of perforation if performed after 48 hours. For patients who have evidence of esophageal injury, the administration of corticosteroids may decrease inflammation and reduce subsequent scarring, but remains controversial.[28]

Cholinergic Syndromes

Sources of Exposure

Agents commonly identified as sources of cholinergic intoxication in children include organophosphates, insecticides, nicotine, and carbamates.

Mechanism of Action

These compounds are absorbed readily through the skin, respiratory tract, and GI tract. Organophosphates bind irreversibly to the acetylcholinesterase enzyme with 150 times the affinity of acetylcholine. This leads to accumulation of the neurotransmitter acetylcholine, and continued stimulation of the receptors. Acetylcholine is released in nicotinic and muscarinic synapses. The subsiding of the stimulus, cessation of acetylcholine release, and rapid degradation of the acetylcholine by acetylcholinesterases normally stops transmission. Carbamates differ from organophosphates in that they only transiently inactivate acetylcholinesterase and have decreased CNS penetration.[29]

Toxic Signs and Symptoms

The effects of these poisonings can be subclassified on the basis of the receptors, as muscarinic, nicotinic, and central (or CNS). The muscarinic effects can be remembered by the acronym "SLUDGE": salivation, lacrimation, urination, defecation, GI distress, and emesis. Nicotinic symptoms include pupillary dilatation, pallor, arrhythmias, hypertension, weakness, paralysis, areflexia, and fasciculations. The central manifestations are variable, but include headache, confusion, irritability, ataxia, seizures, psychosis, and coma. Carbamate poisonings usually lack the central signs of toxicity that can be seen with organophosphate ingestions.

Special Considerations in Treatment

Supportive care and observation is usually adequate in most cases of cholinergic intoxication. Decontamination by removing all clothing and cleansing the skin is imperative. For severe cases, administration of atropine, the classic antidote, starts with 0.05 mg/kg intravenously, with repeat doses, at increased amounts, every 5 minutes until the oral mucosa becomes dry and the heart rate is greater than 80 to 140 beats per minute, depending on the patients age. Atropine binds to the acetylcholine receptor to block further muscarinic stimulation and thereby reduce symptoms. The dose should be repeated every 30 to 60 minutes for 12 to 24 hours. Some authors advocate continuous atropine infusions at 0.02 to 0.08 mg/kg/h intravenously in the setting of severe cholinergic intoxications. With organophosphate intoxication, pralidoxime (25 mg/kg to a maximum of 1 gram) may be beneficial by hastening the recovery of acetylcholinesterase by binding with the phosphate moiety of the organophosphate. As the organophosphates eventually irreversibly bind to the acetylcholinesterase, therapy must be initiated within 24 to 48 hours of exposure. Pralidoxime is most effective in restoring function at nicotinic receptors. A rapid improvement in strength may be observed within 10 to 15 minutes of administration.[30]

Cyanide

Sources of Exposure

A child can develop cyanide poisoning in a variety of settings including inhalation exposure during household fires, the ingestion of cosmetics, silver polish, rodenticides, insecticides, plant and fruit pits, laetrile tablets, or during the therapeutic administration of sodium nitroprusside.[31,32]

Mechanism of Action

Cyanide inhibits oxidative phosphorylation by binding with cytochrome oxidase and creating a "biochemical" asphyxia by uncoupling electron transport and inhibiting oxygen use by the mitochondria.

Toxic Signs and Symptoms

The "classic" smell of bitter almonds is not always present. Other symptoms such as dizziness, headache, acute mental status changes, tachypnea, and hypertension are variable and nonspecific. Laboratory tests may reveal an elevated lactic acid level and widened anion gap resulting from tissue hypoxia. Diagnosis can be made by obtaining a blood cyanide level.

Special Considerations in Treatment

The child should receive a fraction of inspired oxygen (FiO_2) of 1.0 via a high flow or a nonrebreathing system as soon as cyanide poisoning is suspected. Inhaled amyl nitrate followed by intravenous sodium nitrite should be administered to begin the oxidation of iron in hemoglobin from the ferrous (Fe^{++}) state to the ferric (Fe^{+++}) state. This oxidation forms methemoglobin (MetHb), which actively binds cyanide thereby preventing its binding to cytochrome oxidase. The goal is to achieve a MetHb level of 20% to 25%. MetHb in itself is toxic since it does not effectively carry oxygen and can cause inadequate oxygen delivery to the tissues if levels exceed 30%. MetHb has a greater affinity for cyanide and readily binds it, creating cyanomethemoglobin. This first step only reduces the bioavailability of cyanide; another step must occur for its elimination. In the second step, the hepatic rhodanese enzyme system combines cyanide with a sulfur group from thiosulfate to form thiocyanate. Intravenous sodium thiosulfate should be administered along with sodium nitrite to increase the efficiency of this reaction and provide the necessary sulfur substrate for the rhodanese enzyme system. Thiocyanate is then filtered into the urine by the kidneys.[33]

Digoxin

Sources of Exposure

Unlike many poisonings, the majority of digoxin intoxications result from errors in drug administration. However, with the number of adults receiving this medication, accidental ingestions do occur. "Digoxin-like" drugs and compounds are present in other medicines (eg, digitoxin, ouabain) and in some herbal and plant remedies (dogbane, foxglove, lily of the valley, oleander, and red squill).[34]

Mechanism of Action

Digoxin is a cardiac glycoside that acts on the myocardium to increase conduction and inotropy through inhibition of the Na^+-K^+-ATPase pump. Inhibition results in increased intracellular sodium, increased intracellular calcium, and an increased inotropic response.

Toxic Signs and Symptoms

Blood digoxin levels of greater than 2.0 ng/mL in children and adolescents can result in toxicity. Regardless of the level, if symptoms are present, even in chronic users, toxicity should be suspected. Typical GI manifestations include nausea, vomiting, and abdominal pain. CNS changes are often characterized by lethargy, weakness, and behavioral changes. The cardiovascular effects involve various arrhythmias, with a prolongation of the PR interval and a shortened QT interval. Laboratory tests should assess potassium, calcium, and magnesium, as abnormalities of these electrolytes can exacerbate digoxin toxicity and require additional treatment. An ECG should be obtained and compared to prior tracings, if available, to detect subtle signs of toxicity.

Special Considerations in Treatment

If no symptoms are present, simply holding the subsequent doses of digoxin may be satisfactory therapy. If symptoms are present and the amount ingested is likely to produce significant toxicity (eg, a suicide attempt or multiple pills), then aggressive gastric decontamination should occur, along with continuous cardiac monitoring and serial ECGs. Repetitive dosing of activated charcoal with a cathartic is advocated for binding residual digoxin in the GI and preventing further absorption. If symptoms are non-life-threatening, then electrolyte abnormalities such as hypokalemia and hypomagnesemia should be corrected and the patient monitored with a continuous ECG. However, if hypotension, arrhythmias, and hyperkalemia are present, purified digoxin Fab fragment (antibody to digoxin) should be administered. Digoxin Fab will bind 0.5 mg of digoxin for every 40-mg vial administered. The dosage of this antidote can be based on the serum concentration of the digoxin or the estimated amount that has been ingested.[35]

The dose (mg) of digoxin Fab based on the serum digoxin level is:

$$\text{digoxin level (ng/mL)} \times 5.6 \times \text{weight (kg)}/1000$$

The dose (mg) of digoxin Fab based on the amount ingested is:

$$\text{amount of digoxin ingested (mg)} / 0.5 \text{ mg per vial} = \# \text{ of vials}$$

If oral elixir or capsules are ingested, multiply the amount ingested by 0.8 to account for the reduced absorption of the digoxin. If an unknown quantity of digoxin has been ingested and no serum level is available, administer 10 vials of digoxin Fab. In the event that digoxin Fab is not available or if there will be a delay in administration, arrhythmias should be managed with atropine, phenytoin, and lidocaine.

Hemoglobinopathies: Carboxyhemoglobinemia and Methemoglobinemia

Carbon monoxide (CO) is the leading cause of poisoning/toxic deaths in the US for adults and children, resulting in up to 3500 fatalities per year. An additional 10,000 people each year are evaluated in the emergency department because of minor CO toxicity. Methemoglobinemia is a less frequent occurrence, but still occurs in the US from hereditary and environmental exposures.[36,37]

Sources of Exposure

CO is produced by combustion engines, fires, gas furnaces, and propane stoves. Poisonings occur most often in closed settings, automobiles, homes, boat cabins, and house fires. Unenclosed (open-air) CO poisonings do occur, but are rare.

Methemoglobinemia is caused by either hereditary predisposition (abnormal hemoglobins due to amino acid alterations such as hemoglobin M or hereditary deficiencies of enzyme systems such as MetHb reductase) or environmental exposure to nitrogenous compounds. Common sources of environmental oxidants include local anesthetic agents (prilocaine, benzocaine), contaminated well water supplies or foods, house fires, naphthalene (moth balls), nitroglycerin, nitroprusside, and inhaled nitric oxide. Due to the decreased resistance to oxidant stresses of fetal hemoglobin and the decreased efficiency of hepatic enzyme systems such as MetHb reductase, neonates and infants are more prone to develop methemoglobinemia following exposure to specific pharmacologic agents.

Mechanism of Action

CO binds to hemoglobin with 200 times the affinity of oxygen, forming carboxyhemoglobin (COHb). As the percentage of COHb ($\geq 10\%$ to 15%) increases, the oxygen-carrying capacity of the blood is significantly reduced. This results in tissue hypoxia.

MetHb is formed by oxidation of the iron moiety in hemoglobin from the Fe^{++} form to the Fe^{+++} form. This change results in a decreased affinity for oxygen, a shifting of the oxygen-hemoglobin saturation curve to the left, and an overall reduction in oxygen delivery to the tissues with cellular hypoxia. Normal levels of MetHb in the body range from 0% to 3%, with toxic manifestations (tissue hypoxia) beginning at concentrations of $\geq 30\%$.

Both conditions can be detected by co-oximetry from either venous or arterial blood. Many standard blood gas machines do not actually measure the different hemoglobin species. Rather, the oxygen saturation is estimated based on the partial pressure of arterial oxygen (PaO_2). Monitoring, such as pulse oximetry, is also inaccurate (see above). Therefore, clinical suspicion is of paramount importance. In the setting of methemoglobinemia, drawn blood can have a classic "chocolate" appearance. The diagnosis is confirmed by measurement of the hemoglobin species using co-oximetry.

Toxic Signs and Symptoms

Physical findings in CO poisoning can be significant for "cherry red" mucous membranes, tachypnea, tachycardia, and dizziness. However, children most often present with mental status changes, coma, syncope, vomiting, and headache. Diagnosis is made on clinical suspicion and venous/arterial co-oximetry demonstrating an elevated COHb level. Normal COHb levels do not rule out or correlate with the severity of CO poisoning.

Methemoglobinemia will classically present with a cyanotic to grey appearing child with an oxygen saturation measured by pulse oximetry in the low 90% to mid 80% range. Systemic symptoms are seen with more severe intoxication including dyspnea, headache, fatigue, weakness, tachycardia, lactic acidosis, seizures, coma, and death.

Special Consideration in Treatment

A patient suspected of CO poisoning should receive FiO_2 at 1.0 via a high flow or nonrebreathing system. If the COHb is $\geq 15\%$ to 20% or the patient has or has had significant symptoms such as syncope or coma, consideration should be given to hyperbaric oxygen therapy. Treatment for methemoglobinemia begins with careful assessment of airway and breathing. If the methemoglobinemia results from an ingestion and there are no contraindications, gastric decontamination with induced emesis and/or lavage may be undertaken. If the MetHb level is less than 20% and there are no symptoms other than cyanosis, the clinician should proceed with decontamination and supportive care. However, if more severe symptoms are present and/or the MetHb level is $\geq 20\%$, definitive therapy with methylene blue is indicated. Methylene blue is dosed at 1 to 2 mL/kg administered intravenously over 5 to 10 minutes. An improvement in the patient's cyanosis should occur within 10 to 20 minutes. Methylene blue works to convert MetHb back to the normal Fe^{++} state by inducing MetHb reductase. If no improvement is seen, repeat dosing and repeat measurements of MetHb are suggested. If no benefit is demonstrated, the child should be evaluated for possible sulfhemoglobinemia, glucose-6-phosphate dehydrogenase deficiency, or an inherited hemoglobin M or NADPH-dependent MetHb reductase deficiency. At this point in care, hyperbaric oxygen therapy may be considered until a more definitive diagnosis is made.[38,39]

Hydrocarbons

Sources of Exposure

Hydrocarbon ingestions occur in up to 28,000 children per year, the majority of whom are less than 5 years of age. These substances are associated with a high mortality, ranging from 5% to 25%. They are available in many forms and are found in many commonly used materials including gasoline, turpentine, mineral spirits, kerosene, lubricating oil, and lighter fluid.[40]

Mechanism of Action

The physical properties of the hydrocarbon determine the risk of aspiration. The risk is highest in those with low volatility, low viscosity, and low surface tension. Compounds with the highest aspiration risk are kerosene and mineral spirits. Those with the lowest aspiration risk are gasoline, motor oil, mineral oil, and transmission fluid. Hydrocarbon pneumonitis is thought to occur because of surfactant removal and resultant atelectasis, and inflammation of the alveoli. Associated toxicity from compounds in the fluid, such as heavy metals or pesticide, should be considered. Inhalation abuse, or "sniffing," of hydrocarbons has resulted in "sudden death" from arrhythmias because of increased sensitization of the myocardium by the volatile compounds.

Toxic Signs and Symptoms

Children with hydrocarbon intoxication present with pulmonary symptoms, GI upset, and CNS manifestations. Respiratory symptoms include wheezing, coughing, and dyspnea of rapid onset (<2 hours after ingestion). Rather than direct CNS depression from the compounds, CNS symptoms are primarily a result of aspiration-induced hypoxia. GI symptoms include nausea, vomiting, diarrhea, and abdominal pain.

Special Considerations in Treatment

The majority of children who ingest hydrocarbons do not need evaluation provided that they are and remain asymptomatic. However, those who have any respiratory symptoms, such as coughing, gagging, wheezing, or dyspnea, should be immediately evaluated by a physician. Children with mild or transient symptoms should have an ECG and chest x-ray and should be observed for a minimum of 4 to 6 hours. If symptoms recur, if there is an abnormal ECG, or if additional symptoms develop, then the child should be admitted and placed in a monitored bed, even if the chest x-ray is normal. If the child is asymptomatic during this observation period but abnormalities are noted on chest x-ray, admission is strongly advised. Home observation in this latter scenario can only be undertaken with close physician follow-up and reliable parents.

Iron

Sources of Exposure

The majority of toxic ingestions result from unintentional ingestion of over-the-counter vitamin preparations or prescription-strength iron supplements. The severity of iron toxicity can be quite variable depending on the preparation and the resultant total dose of elemental iron. When taking the history, the preparation ingested and its iron concentration should be determined. The percentage of elemental iron in gluconate, sulfate, and fumarate preparations is 12%, 20%, and 33%, respectively.[41]

Mechanism of Action

The majority of early symptoms seen with iron ingestions are attributable to the direct effects of iron on the gastric mucosa. The exact mechanism accounting for other symptoms, such as cardiovascular instability and coagulopathy, remain unclear. All patients who have ingested more than 20 mg/kg of elemental iron are at risk for moderate to severe symptoms and will require medical treatment.

Toxic Signs and Symptoms

The clinical course of iron poisonings has been divided into four phases. The first phase includes mild to severe symptoms of GI upset. Vomiting, nausea, diarrhea, and abdominal pain are typical. In a severe intoxication, hemorrhagic gastroenteritis, shock, and encephalopathy can occur. Severe intoxications are highly unlikely in the absence of any GI symptoms. During the second phase (6 to 12 hours following ingestion), all symptoms of the first phase can resolve. This is true even of severe intoxication symptoms (ie, shock and encephalopathy). However, this quiet period can give way to the third phase of iron poisoning. This phase is characterized by the return of all first-phase symptoms along with hypoglycemia, coagulopathy, liver failure, and renal failure. Multisystem organ failure and death are possibilities during this phase. Only a small percentage of patients progress to the fourth phase, which occurs 4 to 6 weeks following a severe ingestion and is characterized by GI dysfunction and partial GI obstruction resulting from the healing and scarring of the GI tract.

Serum iron concentrations correlate well with the severity and incidence of toxicity. The peak serum iron level occurs 2 to 6 hours following ingestion. During this time, serum iron concentrations below 300 µg/dL are indicative of mild ingestions, serum iron levels of 300 to 500 µg/dL indicate moderate ingestions, and levels greater than 500 µg/dL are indicative of severe iron intoxications. Those iron ingestions with serum levels greater than 1000 µg/dL are considered lethal.

Special Considerations in Treatment

Once the patient's airway is secure, gastric decontamination can occur. Induced emesis or gastric lavage should be instituted as early as possible. After 6 hours following ingestion, these methods should still be applied, but may be of limited utility. The addition of deferoxamine or sodium bicarbonate to the lavage fluid to bind iron still present in the GI tract and to prevent its subsequent absorption has been suggested. An abdominal radiograph should be obtained to look for iron aggregates and pill fragments. If radio-opaque material is seen, WBI or gastrotomy should be considered. Iron tablets can form a large bezoar in the stomach and can act as a source of continued release of iron. In severe cases, the mass may need to be surgically removed. If the total dosage of elemental iron is estimated to be greater than 15 mg/kg or if the 6-hour serum iron level is greater than 500 µg/dL then antidote therapy with deferoxamine should be initiated. At this level, there is a significant amount of free iron in the serum, as the body's total iron-binding capacity has been exceeded. If the amount ingested is unknown or if serum iron levels are not available, a test dose of deferoxamine may be given. If free iron is present, suggesting that the body's ability to bind iron is inadequate, the urine will turn pink with the iron-deferoxamine complex, suggesting the need to institute therapy. Deferoxamine is an iron-binding ligand that chelates iron to a less toxic form. Deferoxamine is administered at a rate of 15 mg/kg/h until symptoms resolves, the urine is clear (deferoxamine and iron in the urine result in a pink tinge to the urine), and serum iron levels are less than 100 µg/dL. Adverse effects from deferoxamine include tachycardia and hypotension. If these occur, slowing the infusion rate by 20% to 30% usually results in resolution of symptoms.[42]

Opioids

Sources of Exposure

Most pediatric opioid poisonings are either unintentional or suicidal. Recreational abuse/use of these drugs is rare in children, but does occur.

Mechanism of Action

The binding of opioid compounds to their specific receptors is responsible for their activity. The μ_1-receptor activity results in analgesia and CNS depression while the μ_2-receptor is responsible for the respiratory and cardiovascular manifestations. Opioids are rapidly absorbed from the oral and gastric mucosa, and undergo hepatic metabolism and renal excretion.[43]

Toxic Signs and Symptoms

The classic triad of opioid intoxication symptoms includes respiratory depression, coma/lethargy, and miosis. Additional symptoms may include bradycardia, hypotension, and decreased GI motility.

Special Considerations in Treatment

Airway management must be of foremost concern because of CNS and respiratory depression. Due to the rapid onset of action that results in CNS depression, induced emesis should be avoided if the ingestion occurred greater than 1 to 2 hours prior to presentation. Naloxone is an opioid receptor antagonist and acts on the mu, kappa, and delta receptors. Its administration is both diagnostic and therapeutic. Initial doses include 0.05 to 0.1 mg/kg to a maximum of 2.0 mg. The dose can be repeated every 2 to 3 minutes until a total of 10 mg has been administered. If at that point reversal of the CNS depression has not occurred, opioid intoxication is unlikely. Because the half-life of naloxone is shorter (15 to 20 minutes) than most opioids, repeat dosing or a continuous naloxone infusion may be warranted until the opioids have been fully metabolized and excreted.[44,45]

Salicylates

Sources of Exposure

The incidence of salicylate intoxication in children has decreased significantly with the introduction of other commercially available "pain relievers" (ie, ibuprofen and acetaminophen) and the decreased use of aspirin in children because of the fear of Reye's syndrome. However, salicylate intoxication still occurs from adult aspirin preparations and from other compounds that contain significant amounts of salicylates including oil of wintergreen (methyl salicylate) or Pepto Bismol (Procter & Gamble, Cincinnati, OH).

Mechanism of Action

Hyperpyrexia and severe metabolic acidosis result from the uncoupling of oxidative phosphorylation and the depletion of intracellular phosphates. In addition, direct inhibition of several enzymes in the Krebs cycle contributes to the worsening of metabolic acidosis and decreased utilization of carbohydrates with resultant hyperglycemia. Salicylates can act directly on the respiratory center, creating rapid breathing and a respiratory alkalosis early in the ingestion that is followed by the subsequent development of metabolic acidosis. This phenomenon of early respiratory alkalosis occurs most frequently in adolescents and adults.

Toxic Signs and Symptoms

Careful monitoring of the patient's symptoms and laboratory values are the basis for treatment and intervention. Severe symptoms are likely with ingestions of greater than 300 mg/kg, with the potential of mortality with ingestions of greater than 500 mg/kg. Mild intoxication (150 to 300 mg/kg) is characterized by symptoms of hyperpnea, lethargy, vomiting, and tinnitus. Moderate intoxication includes worsening hyperpnea and CNS depression (without coma or convulsions). Severe intoxication is characterized by severe hyperpnea, coma, convulsions, and hyperthermia. Because symptoms correlate with severity of poisoning, they, and not the blood levels or the Done nomogram, which may not accurately predict the severity of the ingestion, should be used as a guideline when initiating treatment.[46]

Special Considerations in Treatment

Supportive care of the child, based on the metabolic abnormalities encountered, is the most important treatment for salicylate intoxication. Alkalinization of the urine with parenteral sodium bicarbonate therapy enhances the elimination of salicylates from the body. If enteric coated aspirin has been ingested, repetitive charcoal dosing and WBI should be considered, with repeated measurement of salicylate levels. Salicylate levels along with serum electrolytes, glucose, calcium, and pH should be monitored every 4 to 6 hours to evaluate the patient's response and the efficacy of ongoing therapy.

Sedatives: Benzodiazepines and Barbiturates

Sources of Exposure

Compounds in these two categories are commonly administered to adults and children for their medicinal values. They are both readily available and are a source of frequent poisoning. Morbidity and mortality from barbiturates and benzodiazepines are negligible if recognized and managed appropriately. Phenobarbital is the most widely used of the barbiturates. Many different benzodiazepines are used, including alprazolam (Xanax®, Upjohn, Kalamazoo, MI), chlordiazepoxide (Librium®, Roche Products, Manati, Puerto Rico), clonazepam (Klonopin®, Roche Laboratories, Nutley, NJ), diazepam (Valium®, Roche Products), and lorazepam (Ativan®, Wyeth-Ayerst, Philadelphia, PA).[47]

Mechanism of Action

The benzodiazepines and the barbiturates act by potentiating the action of the inhibitory neurotransmitter γ-aminobutyric acid (GABA), resulting in decreased chloride conductance across the cell membrane, neuronal hyperpolarization with CNS depression, and respiratory depression. The barbiturates are metabolized by the cytochrome P450 system. The majority of benzodiazepines are oxidized by the liver, with a few undergoing conjugation with glucuronide (eg, lorazepam). Some of these compounds also have active metabolites and undergo enterohepatic recirculation.

Toxic Signs and Symptoms

Symptoms of barbiturate intoxication include ataxia, headache, vertigo, lethargy, increased somnolence, respiratory depression, shock, hypothermia, and bullae of the skin. Similar symptoms are present in benzodiazepine toxicity, including dizziness, ataxia, slurred speech, respiratory depression, coma, and hypotension.

Special Considerations in Treatment

In addition to airway management and supportive care, the child suffering from barbiturate intoxication must be carefully monitored and treated with repetitive doses of activated charcoal to prevent further absorption and to decrease the enterohepatic circulation. In the setting of barbiturate intoxication, consideration should be given to forced diuresis and alkalinization of the urine to enhance elimination. If symptoms are severe and cardiovascular instability predominates, then hemodialysis or hemofiltration should be considered.

Benzodiazepine intoxications should receive the same degree of careful evaluation and support, with protection of the airway. If an isolated ingestion of benzodiazepines can be demonstrated, flumazenil, 0.1 to 0.3 mg (10 µg/kg), can be administrated intravenously to reverse symptoms. The dose can be repeated at 5-minute intervals if a benefit is seen. Flumazenil's duration of action is limited (15 to 20 minutes), and repeated doses may be necessary based on the half-life of the ingested benzodiazepine. Unlike naloxone, flumazenil is contraindicated as a diagnostic tool for benzodiazepines and has been reported to precipitate seizures if the patient has been receiving long-term benzodiazepine therapy or has ingested other compounds that are known to decrease the seizure threshold, such as TCADs.[48] Flumazenil's mechanism of action is competitive inhibition of the action of benzodiazepines at the GABA receptor.

Sympathomimetics: Cocaine, Phencyclidine, Amphetamines, Theophylline

Sources of Exposure

A wide variety of substances can cause "sympathomimetic" symptoms. These substances all cause CNS stimulation and tachycardia. Because of the CNS effects, many of these substances are abused, especially by adolescents. However, children may ingest these substances either accidentally or intentionally. Intentional poisonings are an increasingly recognized form of child abuse.[49,50] Cocaine,[51] PCP,[52] and amphetamines[53] are often manufactured and purchased in illegal and uncontrolled settings. Theophylline, still used for asthma treatment, is usually a prescribed medication and is not usually abused. Toxicities are seen in suicide attempts,[54] with drug dosing errors, and with unintentional ingestions.

Mechanism of Action

Each of the sympathomimetics has a unique mechanism of action. Originally used as a local anesthetic and vasoconstrictor, cocaine has neurologic and cardiovascular stimulant qualities that have led to its abuse and characteristic toxic manifestations. Whether smoked, inhaled, or injected, it has a rapid onset of action. In the bloodstream, it undergoes degradation by serum cholinesterases, esterification, demethylation by the liver, and nonenzymatic hydrolation. Some of its metabolites have additional toxic effects. The metabolites benzoylecognine and ecgonine methyl ester are detected in the blood and urine because of the short half-life of cocaine. Cocaine increases sympathetic tone by blocking reuptake of neurotransmitters, specifically norepinephrine. This overstimulation results in its toxic effects on the cardiovascular system and the CNS.

PCP was originally used as an anesthetic agent. However, because of the hallucinatory effects, its medical usage was discontinued. Like cocaine, PCP can be inhaled, smoked, snorted, eaten, and injected (the latter occurs only rarely). The exact mechanism of action is unknown. The stimulatory effects of PCP on the CNS and cardiovascular system are thought to occur via β-adrenergic and α-adrenergic agonism, in addition to some anticholinergic effects.

Amphetamines (eg, dextroamphetamine, methamphetamine) are a commonly abused CNS stimulant. Routes of administration are oral, smoking, snorting, and, less often, injection. Onset of action is slower than that of cocaine and PCP, with symptoms gradually increasing over 15 to 20 minutes. This class of drugs acts as a CNS and cardiovascular stimulant by increasing neurotransmitter release, directly stimulating postsynaptic catecholamine receptors, and preventing neurotransmitter reuptake.

Theophylline is a methylxanthine. The exact mechanism of action is unknown. Theophylline is metabolized in the liver by the P450 system to its active metabolite 3-methylxanthine. Because 70% of theophylline's pharmacologic activity is dependent on this metabolite, any effects on liver function can dramatically effect theophylline levels and thereby increase the risk of toxicity (eg, viral illnesses, erythromycin, cimetidine, phenobarbital). Once toxic levels are reached, phosphodiesterase inhibition and increased β-adrenergic stimulation may explain or contribute to the observed toxic effects of theophylline. Theophylline has positive inotropic and chronotropic effects on the myocardium, causes increased gastric secretions and motility, and acts on the central nervous system to lower seizure threshold and stimulate the respiratory and emetic centers.

Toxic Signs and Symptoms

Sympathomimetic agents share many of the same signs and symptoms, making their individual identification difficult by clinical examination. All of these drugs can cause agitation, diaphoresis, and tachycardia. There are some signs and symptoms unique to each class. Cocaine abuse is suggested on physical examination by perforation of the nasal septum. Early symptoms of cocaine ingestion are euphoria, hyperalertness, paranoia, dilated pupils, and hypertension. Overdose of cocaine can result in coma, myocardial ischemia, hyperthermia, rhabdomyolisis, stroke, and seizures. Laboratory tests should include serum and urine drug screen, creatine phosphokinase of muscle band (CPK-MB) isoenzymes for myocardial damage, ECG, and renal function studies and urinalysis.

PCP ingestions typically result in hallucinogenic states of euphoria and dysphoria, nystagmus, miosis, and ataxia. With more severe toxicity, additional findings are arrhythmias, hyperthermia, hypersalivation, myoclonus, seizures, muscle rigidity, and "eyes-open" coma. Laboratory tests for PCP intoxication should include drug tests on all available body fluids, serum electrolytes, liver function tests, CPK, renal function tests, and urinalysis.

Amphetamines cause increased alertness, hyperactivity, insomnia, hallucinations (visual, tactile and olfactory), tremors, hypertension, and dry mouth. Overdose with amphetamines can result in hypertensive crisis, stroke, and coma.

Acute overdose of theophylline (at levels of 20 to 40 μg/mL) or other methylxanthines (eg, caffeine) can cause nausea, vomiting, anxiety, and sinus tachycardia. More severe acute toxicity (usually with a serum theophylline level >80 μg/mL) results in hypotension, ventricular arrhythmias, seizures, and metabolic abnormalities including hypokalemia, hyperglycemia, leukocytosis, and metabolic acidosis. Long-term theophylline usage with superimposed acute or chronic overdose usually results in subtle symptoms of anorexia and palpitations, which may be difficult to recognize. Repetitive measurement of theophylline levels to determine rise or fall in serum levels can help to determine treatment efficacy, while monitoring of serum electrolytes and glucose levels can identify associated abnormalities.

Special Considerations in Treatment

In patients with sympathomimetic ingestions, rapid evaluation of the airway, vital signs, and neurologic status are important before additional interventions are undertaken. When possible, the route of drug administration should be determined. If this is not possible, then gastric decontamination should ensue. If the toxic agent was ingested (especially, amphetamines and theophylline), syrup of ipecac can be administered for induced emesis. If gastric lavage is performed, caution should be taken in placing the nasogastric/orogastric tube, as protective airway reflexes will be hyperactive. Once the airway is secure, an orogastric tube has been placed, and gastric decontamination has occurred, additional treatments will depend on the clinical scenario and suspected toxic agent. For cocaine intoxication and overdose, supportive care in an intensive care unit is the mainstay of therapy unless acute neurologic findings, chest pain, or cardiovascular instability mandates additional intervention. Sedation with a benzodiazepine can be useful for controlling agitation and preventing elevations in blood pressure. Wide fluctuations in blood pressure should be avoided because of the increased risk for hemorrhages (both, cerebral and GI). Otherwise, management of hypertension and chest pain (ie, myocardial ischemia) can be achieved with sublingual nitroglycerin or with other direct-acting vasodilators. β-Adrenergic antagonists such as propranolol should not be used alone to control tachycardia and hypertension, as the $β_2$-blockade will lead to unopposed alpha stimulation and can result in marked increases in mean arterial pressure. With cocaine, acute toxic exposures usually subside in 6 to 12 hours.

In the setting of PCP intoxication, repetitive doses of activated charcoal and continuous gastric suctioning have been recommended, even in "noningestion" intoxications (ie, snorted, smoked, or injected), because of gastric secretion and reabsorption of PCP. During mild and moderate PCP intoxications, close monitoring with minimal stimulation and sedation with benzodiazepines, if necessary, allows for toxic symptoms to resolve. Aggressive or combative behavior is best managed with haloperidol or benzodiazepines and restraints. Seizures should be managed with benzodiazepines. Rhabdomyolysis from muscle rigidity or seizures should be managed with diuresis. Urinary alkalinization is contraindicated in PCP ingestions because it may decrease renal clearance of PCP. When severe or prolonged muscle rigidity, hyperthermia, or status epilepticus are present, consideration should be given to management by neuromuscular blocking agents, mechanical ventilation, aggressive anticonvulsant therapy, and continuous electroencephalographic monitoring.

Amphetamine intoxications require mainly supportive care. After gastric decontamination, the patient should be monitored until behavior returns to normal. Problems of hypertension, arrhythmias, and hyperthermia should be managed with the appropriate medical and supportive measures. Although acidification and hemodialysis have been reported to enhance elimination, they should only be used in the most severe cases. As with cocaine, amphetamine overdose is associated with increased risk of cerebral hemorrhage, and changes in mental status require prompt investigation.

Intoxication with theophylline is complicated by the availability of slow-release and long-acting preparations and the possibility of acute overdose versus acute toxicity in the setting of long-term usage. Regardless, aggressive gastric decontamination should be undertaken as soon as possible by emesis, lavage, and activated charcoal. Repetitive dosing with activated charcoal is advocated to facilitate "GI dialysis," as discussed earlier. If theophylline levels increase despite aggressive therapy, consideration should be given to WBI, if a theophylline bezoar has been ruled out. Ingestions that result in serum theophylline levels of greater than 80 to 100 µg/mL in acute (single) ingestions, greater than 40 µg/mL in chronic toxicity, or severe symptoms such as refractory seizures, hypotension, or arrhythmias, may necessitate hemodialysis and/or hemoperfusion to aid in elimination.

Tricyclic Antidepressants

Sources of Exposure

Once a leading cause of childhood fatalities from poisoning, the occurrence of TCAD intoxication has decreased significantly with the increased usage of selective serotonin reuptake inhibitors. These latter agents are markedly less toxic than other TCADs. There are many tricyclic compounds used from this class to treat depression. Some of the more common include amitriptyline, imipramine, nortriptyline, and desipramine.[53]

Mechanism of Action

TCADs are rapidly absorbed, but vary greatly in toxicity and in time before the onset of symptoms. The normal daily therapeutic dose is generally 2 to 4 mg/kg. Toxic ingestions generally include 10 to 20 mg/kg, regardless of the agent. There is limited correlation between the serum level obtained and the severity or probability of severe toxic symptoms. CNS and peripheral nervous system symptoms are related to effects on neurotransmitter reuptake, specifically norepinephrine and serotonin, with additional anticholinergic effects (see section on anticholinergic syndromes). TCADs cause cardiovascular problems, most notably arrhythmias, by blocking the sodium channels (in a quinidinelike effect on the myocardium) and, to a lesser degree, by their blockade of the α-adrenergic system.

α-Adrenergic blockade can lead to more sinus tachycardia, and it creates more myocardial irritation as well as hypotension.

Toxic Signs and Symptoms

Most fatalities in patients with TCAD intoxication are associated with uncontrolled status epilepticus or cardiac arrhythmias. The toxicity of TCADs, CNS versus cardiovascular effects, varies depending on the agent. Patients with conduction delays on the initial ECG, with a QRS interval greater than 100 ms, should be closely monitored for 48 to 72 hours due to the possible occurrence of delayed arrhythmias.

Special Considerations in Treatment

Because of the rapid fluctuations in mental status, induced emesis is contraindicated in favor of airway protection and early gastric lavage and aggressive activated charcoal therapy. Gastric lavage may be indicated even hours after ingestion due to the drug's anticholinergic effects and delayed gastric emptying. Seizure activity is common and should be treated with benzodiazepines and barbiturates. Phenytoin is relatively contraindicated in TCAD overdose because it may precipitate arrhythmias. If conduction delays or a wide QRS complex are evident on the initial ECG, then the administration of sodium bicarbonate to achieve serum alkalinization to a pH of 7.50 is suggested. This decreases the cardiac toxicity of the TCADs by decreasing the free fraction of the drug and speeding the recovery of sodium channels by neutralizing the protonation of the drug-receptor complex. Neutralization facilitates the egress of the drug from the channel and lowers the serum potassium, resulting in decreased blockage of the voltage-dependent sodium channel. Ventricular arrhythmias that do not respond to alkalinization should be treated with lidocaine, bretylium, amiodarone, or magnesium. Class Ia antiarrhythmics are contraindicated. The use of amiodarone and bretylium remains controversial, as both drugs prolong the QT interval. If TCAD ingestion is documented but no major signs of toxicity occur, observation in a monitored bed for 24 hours is still warranted. If CNS depression, seizures, and/or conduction abnormalities occur, the patient should be carefully monitored with serial ECGs for a full 24 hours following discontinuation of therapy and resolution of all symptoms.[55,56]

Summary

In the event of a poisoning, prompt and effective therapy is mandatory to ensure a successful outcome. The primary goals of therapy include stabilization of the airway and resuscitation of the cardiovascular system. Identification of the offending agent can be achieved through the patient's history, physical exam, and drug screen. In most cases, GI decontamination is indicated to decrease the load of the poison. In some cases, an effective antidote may be present. As with many other diseases, the primary care for poisoning remains treatment of the physiologic derangements induced by the poison/toxin and general supportive care of the patient.

References

1. Locket S. Evaluation of various forms of treatment administered in poisoning. *Practitioner* 1973;210:709–714.
2. Trinkoff AM, Baker SP. Poisoning hospitalizations and deaths from solids and liquids among children and teenagers. *Am J Public Health* 1986;76:657–660.
3. Lacroix J, Gaudreault P, Gauthier M. Admission to a pediatric intensive care unit for poisoning: A review of 105 cases. *Crit Care Med* 1989;17:748–750.
4. Fazen LE III, Lovejoy FH Jr, Crone RK. Acute poisoning in a children's hospital: A 2 year experience. *Pediatrics* 1986;77:144–151.
5. Chabali R. Diagnostic use of anion and osmolal gaps in pediatric emergency medicine. *Pediatr Emerg Care* 1997;13:204–210.
6. Sugarman JM, Rodgers GC, Paul RI. Utility of toxicology screening in a pediatric emergency department. *Pediatr Emerg Care* 1997;13:194–197.
7. Tenenbein M, Cohen S, Sitar DS. Efficacy of ipecac-induced emesis, orogastric lavage, and activated charcoal for acute drug overdose. *Ann Emerg Med* 1987;16:838–841.
8. Krenzelok EP, McGuigan M, Lheur P. Position statement: Ipecac syrup. American Academy of Clinical Toxicology; European Association of Poisons Centres and Clinical Toxicologist. *J Toxicol Clin Toxicol* 1997;35:699–709.
9. Vale JA. Position statement: Gastric lavage. American Academy of Clinical Toxicology; European Association of Poisons Centres and Clinical Toxicologist. *J Toxicol Clin Toxicol* 1997;35:711–719.
10. Chyka PA, Seger D. Position statement: Single-dose activated charcoal. American Academy of Clinical Toxicology; European Association of Poisons Centres and Clinical Toxicologist. *J Toxicol Clin Toxicol* 1997;35:721–741.
11. James LP, Nichols MH, King WD. A comparison of cathartics in pediatric ingestions. *Pediatrics* 1995;96:235–238.
12. Farley TA. Severe hypernatremic dehydration after use of an activated charcoal-sorbitol suspension. *J Pediatr* 1986;109:719–722.
13. Jones J, Heiselman D, Dougbert J, Eddy A. Cathartic-induced magnesium toxicity during overdose management. *Ann Emerg Med* 1986;15:1214–1218.
14. Tenebein M. Position statement: Whole bowel irrigation. American Academy of Clinical Toxicology; European Association of Poisons Centres and Clinical Toxicologist. *J Toxicol Clin Toxicol* 1997;35:753–762.
15. Pond SM. Diuresis, dialysis, and hemoperfusion. *Emerg Med Clin North Am* 1982;2:29–45.
16. Bolgiano EB, Barish RA. Use of new and established antidotes. *Emerg Med Clin North Am* 1994;12:317–334.
17. Anker AL, Smilkstein MJ. Acetaminophen: Concepts and controversies. *Emerg Med Clin North Am* 1994;12:335–349.
18. Rumack BH, Matthew H. Acetaminophen poisoning and toxicity. *Pediatrics* 1975;55:871–876.
19. Tobias JD, Gregory D, Deshpande JK. Ondansetron to prevent emesis following N-acetylcysteine for acetaminophen overdose. *Pediatr Emerg Care* 1992;8:345–346.
20. Jacobsen D, McMartin KE. Methanol and ethylene glycol poisonings-mechanism of toxicity, clinical course, diagnosis, and treatment. *Med Toxicol* 1986;1:309–334.
21. Eden AF, McGrath CM, Dowdy YG, et al. Ethylene glycol poisoning: Toxicokinetic and analytic factors affecting laboratory diagnosis. *Clin Chem* 1998;44:168–177.
22. Shannon M. Toxicology review: Fomepizole-a new antidote. *Pediatr Emerg Care* 1998;14:170–172.
23. Goldfrank L, Flomenbaum N, Lewin N, et

al. Anticholinergic poisoning. *J Toxicol Clin Toxicol* 1982;19:17–25.
24. Mofenson HC, Caraccio TR, Schauben J. Poisoning by antidysrhythmic drugs. *Pediatr Clin North Am* 1986;33:723–738.
25. Tobias JD. Central nervous system depression following accidental ingestion of Visine eye drops. *Clin Pediatr* 1996;35:539–540.
26. Friedman EM, Lovejoy FH. The emergency management of caustic ingestions. *Emerg Clin North Am* 1984;2:77–86.
27. Thompson N, Lowe-Ponsford F, Mant TGK, Volans GN. Button battery ingestion: A review. *Adv Drug React Actur Pois Rev* 1990;9:157–182.
28. Rothstein FC. Caustic injuries to the esophagus in children. *Pediatr Clin North Am* 1986;33:665–674.
29. Zwiener FM, Ginsburg CM. Organophosphate and carbamate poisoning in infants and children. *Pediatrics* 1988;81:121–126.
30. Bardin PG, Van Eeden SF. Organophosphate poisoning grading the severity and comparing treatment between atropine and glycopyrrolate. *Crit Care Med* 1990;18:956–960.
31. Yoshida M, Adachi J, Watabiki T, et al. A study on house fire victims: Age, carboxyhemoglobin, hydrogen cyanide and hemolysis. *Forensic Sci Int* 1991;52:13–20.
32. Vogel SN, Sultan TR, Ten Eyck RP. Cyanide poisoning. *Clin Toxicol* 1981;18:367–383.
33. Hall AH, Doutre WH, Ludden T, et al. Nitrite/thiosulfate treated acute cyanide poisoning: Estimated kinetics after antidote. *J Toxicol Clin Toxicol* 1987;25:121–133.
34. Lewander WJ, Gaudreault P, Einhorn A, et al. Acute pediatric digoxin ingestion: A ten year experience. *Am J Dis Child* 1986;140:770–773.
35. Woolf AD, Wenger T, Smith TW, Lovejoy FH. The use of digoxin-specific Fab fragments for severe digitalis intoxication in children. *N Engl J Med* 1992;326:1739–1744.
36. Binder JW, Roberts RJ. Carbon monoxide intoxication in children. *Clin Toxicol* 1980;6:287–295.
37. Curry S. Methemoglobinemia. *Ann Emerg Med* 1982;11:214–221.
38. Jaffe FA. Pathogenicity of carbon monoxide. *Am J Forensic Med Pathol* 1997;18:406–410.
39. Rosen PJ, Johnson C, McGehee WB, Beutler E. Failure of methylene blue treatment in toxic methemoglobinemia. *Ann Intern Med* 1971;76:83–86.
40. Victoria MS, Nangia BS. Hydrocarbon poisonings: A review. *Pediatr Emerg Care* 1987;3:184–186.
41. Anderson AC. Iron poisoning in children. *Curr Opin Pediatr* 1994;6:289–294.
42. Henetrig FM, Karl SR, Weintraub WH. Severe iron poisoning treated with enteral and intravenous deferoxamine. *Ann Emerg Med* 1983;12:306–309.
43. Vernon DD, Gleich MC. Poisoning and drug overdose. *Crit Care Clin* 1997;13:647–667.
44. Chamberlain JM, Klein BL. A comprehensive review of naloxone for the emergency physician. *Am J Emerg Med* 1994;12:650–660.
45. Tenebein M. Continuous naloxone infusion for opiate poisoning in infancy. *J Pediatr* 1984;105:645–648.
46. Yip L, Dart RC, Gabow PA. Concepts and controversies in salicylate toxicity. *Emerg Med Clin North Am* 1994;12:351–364.
47. Bertino JS Jr, Reed MD. Barbiturate and nonbarbiturate sedative hypnotic intoxication in children. *Ped Clin North Am* 1986;33:703–722.
48. McDuffe AD, Tobias JD. Seizure after flumazenil administration in a pediatric patient. *Pediatr Emerg Care* 1995;11:186–187.
49. Hickson GB, Altemeier WA, Martin ER, Campbell PW. Parental administration of chemical agents: A cause of apparent life threatening events. *Pediatrics* 1989;143:772–776.
50. Meadows R. ABC of child abuse-poisoning. *BMJ* 1989;298:1445–1446.
51. Mueller PD, Benowitz NL, Olson KR. Cocaine. *Emerg Med Clin North Am* 1990;8:481–493.
52. Karp HN, Kaufman ND, Anand SK. Phencyclidine poisoning in young children. *J Pediatr* 1982;97:1006–1009.
53. King P, Coleman JH. Stimulant and narcotic drugs. *Ped Clin North Am* 1987;34:349–362.
54. Shannon M, Lovejoy FH. Effect of acute versus chronic intoxication on clinical features of theophylline poisoning in children. *J Pediatr* 1992;121:125–130.
55. Frommer DA, Kulig KW, Marx JA, Rumack B. Tricyclic antidepressant overdose: A review. *JAMA* 1987;257:561–562.
56. Shannon M, Liebelt EL. Targeted management strategies for cardiovascular toxicity from tricyclic antidepressant overdose: The pivotal role for alkalinization and sodium loading. *Pediatr Emerg Care* 1998;14:293–298.

Chapter 21

Gastrointestinal Tract Disorders in the Pediatric Intensive Care Unit Patient

Joseph D. Tobias, MD

Introduction

Although disorders of the gastrointestinal (GI) system are seldom the primary derangement necessitating admission to the pediatric intensive care unit (PICU), disorders of or problems related to the GI tract can lead to significant morbidity and even mortality in the PICU patient. Nutrition and related issues (see also chapter 14) are integral components of the care of the critically ill patient. Nutritional deficiencies can lead to inadequate healing and/or breakdown of the normal protective barriers that are provided by the integumentary system. Prolonged withholding of enteral feedings can lead to villous atrophy of the GI mucosa, with the risk of translocation of bacteria and endotoxin leading to multisystem organ failure and sepsis, which remain leading causes of secondary morbidity and mortality in the PICU patient.

GI, hepatic, and pancreatic functions may be compromised as a component of multisystem organ failure or during hypoperfusion states related to shock or cardiopulmonary bypass. Alterations in the normal protective barrier of the stomach can lead to stress ulceration and GI bleeding. Alternatively, the GI system may be the primary organ system involved that necessitates PICU admission, whether from GI bleeding or from hepatic failure. This chapter reviews four distinct issues related to the GI tract, including primary GI bleeding (upper and lower), the prevention of stress ulceration, and control of gastric pH, hepatic failure, and pancreatitis.

Gastrointestinal Bleeding

GI bleeding may be the primary disorder necessitating admission and treatment in the PICU, or may originate as a secondary phenomenon in patients with other underlying disorders such as multisystem organ failure. GI bleeding may occur from either the upper or the lower GI tract. Upper GI bleeding occurs from sources proximal to the ligament of Trietz while lower GI bleeding is classified as that which occurs distal to the ligament. While the initial resuscitation and stabilization are similar regardless of the source of bleeding, the etiologies of the bleeding, (Table 1) as well as the therapies, vary markedly according to the source.

The treatment for upper GI bleeding is outlined in Table 2. The initial treatment fo-

From: Tobias JD (ed): *Pediatric Critical Care: The Essentials.* ©Futura Publishing Co., Inc., Armonk, NY, 1999.

Table 1

Etiology of Upper Gastrointestinal Bleeding in Infants and Children

Neonates/Infants	Toddlers/Children/Adolescents

swallowed blood:
  maternal
  from upper respiratory tract
esophagitis
gastritis
gastric ulcer
vascular malformation
coagulation disturbances:
  vitamin K deficiency
	swallowed blood:
	  Mallory-Weiss tear
	gastritis
	esophagitis
	peptic ulcer
	infection with *H. pylori*
	vascular malformation
	esophageal varices
	gastric varices
	hemobilia

Table 2

Treatment of Upper Gastrointestinal Bleeding in Children

Stabilization of the airway, breathing, and circulation
Establishment of 2 large-bore intravenous infusions
Laboratory evaluation:
  complete blood count with platelet count
  PT, PTT, fibrinogen level
  liver function tests
  electrolytes, BUN, creatinine, glucose
  type and crossmatch
Placement of nasogastric tube
Lavage with room temperature saline:
  consider addition of norepinephrine (5 mg/L) or phenylephrine (10 mg/L)
H_2-antagonists
Somatostatin or octreotide.
Identify source of bleeding:
  endoscopy (also useful for sclerotherapy or banding of varices)
  radionuclide scans
  arteriography
Surgery

BUN = blood urea nitrogen; PT = prothrombin time; PTT = partial thromboplastin time.

cuses on maintenance of the airway and provision of adequate oxygenation/ventilation followed by cardiovascular resuscitation. Adequate intravenous access is mandatory, as large volumes of blood may need to be rapidly transfused. Additionally, blood warmers and means of rapidly infusing blood, such as pressure bags and blood pump tubing, should be available. The reader is referred to chapter 15 for a full discussion of the use of blood products and devices for its rapid administration. Upon arrival in the emergency department or the PICU, venous access is obtained and blood sent for type and crossmatch, coagulation parameters, and hemoglobin and hematocrit with platelet count, in addition to routine blood chemistries including liver function tests. With acute blood loss and prior to intravascular resuscitation with crystalloid, the hemoglobin and hematocrit may be relatively normal. Once adequate venous access is obtained and laboratory parameters obtained, cardiovascular resuscitation is provided using isotonic crystalloid and packed red blood cells. Although most cases of GI bleeding are not related primarily to abnormalities in coagulation function, large amounts of blood loss can lead to dilutional coagulopathies related to the dilution of both platelets and coagulation factors. Additionally, associated hepatic dysfunction may provide another etiology for coagulation disturbances.

Further therapies (see below) will then depend on the cause and location of the GI bleeding. In the pediatric patient, unlike the adult patient, GI bleeding may be related to congenital or hereditary anomalies of the GI tract. The age of presentation of the patient and the location (upper versus lower) may provide clues to the etiology of the GI bleeding (Table 1). The differentiation between upper and lower GI bleeding may be difficult. Passage of bright red blood from the rectum may occur with rapid bleeding from any site of the GI tract including the esophagus, stomach, and proximal duodenum. However, melanotic stools or emesis of bright red blood are indicative of upper GI bleeding. The use of the blood urea nitrogen (BUN)/creatinine ratio has been suggested as means of localizing the site of bleeding. With upper GI bleeding, the blood enters the small bowel and the protein is digested and absorbed, resulting in a rise in the BUN/creatinine ratio (≥ 20). The latter is related to a relative rise of the BUN to 15 to 25 mg/dL in relation to a normal creatinine of 0.5 to 0.7 mg/dL. No absorption or digestion of blood occurs with lower GI bleeding and therefore no change in the BUN/creatinine ratio is noted.

Additional therapy for upper GI bleeding includes placement of a nasogastric (NG) tube followed by saline lavage. NG placement can also be helpful in differentiating between upper and lower GI bleeding in the majority of patients. Although iced saline has been suggested to provide superficial vasoconstriction of the gastric mucosa and perhaps decrease gastric bleeding, iced saline lavage is not recommended in children, due to the risks of hypothermia. Rather, room temperature saline lavage is suggested. While there are no randomized studies demonstrating its efficacy, the addition of a vasoconstrictor agent to the saline lavage solution makes theoretical sense. Norepinephrine (5 mg) or phenylephrine (10 mg) can be added to each liter of lavage fluid in attempt to attain a local vasoconstrictor effect. There is limited to no absorption of these agents across the gastric mucosa.

Pharmacologic therapy may be indicated for patients with ongoing or recurrent upper GI bleeding. Agents to control gastric pH should be instituted (see next section). Initially the synthetic posterior pituitary hormone, vasopressin, was used to provide increased resistance in the splanchnic circulation and thereby decrease splanchnic blood flow and GI bleeding. Dosing of vasopressin includes 0.2 to 0.4 U/1.73 m^2/min. However, significant adverse effects may occur, including hypertension, cardiac arrhythmias, seizures, and oliguria related to its nonspecific vasoconstricting effects, which lead to systemic hypertension.[1] Additionally, as a result of its antidiuretic effects, free water retention with hyponatremia may occur. The direct intra-arterial infusion of vasopressin has been suggested as a means of limiting the dose and thereby limiting the systemic side effects. However, this therapy requires precise placement of the infusion catheter by use of invasive radiologic techniques in the catheterization laboratory—a procedure that may not be readily available or feasible for the pediatric patient.

Alternatively, somatostatin and its analogues have replaced vasopressin as a pharmacologic aid in decreasing upper GI bleeding.[2] Somatostatin and its analogues may be effective for the treatment of upper GI bleeding related to peptic ulcer disease, diffuse gastritis, esophageal or gastric varices, Mallory-Weiss tears, and hepatic and prehepatic portal hypertension. Somatostatin's effects are twofold, including a reduction in splanchnic blood flow as well as a decrease in gastric acid production. The decrease in splanchnic blood flow is related to venous dilation and a decrease in portal venous pressure. The latter occurs without alterations in cardiac output or mean arterial pressure. Dosing regimens for somatostatin include continuous infusions of 250 µg/h. More recently, the somatostatin analogue octreotide has become available for clinical use.[3] Octreotide has a half-life of 90 minutes, roughly 30 times that of somatostatin. Due to its longer half-life, it can be administered twice daily by the intravenous or subcutaneous route. There are limited data concerning dosing regimens for octreotide in children. Siafakas et al[3] reported the use of octreotide in seven children with upper GI bleeding. The dosing regimen included a bolus of 1 to 2 μg/kg followed by a continuous infusion starting at 1 μg/kg/h. The authors suggest increasing the dose in increments of 1 μg/kg/h if bleeding continues. The maximum infusion rate in their study was 5 μg/kg/h. If the bleeding ceases and does not recur, the dose is decreased in a similar fashion. Due to octreotide's longer half-life of 90 minutes, compared to that of somatostatin, intermittent dosing with 1 μg/kg every 8 hours is also possible. Adverse effects related to octreotide have been uncommon and include temporary nausea/vomiting with bolus administration and alterations of glucose homeostasis including hyper- and hypoglycemia.

Once the acute bleeding is controlled and the patient's cardiorespiratory system stabilized, attention is directed to the identification of the site of the bleeding.[4] For upper GI bleeding, this is accomplished with upper GI endoscopy, which also allows for therapeutic treatment of various lesions including cauterization of gastric/duodenal ulcers, sclerotherapy, or banding of esophageal varices. If endoscopy does not adequately identify the source of bleeding, other more invasive procedures including arteriography may be required. Routine barium studies are not indicated in patients with upper GI bleeding.

Radioisotope studies may be used to locate the site of bleeding. The ^{99m}technetium-sulfur colloid (Tc-SC) scan can detect rates of bleeding down to 0.1 mL/min.[4] Tc-SC is a radioisotope with a half-life of 2.5 minutes that is cleared and concentrated in the reticuloendothelial system. The compound is cleared rapidly by the liver and spleen. Any extravascular bleeding that occurs allows the compound to accumulate outside of the vascular system, where it cannot be rapidly cleared and thereby shows up as an area of increased activity during the scan. The disadvantage of the test is that it is positive only if there is active bleeding during the scan. ^{99m}Tc-labeled red blood cells can also be used to identify the site of bleeding. The labeled red blood cells remain in the circulation for up to 24 hours and hence are more accurate for identifying intermittent bleeding. However, repeated imaging is required to identify sites of intermittent bleeding.

With the above mentioned studies and improvements in upper GI endoscopy, the need for arteriography has decreased. However, if bleeding continues and its source cannot be identified, arteriography may be required. Arteriography can identify sites of bleeding as little as 0.5 mL/min. As with other studies, active bleeding is generally required for arteriography to be positive; however, abnormal vascular formations can be identified by arteriography even when active bleeding is not occurring. With arteriography, therapeutic interventions such as embolization may be possible.

The final therapy that has been recommend for upper GI bleeding, especially that due to esophageal and gastric varices, is placement of a Sengstaken-Blakemore (SB) tube. The SB tube has a gastric and an esophageal balloon. It is placed into the esophagus and stomach, then the gastric balloon is inflated and the tube pulled partially out to tamponade the gastric balloon against the upper portion of the stomach. If bleeding does not cease, the esophageal balloon is inflated. Although the device is available in a pediatric size, due to its high incidence of complications including gastric/esophageal necrosis and perforation, its use is no longer recommended. Airway protection with endotracheal intubation is suggested prior to placement of the SB tube.

In the patient with uncontrolled hemorrhage, surgical intervention may be required to identify and control the source of bleeding. However, in the majority of cases, the acute bleeding episode can be controlled and investigations carried out to define the cause of the bleeding. Patients with upper GI bleeding related to peptic ulcer disease may respond to conservative therapy with H_2-antagonists and therapy directed at eradication of *H. pylori,* an organism which has gained recent attention as a prominent factor associated with peptic ulcer disease. The course in patients with esophageal varices is dependent on the site of obstruction. Patients with preportal hypertension and normal hepatic function tend to have progressively fewer episodes of acute bleeding and therefore conservative, nonsurgical therapy has been suggested for such patients.[5] However, patients with hepatic disease and portal hypertension tend to have progressively more problems with upper GI bleeding. For these patients, portal-to-systemic shunting procedures may be indicated. The exact timing and indications of such procedures are somewhat controversial in the pediatric patient. Portal-to-systemic shunting generally includes a spleno-renal shunt rather than a porto-caval shunt due to the higher incidence of hepatic encephalopathy with the latter procedure. Additional problems relate to the smaller size of these vessels in children and the resultant increased incidence of postoperative thrombosis of the shunts. Previous shunt surgery also disrupts the normal anatomic relationships of the hepatic and portal vascular systems, making future hepatic transplantation technically more difficult and time consuming.

Additional therapy for patients with esophageal varices includes endoscopic procedures such as sclerosis with hypertonic saline or banding of the esophageal varices.[6] These procedures may be used following an acute bleeding episode to provide some time for stabilization so that porto-systemic surgical shunting procedures can be performed in the nonemergent setting.

Pharmacologic measures to reduce recurrent bleeding have shown some promise. Agents, such as propranolol, that decrease portal venous pressure have been shown to reduce recurrent bleeding in both the adult and the pediatric population.[7,8] Ozsoylu et al[8] administered propranolol to 13 children with portal hypertension. They started propranolol dosing at 2 mg/kg/day and doubled it every other day to achieve a reduction in the resting heart rate to 75% of baseline. They noted a reduction in splenic pulp pressure of ≥ 50 mm H_2O in 2 weeks. No long-term follow-up was performed to determine the incidence of GI bleeding.

While lower GI bleeding is more common in children than upper GI bleeding, it tends to be less likely to be of a quantity that is great enough to result in hemodynamic compromise and the need for PICU admission. However, circulatory collapse can result from lower GI bleeding. As with upper GI bleeding, the immediate treatment of lower GI bleeding involves resuscitation and stabilization of the airway and cardiorespiratory systems. The differential diagnosis varies depending on the age of the child (Table 3). An important consideration when determining the etiology is that excessive upper GI bleeding can lead to a rapid GI transit time, an inadequate time for enzymatic digestion of the blood, and hematochezia instead of melena. Diagnostic investigations for lower GI bleeding include

Table 3

Lower Gastrointestinal Bleeding in Infants and Children

Neonates/Infants	Toddlers/Children/Adolescents
swallowed blood:	swallowed blood:
upper respiratory tract	upper respiratory tract
maternal	polyps
upper GI bleeding	intussusception
milk-protein intolerance	antibiotic-associated colitis
necrotizing enterocolitis	Meckel's diverticulum
hirschsprung's disease with enterocolitis	ectopic gastric mucosa
intussusception	hemolytic-uremic syndrome
volvulus	Henonch-Schonlein purpura
infection	infection
	inflammatory bowel disease
	vascular malformation

GI = gastrointestinal.

barium contrast studies, radionuclide scanning including a Meckel's scan, stool cultures, assay for *Clostridium difficile* toxin, arteriography, and/or endoscopic procedures (sigmoidoscopy, colonoscopy). The need for the various diagnostic tests is based on the patient's history, the presumed diagnosis, the presence or absence of bowel obstruction, and the severity of the bleeding (Fig. 1). Patients with life-threatening or recurrent GI bleeding require consultation with a pediatric gastroenterologist and a pediatric surgeon.

Ulcer Prophylaxis in the Pediatric Intensive Care Unit Patient

One of the more controversial areas of PICU care is the prophylaxis of stress ulcers. The issues of controversy include not only who should receive prophylaxis, but also which agent or agents are most effective. Patients with acute illness are prone to develop stress ulcers or, more accurately, stress gas-

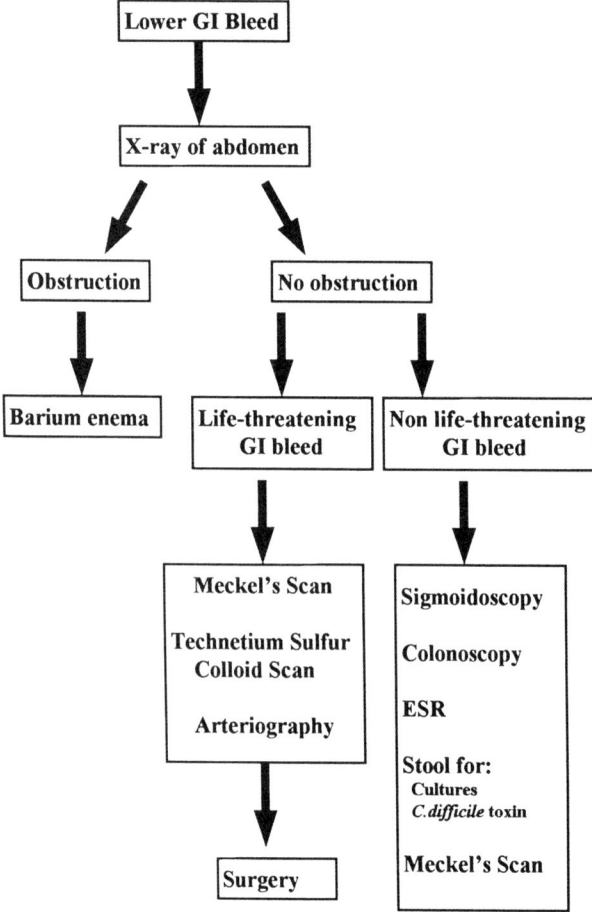

Figure 1. Suggested scheme for evaluation of patient with lower gastrointestinal (GI) bleeding. The differential diagnosis must always include a large upper GI bleed, which can result in hematochezia. The diagnostic work-up will depend on certain patient factors such as the severity of the bleeding and the presence or absence of bowel obstruction as well as the past and current medical history, which will aid in deciding on the appropriate diagnostic text to arrive at the correct diagnosis. ESR = erythrocyte sedimentation rate.

tritis, which is characterized by a diffuse, inflammatory process of the gastric mucosa. Discrete areas of ulceration can also be seen. The pathophysiology of stress ulcers/gastritis is distinctly different from peptic ulcer disease in that the process is not related to overproduction of acid, but rather to a disruption of the normal mucosal protective barrier. Several factors may play a role in the disruption of the mucosal integrity, including hypoxia and decreased perfusion, both of which impair the ability of the gastric mucosa to produce the protective mucous layer.

Stress ulcers can present anywhere on the continuum from occult bleeding manifested as Hemoccult-positive NG drainage to rapid exsanguination with the emesis of bright red blood. Various studies have attempted to define not only the incidence of significant upper GI bleeding in the PICU patient, but also its risk factors. Lacroix et al[9] prospectively determined the incidence of GI bleeding, defined as grossly visible blood in the NG aspirate or hematemesis, in the PICU population over a 55-week period. Sixty-three of 984 patients (6.4%) had documented upper GI bleeding. Identifiable risk factors included a high Pediatric Risk of Mortality Score, underlying coagulopathy, pneumonia, and multitrauma. A significant GI bleed, defined as a GI bleed resulting in hypotension or the need for a transfusion, occurred in 4 of the 984 patients. Coagulopathy was present and contributed in some degree to the bleed in these four patients. No deaths attributed to GI bleeding were noted.

Based on the studies of Lacroix et al and others, several risk factors for GI bleeding in the PICU patient have been identified (Table 4). The debate continues as to whether all patients admitted to the PICU require prophylaxis against GI bleeding.[10] Lopez-Herce et al[11] prospectively evaluated the efficacy of one of three regimens, an antacid, sucralfate, or an H_2-antagonist (ranitidine), in decreasing microscopic and significant GI bleeding in the PICU population. Significant GI bleeding was defined as a decrease of the hematocrit of $\geq 15\%$, hypotension, or need for a transfusion. The incidence of significant GI bleeding was statistically significantly greater in the control group (7 of 35, 20%) than in the other three groups combined (6 of 105 or 5.7%, $P<0.05$). When the three prophylaxis regimens were compared, there was no difference in the incidence of GI bleeding. Of the 13 patients who had a significant GI bleed, 9 experienced the bleeding following cardiovascular surgery, 3 had meningococcemia, and 1 had hepatic failure. The authors noted, as did Lacroix et al,[10] that the incidence of GI bleeding was highest in patients with the highest severity-of-illness scores. There were two deaths attributed to upper GI bleeding in the study. Although its consequences may be mild and it is generally self-limited, significant GI bleeding does occasionally occur in the PICU population, and some form of prophylaxis seems warranted for patients with identifiable risk factors.

The final question concerning prophylaxis for stress gastritis/ulcer formation in the PICU patient is that of which agent or agents should be used (Table 5). The time-honored therapies for prevention of gastritis and ulcer formation have been antacids and the H_2-antagonists. These agents both act, albeit via different mechanisms, to raise the gastric pH. It has been suggested that the optimal gastric pH for the prevention of stress ulceration ranges from 4 to 5.[12] A gastric pH greater than 5 signifies that 99.9% of the gastric acid has been neutralized and that the activity of the proteolytic enzyme pepsin is minimal.

Antacids react with hydrochloric in stomach acid to form salt and water. Antacids contain magnesium hydroxide, magnesium trisilicate, aluminum hydroxide, or calcium carbonate. Regardless of the agent used, the effects on gastric pH are brief, requiring redosing at 2- to 3-hour intervals. Additional concerns relate to the absorption of the cation in the antacid (aluminum, magnesium, or calcium). A concern regarding the use of antacids that contain calcium is acid rebound with the sustained hypersecretion of gastric acid after the stomach has emptied. Additional issues concerning conventional antacid formulations involve the high sodium content of most preparations and the binding of other oral medications with the formation of unabsorbable complexes. Because of these issues, there is limited enthu-

Table 4

Potential Risk Factors for Gastrointestinal Bleeding in the Pediatric ICU Patient

High severity of illness score
Multisystem organ failure
Major surgical procedure
Prolonged hypoperfusion
Coagulopathy
Multitrauma
Intracranial disease
Respiratory failure requiring mechanical ventilation
Thermal injury ($\geq$ 15%–20% body surface area)
Organ transplant recipient
Glucocorticoid administration
History of peptic ulcer disease

ICU = intensive care unit.

Table 5

Agents for Prophylaxis of Gastrointestinal Bleeding in the Pediatric ICU Patient

H_2-antagonists
   cimetidine (20–30 mg/kg/day i.v. divided, every 4-hour dosing interval)
   ranitidine (1.5–2.0 mg/kg i.v. every 6 hours or 6–8 mg/kg/day by continuous infusion)
   famotidine (0.5 mg/kg/dose i.v. every 8–12 hours)
Antacids (1 mL/kg NG every 2 hours for pH $\leq$ 4.0)
Sucralfate (10–15 mg/kg/dose NG every 4–6 hours)
Omeprazole (0.5 mg/kg/dose NG every 12–24 hours)
Prostaglandin analogs:
   enprostil (no pediatric data, adult dosing 50–100 μg/day administered once or twice daily)
   misoprostol (no pediatric data, adult dosing 200 μg administered every 6 hours)

ICU = intensive care unit; NG = nasogastrically.

siasm for the use of these agents as sole therapy for prevention of stress gastritis. However, they may have a role, in conjunction with H_2-antagonists, for treatment of the patient with an occasional NG aspirate pH of $\leq$4. In this setting, as-needed doses of 1 mL/kg of an antacid can be administered. The antacid to be used should be determined based on the patient's status and the potential toxicity of the cation (calcium, magnesium, aluminum) in the antacid.

In many PICUs, H_2-antagonists remain the mainstay for the prevention of stress gastritis. Cimetidine was licensed for use in the United States in 1978. Lacroix et al[13] demonstrated the efficacy of cimetidine (20 mg/kg/day, maximum dose 1000 mg, administered at 6-hour intervals) in raising gastric pH above 4.0 in the PICU. In a prospective study of 30 children receiving cimetidine (20 mg/kg/day, administered every 6 hours), Lloyd et al[14] demonstrated a gastric pH of 2.2, 6 hours after a cimetidine dose, and suggested that the daily dose of 20 to 30 mg/kg/day should be administered at 4-hour intervals.

Issues concerning cimetidine include its cardiovascular effects (bradycardia, hypotension) when administered too rapidly and its impairment of the P_{450} hepatic system that results in the alteration of metabolism of several pharmacologic agents including midazolam, diazepam, phenytoin, theophylline, and propranolol.[15,16] Because of such issues, recent attention has focused on the newer H_2-antagonists such as ranitidine. Ranitidine has limited effects on the hepatic P_{450} system and has been demonstrated to have minimal effects on cardiovascular function in the ICU patient.[17]

Lopez-Herce et al[18] compared four dosing regimens for ranitidine in the pediatric population. Patients were randomized to receive either 2 mg/kg NG every 12 hours, 4 mg/kg NG every 12 hours, 0.75 mg/kg i.v. every 6 hours, or 1.5 mg/kg i.v. every 6 hours. The fourth group had a higher mean gastric pH than the other three groups, and only the dose of 1.5 mg/kg i.v. every 6 hours maintained gastric pH ≥4.0 for greater than 80% of the time.

A more recent addition to the H_2-antagonist group is famotidine. Like ranitidine, it has minimal effects on cardiovascular function and the P_{450} system. However, its half-life is somewhat longer than ranitidine, suggesting that its dosing interval can be extended to every 8 to 12 hours.[19]

An additional question concerning H_2-antagonists is, does the use of a continuous infusion rather than intermittent dosing provide more effective control of gastric pH? Due to the short duration of effect of H_2-antagonists such as ranitidine and cimetidine, frequent dosing at 4- to 6-hour intervals is necessary to maintain gastric pH at the desired level. While continuous infusions may be more effective in maintaining gastric pH, logistic problems including drug incompatibilities and limited intravenous access may lead to frequent disruptions of the continuous infusion, thereby negating its effect.[20] However, ranitidine and the other H_2-antagonists can be mixed in parenteral nutrition solutions. The practice in our PICU is to use continuous ranitidine infusions when patients are receiving parenteral nutrition solutions, by adding the ranitidine into the solution. However, when this is done, it must be remembered that alterations in the rate of administration of the parenteral nutrition will also result in changes in the ranitidine dose. This is particularly important as the parenteral nutrition solution is decreased and enteral feedings are increased.

Issues with the H_2-antagonists are: 1) what to do when the gastric pH remains low despite maximum dosing, and 2) the concerns of an increased risk of nosocomial pneumonia in patients receiving H_2-antagonists. If the gastric pH is persistently ≤4.0, the first step is to ensure maximum dosing of the H_2-antagonist. This may include doses of ranitidine of up to 2 mg/kg/dose every 6 hours or 8 mg/kg/day by continuous infusions. Intravenous administration is suggested for the critically ill patient, as alterations in splanchnic blood flow may affect absorption of any enteral medication. Enteral dosing is possible and is certainly cheaper than intravenous administration once the acute phase of the illness has resolved, and enteral feedings are initiated and well tolerated.

Even with effective dosing regimens, occasional patients will have a gastric pH ≤4.0. Intermittent doses of either an antacid or sucralfate are suggested if the low pH occurs once or twice a day. In patients with a persistently low gastric pH, our practice is to add omeprazole (0.5 mg/kg/dose NG every 12 to 24 hours). At the time of the writing of this chapter, omeprazole is not available for intravenous administration in the United States.[21]

Recent concerns have been raised about the use of agents that raise gastric pH and their effects on the incidence of nosocomial pneumonia.[22,23] Driks et al[22] evaluated the incidence of nosocomial pneumonia in 130 adults who required mechanical ventilation. GI prophylaxis included agents that raise gastric pH (H_2-antagonists, antacids, or both) or sucralfate. Patients who received sucralfate had a greater percentage of gastric aspirates with a pH ≤4.0 and a lower concentration of gram-negative bacilli than patients who received H_2-antagonists/antacids. The incidence of nosocomial pneumonia was twice as high and the mortality rate was 1.6 times higher in the H_2-antagonist/antacid group compared to the sucralfate group. Although the results fell short of being statistically significant, the authors suggested the use of barrier agents such as sucralfate rather than agents that raise gastric pH for GI prophylaxis during mechanical ventilation. A follow-up study in the adult population by Apte et al[23] compared 16 patients who received H_2-antagonists with 18 patients who received no GI prophylaxis. They noted a higher incidence of nosocomial pneumonia (13 of 16; 81%) in patients who received H_2-antagonists for GI prophylaxis versus those who received no prophylaxis (9 of 18,

$P<0.05$). Although the methodologies of these two studies[22,23] have been questioned, including concerns of the definition of nosocomial pneumonia, future studies are needed to fully address the issue of the association of nosocomial pneumonia and the H_2-antagonists. From a theoretical point of view, although raising gastric pH may prevent stress ulceration, the higher pH may also provide a more hospitable milieu for the growth of pathogenic bacteria.

In summary, significant GI bleeding rarely occurs in the PICU population. However, it can have a significant impact on mortality and is on occasion the primary cause of mortality. The incidence of GI bleeding is highest in patients with the highest severity of illness scores and in those with specific risk factors (Table 4). In these patients, measures to maintain gastric pH ≥ 4.0 seem justified. Several options are appropriate for raising gastric pH (Table 5), each with its own adverse effect profile. None has been shown to be statistically superior to the others in the prevention of GI stress ulceration. Our current regimen includes the intermittent intravenous administration of an H_2-antagonist or its continuous infusion in patients receiving parenteral nutrition. Gastric pH should be monitored every 2 to 4 hours, and an antacid or sucralfate administered for a pH ≤ 4.0. Omeprazole may be an option for patients with a persistently low gastric pH despite maximum dosing of an H_2-antagonist. The most effective way to prevent stress ulceration of the GI tract may be to provide enteral feedings. However, this may not be possible based on the patient's underlying status. Although transpyloric feedings are being used more frequently for the critically ill patient (see also chapter 14), these will not control gastric pH, and prophylaxis is still indicated in such patients.

Hepatic Function and Failure

Hepatic failure may be the primary disorder necessitating PICU admission or may be a component of multisystem organ failure occurring as a secondary sequela of the primary insult (eg, hypoperfusion state from sepsis or cardiorespiratory failure). Regardless of the etiology of hepatic failure, the support and care of affected patients requires, whenever possible, reversal of the factors responsible for hepatic failure and support of the patient to provide time for the liver to recover function. When the latter does not occur, hepatic transplantation must be considered.

The liver is responsible for several synthetic and metabolic functions including the production of cholesterol, bile salts, albumin, and coagulation factors, as well as metabolic processes including glycogen synthesis/breakdown, oxidative phosphorylation, fatty acid oxidation, bilirubin conjugation, and conversion of ammonia to urea nitrogen. The support of patients with hepatic failure requires, whenever possible, taking over the above mentioned list of hepatic functions.

Several etiologies are possible for hepatic failure in the PICU patient (Table 6). Many are readily apparent from the patient's previous medical history or the history of present illness. Little diagnostic work-up is needed for the adolescent who presents with hepatic failure 72 hours after admitting to the ingestion of a large quantity of acetaminophen, or for the patient with a previous history of biliary atresia who presents with worsening jaundice. However, an exhaustive work-up may be required in the previously healthy 2-year-old child presenting with the acute onset of jaundice and hepatic failure. In the pediatric age range, viral infections, drug toxicity, congenital malformations, and metabolic disorders are the four most likely etiologies of hepatic failure (Table 6). In the PICU, a hypoperfusion injury must be added to the list of most likely etiologies for hepatic failure.

The diagnosis may be readily apparent based on the onset of hyperbilirubinemia and jaundice or may be more subtle, reached only when a high ammonia level is detected in a patient with altered mental status, when an abnormal coagulation profile is found in a patient who develops unexplained bleeding, or an increase in liver function tests obtained during routine laboratory evaluation. Although the increase in

Table 6

Possible Etiologies of Hepatic Failure

Infectious agents:
  hepatitis A, B, C, D
  Epstein-Barr virus
  herpes simplex
  cytomegalovirus
  enterovirus
  nonspecific response to bacteremia/sepsis
Toxins/drugs:
  acetaminophen
  phenytoin
  valproic acid
  isoniazid
  carbon tetrachloride
  halothane
  sulfamethoxazole
  sulfasalazine
  carbamazepine
  iron
  vitamin A
Congenital biliary tree anomalies:
  biliary atresia
Metabolic disorders:
  cystic fibrosis
  hereditary fructose intolerance
  α-antitrypsin deficiency
  galactosemia
  tyrosinemia
  Wolman's disease
  Wilson's disease
  Niemann-Pick disease
Vascular malformations:
  Budd-Chiari syndrome
  veno-occlusive disease following bone
    marrow transplantation
Reye's syndrome
Multisystem organ failure
Hypoperfusion injury

liver function tests such as the transaminases (ALT/SGPT or AST/SGOT) may indicate the presence of hepatic dysfunction, they are merely bystanders of hepatocyte death and are of little clinical significance.

Care of the patient with hepatic failure requires identification of the etiology, reversal of the underlying process, and support of the individual organ systems that are secondarily deranged by hepatic failure. Initial support includes stabilization and resuscitation of the airway and cardiorespiratory systems. The diagnostic work-up is guided by the patient's medical history and history of current illness. In patients with chronic hepatic disorders, acute infectious processes leading to sepsis can tip the scales, resulting in hepatic failure. Patients with chronic hepatic dysfunction have a significantly higher incidence of infectious problems than other children.[24] These infectious problems relate to defective hepatic clearance of endotoxins and bacteria that gain access to the portal blood from the gut, and to spontaneous infection of ascitic fluid, pneumonia, and urinary tract infections. A thorough search for an infectious process including cultures of blood, urine, and ascitic fluid with the administration of broad-spectrum antibiotics is suggested. The empiric antibiotic regimen should include coverage for the most likely gram-positive (*S. aureus, S. pneumoniae,* and group A β-hemolytic streptococcus) and gram-negative organisms (*E. coli*). The semisynthetic penicillins such as ticarcillin or piperacillin provide coverage for most aerobic organisms, and also provide anaerobic coverage. The addition of vancomycin is suggested if infection with *S. aureus* or a penicillin-resistant strain of *S. pneumoniae* is suspected.

As several organ systems can be secondarily deranged by hepatic failure, a systematic organ system approach is suggested when dealing with affected patients. Airway control may be required for patients with altered mental status due to hyperammonemia or to control intracranial pressure (ICP) in patients developing cerebral edema (see below). Respiratory function may be compromised by neurogenic pulmonary edema, by noncardiogenic edema from multisystem organ failure, by increased intravascular volume related to blood product administration to correct coagulation disturbances and sodium/fluid retention that are due to ineffective hepatic clearance of aldosterone and other antidiuretic compounds, and by intrapulmonary shunting from the release of vasoactive compounds.

Neurologic function can be significantly compromised as a result of hepatic failure. This may be related to hepatic encephalopathy with hyperammonemia or cerebral edema. The exact agent(s) responsible for hepatic encephalopathy remain controversial. While it is frequently assumed to be related to hyperammonemia, some patients with obvious hepatic encephalopathy have normal serum ammonia levels. Therefore, others suggest that hepatic encephalopathy is related to other chemical mediators. Treatment for or prevention of hepatic encephalopathy in patients with hepatic failure includes protein restriction (0.5 to 1.0 g/kg/day). An adequate amount of protein based on the age of the patient must be administered to prevent endogenous protein catabolism (see chapter 14 for more information concerning nutrition in the patient with hepatic failure). The use of branched-chain amino acids has been suggested as a means of decreasing or reversing hepatic encephalopathy. Arginine, a branched-chain amino acid, plays a crucial role in the removal of ammonia. It has also been suggested that the addition of branched-chain amino acids by competing for a common transport system decreases the central nervous system (CNS) penetration of methionine and mercaptans, mediators thought to play a role in the pathogenesis of hepatic encephalopathy. Despite the theoretical advantage of the branched-chain amino acids, their use has not been shown to consistently alter the course of hepatic encephalopathy.

The mainstay of therapy for hepatic encephalopathy includes protein restriction and use of agents to decrease the production of ammonia by the GI flora. Neomycin (50 to 100 mg/kg/day administered at 6-hour intervals) is not absorbed when administered orally, and serves to inhibit the growth of urea-splitting GI flora, allowing for the overgrowth of lactobacillus species. Lactulose is a nonabsorbable synthetic disaccharide that produces an osmotic diarrhea also resulting in the loss of urea-splitting organisms and the overgrowth of lactobacillus species. Additionally, the production of an acid pH from the metabolism of lactulose traps ammonia in the GI lumen by converting ammonia (NH_3) to NH_4^+.

More recently, it has been suggested that the pathogenesis of hepatic encephalopathy is in part related to the overproduction of γ-aminobutyric acid (GABA), an inhibitory neurotransmitter in the CNS. GABA increases the chloride conductance of the neuronal cell membranes, leading to hyperpolarization.[25] Based on these findings, the use of GABA antagonists such as flumazenil has been suggested to improve the encephalopathy of hepatic failure. However, because of the rapid half-life of flumazenil, these effects are generally short-lived.[26] Despite the recent information concerning the pathogenesis of hepatic encephalopathy, there have been no significant additions to its treatment, other than protein restriction and methods to decrease the production of ammonia by the GI flora.

An additional CNS issue during hepatic failure is the development of cerebral edema, which may account for death in up to 50% of patients. As with hepatic encephalopathy, the exact mechanisms responsible for cerebral edema have not been identified. The development of hepatic encephalopathy and cerebral edema may be related, as patients who develop higher grades of hepatic encephalopathy have a higher incidence of cerebral edema. One mechanism that has been postulated is an alteration in the permeability of the blood-brain barrier due to toxic products such as ammonia or mercaptans. The treatment of increased ICP with hepatic failure is similar to the control of increased ICP from other causes (see chapter 10). ICP monitoring is suggested for patients with grade III or IV hepatic encephalopathy (Table 7).

Fluid management in the patient with hepatic encephalopathy is adjusted to maintain euvolemia. This adjustment may be difficult when relying solely on physical findings, and invasive hemodynamic monitoring may be indicated especially in patients with associated renal dysfunction (see below). Significant hypoglycemia may occur due to defective hepatic breakdown of glycogen. Hypoglycemia may require the administration of glucose concentrations of 20% to 25% to maintain normoglycemia. Most patients with hepatic failure will be slightly hyponatremic due to alterations in renal clearance of sodium and free water; however, total-body sodium content is generally high and sodium restriction is generally indicated. Significant potassium wasting is present due to high levels of aldosterone.

Ascites frequently complicates the man-

Table 7

Clinical Grades of Hepatic Encephalopathy

Grade 0: No evidence of CNS involvement
Grade I: Altered proprioception, abnormal sleep pattern, abnormal mood and affect, intention tremor.
Grade II: Lethargy, combative, disorientation, slurred speech, asterixis, dysarthria, increased muscle tone, hyper-reflexia, hyperpnea
Grade III: Stuporous, intention tremor, incoherent
Grade IV: Unarouseable, no spontaneous activity, irregular respiratory pattern, sluggish pupillary response, decorticate/decerebrate posturing.

agement of patients with hepatic failure. The accumulation of peritoneal fluid may be great enough to compromise respiratory function or renal perfusion. The pathogenesis involves high hepatic resistance, low serum oncotic pressure, and altered aldosterone secretion. Treatment includes a diagnostic paracentesis if an infectious process is suspected. Attempts at a therapeutic paracentesis are indicated only if respiratory or renal function is compromised. The removal of a large volume of peritoneal fluid may result in its rapid reaccumulation and intravascular volume depletion. When large volumes of ascitic fluid are removed, the intravenous infusion of albumin may be used to prevent intravascular volume depletion. Treatment for ascites includes sodium restriction, aldosterone antagonists such as spironolactone, and a slow diuresis. The latter may include intermittent doses of 25% albumin and a loop diuretic.

Coagulation disturbances are common in hepatic failure, due to defective hepatic synthesis of factors II, V, VII, IX, and X. Factor replacement with fresh frozen plasma or cryoprecipitate is indicated in patients with ongoing bleeding. Attempts to correct abnormal laboratory values of prothrombin time and partial thromboplastin time are generally not indicated in the absence of bleeding. Such attempts may require large volumes of fluid, and may result in little or no significant clinical gain. Vitamin K in doses of 0.2 mg/kg to a maximum of 10 mg/day can be helpful in addition to fresh frozen plasma in correcting the coagulopathy. The differentiation of abnormal coagulation function of hepatic failure from disseminated intravascular coagulation (DIC) may be difficult. Assays of factors VII and VIII can help to differentiate the two. With DIC, consumption of factors occurs with a decreased level of both factor VII and factor VIII. When hepatic dysfunction occurs, levels of factor VII are low while levels of factor VIII, which is synthesized by endothelial cells, are normal.

In the setting of hepatic failure, platelet numbers and function may be defective. Thrombocytopenia may be related to bone marrow suppression or increased consumption. Platelet dysfunction may be improved by the use of desmopressin (0.2 to 0.3 μg/kg i.v. over 20 to 30 minutes). Upper and lower GI bleeding are treated as outlined above.

Hepatic failure can subsequently result in renal dysfunction, also known as the hepatorenal syndrome. The exact pathogenesis remains controversial and is thought to result from alterations in intravascular volume as well as from a redistribution of renal blood flow perhaps related to altered concentrations of prostaglandin. A diagnosis of the hepatorenal syndrome should be suspected in patients with hepatic dysfunction and previously normal renal function who develop oliguria and an increasing serum concentration of BUN and creatinine. Treatment involves restoring intravascular volume, a process that generally involves central venous pressure monitoring with fluid administration to maintain a central venous pressure of 8 to 10 mm Hg. Potentially nephrotoxic agents such as aminoglycoside antibiotics and nonsteroidal anti-inflammatory drugs should be discontinued. Once intravascular volume is restored, osmotic diuretics such as mannitol and loop diuretics can be used in combination to increase urine output.

For the majority of pediatric patients with hepatic failure, PICU care involves support of the various organ systems that are affected by either the primary disorder that led to hepatic failure or of those that fail as a result of hepatic failure. Extracorporeal techniques such as porcine hepatocytes grafted to synthetic membranes as a means of providing temporary support and detoxification of the factors causing hepatic encephalopathy remain controversial and experimental. For patients with progressive hepatic failure, transplantation should be considered and offers a viable option for long-term survival.

Pancreatitis

The most common disorder of pancreatic function that necessitates PICU admission is diabetic ketoacidosis. The treatment and management of patients with diabetic ketoacidosis are outlined in chapter 17. Unlike in the adult population, pancreatitis is an uncommon reason for PICU admission, although pancreatitis may develop in the pediatric population as a consequence of the primary disease process or in relation to the various pharmacologic agents administered to the critically ill child. In the PICU patient, the presentation of pancreatitis may be vague. Therefore, a high index of suspicion is necessary as many of the classic signs and symptoms may be absent (Table 8). Isolated episodes of nausea, vague complaints of abdominal pain, or an ileus with feeding intolerance may be the only signs and symptoms noted.

The etiology of pancreatitis is varied (Table 9) and many times the exact causes cannot be established in the PICU patient. However, a review of the current drug therapy is indicated in order to attempt to identify those agents that may play a role. The diagnosis is suggested by the physical signs and symptoms, and is confirmed by elevated serum concentrations of amylase and lipase. Amylase levels may decline rapidly resulting in a normal serum concentration. A 4-hour urine collection for an amylase/creatinine ratio (≥4 suggests the diagnosis) can aid in the diagnosis in patients who are rapidly clearing amylase from the serum. The latter is especially common in the pediatric age range, due to the rapid clearance of amylase by the kidneys. Amylase levels in the fluid should be measured if ascitic or pleural fluid is obtained for diagnostic purposes. The remainder of the diagnostic work-up is based on the patient's history and the likely etiologic factors. All patients should have an ultrasound examination. An ultrasound may help to establish the diagnosis by demonstrating pancreatic edema/increased hypoechogenicity as well as ruling out congenital malformations of the biliary tree and cholelithiasis.

Treatment is generally supportive in addition to surgery as indicated for congenital malformations or cholelithiasis. The mainstay of therapy remains bowel rest. The need for NG decompression and drainage, once standard therapy, has recently been questioned. NG decompression is indicated in patients with ileus and vomiting. The efficacy of H_2-antagonists has been questioned; however, their use makes sound physiologic sense as the release of acidic gastric secretions into the duodenal lumen is a potent stimulus for pancreatic contraction. Parenteral nutrition may be required for prolonged periods of time while the pancreatitis resolves. Enteral feedings are held until the patient is afebrile, the white blood cell count has returned to normal, and the pain has resolved. When enteral feedings are restarted, carbohydrates are administered

Table 8

Signs, Symptoms, and Laboratory Findings of Pancreatitis

Abdominal pain
Nausea
Vomiting
Fever
Ileus
Feeding intolerance
Pleural effusion
Ascites
Tachycardia
Hypotension
High serum amylase
High serum lipase
Hypocalcemia
Hyperglycemia
Hypoglycemia
Leukocytosis

Table 9

Etiology of Pancreatitis

Drugs and toxins:
  thiazide diuretics
  loop diuretics
  corticosteroids
  azathioprine
  valproic acid

Infectious agents:
  mumps
  coxsackie
  rubella
  hepatitis A,B
  Influenza
  Epstein Barr virus
  echovirus

Congenital abnormalities of the biliary tree:
  choledochal cyst
  duodenal duplications
  anomalous insertion of the bile duct
  annular pancreas

Biliary tract disease:
  cholelithiasis

Trauma

Reye syndrome

Metabolic disorders:
  cystic fibrosis
  defects of amino acid metabolism
  hyperlipoproteinemia (types I, IV, V)
  hyperparathyroidism

Systemic vasculitis:
  collagen vascular disorders
  Henoch-Schonlein purpura
  hemolytic-uremic syndrome

Hypoperfusion injury

Multisystem organ failure

---

first, followed by the slow and cautious addition of protein and fat (see also chapter 14 for feeding in patients with pancreatitis).

Recent reports in the adult literature in patients with alcoholic pancreatitis suggest the efficacy of somatostatin and its analog, octreotide, in hastening the resolution of pancreatitis.[2] These latter agents have been suggested to decrease the pancreatic production of proteolytic enzymes which may play a role in the production of ongoing pancreatic damage and inflammation.

Although pancreatitis is generally self-limited, progression to multisystem involvement and failure may occur. In the adult population, hypocalcemia, a white blood cell count greater than 20,000/mm^3, a room-air PaO$_2$ less than 60 mm Hg, and a BUN greater than 20 mg/dL are associated with a greater incidence of morbidity and mortality. Complications related to pancreatitis include the development of end-organ failure (multisystem organ failure, renal failure, adult respiratory distress syndrome, DIC), abscess/pseudocyst formation, pleural/peritoneal fluid collections, glucose intolerance, and GI bleeding. Early identification and treatment of these problems is necessary to limit their impact on morbidity and mortality.

References

1. Resnick RH. Intra-arterial vasopressin: A continuing challenge. *Gastroenterology* 1975;68:411–412.
2. Mulvihill S, Pappas TN, Passaro E Jr, Debas HT. The use of somatostatin and its analogs in the treatment of surgical disorders. *Surgery* 1986;100:467–476.
3. Siafakas C, Fox VL, Nurko S. Use of octreotide for the treatment of severe gastrointestinal bleeding in children. *J Pediatr Gastroent Nutr* 1998;26:356–359.
4. Hyams JS, Leichtner AM, Schwartz AN. Recent advances in diagnosis and treatment of gastrointestinal hemorrhage in infants and children. *J Pediatr* 1985;106:1–9.
5. Mitra SK, Kumar V, Datta DV, et al. Extrahepatic portal hypertension: A review of 70 cases. *J Pediatr Surg* 1978;13:51–55.
6. Besson I, Ingrand P, Person B, et al. Sclerotherapy with or without octreotide for acute variceal bleeding. *N Engl J Med* 1995;333:555–560.
7. Burroughs AK, Jenkins WJ, Sherlock S, et al. Controlled trial of propranolol for the prevention of recurrent variceal hemorrhage in patients with cirrhosis. *N Engl J Med* 1983;309:1539–1542.
8. Ozsoylu S, Kocak N, Yuce A. Propranolol therapy for portal hypertension in children. *J Pediatr* 1985;106:317–321.
9. Lacroix J, Nadeau D, Laberge S, et al. Frequency of upper gastrointestinal bleeding in a pediatric intensive care unit. *Crit Care Med* 1992;20:35–42.
10. Lacroix J, Infante-Rivard C, Jenicek C, et al. Prophylaxis of upper gastrointestinal bleeding in intensive care units: A meta-analysis. *Crit Care Med* 1989;17:862–869.
11. Lopez-Herce J, Dorao P, Elola P, et al. Fre-

quency and prophylaxis of upper gastrointestinal hemorrhage in critically ill children: A prospective study comparing the efficacy of almagate, ranitidine, and sucralfate. *Crit Care Med* 1992;20:1082–1089.
12. Rovers JP, Souney PF. A critical review of continuous infusion H_2 receptor therapy. *Crit Care Med* 1989;17:814–821.
13. Lacroix J, Infante-Rivard C, Gauthier M, et al. Upper gastrointestinal tract bleeding acquired in a pediatric intensive care unit: Prophylaxis trial with cimetidine. *J Pediatr* 1986;108:1015–1018.
14. Lloyd CW, Martin WJ, Taylor BD, et al. Pharmacokinetics and pharmacodynamics of cimetidine and metabolites in critically ill children. *J Pediatr* 1985;107:295–300.
15. Byrne WJ. Diagnosis and treatment of peptic ulcer disease in children. *Pediatr Rev* 1985;7:182–190.
16. Deutsch PH. Cimetidine: The interactions. *Res Staff Phys* 1984;30:46–55.
17. Goelzer SL, Farin-Rush C, Coursin DB. Ranitidine produces minimal hemodynamic depression in stable intensive care unit patients: A double-blind, prospective study. *Crit Care Med* 1988;16:8–10.
18. Lopez-Herce J, Velasco LA, Codoceo R, et al. Ranitidine prophylaxis in acute gastric mucosal damage in critically ill pediatric patients. *Crit Care Med* 1988;16:591–593.
19. James LP, Kearns GL. Pharmacokinetics and pharmacodynamics of famotidine in pediatric patients. *Clin Pharmacokinet* 1996;31:103–110.
20. Rovers JP, Souney PF. A critical review of continuous infusion H_2 receptor therapy. *Crit Care Med* 1989;17:814–821.
21. Atanassoff PG, Alon E, Pasch T. Effects of single-dose intravenous omeprazole and ranitidine on gastric pH during general anesthesia. *Anesth Analg* 1992;75:95–98.
22. Driks MR, Craven DE, Celli BR, et al. Nosocomial pneumonia in intubated patients given sucralfate as compared with antacids of histamine type 2 blockers. *N Engl J Med* 1987;317:1376–1382.
23. Apte NM, Karnad DR, Medhekar TP, et al. Gastric colonization and pneumonia in intubated critically ill patients receiving stress ulcer prophylaxis: A randomized, controlled trial. *Crit Care Med* 1992;20:590–593.
24. Gradual N, Milman N, Kirkegaard E, et al. Bacteremia in cirrhosis of the liver. *Liver* 1986;6:297–301.
25. Schafer DF, Jones EA. Potential neural mechanisms in the pathogenesis of hepatic encephalopathy. *Prog Liver Dis* 1982;7:615–620.
26. Bansky G, Meier PJ, Riedere E, et al. Effects of the benzodiazepine receptor antagonist flumazenil in hepatic encephalopathy in humans. *Gastroenterology* 1989;97:744–748.

Index

Page numbers in italics indicate figures; page numbers followed by "t" indicate tables.

Aberrant origin of left coronary artery, 168–169
ACE inhibitors, 384
Acetaminophen, toxic ingestion of, 421, *422*, 423
Acid-base disturbances, 303–305
Acidosis
  metabolic, 25, 303–304, 372
  respiratory, 303
Acids, ingestion of, 425–426
Acute renal failure. *See* Renal failure, acute
Acute respiratory distress syndrome
  clinical course, 141
  diagnosis, 137–138, 139t, 141
  fluid management in, 24, 149
  mechanical ventilation in, 86–88, 145–147
  mechanisms, 142–143
  multiple organ dysfunction syndrome, 144–145
  pathology, 141–142
  permissive hypercapnia, use of, 87–88, 147–148
  pneumonia associated with, 143–144
  pulmonary function, long-term outcome, 151–152
  risk factors, 139–140
  severity of, 140
  surfactant replacement, use of, 114
  therapies, 113, 114, 145–152
Adrenergic agonists
  in postoperative cardiac care, 189
  in shock, 26–29
  in status asthmaticus, 45–50
Adult respiratory distress syndrome. *See* Acute respiratory distress syndrome
Airway management. *See also* Intubation, endotracheal
  in abnormal airways, 13–14
  in burns, 282–283
  in increased intracranial pressure, 230–231
  in normal airways, 5–12
  relieving obstructions, 1–2
  in shock, 21–22
  in traumatic injuries, 273–274, 275–276
Airway obstructions, lower. *See* Status asthmaticus
Airway obstructions, upper
  acute, 37–40
  antibiotic therapy, 39
  differential diagnosis of, 38t

  management of, 1–2
  mild to moderate, 40
  surgery in, 37–38
  use of helium/oxygen therapy, 41–43
Airways
  laryngeal mask, 8–12
  oral, 2
Albumin 5%, 22–23, 278
Albuterol, 45
Alcohol ingestions, 423
Alkalis, ingestion of, 425–426
Alkalosis
  metabolic, 304–305
  respiratory, 303
Alveolar distention. *See* Volutrauma
Alveolar gas equation, 58
Alveolar ventilation, 59
Amnestic/analgesic agents, 5t, 6–7. *See also* Sedation/analgesia; Sedative/analgesic agents
Amphetamines, toxic ingestion of, 433–436
Amrinone, 27, 28, 190
Analgesia. *See* Amnestic/analgesic agents; Sedation/analgesia; Sedative/analgesic agents
Anemia, postoperative, 200
Anesthesia
  in airway management, 6–7, 13
  inhalation, 53–54, 243–245
Antacids, 445–446
Anthropometric measurements, 327–329
Antibiotics
  in ARDS, 149
  in burns, 284–285
  in meningitis, 400–402
  in postoperative cardiac care, 201
  in sepsis/septic shock, 390–394, 395t, 396
  in upper airway obstructions, 39, 40
Anticholinergic drugs
  in status asthmaticus, 45–47
  toxic ingestions, 424
Antidotes for toxic ingestions, 420
Anti-inflammatory agents, 401–402
Antimicrobial agents, topical, 284–285
Anuria, 349. *See also* Renal failure, acute
Anxiety, in PICU patients, 241–243
Aorta
  coarctation, severe, 157–158, 196
  transposition of, 159–160

Aortic arch, interrupted, 157–158
Aortic stenosis, 157
Aprotinin, 345
ARDS. *See* Acute respiratory distress syndrome
ARF. *See* Renal failure, acute
Arrhythmias, 169–179. *See also specific arrythmias*
  in diabetic ketoacidosis, 375
  diagnosis of, 169–170
  medications, 178–179
Arterial switch procedure, 160, 203
Arteries, great, transposition of, 169–169
Artificial lungs, 118–119
Ascites, 450–451
Aspiration during intubation, 4
Assist control mode (ventilation). *See* Supported ventilation
Asthma, 43, 88–90. *See also* Status asthmaticus
Asystole, 176–177
Atrial flutter/fibrillation, 170–172
Atropine, 47
AV block, 176, 187–188
Awake intubations, 13–14

Bacterial tracheitis, 38, 39–40, 407
BAL. *See* Bronchoalveolar lavage
Barbiturates
  in increased intracranial pressure, 233–234
  for sedation, 250–251
  toxic ingestion of, 432–433
Barotrauma, 95, 96t, 107. *See also* Ventilator-induced lung injury; Volutrauma
Benzodiazepines
  agents for sedation, 246–247
  toxic ingestion of, 432–433
β-adrenergic agonist therapy
  inhaled, 45–47
  intravenous, 49–50
  in postoperative cardiac care, 189
β-adrenergic antagonists, toxic ingestion of, 424–425
Bioelectric impedance analysis, 329
Blalock-Taussig shunt, 161, 203, 204
Bleeding, excessive, 199–200
Blood component therapy. *See* Transfusions
Blood filters, 340
Blood/hemoglobin substitutes, 338–340
Blood loss, in traumatic injuries, 276, 277t
Blood transfusions. *See* Transfusions
Bradyarrhythmias, 175–176
Brain edema, 225–226, 373–374, 450
Breathing mechanics, 65–66, 67
Bronchoalveolar lavage, 138, 139t, 143–144
Bronchodilator therapy, 45
Bullard laryngoscope, 14
Burns, 282–285

Calcium, 299
  exogenous administration, 189
  hypercalcemia, 300
  hypocalcemia, 25, 299–300, 358
Calcium channel blockers, 424
Cannulae, ECLS, 117–118
Capnography, 7, 98–99
Carbon dioxide
  alveolar partial pressure, 58, 59
  and cerebral blood flow, 228
  monitoring, 98–99
Carbon monoxide poisoning, 428–429
Carboxyhemoglobinemia, 428–429
Cardiac care, postoperative
  analgesia/sedation, 202–203
  cardiovascular system, 185–191
  central nervous system, 195–196
  electrolytes and fluids, 197–199
  gastrointestinal and hepatic systems, 196–197
  hematologic issues, 199–200
  infectious diseases, 200–201
  initial evaluation, 184–185
  renal system, 201–202
  respiratory system, 191–195
Cardiac ECLS, 126–130
Cardiac lesions, obstructive left-side, 20–21
Cardiac output
  assessment of, 17–18, 29–35
  in hypertensive emergencies, 378
  in postoperative cardiac patients, 185–188
Cardiac rhythm, alterations, 187
Cardiogenic shock
  fluid resuscitation, 24
  physiologic changes in, 19, 20
  in postoperative cardiac care, 190
  treatment with inotropic agents, 28
Cardiomyopathy, 165–168
Cardiopulmonary bypass, 182–184. *See also* Cardiac care, postoperative
Cardiorespiratory failure, 186
Cardiovascular physiology
  cardiac output and vascular tone, 17–19
  changes in mechanical ventilation, 95–96
  changes in shock, 19t, 20
Cardiovascular resuscitation
  crystalloid *vs.* colloid fluids, 22–24
  in traumatic injuries, 276–280
  in treatment of shock, 22–26
Cathartics, 418, 419
Caustic agents, toxic ingestion of, 425–426
CBF. *See* Cerebral blood flow
Central line infections, 409
Central nervous system
  injuries and mechanical ventilation, 85
  in postoperative cardiac care, 195–196
Central venous pressure, monitoring, 29, 186
Cerebral blood flow
  and carbon dioxide, 228
  metabolism, 227–228
  and oxygen, 228–229

pressure-flow autoregulation, 227
    regulation of, 226–230
    SjO₂ monitoring, 229–230
Cerebral edema, 225–226, 373–374, 450
Cerebral perfusion pressure, 223, 227
Cerebrospinal fluid drainage, 233
Cervical spine
    injuries in trauma patients, 274–275
    protection in airway management, 1, 2, 13, 14
Charcoal, activated, 418–419
Cholinergic syndromes, 426–427
Circulatory pump failure, 85
Clonidine, 424–425
Coagulation abnormalities
    in hepatic failure, 451
    postoperative, 199–200
Coagulation cascade, modifiers, 343–345
Coagulation factors
    in blood transfusions, 279–280
    concentrates, use of, 342–343
Coarctation of the aorta, 157–158, 196–197
Cocaine, 433–436
Colloidal fluids, 22–24, 278
Congenital adrenal hyperplasia, 20–21
Congenital heart diseases. *See* Heart diseases, congenital
Congestive heart failure
    aberrant origin of left coronary artery, 168–169
    myocarditis/cardiomyopathy, 165–168
Continuous arteriovenous hemofiltration, 202
Continuous positive airway pressure, 80–81
Continuous venous-venous hemofiltration, 202
Controlled (mandatory) ventilation, 71
Coronary artery, left, aberrant origin, 168–169
Corticosteroids
    in ARDS, 150–151
    in increased intracranial pressure, 235
    in invasive meningococcal disease, 394, 397
    in status asthmaticus, 47–48
CPAP (Continuous positive airway pressure), 80–81
CPB. *See* Cardiopulmonary bypass
CPP (Cerebral perfusion pressure), 223, 227
Craniectomy, decompressive, 235
Cricoid pressure (Sellick's maneuver), 4, 10
Cricothyrotomy, needle, 8, 12
Critical aortic stenosis, 157
Croup, 38t, 39–41, 407
Cryoprecipitate, 341
Crystalloid fluids, 22–24, 278–279
CVP (Central venous pressure) monitoring, 29, 186
Cyanide, ingestion of, 427
Cyanosis, 159
Cyanotic heart disease. *See* Heart diseases, congenital

Decompressive craniectomy, 235
Dehydration, 289–290, 368, 370
Desmopressin, 343–344
Dexamethasone, 401–402
Dextran, 22
Diabetes mellitus, insulin-dependent, 368
Diabetic ketoacidosis
    assessment and management, 368–373
    clinical presentation, 368
    complications, 373–375
    and pancreatitis, 452
    pathophysiology, 367–368
Dialysis
    hemodialysis, 202, 360–362
    hemofiltration with, 362–363
    hemoperfusion, 363
    peritoneal, 202, 360–362
    replacement fluids in, 363
Diazepam, 246
Diazoxide, 384
DiGeorge syndrome, 158, 163, 164
Digoxin, toxic ingestion of, 427–428
Distributive shock, 19, 20, 24, 28
Diuretics
    in poisonings/toxic ingestions, 419–420
    in postoperative cardiac care, 198
    use in acute renal failure, 359
DKA. *See* Diabetic ketoacidosis
Dobutamine, 27, 28
Dopamine, 26, 28, 359
Drugs. *See specific drugs*
Drug screens, 415
Dynamic hyperinflation, 88–89
Dysrhythmias, 187–188

Ebstein's anomaly of the tricuspid valve, 161
ECLS. *See* Extracorporeal life support
ECMO (Extracorporeal membrane oxygenation), 190
Edema
    brain (cerebral), 225–226, 373–374, 450
    pulmonary, 375
Eisenmenger syndrome, 175–176
Electrocardiogram
    in congenital heart disease, 169, 170, *171*
    in hyperkalemia, 297, *298*
Electrolytes
    in acute renal failure, 357
    in cardiac care, 197–199
    maintenance of, 288, 289t
    in myocarditis/cardiomyopathy, 167
Electromechanical dissociation, 177
ELV (End-expiration lung volume), 65, 84
Emergence phenomena, 248–249
Emesis, induced, 417–418
EN. *See* Enteral nutrition
Enalapril, 384
Encephalitis, 403–404, 405t

Encephalopathy
  hepatic, 449–450, 451t
  hypertensive, 377–378
End-expiration lung volume, 65, 84
Endotracheal intubation. *See* Intubation, endotracheal
Endotracheal tubes, 2–4, 14
End-tidal carbon dioxide devices, 7–8, 15
Enteral nutrition
  advantages/disadvantages, 311–312
  complications of, 316–317
  formulas, 315–316
  guidelines, 315t
  indications for, 312
  monitoring, 328
  in postoperative cardiac care, 196–197
  transpyloric tube feeding, 312–315
Enterocolitis, necrotizing, 196–197
Epiglottitis
  diagnosis and treatment, 406–407
  and endotracheal intubation, 38–39, 406
  surgery for, 37–38
  vs. croup, 38t
Epilepsy. *See* Status epilepticus
Epinephrine
  in postoperative cardiac care, 189
  racemic, 41
  in shock, 27, 28
ε-aminocaproic acid, 344–345
Equation of motion, 61, 62
Esophageal varices, 442, 443
$ETCO_2$ (End-tidal carbon dioxide) devices, 7–8, 15
ETTs (Endotracheal tubes), 2–4, 14
Extracorporeal life support, 115–130
  artificial lungs/membrane oxygenators, 118–119
  cannulae, 117–118
  cardiac, 126–130
  classification of, 116–117
  heat exchangers, 119
  history of, 115
  in neonates, 119–125
  in pediatric population, 125–127
  pumps, 118
  safety devices, 119
  selection criteria, 120–121, 122t, 123, 125–126, 127t
  survival rates, 124–125, 126, 130
  "trial off," 123–124
  venoarterial and venovenous, 116, 123–124
Extracorporeal membrane oxygenation, 190
Extravascular lung water, 95
Extubation, 93, 192–193. *See also* Intubation, endotracheal

Fenoldopam, 385
Fever, in immunocompromised patients, 407–408

Fiber optic brochoscopy, use of LMA in, 11
Fluid, body compartments, 287–288
Fluid management
  in ARDS, 149
  in burns, 284
  in cardiac care, 188, 197–199
  crystalloid *vs.* colloid, 22–24
  in dehydration, 289–290
  in diabetic ketoacidosis, 368, 370
  in hepatic encephalopathy, 450
  in renal failure, acute, 357–359
  in renal replacement therapy, 363
  in traumatic injuries, 276–280
  in treatment of shock, 22–26
  water and electrolyte maintenance, 288, 289t
Flumazenil, 247
Fontan procedure, 161, 192, 194, 203
Foreign body aspiration, 37, 38
Fresh frozen plasma, 340–341
Functional residual capacity (FRC), 65, 84
Fungal infections, 409–410

Gastric lavage, 418
Gastritis, stress, 444–445
Gastrointestinal bleeding. *See also* Ulcer prophylaxis
  lower, 443–444
  prophylaxis, 445
  risk factors, 445, 446
  upper, 439–443
Gastrointestinal system
  in postoperative cardiac care, 196–197
GI bleeding. *See* Gastrointestinal bleeding
Glasgow coma score, 273, 280
Glenn shunt, 192, 194, 203
Glucose, serum
  in diabetic ketoacidosis, 367–368
  in shock, 26
  in traumatic injuries, 280
Great arteries, transposition of, 159–160
Gum elastic bougie, 10

Halothane, 53, 244
H_2-antagonists, 446–448
HD (Hemodialysis), 202, 360–362
Heart block, 176
Heart diseases, congenital
  coarctation of the aorta/interrupted aortic arch, 157–158, 196
  critical aortic stenosis, 157
  Ebstein's anomaly, 161
  hypoplastic left heart syndrome, 155–157
  ketamine use, 248
  medications, 178–179
  tetralogy of Fallot, 161–163
  total anomalous pulmonary venous return, 164–165
  transposition of the great arteries, 159–160

tricuspid valve and pulmonary valve atresia, 160–161
truncus arteriosus, 163–164
Heart failure, congestive, 165–169
Heart rates, 187
Heat exchangers, ECLS, 119
Helium/oxygen therapy, 41–43, 51–53
Hematocrit, postoperative, 200
Hematologic issues, postoperative, 199–200
Hemodialysis, 202, 360–362
Hemodynamic monitoring
 in cardiac patients, 185
 CVP monitoring, 29
 in increased intracranial pressure, 231–232
 mixed venous oxygen saturation, 31
 PA catheters (Swan-Ganz), 29, 30, 31–35
Hemofiltration, 362–363
Hemoglobinopathies, 428–429
Hemoglobin substitutes, 338–340
Hemoglobinuria, 355
Hemolysis, postoperative, 200
Hemolytic uremic syndrome, 354–355
Hemoperfusion, 363
Hepatic encephalopathy, 449–450, 451t
Hepatic failure
 ascites in, 450–451
 coagulation abnormalities, 451
 diagnosis, 448–449
 etiologies, 448, 449t
 hepatic encephalopathy, 449–450, 451t
 hepatorenal syndrome, 451
 management, 449–452
 nutrition in, 322, 324t, 325
Hepatic function, 196–197, 448
Hepatorenal syndrome, 354, 451
Herpes simplex virus, 404, 405t
HFV. See High-frequency ventilation
High-frequency ventilation
 categories of, 107–108
 flow interrupters, 112
 jet ventilation, 111–112
 oscillatory, 109–111
 positive pressure, 108–109
HIV (Human immunodeficiency virus), 408
HLHS (Hypoplastic left heart syndrome), 155–157
HP (Hemoperfusion), 363
HSV (Herpes simplex virus), 404, 405t
Human immunodeficiency virus (HIV), 408
HUS (Hemolytic uremic syndrome), 354–355
Hydrocarbons, toxic ingestion of, 429–430
Hydroxyethyl starch, 22, 23, 278
Hyperammonemia
 in cardiogenic shock, 20
 diagnosis, 305–307
 treatment, 307–308
Hypercalcemia, 300
Hypercapnia, permissive, 87–88, 147–148

Hyperglycemia, 367–368. See also Diabetic ketoacidosis
Hyperkalemia
 in acute renal failure, 357–358, 359t
 in diabetic ketoacidosis, 371
 diagnosis and treatment, 297–299
Hypermagnesemia, 302
Hypernatremia, 294–296, 371
Hyperphosphatemia, 301, 358
Hypertensive emergencies
 defined, 377
 drug therapy, 382–386
 evaluation, 379–381
 management, 381–382
 signs and symptoms, 377–378
Hypertensive encephalopathy, 377–378
Hypertonic crystalloids, 23–24
Hyperventilation, 234–235
Hypocalcemia
 in acute renal failure, 358
 diagnosis and treatment, 299–300
 in traumatic injuries, 280
 in treatment of shock, 25
Hypoglycemia, 26, 374
Hypokalemia, 296, 297t, 374–375
Hypomagnesemia, 25–26, 301–302
Hyponatremia, 290–294, 358
Hypophosphatemia, 301
Hypoplastic left heart syndrome, 155–157
Hypotension, systemic, 50–51
Hypothermia
 in increased intracranial pressure, 234
 in postoperative cardiac patients, 184–185
 in transfusions, 336–337
 in traumatic injuries, 279, 280
Hypoventilation, 92
Hypovolemic shock, 19, 24
Hypoxemia
 in ARDS, 137, 143
 etiologies, 58–59
 in pulmonary disease, 86, 90
 during weaning from ventilator, 92

IABP (Intra-aortic balloon pump), 190–191
ICP. See Intracranial pressure, increased
Immunocompromised patients, 407–408, 408
IMV (Intermittent mandatory ventilation), 76–77
Infections, nosocomial, 408–409
Infectious diseases, 200–201. See also Sepsis/septic shock; specific infectious diseases
Inhalation anesthetic agents, 53–54, 243–245
Inotropic agents
 in HLHS, use, 157
 mixing infusions, 28–29
 in myocarditis, 167–168
 in postoperative cardiac care, 188–190
 in shock, treatment of, 24, 26–29
Inspiratory times, 83, 191

Insulin therapy, 371–372, 373
Intermittent mandatory ventilation, 76–77
Interrupted aortic arch, 157–158
Intestinal failure, nutrition in, 325
Intra-aortic balloon pump, 190–191
Intracranial pressure, increased
   airway management, 230–231
   analgesia/sedation/neuromuscular blockades, 232–233
   head positioning, 232
   hemodynamic management, 231–232
   management, 230–233
   monitoring, 223–224
   pathophysiology, 224–226
   seizure management, 232
   temperature control, 232
   therapies, 233–235
   therapy integration, 235–237
   ventilator management, 231
Intracranial vault, 224–225
Intrapulmonary shunt fraction, 33–34
Intubation, endotracheal
   aspiration during, 4
   contraindications, 2
   correct tube placement, 7–8
   in croup, 40–41
   drugs and doses, 5–7
   equipment, 2–4, 7–8
   extubation, 93, 192–193
   failed, 8–13
   fiber optic guided, 14
   Gum elastic bougie, use of, 10, *11*
   LMA, use of, 9–11
   oral *vs.* nasal, 2
   rapid-sequence, 4–8
   respiratory function following, 14–15
   in status asthmaticus, 50–51
   in traumatic injuries, 275–275
   upper airway obstruction, use in, 38–39
Intubations, awake, 13–14
Ipratropium, 47
Iron, toxic ingestion of, 430–431
Irradiation of blood products, 158, 164, 338
Isoflurane, 54, 244–245
Isoproterenol, 28
Isradipine, 385

Jet ventilation, 12–13

Ketamine, 247–249
Ketoacidosis, diabetic. *See* Diabetic ketoacidosis

Labetalol, 384
Laryngeal mask airway, 8–12
Laryngoscopes, 2, *3*, 3t
Laryngoscopy, 2–3, 13–14
Laryngotracheobronchitis, 39–41, 407
Left-sided obstructive heart disease. *See* Heart diseases, congenital

Left ventricle at the end of diastole, 18, 29, 31–32
Light wand, 14
Liquid ventilation, 114–115, 148
LMA (Laryngeal mask airway), 8–12
Lorazepam, 246–247
Lower airway obstruction. *See* Status asthmaticus
Lung injury. *See* Acute respiratory distress syndrome; Ventilator-induced lung injury
LVEDV (Left ventricle at the end of diastole), 18, 29, 31–32

Magnesium
   and cardiac function, 199
   hypermagnesemia, 302
   hypomagnesemia, 301–302
   in shock, 25–26
Magnesium sulfate, 48–49
Mandatory ventilation, 71
Mannitol, 233, 359
Mean airway pressure, 59
Mechanical assist devices
   in cardiomyopathy/myocarditis, 168
   extracorporeal membrane oxygenation, 190
   intra-aortic balloon pump, 190–191
   ventricular assist device, 190
Mechanical ventilation. *See* Ventilation, mechanical
Medications. *See specific medications*
Membrane oxygenators, 118–119
Membranous laryngotracheobronchitis. *See* Bacterial tracheitis
Meningitis
   antibiotic treatment, 400–401, 402
   and anti-inflammatory agents, 401–402
   laboratory work-up, 398, 399t, 400
   mechanisms of infection, 397–398
   microorganisms associated with, 397
   risk factors, 397
   symptoms, 398, 399t
   tuberculous, 402–403
   viral, 397
Meningococcal disease, invasive, 394–397
Metabolic acidosis, 25, 280
Metabolic alkalosis, 304–305
Methemoglobinemia, 428–429
Midazolam, 246
Milrinone, 190. *See also* PDE inhibitors
Minoxidil, 385
Mixed venous oxygen saturation, 31, 186
MODS (Multiple organ dysfunction syndrome), 144–145
Morbidity/mortality
   in acute renal failure, 349
   in ARDS, 140, 141, 144
   in cardiac care, postoperative, 186, 191, 200
   in ECLS, 124–125, 126, 130
   in sepsis/septic shock, 389, 390, 394
   in status asthmaticus, 43, 88–89

in status epilepticus, 209–210
in traumatic injuries, 273
Multiple organ dysfunction syndrome, 144–145
Myocardial contractility, 18
Myocardial failure, 186
Myocardial oxygen delivery, 187
Myocarditis, 165–168
Myoglobinuria, 355

Nebulization treatments, 45
Necrotizing enterocolitis, 196–197
Needle cricothyrotomy, 8, 12
Neurologic evaluation, in traumatic injuries, 280
Neurologic injury, mechanical ventilation in, 85
Neuromuscular blockades, 4
  in abnormal airway, 13–14
  agents, 5–6, 257–262
  dosing guidelines, 264–266
  in increased intracranial pressure, 232–233
  indications for use, 257–258
  monitoring blockade, 262–263
  in normal airway, 5–13
  in pediatric intensive care unit, use, 263–266
  reversal of blockade, 263
  in status asthmaticus, 50
  in upper airway obstructions, 38–39
Neutropenia, 407–408
Nicardipine, 383
Nifedipine, 385
Nitric oxide, 112–114
  in ARDS, 148
  complications, 114
  in PVR treatment, 195
  uses, 113–114
Nitrous oxide, 245–246
Norepinephrine, 27–28, 189
Norwood procedures, 157, 191, 203–204
Nosocomial infections, 408–409
Nutrition, 311. *See also* Enteral nutrition; Parenteral nutrition
  in acute renal failure, 360
  assessment and monitoring, 327–329
  in burns, 284
  estimating caloric needs, 321
  future directions, 329
  in hepatic failure, 322, 324t, 325
  in intestinal failure, 325
  in postoperative cardiac care, 196–197
  in renal failure, 322, 323t, 324t
  in respiratory failure, 194
  in skin failure, 325–327

Obstructions
  lower airway (*See* Status asthmaticus)
  upper airway (*See* Airway obstructions, upper)
Obstructive left-side cardiac lesions, 20
Obstructive lung disease, 88–90

Obstructive shock, 19, 20t
Octreotide, 441–442
Oliguria, 349, 353t. *See also* Renal failure, acute
Opioids
  administration of, 251–253
  agents, 252–257
  toxic ingestion of, 431–432
  withdrawal and addiction, 255–256
Oral airways, 2
Organ failure, nutrition in, 322–327
Oxygen
  administration of, 1, 15, 21–22, 37
  alveolar partial pressure of 57–58
  and cerebral blood flow, 228–229
  consumption of, 34, 187
  content of, calculating, 33
  delivery of, 34, 151, 187
  saturation, mixed venous, 31
  toxicity of, 96–97, 148–149
Oxygenation, maintenance, 57–59
Oxygen therapy, 148–149

PA catheters. *See* Pulmonary artery catheters
Pacemaker failure, 177
$PACO_2$ (Partial pressure of alveolar carbon dioxide), 58, 59
Pain management, 241–243
Pancreatitis, 452–453
Pancuronium, 6, 260–261, 264
PAO_2 (Partial pressure of alveolar oxygen), 57–58
Parenteral nutrition
  administration of, 318–319
  and central line infections, 409
  complications, 321
  indications for, 317–318
  monitoring, 328–329
  in postoperative cardiac care, 196–197
Partial pressure of alveolar carbon dioxide, 58, 59
Partial pressure of alveolar oxygen, 57–58
Patent ductus arteriosus, 155–160
Patient-controlled analgesia, 251, 252–253
P_{aw} (Mean airway pressure), 59
PCA (Patient controlled analgesia), 251, 252–253
PCV *See* Pressure-controlled ventilation
PCWP (Pulmonary capillary wedge pressure), 31–32
PDA (Patent ductus arteriosus), 155–160
PDE inhibitors, 27, 28, 189, 190
PD (Peritoneal dialysis), 202, 360–362
PEEP (Positive end-expiratory pressure)
  in hypoplastic left heart syndrome, 156
  and mechanical ventilation, 80–81
  in postoperative cardiac care, 191–192
  and spontaneous ventilation, 80–81
  in treatment of ARDS, 32–33, 86–87, 145–146
  trials, 86–87
Perfluorocarbons, 338–339

Peritoneal dialysis, 202, 360–362
Peritonsillar abscesses, 40
Permissive hypercapnia, 87–88, 147–148
Persistent pulmonary hypertension of the newborn, 113
$P_{et}CO_2$ (Peak carbon dioxide during expiration) monitoring, 98–99
Phencyclidine, toxic ingestion of, 433–436
Phenylephrine, 27–28
Phosphorus/phosphate, 301, 358
Pipecuronium, 261
Plasma derivatives, 342–343. See also Transfusions
Plasmalyte, 23
Platelets
  concentrates, 341–342
  thrombocytopenia, 199–200
PN. See Parenteral nutrition
Pneumonia
  associated with ARDS, 143–144
  bacterial, 406
  nosocomial, 447–448
Pneumothorax, tension, 51
Poisonings/toxic ingestions. See also Poisons/toxic agents
  activated charcoal, 418–419
  antidotes, 420
  cathartics, 418, 419
  enhanced elimination of poisons/toxins, 419–420
  evaluation and stabilization, 413–417
  gastric lavage, 418
  induced emesis, 417–418
  laboratory tests, 414–415, 417t
  management, 417–420
  medical history, importance of, 413–414
  physical examination in, 414, 415, 416t
  whole-bowel irrigation, 418, 419
Poisons/toxic agents
  acetaminophen, 421, 422, 423
  alcohols, 423
  anticholinergic syndromes, 423
  calcium channel blockers/ β-Adrenergic antagonists/clonidine, 424–425
  carbon monoxide, 428–429
  caustic agents, 425–426
  cholinergic syndromes, 426–427
  cyanide, 427
  digoxin, 427–428
  hemoglobinopathies, 428–429
  hydrocarbons, 429–430
  iron, 430–431
  opioids, 431–432
  salicylates, 432
  sedatives, 432–433
  sympathomimetics, 433–436
  tricyclic antidepressants, 436–437
Positive end-expiratory pressure. See PEEP

Postoperative care, cardiac patients. See Cardiac care, postoperative
Postsurgical stress response, 241–242
Potassium
  in acute renal failure, 357–358, 359t
  hyperkalemia, 297–299
  hypokalemia, 296, 297t
Potts shunt, 204
Pressure-controlled ventilation, 61, 73–75, 83, 90–91
Pressure-flow autoregulation, 227
Pressure-regulated volume controlled ventilation, 75–76
Pressure-supported ventilation, 77–80
Prone positioning, in ARDS, 149
Propofol, 249–250
Prostaglandin E
  in cyanotic heart disease, 159, 160, 164
  in obstructive heart disease, 156–157, 158
  use in shock, 19, 22
PRVC (Pressure-regulated controlled ventilation), 75–76
PSV (Pressure-supported ventilation), 77–80
Pulmonary artery, transposition of, 159–160
Pulmonary artery catheters
  complications, 34–35
  data provided, 31–34
  in monitoring cardiac output, 29–35
  use in diagnosis of ARDS, 138
Pulmonary capillary wedge pressure, 31–32
Pulmonary disease, restrictive, 85–88, 91
Pulmonary edema, 375
Pulmonary hypertension, 194–195
Pulmonary injury. See Acute respiratory distress syndrome; Ventilator-induced lung injury
Pulmonary valve atresia, 160–161
Pulmonary vascular resistance
  calculating, 32–33
  in mechanical ventilation, 191–192, 194–195
Pulmonary vasculature abnormalities, 142
Pulmonary vasospasm, 194–195
Pulseless electrical activity, 177
Pulse oximetry, 4, 97–98, 158
Pumps, ECLS, 118
PVR. See Pulmonary vascular resistance

Racemic epinephrine, 41
Rapid sequence intubation, 4–8
Red blood cells. See Transfusions
Refractory status epilepticus, 218–219
Renal failure, acute
  classification, 350–354
  complications, 365
  defined, 349
  epidemiology, 349–350
  evaluation/diagnosis, 356–357
  hemolytic uremic syndrome, 354–355

hepatorenal syndrome, 354, 451
  management and treatment, 357–360
  myoglobinuria/hemoglobinuria, 355
  nutrition in, 322, 323t, 324t
  pathophysiology/causes, 350–354
  renal replacement therapy, 360–364
  renal transplantation, 355–356
Renal replacement therapy, 360–363, 364
  hemodialysis, 202, 360–362
  hemofiltration, 362–363
  hemoperfusion, 363
  peritoneal dialysis, 360–362
  replacement fluid, 363
Renal system. See also Renal failure, acute; Renal replacement therapy
  diseases with hypertension, 379
  function in postoperative cardiac care, 201–202
  transplantation, 355–356
Respiratory acidosis/alkalosis, 303
Respiratory distress syndrome, acute. See Acute respiratory distress syndrome
Respiratory failure. See also Acute respiratory distress syndrome
  in airway obstruction, 37, 40
  as a cause of death, 191
  indication for mechanical ventilation, 81
  mechanisms, 193–194
Respiratory infections, 406–407
Respiratory monitoring
  carbon dioxide monitoring, 98–99
  in cardiac patients, postoperative, 191–195
  and helium administration, 43
  intubation, following, 14–15
  pulse oximetry, 97–98
  respiratory mechanics monitoring, 99–101
Respiratory muscle load, increased, 92
Respiratory physiology
  abnormal mechanics and physiology, 85–90
  alveolar ventilation, 59
  breathing mechanics, 65–66, 67
  developmental aspects, 67–68
  and mechanical ventilation, 82t
  oxygenation, maintenance of, 57–59
  ventilation mechanics, 59–65
Respiratory pump (muscle) failure, 85, 92
Respiratory support, alternatives
  extracorporeal life support, 115–130
  high-frequency ventilation, 107–112
  liquid ventilation, 114–115
  nitric oxide, 112–114
  surfactant replacement, 114
Restrictive pulmonary disease, 85–88, 91
Retropharyngeal abscesses, 40
Reynolds' number, 51
Rifampin, 403
Ringer's lactate, 23
Rocuronium, 6, 260, 261
Ross procedure, 204

Safety devices, ECLS, 119
Salicylates, toxic ingestion, 432
Saline, normal, in treatment of shock, 23
Sedation/analgesia
  in ARDS, 150
  dosing recommendations, 5t, 243, 265t
  duration of, 243
  importance of, in PICU patients, 241–243
  in increased intracranial pressure, 232–233
  in intubation, 6–7
  during mechanical ventilation, 243
  patient-controlled, 251, 252–253
  postoperative, 202–203
  toxic ingestion of, 432–433
  use in ARDS, 150
Sedative/analgesic agents
  barbiturates, 250–251
  benzodiazepines, 246–247
  inhalational anesthesia, 243–245
  ketamine, 247–249
  miscellaneous agents, 256–257
  nitrous oxide, 245–246
  opioids, 251–256
  propofol, 249–250
Seizures, 196, 232. See also Status epilepticus
Sellick's maneuver (cricoid pressure), 4
Sengstaken-Blakemore tube, 442
Sepsis/septic shock
  antibiotic therapy, 390–394, 395t, 396
  in burns, 285
  fluid treatments, 24
  and inotropic agents, 28
  laboratory evaluation, 389–390
  management, 392–397
  microorganisms involved, 391–392
  morbidity/mortality, 389, 390, 394
  and oxygen consumption, 34
  physiologic changes in, 19, 20
  postoperative, 201
  signs/symptoms, 390t
Severe coarctation of the aorta, 157–158, 196
Shock. See also specific types of shock
  airway management, 21–22
  cardiovascular resuscitation and fluid management, 22–24
  classifications of, 19–21
  hemodynamic monitoring, 29–35
  and inotropic agents, 26–29
  laboratory evaluations, 25–26
  metabolic abnormalities, 25–26
  physical exam, 21
  symptoms in HLHS, 156
  treatment of, 21–29
SIADH (Syndrome of inappropriate antidiuretic hormone secretion), 291–292
Sickle cell disease, 408
Silver sulfadiazine, 285

SIMV (Synchronized intermittent mandatory ventilation), 76–77, 79, 93–94
Sinus tachycardia, 170
SjO$_2$ monitoring, 229–230
Skin failure, nutrition in, 325–327
Sodium
 in acute renal failure, 358
 hypernatremia, 294–296
 hyponatremia, 290–294
Sodium bicarbonate, 25, 280
Sodium nitroprusside, 383–384
Somatostatin, 441
Spinal shock, 276–278
Spontaneous ventilation, 80–81
Status asthmaticus
 endotracheal intubation and ventilation, 50–51
 helium administration, 51–53
 initial evaluation and therapy, 43–44
 morbidity/mortality, 43, 88–89
 prehospital care, 44–45
 treatments, 45–50
 use of mechanical ventilation, 88–90
Status epilepticus
 defined, 207
 diagnostic evaluation, 219
 drug treatments, 214–216
 etiology, 207–209
 morbidity/mortality, 209–210
 pathophysiology, 210–212
 refractory status, 218–219
 stabilization, initial, 212–214
 therapeutic goals and strategies, 212, 216–218
Stress ulcers. *See* Ulcer prophylaxis
Stridor. *See* Airway obstructions, upper
Stroke volume, 18, 187
Stylet, intubating, 10, *11*
Succinylcholine, 5, 258–260
Supported ventilation (PSV and VSV), 77–80, 89
Supraventricular tachycardia, 172–173
Surfactant replacement, 114, 149–150
Surgery
 cardiac techniques, 182
 in gastrointestinal bleeding, 442–443
 in intracranial pressure evaluation, 233
 postsurgical stress response, 241–242
 in transposition of great arteries, 160
 for upper airway obstruction, 37–38
Survival rates in ECLS, 124–125, 126, 130
SVR (Systemic vascular resistance), 19, 32
SVT (Supraventricular tachycardia), 172–173
Swan-Ganz catheters. *See* Pulmonary artery catheters
Sympathomimetics, toxic ingestion of, 433–436
Synchronized intermittent mandatory ventilation, 76–77, 79, 93–94
Syndrome of inappropriate antidiuretic hormone secretion, 291–292

Systemic hypotension, 50–51
Systemic vascular resistance, 19, 32

Tachycardias
 sinus, 170
 supraventricular, 172–173
 ventricular, 173–175
TAVPR (Total anomalous pulmonary return), 164–165
Tension pneumothorax, 51
Tetralogy of Fallot, 161–163
Theophylline
 in status asthmaticus, 48
 toxic ingestion of, 433–436
Thermal injuries. *See* Burns
Thermodilution catheters. *See* Pulmonary artery catheters
Thrombocytopenia, 199–200
Tidal volumes, 67–68, 83–84
TOF (Tetralogy of Fallot), 161–163
Tonsillitis, 40
Total anomalous pulmonary venous return, 164–165
Total parenteral nutrition. *See* Parenteral nutrition
Toxic ingestions/agents. *See* Poisons/toxic agents
Toxic shock syndromes, 394
TPN. *See* Parenteral nutrition
TPT (Transpyloric tube) feeding, 312–315
Train-of-four monitoring, 262–263
Tranexamic acid, 344–345
Transfusion reactions, 334–335
Transfusions
 adverse effects, 333–335, 337–338
 blood filters, 340
 blood/hemoglobin substitutes, 338–340
 cryoprecipitate, 341
 fresh frozen plasma, 340–341
 in invasive meningococcal disease, 396
 plasma derivatives, other, 342–343
 platelet concentrates, 341–342
 red blood cells, 336–338
 in traumatic injuries, 279–280
 type and screen *vs.* type and crossmatch, 335
 washed and irradiated products, 158, 164, 338
Transplantation, renal, 355–356
Transposition of the great arteries, 159–160
Transpyloric tube feeding, 312–315
Traumatic injuries
 airway management, 273–274, 275–276
 cardiovascular stabilization, 276–280
 cervical spine injuries, 274–275
 metabolic abnormalities, 280
 neurologic evaluation, 280
 secondary survey, 281–282
 ventilation and oxygenation, 276

Tricuspid valve
  atresia, 160–161
  Ebstein's anomaly, 161
Tricyclic antidepressants, toxic ingestion of, 436–437
Triple airway maneuver, 2
Truncus arteriosus, 163–164
Tuberculosis, 402
Tumor lysis syndrome, 302–303
Type and screen/type and crossmatch, 335

Ulcer prophylaxis, 444–448
Upper airway obstructions. See Airway obstructions, upper

Valvular heart diseases
  Ebstein's anomaly, 161
  pulmonary valve atresia, 160–161
  trucuspid valve atresia, 160–161
Vascular tone, 17, 18. See also Systemic vascular resistance
Vasopressin, 441
VCV. See Volume-controlled ventilation
Vecuronium, 6, 261
Vein cannulation, percutaneous peripheral, 22, 277–278
Venoarterial/Venovenous ECLS, 116, 123–124
Ventilation, alveolar, 59
Ventilation, high-frequency. See High-frequency ventilation
Ventilation, liquid, 114–115, 148
Ventilation, mechanical
  with abnormal respiratory mechanics, 85–90
  in ARDS, 145–147
  in circulatory pump failure, 85
  complications of, 94–97
  controlled (mandatory), 71
  controversies of, 90–97
  duration of, 192–193
  following intubation, 15
  goals, 57–59
  in increased intracranial pressure, 231
  indications for, 81–84, 90
  intermittent mandatory, 76–77
  mechanics of, 59–65
  modes, 71, 72t, 73–81, 82
  in neurological injury, 85
  in postoperative patients, 84, 191–192
  pressure-controlled, 61, 73–75, 83, 90–91
  pressure limited vs. volume-limited, 90–91
  pressure-regulated volume-controlled, 75–76
  prolonged, postoperative, 193–194
  in respiratory pump failure, 85
  spontaneous, 81
  in status asthmaticus, 50–53
  supported, 77–80
  in traumatic injuries, 276
  volume-controlled, 61, 71, 73, 82–83, 90–91
  weaning from, 78–79, 91–94
Ventilation-perfusion matching, 51
Ventilator-induced lung injury, 107, 145
Ventilators, mechanical, 69–71. See also Ventilation, mechanical
Ventricular assist devices, 190
Ventricular fibrillation, 175
Ventricular tachycardia, 173–175
Volume-controlled ventilation, 61, 71, 73, 82–83, 90–91
Volume-support ventilation, 77, 79–80
Volutrauma, 87, 90, 91, 94–95
VSV (Volume-support ventilation), 77, 79–80

Waterston shunt, 204
Weaning, from mechanical ventilation, 78–79, 91–94
Whole-bowel irrigation, 418, 419
Wound management, 284–285

X-rays, chest
  in ARDS, 138, *139*, 141
  in heart disease, 155, 156t, 160
  in upper airway obstruction, 40